Fecal Incontinence

Diagnosis and Treatment

Carlo Ratto • Giovanni B. Doglietto

Fecal Incontinence
Diagnosis and Treatment

Forewords by
A.C. Lowry • L. Påhlman • G. Romano

Springer

EDITORS

CARLO RATTO
Department of Surgical Sciences
Division of Digestive Surgery
Catholic University
Rome, Italy

GIOVANNI B. DOGLIETTO
Department of Surgical Sciences
Division of Digestive Surgery
Catholic University
Rome, Italy

ISBN 978-88-470-5799-9 Springer Milan Berlin Heidelberg New York
DOI 10.1007/978-88-470-0638-6

Springer is a part of Springer Science+Business Media
springer.com

Softcover re-print of the Hardcover 1st edition 2007

Cover image: Simona Colombo, Milan, Italy
Typesetting: Compostudio, Cernusco s/N, Italy
Printing: Arti Grafiche Nidasio, Assago, Italy

Springer-Verlag Italia S.r.l., Via Decembrio 28, I-20137 Milan, Italy

Foreword

by Ann C. Lowry

Several years ago, the American media presented urinary incontinence as the "last closet issue". Arguably, that designation really belongs to fecal incontinence. Even today, only a third of patients suffering with the condition discuss it with their physicians. This is particularly unfortunate, as the condition affects a significant portion of the population and is a significant burden to patients, their families, and society.

This situation exists for a number of reasons. The social stigma of incontinence of stool is the primary reason. Early on, children are taught to avoid "bathroom talk", and that admonishment continues into adulthood. However, there are other reasons as well. Continence of flatus and stool is an extremely complex process involving feces consistency and transit time, the sensory capability of the rectum, and the neurological and muscular function of the sphincter muscle. Despite years of research on the pathophysiology, it is hard to explain how a patient with an intact sphincter has daily episodes of incontinence while a patient with a cloaca has none. Inconsistent presentations of the condition make it baffling to health care providers. Partially because of the complexity of the condition, a number of different providers are interested in fecal incontinence. Each specialty focuses upon a different aspect of the disorder. For instance, pediatricians focus largely on congenital abnormalities associated with incontinence and treatment options applicable to children. Gerontologists concern themselves with the opposite age spectrum, where the etiology and appropriate treatment options are different. In most institutions, there is little communication among specialties about the disorder, which limits progress in diagnosis and treatment. Finally, incontinence is not a life-threatening process; there is thus less pressure to overcome the natural tendency of patients and providers to avoid discussing the situation.

In view of all of the above, this book, *Fecal Incontinence: Diagnosis and Treatment,* is a significant contribution to the medical profession. Discussion of all aspects of incontinence is presented in a clear, concise manner. The contributors represent distinguished experts from multiple disciplines and continents; these authors are the leaders and innovators in their fields. The book is especially timely, as understanding of the disorder and treatment options have progressed significantly within the past few years.

In this one volume, the reader will find information about all elements of the incontinence of stool, starting with the current understanding of continence and the pathophysiology of incontinence. The burden of the illness on patients and their families, including its economic and psychological consequences, is empathetically covered. Appropriate diagnosis and evaluation is thoroughly reviewed. Traditional medical and surgical treatment alternatives as well as innovative treatment options and their outcomes are critically analyzed. Following that section, specific conditions and their currently recommended management are presented. Hours of library research would be required to obtain equivalent knowledge.

Armed with this information about the impact on patients and available treatment options, providers hopefully will be more likely to ask patients about the symptom. That opens the possibility of more evaluation and treatment, which should reduce the burden on patients and their families. The editors and contributors are to be congratulated for this excellent presentation of their consolidated knowledge.

Minneapolis, April 2007

Ann C. Lowry, MD, FASCRS, FACS
Past President
American Society of Colon and
Rectal Surgeons (ASCRS)

Foreword

by Lars Påhlman

Faecal incontinence (FI) has been evaluated and treated for many years. Awareness of its incidence, particularly among women, has seen enormous changes over the last two to three decades and research into and the understanding of FI has improved during the same time period. This is a rapidly developing area of expertise in which different surgical techniques have been challenged and new ones have been approached, mainly based upon the understanding of the problem. In this volume edited by Drs. Ratto and Doglietto, the entire spectra within the field of incontinence are covered. Moreover, most of the expertise gained in the new century is expressed in this volume, placing a quality stamp on most of the chapters.

Section I, regarding structure and function in continence and incontinence, is very instrumental and easily read. Even for those with minor knowledge about pathophysiology, this part of the book is important and not difficult to understand.

Section II, how to diagnose FI, provides a more "hands-off" description of how to address patients with incontinence. Numerous different tests are described, and one can argue whether or not the entire spectrum of investigation should be used when diagnosing FI. Again, this volume evaluates the important aspects of the diagnostic procedure, and its place in clinical practice is established.

Regarding Section III, the treatment section, enormous developments have occurred over the last 10–15 years. Important options such as biofeedback and normal care are well evaluated and described here. Moreover, the more or less simple reconstruction with an overlap repair to the more sophisticated treatment options after sphincter-damaging injuries, such as dynamic graciloplasty and artificial bowel sphincter, are described, although the place for those rather advanced techniques is yet to be defined. The latest treatment option, sacral nerve stimulation, is also elegantly discussed. Bulking agents is a totally new area in which advanced techniques have yet to be employed. This developing area is difficult to evaluate, and evidence determining how to best use it is still lacking.

The optimal ways in which to use the entire list of treatment options in FI is difficult to establish, and an algorithm taking the readers through all the different options, with their pros and cons, is important but is actually omitted from this book. After descriptions of different treatment options, entities in which bowel function can be altered in terms of incontinence are presented and clearly described in Section IV. This makes the entire volume more valuable, and it is possible for readers to ascertain essential knowledge, particularly regarding how to use the different treatment options according to a patient's history.

In summary, this is a very well-written and well-presented book about FI that addresses the different aspects on how to diagnose the problem, how to treat it, and what diseases lie behind the treatment options. The future in diagnosing and treating FI is demanding, as the incidence of FI is probably underreported; thus, many patients are suffering in silence. Once new techniques for diagnosing and treating those patients is readily available, demands for such treatment will increase enormously, as will the consequent advantages to society.

Uppsala, April 2007

Lars Påhlman, MD, PhD, FRCS
President
European Society of
Coloproctology (ESCP)

Foreword

by Giovanni Romano

There are very few topics in the field of coloproctology like faecal incontinence for which such an impressive progress in understanding pathophysiology and treatment has been achieved in recent years. This opinion, derived from the comparison between my previous book published in 2000 on *Diagnosis and Treatment of Faecal Incontinence* and this book, is confirmed by the significant changing attitudes of outstanding researchers all over the world towards modern treatment of the disorder. Whereas a few years ago aggressive surgical treatment was advised not only for patients with proven postobstetric or traumatic sphincter defects but also for neurogenic faecal incontinence, today, more conservative measures are indicated as a consequence of the very good results reported with advanced rehabilitation techniques and sacral neuromodulation.

It is becoming clear that the promising results first enthusiastically reported after complex surgical operations such as sphincteroplasty, dynamic graciloplasty or artificial bowel sphincters inevitably deteriorate with longer follow-up. This is not unusual whenever surgery is applied to "functional" disorders, and many examples come to mind: the Nissen operation for gastroesophageal reflux or, in the field of coloproctology, postanal repair for idiopathic faecal incontinence. Nevertheless, it seems a hard lesson to learn, even today: surgery is advocated as an absolute indication in the treatment of a number of functional diseases and many authors claim 100% positive results, which in my opinion does not make sense. An outstanding merit of this book is that it stresses the complexity of the disorder and invites physicians to be cautious about proposing distressing operations without proper assessment and indication.

On the other hand, appropriate surgery with skilled operative technique still has an important role in the management of specific conditions. Immediate sphincter repair due to postdelivery injury, or even late repair, by experienced colorectal surgeons has a very good outcome in about 60% of cases, which is relatively good for a "low-tech", "low-cost" technique. Attention to surgical details has too often been neglected in recent times, although it has been proven without doubt that the surgeon is the most important independent variable when assessing results of any surgical operation. This simple concept is appropriately outlined in many chapters of the book.

Another issue emerging from the literature and from congressional debates is the need for cooperation between pelvic floor specialists. It is a fact that when the patient is assessed and operated by the gynaecologist and the urologist in collaboration, the treatment results show a much better outcome. This attitude is well illustrated in specific sections of the book, thus contributing to a future in which pelvic floor units will be established in any specialised institution.

If quality of treatment has undoubtedly improved, the emerging problem is the cost of the cures: new technology is very expensive, and even when its use is appropriate, its widespread use must be balanced with the socioeconomic impact that follows. Distribution of financial resources is crucial for the survival of a modern society, and it is a duty of the scientific community to provide the political authority with a proper assessment of the cost–benefit ratio for any kind of therapy. This topic is specifically addressed in one chapter and is often referred to in many other chapters of the book.

Finally, I was impressed by what I dare to call the "leading philosophy" of this book: the patient is not in the background but at centre stage. Too often in the past, assessment of result has been surgeon oriented, with an underestimation of patients' real needs. The introduction of quality of life scores, although difficult to use in clinical practice and sometimes questionable, has definitely changed this attitude. Great effort has been made by the editors to give this issue the importance it deserves, and this effort in time will undoubtedly improve treatment quality.

There is no question that this book represents a great contribution for young and even experienced colorectal surgeons willing to deal with such difficult patients. One only needs to read the general index and the names of the authors who have written the chapters or the invited commentaries to understand the truth of this statement.

As president of the Italian Society of Colorectal Surgeons (SICCR), I can only congratulate Carlo Ratto–whom I have known for many years and who is current secretary of the SICCR–and Giovanni B. Doglietto for their splendid work. The entire Italian scientific community has reason to be proud that such outstanding personalities from all over the world were willing to contribute to this book, thus showing interest and respect for the work of so many Italian surgeons and researchers.

Avellino, March 2007

Giovanni Romano, MD
Past President
Italian Society of
Colorectal Surgeons (SICCR)

Preface

by Carlo Ratto, Giovanni B. Doglietto

Fecal incontinence (FI) is a frequent, distressing condition that has a devastating impact on patients' lives. However, patients are typically embarrassed and reluctant to acknowledge this disability, so they relinquish the possibility of being cured and remain socially isolated. They become housebound and prefer to pass the day very close to the toilet to avoid losing feces. The exact incidence of FI is uncertain because of patients' hesitation to seek help from their physicians. Most epidemiological studies suggest a prevalence as high as 2% of the general population, but when an interview specifically in relation to FI is conducted, this rate is usually significantly higher. Women seem to be at higher risk, mostly due to obstetric damage to the anal sphincters; however, during the last decade, an increasing interest has been dedicated to those forms of FI related to nontraumatic factors, which reach a relevant incidence. Older subjects are at very high risk, especially those with disabilities and those who are institutionalized. Moreover, young people are often affected. These factors create a significant economic impact for society, not only due to direct and indirect costs, but also due to intangible costs.

FI may result from a variety of pathophysiological situations, and various risk factors can cause a wide range of inability to control feces passage. Therefore, an accurate diagnostic workup of each patient is fundamental. Although not fully agreed upon by all physicians, a multimodal diagnosis, using a multiparametric evaluation, seems to allow the most thorough understanding of FI pathophysiology and to indicate optimal treatment. These are really the most important and challenging aspects of FI management. Indeed, a wide range of therapeutic options is available, including conservative, rehabilitative, and surgical procedures.

The aim of surgery may be to correct a defect or to improve a dysfunction in continence control while the sphincter complex is intact, or it may be to replace a largely fragmented or nonfunctioning sphincter. Making the correct choice is pivotal to the successful management of this condition. Although a number of reports are available regarding results of different surgical procedures, the lack of sufficient evidence from randomized controlled studies makes choosing the type of surgery very difficult. This has been confirmed in the very recent Cochrane Review: all randomized or quasirandomized trials of surgery in the management of adult FI (other than surgery for rectal prolapse) were analyzed, and nine trials were selected with a total sample size of 264 participants. The authors concluded: "it was impossible to identify or refute clinically important differences between the alternative surgical procedures. Larger rigorous trials are still needed. However, it should be recognised that the optimal treatment regime may be a complex combination of various surgical and non-surgical therapies" [Brown S, Nelson R (2007) Surgery for faecal incontinence in adults. Cochrane Database Syst Rev 2:CD001757].

This book is aimed at all physicians involved in the assessment and treatment of FI. Its main purpose is to review the latest advances in the epidemiologic, socioeconomic, psychologic, diagnostic, and therapeutic aspects of FI in order to establish guidelines for effective treatment. We hope this book may help physicians to relieve or solve FI in the many individuals suffering from this disabling condition and, through their positive results, encourage other incontinent people to receive effective treatment.

Rome, April 2007

Carlo Ratto
Giovanni B. Doglietto

Contents

Section IV SELECTED CLINICAL CONDITIONS

Section V FUTURE PERSPECTIVES

List of Contributors

SALEH M. ABBAS
Department of Surgery
Auckland Hospital
University of Auckland
Auckland, New Zealand

DONATO F. ALTOMARE
Department of Emergency
and Organ Transplantation
General Surgery and Liver
Transplantation Unit
University of Bari
Bari, Italy

CORNELIUS G.M.I. BAETEN
Department of Surgery
University Hospital Maastricht
Maastricht, The Netherlands

DAVID C.C. BARTOLO
Colorectal Unit
Western General Hospital
Edinburgh, Scotland, UK

ADIL E. BHARUCHA
Clinical Enteric Neuroscience
Translational
and Epidemiological Research
(CENTER) Program
Division of Gastroenterology
and Hepatology
Mayo Clinic College of Medicine
Rochester, MN, USA

IAN P. BISSETT
Department of Surgery
Auckland Hospital
University of Auckland
Auckland, New Zealand

ROBERTA E. BLANDON
Division of Female Pelvic Medicine
and Reconstructive Surgery
Department of Obstetrics and
Gynecology
Mayo Clinic Rochester
Rochester, MN, USA

MAURO CERVIGNI
Urogynecological Department
S. Carlo – IDI Hospital
Rome, Italy

MARIA CIARLEGLIO
Division of Biostatistics
Yale University School of Medicine
New Haven, CT, USA

MIGUEL A. CIGA
Department of General Surgery
Coloproctology Unit
Virgen del Camino University Hospital
Pamplona, Spain

MARIO DE MIGUEL
Department of General Surgery
Coloproctology Unit
Virgen del Camino University Hospital
Pamplona, Spain

GIOVANNI B. DOGLIETTO
Department of Surgical Sciences
Division of Digestive Surgery
Catholic University
Rome, Italy

LORENZA DONISI
Department of Surgical Sciences
Division of Digestive Surgery
Catholic University
Rome, Italy

RICHARD A. FALCONE JR.
Department of Pediatric Surgery
Colorectal Center for Children
Cincinnati Children's Hospital
University of Cincinnati
Cincinnati, OH, USA

RICHELLE J.F. FELT-BERSMA
Department of Gastroenterology and Hepatology
VU University Medical Center
Amsterdam, The Netherlands

JILL C. GENUA
Department of Colorectal Surgery
Cleveland Clinic Florida
Weston, FL, USA

FRANC H. HETZER
Department of Surgery
Hospital of St. Gallen
St. Gallen, Switzerland

MICHAEL HOROWITZ
Department of Medicine
University of Adelaide and
Royal Adelaide Hospital
Adelaide, SA, Australia

TRACY L. HULL
Department of Colon and
Rectal Sugery
Cleveland Clinic Foundation
Cleveland, OH, USA

C. SCOTT HULTMAN
Division of Plastic and
Reconstructive Surgery
University of North Carolina
Chapel Hill, NC, USA

MICHAEL E.D. JARRETT
Colorectal Department
John Radcliffe Hospital
Oxford, UK

OLIVER M. JONES
Department of Colorectal Surgery
John Radcliffe Hospital
Oxford, UK

MARIE-FRANCE KONG
Department of Diabetes
and Endocrinology
Leicester General Hospital
University Hospitals of Leicester
Leicester, UK

FILIPPO LA TORRE
Department of Surgical Sciences
Rome University "La Sapienza"
Rome, Italy

SOEREN LAURBERG
Department of Surgery
University Hospital of Aarhus
Aarhus, Denmark

PAUL-ANTOINE LEHUR
Clinique Chirurgicale II - Pôle Digestif
University Hospital of Nantes
Nantes, France

ANNE-MARIE LEROI
Digestive Tract Research Group
Rouen University Hospital
Rouen, France

MARC A. LEVITT
Department of Pediatric Surgery
Colorectal Center for Children
Cincinnati Children's Hospital
University of Cincinnati
Cincinnati, OH, USA

IAN LINDSEY
Department of Colorectal Surgery
John Radcliffe Hospital
Oxford, UK

FRANCESCO LITTA
Department of Surgical Sciences
Division of Digestive Surgery
Catholic University
Rome, Italy

ANN C. LOWRY
Division of Colon and Rectal Surgery
University of Minnesota
Minneapolis, MN, USA

Peter J. Lunniss
Centre for Academic Surgery and
GI Physiology Unit
The Royal London Hospital
Academic Department of Medical
and Surgical Gastroenterology
Homerton Hospital
London, UK

Alexandra K. MacMillan
School of Population Health
University of Auckland
Auckland, New Zealand

Robert D. Madoff
Department of Surgery
Division of Colon and Rectal Surgery
University of Minnesota
London, MN, USA

Yasuko Maeda
Physiology Unit
St. Mark's Hospital
London, UK

Andrea Maier
Department of Radiology
University of Vienna
Vienna, Austria

Albert Mako
Urogynecological Department
S. Carlo - IDI Hospital
Rome, Italy

Klaus E. Matzel
Chirurgische Klinik der
Universität Erlangen
Erlangen, Germany

Lindsee McPhail
Division of Plastic and
Reconstructive Surgery
University of North Carolina
Chapel Hill, NC, USA

Jarno Melenhorst
Department of Surgery
University Hospital Maastricht
Maastricht, The Netherlands

Anders F. Mellgren
Division of Colon and Rectal
Surgery
University of Minneapolis
Minneapolis, MN, USA

Arend E.H. Merrie
Division of Surgery
University of Auckland
Auckland, New Zealand

Guillaume Meurette
Clinique Chirurgicale II - Pôle Digestif
University Hospital of Nantes
Nantes, France

Franca Natale
Urogynecological Department
S. Carlo - IDI Hospital
Rome, Italy

James W. Ogilvie Jr.
Department of Surgery
Division of Colon and Rectal Surgery
University of Minnesota
Minneapolis, MN, USA

Héctor Ortiz
Department of General Surgery
Coloproctology Unit
Virgen del Camino University Hospital
Pamplona, Spain

Angelo Parello
Department of Surgical Sciences
Division of Digestive Surgery
Catholic University
Rome, Italy

Giuseppe Pelliccioni
Neurology Unit
Geriatric Hospital
Italian National Research
Centre on Aging (INRCA)
Ancona, Italy

Alberto Peña
Department of Pediatric Surgery
Colorectal Center for Children
Cincinnati Children's Hospital
University of Cincinnati
Cincinnati, OH, USA

Patrizia Ponzi
Department of Health Economics
Medtronic Italia S.p.A.
Sesto San Giovanni, Italy

Filippo Pucciani
Department of Surgery
University of Florence
Florence, Italy

Satish S. Rao
Department of Gastroenterology and Hepatology
University of Iowa Carver College of Medicine
Iowa City, IA, USA

Carlo Ratto
Department of Surgical Sciences
Division of Digestive Surgery
Catholic University
Rome, Italy

Marcella Rinaldi
Department of Emergency and Organ Transplantation
General Surgery and Liver Transplantation Unit
University of Bari
Bari, Italy

Todd H. Rockwood
Division of Health Policy and Management
Center for Survey Research in Public Health
University of Minnesota
Minneapolis, MN, USA

Harald R. Rosen
Department of Surgery
St. Vincent Hospital, Vienna
Vienna, Austria

Giulio A. Santoro
Section of Anal Physiology and Ultrasound
Coloproctology Service
Department of Surgery
Regional Hospital
Treviso, Italy

Osvaldo Scarpino
Neurology Unit
Geriatric Hospital
Italian National Research Centre on Aging (INRCA)
Ancona, Italy

S. Mark Scott
Centre for Academic Surgery and GI Physiology Unit
The Royal London Hospital
London, UK

Junaid Siddiqui
Department of Gastroenterology and Hepatology
University of Iowa Carver College of Medicine
Iowa City, IA, USA

Mette M. Soerensen
Department of Surgery
University Hospital of Aarhus
Aarhus, Denmark

Marco Soligo
Urogynecology Service
Obstetrics and Gynecology Department
San Carlo Borromeo Hospital
Milan, Italy

Jenny Speranza
Department of Colorectal Surgery
Cleveland Clinic Florida
Weston, FL, USA

Francesca Di Stasi
Department of Health Economics
Medtronic Italia S.p.A.
Sesto San Giovanni, Italy

Scott R. Steele
Madigan Army Medical Center
Department of Surgery
Fort Lewis, WA, USA

Julian M. Stern
St. Mark's Hospital
Harrow, UK

Eddie H.M. Sze
Division of Urogynecology and Reconstructive Pelvic Surgery
Department of Obstetrics and Gynecology
West Virginia University School of Medicine
Morgantown, WV, USA

Joe J. Tjandra
Epworth and Royal Melbourne Hospitals University of Melbourne
Melbourne, VIC, Australia

Carolynne J. Vaizey
Physiology Unit
St. Mark's Hospital
London, UK

Arnold Wald
Section of Gastroenterology and Hepatology
University of Wisconsin School of Medicine and Public Health
Madison, WI, USA

Steven D. Wexner
Department of Colorectal Surgery
Cleveland Clinic Florida
Weston, FL, USA

Luigi Zorcolo
Colorectal Unit
University of Cagliari
Cagliari, Italy

SECTION I

Structure and Function in Continence and Incontinence

Anatomy and Physiology of Continence

1

Adil E. Bharucha, Roberta E. Blandon

Introduction

Webster's dictionary defines continence as "the ability to retain a bodily discharge voluntarily". The word has its origins from the Latin *continere* or *tenere*, which means "to hold". The anorectum is the caudal end of the gastrointestinal tract, and is responsible for fecal continence and defecation. In humans, defecation is a viscero somatic reflex that is often preceded by several attempts to preserve continence. Any attempt at managing anorectal disorders requires a clear understanding of the anatomy and the integrated physiologic mechanisms responsible for maintaining continence.

Embryology

The primitive gut is formed during the third week of gestation. The anorectal region in humans derives from four separate embryological structures: the hindgut, the cloaca, the proctodeum, and the anal tubercles [1]. The hindgut forms the distal third of the transverse colon, the descending colon, the sigmoid, the rectum, and the upper part of the anal canal to the level of the anal valves [2]. The end of the hindgut enters into the cloaca, an endoderm-lined cavity that is in direct contact with the surface ectoderm. The cloaca is initially a single tube that is subsequently separated by caudad migration of the urorectal septum into anterior urogenital and posterior intestinal passages. During the 10th week of development, the external anal sphincter is formed from the posterior cloaca as the descent of the urogenital septum becomes complete. By the 12th week, the internal anal sphincter is formed from a thickened extension of rectal circular muscle [3]. The proctodeal portion of the cloacal membrane disintegrates to form the anal tubercles that join posteriorly and migrate ventrally to encircle a depression, known as the anal dimple or proctodeum. The anal tubercles join the urorectal septum and genital tubercles to form the perineal body, completing the separation between the rectum and the urogenital tract. The upper portion of the anal canal is derived from endoderm and is supplied by the inferior mesenteric artery, which supplies the hindgut. The lower third of the anal canal has ectodermal origins and is supplied by the rectal arteries, which are branches of the internal pudendal artery [2].

Anatomy

Pelvic Floor

The pelvic floor is a dome-shaped muscular sheet [4] that predominantly contains striated muscle and has midline defects enclosing the bladder, the uterus, and the rectum. These defects are closed by connective tissue anterior to the urethra, anterior to the rectum (i.e., the perineal body), and posterior to the rectum (i.e., the postanal plate). Together with the viscera (i.e., the bladder and anorectum), the pelvic floor is responsible for storing and evacuating urine and stool.

The levator ani and the coccygeus muscle comprise the two muscular components of the pelvic floor or pelvic diaphragm. The muscles that constitute the levator ani complex are the puborectalis, the pubococcygeus, and the ileococcygeus. These muscles originate at different levels of the pubic bone, the arcus tendineus fascia pelvis (condensation of the obturator internus muscle fascia), and the ischial spine. These muscles are inserted at the level of the rectum, the anococcygeal raphe (levator plate), and the coccyx (Fig. 1).

It is unclear whether the puborectalis should be regarded as a component of the levator ani complex or the external anal sphincter. Based on developmental evidence, innervation, and histological studies, the puborectalis appears distinct from the majority of the levator ani [1]. On the other hand, the puborectalis and external sphincter complex are innervated by separate nerves originating from S_{2-4} (see below), suggesting phylogenetic differences between these two muscles [5].

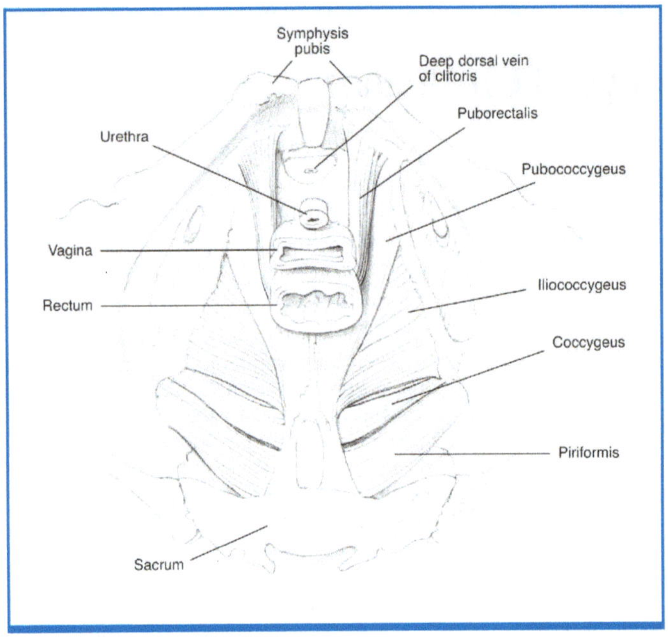

Fig. 1. Pelvic view of the levator ani demonstrating its four main components: puborectalis, pubococcygeus, iliococcygeus, and coccygeus. Reprinted with permission from [6]

Rectum and Anal Canal

The rectum is 15- to 20-cm long and extends from the recto sigmoid junction at the level of third sacral vertebra to the anal orifice (Fig. 2). The upper and lower rectums are separated by a horizontal fold. The upper rectum is derived from the embryological hind gut, generally contains feces, and can distend toward the peritoneal cavity [7]. The lower part, derived from the cloaca, is surrounded by condensed extra peritoneal connective tissue and is generally empty

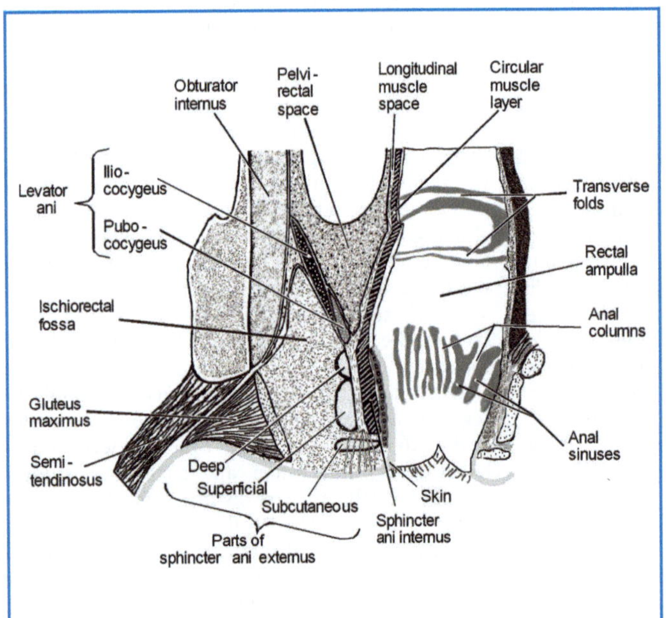

Fig. 2. Diagram of a coronal section of the rectum, anal canal, and adjacent structures. The pelvic barrier includes the anal sphincters and the pelvic floor muscles. Reprinted with permission from [8]

in normal subjects, except during defecation. In humans, there are fewer enteric ganglia in the rectum compared with the colon and very few ganglia in the anal sphincter [9, 10].

The anal canal is an anteroposterior slit, with its lateral walls in close contact. The literature describes a longer (approximately 4.0–4.5 cm) "surgical" or "clinical" anal canal and a shorter (approximately 2.0 cm) "anatomical" or "embryological" anal canal. The anal valves and the distal end of the ampullary part of the rectum mark the proximal margin of the "short" and "long" anal canal, respectively. The proximal 10 mm of the anal canal is lined by columnar, rectal-type mucosa. The next 15 mm (which includes the valves) is lined by stratified, or a modified columnar, epithelium. Distal to that is about 10 mm of thick, non hairy, stratified epithelium (i.e., the pecten). The most distal 5–10 mm is lined by hairy skin.

The anal canal is surrounded by the internal and external anal sphincters. The internal sphincter is a thickened extension of the circular smooth muscle layer surrounding the colon that contains discrete muscle bundles separated by large septa [11]. In the rectum, the interstitial cells of Cajal (ICC) are organized in dense networks along the submucosal and myenteric borders. In the internal anal sphincter, the ICCs are located along the periphery of the muscle bundles within the circular layer.

The external sphincter is composed of superficial, subcutaneous, and deep portions; the deep portion blends with the puborectalis [7]. In men, this trilaminar pattern is preserved around the sphincter circumference. In contrast, the anterior portion of the external sphincter in women is a single muscle bundle. External sphincter fibers are circumferentially oriented, very small, and separated by profuse connective tissue [12].

Nerve Supply to the Pelvic Floor

Autonomic Innervation

The anorectum and pelvic floor are supplied by sympathetic, parasympathetic, and somatic fibers [13]. Sympathetic pre ganglionic fibers originate from the lowest thoracic ganglion in the paravertebral sympathetic chain and join branches from the aortic plexus to form the superior hypogastric plexus. Because the superior hypogastric plexus is not a single nerve, the alternative term for this plexus, i.e., "presacral nerve", should be avoided. The superior hypogastric plexus provides branches to the uteric and ovarian (or testicular) plexus, and divides into right and left hypogastric nerves. The hypogastric nerves unite with preganglionic parasympathetic fibers originating from ventral rami of the second, the third, and often the fourth sacral nerves to form the inferior hypogastric plexus, which is located posterior to the urinary bladder. The inferior hypogastric plexus gives rise to the middle rectal plexus, the vesical plexus, the prostatic plexus, and the uterovaginal plexus. The nerve supply to the rectum and anal canal is derived from the superior, middle, and inferior rectal plexus. Parasympathetic fibers in the superior and middle rectal plexuses synapse with postganglionic neurons in the myenteric plexus in the rectal wall. In addition, ascending fibers from the inferior hypogastric plexus travel via superior hypogastric and aortic plexuses to reach the inferior mesenteric plexus, ultimately innervating the descending and sigmoid colon. After entering the colon, these fibers form the ascending colonic nerves, traveling cephalad in the plane of the myenteric plexus to supply a variable portion of the left colon.

Sacral parasympathetic pathways to the colon have excitatory and inhibitory components [14]. Excitatory pathways play an important role in colonic propulsive activity, especially during defecation. In other species (e.g., guinea pig), feces transport may be entirely organized by the enteric nervous system; spinal and supraspinal reflexes are also involved in the process [15]. Inhibitory pathways allow colonic volume to adapt to its contents, and they also mediate descending inhibition that initiates colonic relaxation ahead of a fecal bolus.

Somatic Motor Innervation

Cortical mapping with transcranial magnetic stimulation suggests that rectal and anal responses are bilaterally represented on the superior motor cortex, i.e., Brodmann area 4 [16]. There are subtle differences in the degree of bilateral hemispheric representation between subjects. Motor neurons in Onuf's nucleus, which is located in the sacral spinal cord, innervate the external anal and urethral sphincters. Though they supply striated muscles under voluntary control, these motor neurons are smaller than usual α-motor neurons and resemble autonomic motor neurons [17]; however, the conduction velocity in pudendal nerve fibers is comparable with that of peripheral nerves. In contrast to other somatic motor neurons in the spinal cord, these neurons are relatively spared in amyotrophic lateral sclerosis but are affected in Shy-Dräger syndrome [18, 19]. Somatic branches originating from Onuf's nucleus travel in the pudendal nerve, the muscular branches, and the coccygeal plexus. The pudendal nerve branches into inferior rectal and perineal and posterior scrotal nerves. The inferior rectal nerve conveys motor fibers to the external anal sphincter and sensory input from the lower anal canal and the skin around the anus. The perineal nerve divides into posterior scrotal (or labial) branches and muscular branches. The posterior scrotal branches innervate the skin, while muscular branches are distributed to the transverse perinei, the bulbospongiosus, the ischiocavernosus, the urethral sphincter, the anterior part of the external anal sphincter, and the levator ani.

Motor fibers of the right and left pudendal nerves have overlapping distributions within the external anal sphincter. Sherrington observed that stimulation of the right pudendal nerve caused circumferential contraction of the external anal sphincter [20]. Conversely, tonic external sphincter activity, sphincter inhibition during colonic distention, and the cutaneo anal reflex were not affected by sectioning either pudendal nerve.

The nerve supply to the puborectalis has been the subject of controversy. The early literature based on dissections by several workers suggested that the puborectalis was innervated from below by the pudendal nerve, or jointly by the inferior rectal and perineal branches of the pudendal nerve. Therefore, the puborectalis was regarded as being derived not from the levator ani but from the external anal sphincter. However, an electrophysiological study that preoperative stimulation of the sacral nerves above the pelvic floor invariably (i.e., 19 of 20 experiments) resulted in electromyogram (EMG) activity in the ipsilateral puborectalis, but not in the external anal sphincter [5]. Gross dissection studies in humans, rats, and squirrel monkeys demonstrate that the anal sphincter and levator ani muscle are innervated by separate nerves [21–23].

Somatic Sensory Innervation

Rectal distention is perceived as a more localized sensation of rectal fullness, interpreted by the patient as a desire to pass wind or motion. Colonic distension, on the other hand, causes ill-defined discomfort and eventually pain. The anal canal responds to distention and to innocuous mucosal proximo distal mechanical shearing stimuli [24]. In addition to mucosal nerve endings, there are also low threshold, slowly adapting mechanoreceptors in the guinea pig rectum. These intraganglionic laminar endings (IGLEs) detect mechanical deformation of the myenteric ganglia [25, 26]. The anal canal is lined by numerous free and organized nerve endings (i.e., Meissner's corpuscles, Krause end-bulbs, Golgi-Mazzoni bodies, and genital corpuscles), perhaps explaining why it is exquisitely sensitive to light touch, pain, and temperature. Sensory traffic is conveyed by unmyelinated small C fibers and larger Aδ myelinated fibers that have slow and fast conduction velocities, respectively [27].

Animal models and clinicopathological findings in humans suggest that pelvic nerves traveling to the sacral segments are more important for conveying non-noxious and noxious colonic sensations than are lumbar colonic (sympathetic) nerves [12, 28–30]. There are more afferent neurons supplying the colon in the sacral, compared with lumbar segments in the cat, i.e., 7,500 versus 4,500 neurons [31, 32]. However, the number of spinal visceral afferent neurons is relatively small, i.e., only 2.5% or less of the total number of spinal afferent neurons supply skin and deep somatic structures [33].

In general, sacral afferents may be better suited for conveying afferent information than are lumbar afferents, as they are more likely to lack resting activity and respond to pressure increments with a wider range of discharge frequency [34, 35]. Janig and Morrison identified three different classes of mechanosensitive visceral afferents in the cat colon [33]. Tonic afferents fired throughout colonic distention and accurately encoded the intensity of distention between 20 and 100 mmHg. Phasic colonic afferents generally discharged at the onset and occasionally at the cessation of a distention stimulus. Tonic afferents were predominantly unmyelinated, slowly conducting C fibers, while most phasic afferents were faster-conducting myelinated Aδ fibers. The afferents innervating the anal canal responded to shearing stimuli, but not colonic or anal distention.

Two different theories have been proposed to explain visceral pain perception. Proponents of the specificity theory suggested that pain was a distinct sensory modality, mediated by sequential activation of visceral nociceptors and central pain-specific neurons in the spinal dorsal horn. However, in the cat colon, Janig and Koltzenburg found no afferent fibers that were selectively activated by noxious stimuli, arguing against the specificity theory. The alternative hypothesis for pain perception, i.e., pattern or intensity theory, attributes pain perception to spatial and temporal patterns of impulses generated in non specific visceral afferent neurons [24]. However, electrophysiological studies of visceral afferent fibers in other organs, including the colon, have documented high-threshold visceral afferent fibers that only respond to noxious mechanical stimuli. Subsequently, Cervero and Janig reconciled these opposing concepts in a convergence model wherein input from low- and high-threshold mechanoreceptors converge on spinothalamic and other ascending tract cells [36]. Physiological processes are generally accompanied by low- level activity, mediation of regulatory reflexes, and transmission of nonpainful sensations.

High-intensity stimuli increase firing of low-threshold afferents and also activate high-threshold afferents, thereby activating nociceptive pathways and triggering pain [36].

More than 90% of all unmyelinated pelvic afferents are silent, being activated by electrical stimulation, but not even by extreme noxious stimuli [33]. Silent afferents can respond to chemical stimuli or tissue irritation, becoming responsive to even innocuous mechanical stimuli after sensitization [37]. These neurophysiological changes are detectable within minutes after tissue irritation, are likely to persist for the duration of irritation, and have been implicated in explaining visceral hypersensitivity.

Anal Sphincter Tone and Reflexes

Internal Anal Sphincter

The internal sphincter is primarily responsible for ensuring that the anal canal is closed at rest [14, 38]. The other contributors to anal resting tone include the external anal sphincter, the anal mucosal folds, and the puborectalis muscle. Penninckx et al. [39] estimated that anal resting tone was generated by nerve-induced activity in the internal sphincter (45% of anal resting tone), myogenic tone in the internal sphincter (10%), the external sphincter (35%), and the anal hemorrhoidal plexus (15%). These figures should be regarded as estimates, because they were obtained, in part, from complex studies in which anal resting pressure was sequentially recorded before surgery (i.e., abdomino perineal resection), after curarization, and in the resected specimen before and after verapamil. Moreover, the relative contributions of these factors to anal resting tone are influenced by several factors, including the size of the probe and the location at which pressure was measured.

Frenckner and Ihre investigated the contribution of myogenic tone and the extrinsic (sympathetic and parasympathetic) nerves to anal resting tone by assessing anal pressure at rest and in response to rectal distention under baseline conditions after low spinal anesthesia (L_5–S_1), and after high spinal anesthesia (T_6–T_{12}) [38]. A separate study assessed anal pressures before and after pudendal nerve blockade. The decline in anal resting pressure was significantly greater after high (32±3.2 mm Hg) than low (11±7.1 mm Hg) anesthesia or after pudendal nerve blockade (10±3.9 mmHg), suggesting there is a tonic excitatory sympathetic discharge to the internal anal sphincter in humans. However, the anal pressure during rectal distention was similar among the three groups, suggesting that this excitatory sympathetic discharge does not contribute to anal pressure during rectal distention. Conversely, sympathetic stimulation either evoked internal anal sphincter relaxation, [40, 41] or contraction followed by relaxation [42].

Anal resting pressure is not stationary but varies during the day. In addition to spontaneous relaxation of the internal sphincter, circadian variations that are dependent on the sleep/wake cycle and ultradian (~20 to 40 min in length) rhythms that are independent of the sleep/awake cycle have also been described [43].

Anal relaxation induced by rectal distention [i.e., the recto anal inhibitory reflex (RAIR)] is mediated by intrinsic nerves. This reflex is absent in Hirschsprung's disease. The extrinsic nerves are not essential for the reflex, as it is preserved in patients with cauda equina lesions or after spinal cord transection. However, extrinsic nerves may modulate the reflex, as relaxation is more pronounced and prolonged in children with sacral agenesis [44]. The recto anal inhibitory reflex is probably mediated by nitric oxide (NO); morphological studies reveal an efferent descending nitrergic rectoanal pathway [45]. Other nonadrenergic/noncholinergic neurotransmitters, i.e., vasoactive intestinal peptide (VIP) and adenosine triphosphate (ATP), may also participate in the RAIR [46, 47].

External Anal Sphincter

Though resting sphincter tone is predominantly attributed to the internal anal sphincter, studies under general anesthesia or after pudendal nerve block suggest the external anal sphincter generally accounts for ~25% up to 50% of resting anal tone. When continence is threatened, the external sphincter contracts to augment anal tone, preserving continence. This "squeeze" response may be voluntary, or it may be induced by increased intra-abdominal pressure [48] or by merely moving a finger across the anal canal lining [49]. Conversely, the external sphincter relaxes during defecation.

The only other striated muscles that display resting activity are the puborectalis, the external urethral sphincter, the cricopharyngeus, and the laryngeal abductors. Resting or tonic activity depends on the monosynaptic reflex drive, perhaps explaining why resting anal sphincter tone is reduced, but voluntary contraction of the external sphincter is preserved in tabes dorsalis [50]. The fiber distribution also favors tonic activity; type 1 (i.e., fatigue-resistant, slow twitch) fibers predominate in the human anal sphincter [12], while cats and rabbits predominantly contain type 2 or fast-twitch muscle fibers [51].

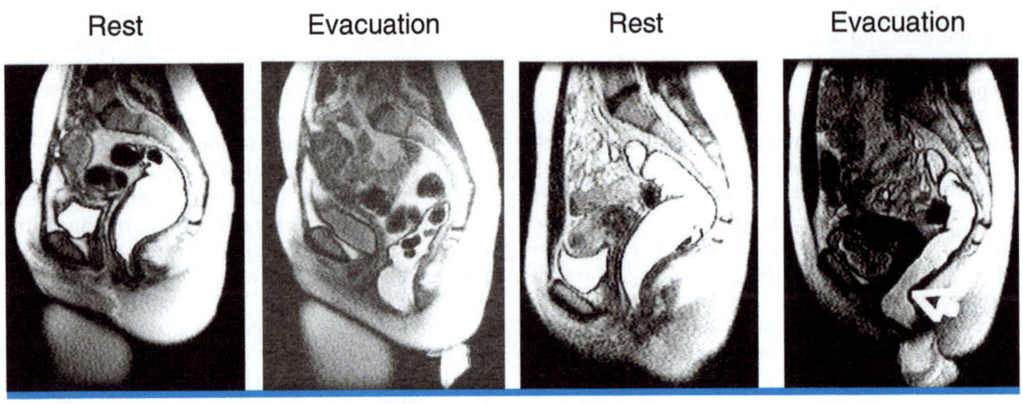

Fig. 3. Sagittal dynamic magnetic resonance images of normal puborectalis relaxation (*left panel*, subject 1) and puborectalis contraction (*arrow*, *right panel*, subject 2) during rectal evacuation. In both subjects, evacuation was associated with perineal descent (2.6 cm in subject 1; 1.7 cm in subject 2) and opening of the anorectal junction. During evacuation, the anorectal angle increased by 36° in subject 1 and declined by 10° in subject 2. Reprinted with permission from [52]

Puborectalis

The tonically active puborectalis muscle maintains the resting anorectal angle. Moreover, puborectalis contraction during a sudden rise in abdominal pressure reduces the anorectal angle, thus preserving continence. As noted earlier, electrophysiological stimulation studies in humans suggest this muscle is supplied, strictly ipsilaterally, by branches originating from the sacral plexus above the pelvic floor [5]. Disruption of the puborectalis inevitably causes significant incontinence, underscoring the importance of this muscle in maintaining continence.

Sacral Reflexes

The pelvic floor striated muscles contract reflexly in response to stimulation of perineal skin, (i.e., a somatosomatic reflex) or anal mucosa (i.e., a viscerosomatic reflex). The cutaneoanal reflex is elicited by scratching or pricking the perianal skin and involves the pudendal nerves and S_4 roots. Sacral reflexes also regulate anal sphincter tone during micturition. Thus, electrical activity of the internal anal sphincter increases during urinary bladder emptying in humans, returning to normal after micturition [53]. Conversely, the external anal sphincter relaxes during micturition in humans, cats, and dogs.

Mechanisms of Continence and Defecation

The mechanisms that maintain fecal continence include anatomical factors (i.e., the pelvic barrier, the rectal curvatures, and the transverse rectal folds), recto anal sensation, and rectal compliance. Stool is often transferred into the rectum by colonic high-amplitude-propagated contractions, which often occur after awakening or meals [54]. Denny-Brown and Robertson observed that rectal distention evoked rectal contraction and anal sphincter relaxation, facilitating evacuation [28]. The pelvic floor, particularly the puborectalis, also generally relaxes during defecation (Fig. 3). Simultaneous assessments of intrarectal pressures and pelvic floor activity (by manometry, EMG, or imaging) reveal that increased intra rectal pressure and anal relaxation are required for normal defecation. However, the relative contributions of increased intra-abdominal pressure generated by voluntary effort [55] and rectal contraction [56] to the "propulsive" force during defecation are unclear, partly because a barostat rather than a manometry is necessary to optimally characterize rectal contractions, which are of relatively low amplitude. Current concepts suggest that minimal straining to initiate defecation is not abnormal, because many asymptomatic subjects strain to initiate defecation [57]. However, excessive straining, and particularly a Valsalva maneuver, may impede evacuation because while a Valsalva maneuver may increase intrarectal pressure, the pelvic floor muscles also contract, increasing outlet resistance [58]. Thus, it is necessary to assess the balance between these two sometimes opposing forces by measuring the net recto anal force during evacuation [59]. One possibility is that the relative contributions of voluntary effort and rectal contraction to defecation vary, depending on the circumstances prior to defecation. For example, the voluntary effort may range from being negligible when stool is soft to considerable when stool is hard and situated in the upper rectum.

If defecation is inconvenient, it can generally be postponed. The rectal contractile response to distention normally subsides as the rectum accommodates or relaxes. The external sphincter and/or puborectalis can be contracted voluntarily. This contractile response requires the ability to perceive stool in the rectum and perhaps also in the anal canal. Indeed, the anal sphincter may also relax independently of rectal distention, allowing the anal epithelium to periodically "sample" and ascertain whether rectal contents are gas, liquid, or stool [60].

These mechanisms underscore that defecation is an integrated somato visceral reflex. Indeed, the central nervous system plays a greater role in regulating anorectal sensomotor functions compared with other regions of the gastrointestinal tract. The elaborate somatic defecation response depends on centers above the lumbo sacral cord, and probably craniad to the spinal cord itself. However, Garry observed that colonic stimulation in cats induced colonic contraction and anal relaxation, even after destruction of the lumbo sacral cord, and concluded that the gut "seems not to have wholly surrendered its independence" [61].

Pharmacological Considerations

In contrast to non sphincteric regions, sympathetic nerves excite while parasympathetic nerves inhibit the sphincters. The internal anal sphincter has dense adrenergic innervation in humans and monkeys. It is also more sensitive to adrenergic compared with cholinergic agonists [62]. Cholinergic agonists either contracted or relaxed internal anal sphincter strips in humans.

Anal administration of exogenous nitrates (i.e., 0.2% glyceryl trinitrate) has been extensively tested and widely used to treat anal fissures, as these are often associated with increased anal resting tone [63]. Topical calcium-channel blockers (e.g., 0.2% nifedipine or 2% diltiazem) are probably more effective than nitrates for treating anal fissures, with a lower incidence of side effects. Bethanecol and botulinum toxin have also been used to treat anal fissures.

The beneficial effects of loperamide in fecal incontinence may be attributable not only to a reduction of diarrhea, but also to an increase of anal resting tone [64]. The α_1 adrenoreceptor agonist phenylephrine applied to the anal canal increased anal resting pressure by 33% in healthy subjects and incontinent patients [65]. However, phenylephrine did not significantly improve incontinence scores or resting anal pressure compared with placebo in a randomized double-blind placebo-controlled crossover study of 36 patients with fecal incontinence [66].

Surgical Considerations

From a therapeutic perspective, an understanding of anatomy is particularly important for managing anal fistulae, preventing nerve injury during surgical dissection, and understanding the consequences of rectal resection. Left-sided colectomy may result in postoperative colonic transit delays in the unresected segment; this likely represents parasympathetic denervation, as ascending intramural fibers travel in a retrograde manner from the pelvis to the ascending colon. The sigmoid colon and rectum are also supplied by descending fibers that run along the inferior mesenteric artery. These nerves may be disrupted during a low anterior resection, leaving a denervated segment that may be short or long depending on whether the dissection line includes the origin of the inferior mesenteric artery [67]. A long denervated segment is more likely to be associated with non-propagated colonic pressure waves and delayed colonic transit than is a short denervated segment. In addition to colonic denervation, a low anterior resection may damage the anal sphincter and reduce rectal compliance [68]; in contrast to anal sphincter injury, rectal compliance may recover with time [69]. Defecation may also be affected after surgical section of pelvic nerves in humans [70, 71].

Denonvilliers' fascia is intimately adherent to the anterior mesorectal fat but only loosely adherent to the seminal vesicles. During anterior rectal dissection, the deep parasympathetic nerves situated in the narrow space between the rectum and the prostate and seminal vesicles may be damaged, leading to impotence [72]. For benign disease, most surgeons will tend to stay posterior to Denonvilliers' fascia in an attempt to protect the pelvic nerves. For malignant disease, the choice is less straightforward, because dissection behind rather than in front of the fascia may, in theory, be associated with incomplete resection and/or local recurrence.

Because vaginal delivery can damage the anal sphincters and the pudendal nerve, up to 10% of women develop fecal incontinence after a vaginal delivery [73]. The incidence of post partum fecal incontinence is considerably higher (i.e., 15–59%) in women who sustain a third-degree (i.e., anal sphincter disruption) or a fourth-degree tear (i.e., a third-degree tear with anal epithelial disruption) [74, 75]. The only prospective study that imaged the anal sphincters before and after vaginal delivery demonstrated that anal sphincter defects and pudendal nerve injury after vaginal delivery were often clinically occult and that forceps delivery was the only independent factor associated with anal sphincter damage during vaginal delivery [76]. A Cochrane Review concluded that restrictive episiotomy policies were beneficial (i.e., less posterior perineal trauma, less suturing, and fewer complications) compared with routine episiotomy policies [77]. However, there is an increased risk of anterior perineal trauma with restrictive episiotomy. Both the external and internal anal sphincters may be damaged during a severe perineal laceration. When possible, lacerations that require complex repair should be carried out in the operating room, under regional or general anesthesia, with appropriate instruments, adequate light, and an assistant [78]. A randomized controlled study demonstrated that compared with end-to-end repair, primary overlapping repair of external anal sphincter defects was associated with a significantly lower incidence of fecal incontinence, fecal urgency, and perineal pain at 12 months [79]. Though some experts have suggested that both the internal and external anal sphincters be repaired, there are no trials comparing concurrent repair of the internal and external anal sphincters to repair of the external sphincter alone after obstetric injury [80, 81].

References

1. Cook TA, Mortensen NJ (2002) Colon, rectum, anus, anal sphincters and the pelvic floor. In: Pemberton JH, Swash M et al (eds) The pelvic floor: its function and disorders. Harcourt, London, pp 61–76
2. Lau ST, Caty MG (2006) Hindgut abnormalities. Surg Clin North Am 86:301–316
3. Mahmoud N, Ross, H; Fry, R (2004) Colon and rectum. In: Towsend CM, Beauchamp RD et al (eds) Sabiston Textbook of Surgery. W.B. Saunders, New York
4. Hjartardottir S, Nilsson J, Petersen C et al (1997) The female pelvic floor: a dome-not a basin. Acta Obstet Gynecol Scand 76:567–571
5. Percy JP, Neill ME, Swash M et al (1981) Electrophysiological study of motor nerve supply of pelvic floor. Lancet 1:16–17
6. Bharucha AE, Klingele CJ (2005) Autonomic and somatic systems to the anorectum and pelvic floor. In: Dyck PJ, Thomas PK, (eds.) Peripheral neuropathy, 4th edn. Elsevier Saunders, Philadelphia, pp 279–298
7. Williams PL, Warwick R (eds) (1980) Splanchnology. Churchill Livingstone, London
8. Bharucha AE (2003) Fecal Iincontinence. Gastroenterology 124(6):1672–1685
9. Hoffman S, Orestano F (1967) Histology of the myenteric plexus in relation to rectal biopsy in congenital megacolon. J Pediatr Surg 2:575–577
10. Weinberg AG (1970) The anorectal myenteric plexus: its relation to hypoganglionosis of the colon. Am J Clin Pathol 54:6370–6420
11. Horiguchi K, Keef KD, Ward SM (2003) Distribution of interstitial cells of Cajal in tunica muscularis of the canine rectoanal region. Am J Physiol Gastrointest Liver Physiol 284:G756–767
12. Schroder HD, Reske-Nielsen E (1983) Fiber types in the striated urethral and anal sphincters. Acta Neuropathol 60:278–282
13. Williams PL, Warwick R (eds) (1980) Neurology. Churchill Livingstone, London
14. Gonella J, Bouvier M, Blanquet F (1987) Extrinsic nervous control of motility of small and large intestines and related sphincters. Physiol Rev 67:902–961
15. Nakayama S, Neya T, Yamasato T et al (1979) Activity of the spinal defaecation centre in the guinea pig. Ital J Gastroenterol 11:168–173
16. Turnbull GK, Hamdy S, Aziz Q et al (1999) The cortical topography of human anorectal musculature. Gastroenterology 117:32–39
17. Holstege G, Tan J (1987) Supraspinal control of motoneurons innervating the striated muscles of the pelvic floor including urethral and anal sphincters in the cat. Brain 110:1323–1344
18. Chalmers D, Swash M (1987) Selective vulnerability of urinary Onuf motoneurons in Shy-Drager syndrome. J Neurol 234:259–260
19. Sung JH, Mastri AR, Segal E (1979) Pathology of Shy-Drager syndrome. J Neuropathol Exp Neurol 38:353–368
20. Sherrington CS (1892) Notes on the arrangement of some motor fibres in the lumbosacral plexus. J Physiol 13:672–675
21. Barber MD, Bremer RE, Thor KB et al (2002) Innervation of the female levator ani muscles. Am J Obstet Gynecol 187:64–71
22. Bremer RE, Barber MD, Coates KW et al (2003) Innervation of the levator ani and coccygeus muscles of the female rat. Anat Rec A Discov Mol Cell Evol Biol 275:1031–1041
23. Pierce LM, Reyes M, Thor KB et al (2003) Innervation of the levator ani muscles in the female squirrel monkey. Am J Obstet Gynecol 188:1141–1147
24. Janig W, Koltzenburg M (1991) Receptive properties of sacral primary afferent neurons supplying the colon. J Neurophysiol 65:1067–1077
25. Lynn PA, Olsson C, Zagorodnyuk V et al (2003) Rectal intraganglionic laminar endings are transduction sites of extrinsic mechanoreceptors in the guinea pig rectum. Gastroenterology 125:786–794
26. Lynn P, Zagorodnyuk V, Hennig G et al (2005) Mechanical activation of rectal intraganglionic laminar endings in the guinea pig distal gut. J Physiol 564:589–601
27. Hulsebosch CE, Coggeshall RE (1982) An analysis of the axon populations in the nerves to the pelvic viscera in the rat. J Comp Neurol 211:1–10
28. Denny-Brown D, Robertson E (1935) An investigation of the nervous control of defaecation. Brain 58:256–310
29. Goligher JC, Hughes ESR (1951) Sensibility of rectum and colon: its role in the mechanism of anal continence. Lancet 1:543–548
30. Ness TJ, Gebhart GF (1990) Visceral pain: a review of experimental studies. Pain 41:167–234
31. Morgan C, Nadelhaft I, de Groat WC (1981) The distri-

bution of visceral primary afferents from the pelvic nerve to Lissauer's tract and the spinal gray matter and its relationship to the sacral parasympathetic nucleus. J Comp Neurol 201:415–440
32. Baron R, Janig W, McLachlan EM (1985) The afferent and sympathetic components of the lumbar spinal outflow to the colon and pelvic organs in the cat. III. The colonic nerves, incorporating an analysis of all components of the lumbar prevertebral outflow. J Comp Neurol 238:158–168
33. Janig W, Morrison JFB (1986) Functional properties of spinal visceral afferents supplying abdominal and pelvic organs, with special emphasis on visceral nociception. In: Cervero F, Morrison JFB (eds) Progress in brain research. Visceral sensation. Elsevier, Amsterdam, pp 87–114
34. Blumberg H, Haupt P, Janig W et al (1983) Encoding of visceral noxious stimuli in the discharge patterns of visceral afferent fibres from the colon. Pflug Arch 398:33–40
35. Bahns E, Halsband U, Janig W (1987) Responses of sacral visceral afferents from the lower urinary tract, colon and anus to mechanical stimulation. Pflugers Arch 410:296–303
36. Cervero F, Janig W (1992) Visceral nociceptors: a new world order? Trends Neurosci 15:374–378
37. Mayer EA, Gebhart GF (1994) Basic and clinical aspects of visceral hyperalgesia. Gastroenterology 107:271–293
38. Frenckner B, Ihre T (1976) Influence of autonomic nerves on the internal and sphincter in man. Gut 17:306–312
39. Penninckx F, Lestar B, Kerremans R (1992) The internal anal sphincter: mechanisms of control and its role in maintaining anal continence. Baillieres Clin Gastroenterol 6:193–214
40. Horgan PG, O'Connell PR, Shinkwin CA et al (1989) Effect of anterior resection on anal sphincter function. Br J Surg 76:783–786
41. Lubowski DZ, Nicholls RJ, Swash M et al (1987) Neural control of internal anal sphincter function. Br J Surg 74:668–670
42. Carlstedt A, Nordgren S, Fasth S et al (1988) Sympathetic nervous influence on the internal anal sphincter and rectum in man. Int J Colorectal Dis 3:90–95
43. Enck P, Eggers E, Koletzko S et al (1991) Spontaneous variation of anal "resting" pressure in healthy humans. Am J Physiol 261:G823–826
44. Morera C, Nurko S (2003) Rectal manometry in patients with isolated sacral agenesis. J Pediatr Gastroenterol Nutr 37(1):47–52
45. Stebbing JF, Brading AF, Mortensen NJ (1996) Nitric oxide and the rectoanal inhibitory reflex: retrograde neuronal tracing reveals a descending nitrergic rectoanal pathway in a guinea-pig model. Br J Surg 83:493–498
46. Nurko S, Rattan S (1988) Role of vasoactive intestinal polypeptide in the internal anal sphincter relaxation of the opossum. J Clin Invest 81:1146–1153
47. Biancani P, Walsh J, Behar J (1985) Vasoactive intestinal peptide: a neurotransmitter for relaxation of the rabbit internal anal sphincter. Gastroenterology 89:867–874
48. Floyd W, Walls E (1953) Electromyography of the sphincter ani externus in man. J Physiol 122:599–609
49. Taverner D, Smiddy FG (1959) An electromyographic study of the normal function of the external anal sphincter and pelvic diaphragm. Dis Col Rectum 2:153–160
50. Melzak J, Porter NH (1964) Studies of the reflex activity of the external sphincter ani in spinal man. Paraplegia 1:277–296
51. Krier J, Adams T, Meyer RA (1988) Physiological, morphological, and histochemical properties of cat external anal sphincter. Am J Physiol: Gastrointest Liver Physiol 255:G772–778
52. Bharucha AE, Fletcher JG, Seide B et al (2005) Phenotypic variation in functional disorders of defecation. Gastroenterology 128(5):1199–1210
53. Salducci J, Planche D, Naudy B (1982) Physiological role of the internal anal sphincter and the external anal sphincter during micturition. In: Wienbeck M (eds) Motility of the digestive tract. Raven, New York, pp 513–520
54. Bassotti G, Crowell MD, Whitehead WE (1993) Contractile activity of the human colon: lessons from 24 hour studies. Gut 34:129–133
55. MacDonald A, Paterson PJ, Baxter JN et al (1993) Relationship between intra-abdominal and intrarectal pressure in the proctometrogram. Br J Surg 80:1070–1071
56. Halpert A, Keck L, Drossman DA et al (2004) Rectal contractions are part of normal defecation. Gastroenterology 126:A-362
57. Heaton KW, Ghosh S, Braddon FE (1991) How bad are the symptoms and bowel dysfunction of patients with the irritable bowel syndrome? A prospective, controlled study with emphasis on stool form. Gut 32:73–79
58. Sapsford RR, Hodges PW, Richardson CA et al (2001) Co-activation of the abdominal and pelvic floor muscles during voluntary exercises. Neurourol Urodyn 20:31–42
59. Bharucha AE, Croak AJ, Gebhart JB et al (2006) Comparison of rectoanal axial forces in health and functional defecatory disorders. Am J Physiol: Gastro Liver Physiol 290: G1164–G1169
60. Miller R, Bartolo DC, Cervero F et al (1988) Anorectal sampling: a comparison of normal and incontinent patients. Br J Surg 75:44–47
61. Garry R (1933) The responses to stimulation of the caudal end of the large bowel in the cat. J Physiol Lond 78:208
62. Parks AG, Fishlock DJ, Cameron JD et al (1969) Preliminary investigation of the pharmacology of the human internal anal sphincter. Gut 10:674–677
63. Madoff RD, Fleshman JW (2003) AGA technical review on the diagnosis and care of patients with anal fissure. Gastroenterology 124:235–245
64. Read M, Read NW, Barber DC et al (1982) Effects of loperamide on anal sphincter function in patients complaining of chronic diarrhea with fecal incontinence and urgency. Dig Dis Sci 27:807–814
65. Cheetham MJ, Kamm MA, Phillips RK (2001) Topical phenylephrine increases anal canal resting pressure in patients with faecal incontinence. Gut 48:356–359
66. Carapeti EA, Kamm MA, Phillips RK (2000) Randomized controlled trial of topical phenylephrine in the

treatment of faecal incontinence. Br J Surg 87:38–42
67. Koda K, Saito N, Seike K et al (2005) Denervation of the neorectum as a potential cause of defecatory disorder following low anterior resection for rectal cancer. Dis Colon Rectum 48:210–217
68. Batignani G, Monaci I, Ficari F et al (1991) What affects continence after anterior resection of the rectum? Dis Colon Rectum 34:329–335
69. Williamson ME, Lewis WG, Finan PJ et al (1995) Recovery of physiologic and clinical function after low anterior resection of the rectum for carcinoma: myth or reality? Dis Colon Rectum 38:411–418
70. Devroede G, Lamarche J (1974) Functional importance of extrinsic parasympathetic innervation to the distal colon and rectum in man. Gastroenterology 66:273–280
71. Scott HWJ, Cantrell JR (1949) Colonmetrographic studies of the effects of section of the parasympathetic nerves of the colon. Bull Johns Hopkins Hosp 85:310–319
72. Lindsey I, Guy RJ, Warren BF et al (2000) Anatomy of Denonvilliers' fascia and pelvic nerves, impotence, and implications for the colorectal surgeon. Br J Surg 87:1288–1299
73. Bharucha AE (2003) Fecal incontinence. Gastroenterology 124:1672–1685
74. Mostwin J BA, Haab F, Koelbl H et al (2005) Pathophysiology of urinary incontinence, fecal incontinence and pelvic organ prolapse. In: Abrams P, Cardozo L et al (eds) Incontinence. Health Publication, Paris, pp 425–484
75. Sultan AH (1999) Obstetrical perineal injury and anal incontinence. Clin Risk 5:193–196
76. Sultan AH, Kamm MA, Hudson CN et al (1993) Anal-sphincter disruption during vaginal delivery. N Engl J Med 329:1905–1911
77. Carroli G, Belizan J (2006) Episiotomy for vaginal birth [systematic review]. Cochrane Database of Systematic Reviews http://www.cochrane.org. Cited 15 Nov 2006
78. Royal College of Obstetricians and Gynaecologists (2001) Management of third- and fourth-degree perineal tears following vaginal deliveries. London
79. Fernando RJ, Sultan AH, Kettle C et al (2006) Repair techniques for obstetric anal sphincter injuries: a randomized controlled trial. Obstet Gynecol 107:1261–1268
80. Sultan AH, Monga AK, Kumar D et al (1999) Primary repair of obstetric anal sphincter rupture using the overlap technique. Br J Obstet Gynaecol 106:318–323
81. Norderval S, Oian P, Revhaug A et al (2005) Anal incontinence after obstetric sphincter tears: outcome of anatomic primary repairs. Dis Colon Rectum 48:1055–1061

Invited Commentary

Peter J. Lunniss, S. Mark Scott

The comprehensive overview of the anatomy and physiology of faecal continence by Drs. Bharucha and Blandon provides an excellent summary of what is increasingly acknowledged to be a highly complex area of human biology. Readers should also direct their attention to Table 1 in Chapter 4 in this book. Historically, both research and clinical interest have focused on the role of the anal sphincter complex in the maintenance of continence and the physiological changes within the sphincters and pelvic floor associated with defecation. This is perhaps not surprising because of both the relative inaccessibility to study of the colorectum itself and the lack of appropriate physiological tools to assess function. However, it is becoming increasingly recognised, principally through the efforts of the Mayo Clinic group [1–3], our own group [4–6], and that of others [7, 8], that the contribution of normal rectal sensorimotor and biomechanical function may be equally crucial to the maintenance of continence, as evident from recent studies showing loss of rectal reservoir function associated with hypersensitivity, hypocompliance, hypercontractility, and hyperreactivity in faecal incontinence [1–8]. Conversely, an appreciation that impaired sensation (*hypo*sensitivity) and *hyper*compliance may underlie (notably, passive) incontinence in a proportion of patients is also gaining momentum [9–14]. Introduction of the barostat and standardised protocols for its use has facilitated this greater understanding of rectal and colonic dynamics, both in health and in disturbed bowel function [2, 8, 13]. Evaluation of colorectal motor function, though still primarily restricted to the research setting, can now be reproducibly determined by a variety of techniques, including the use of long catheters placed either antegrade [15, 16] or retrograde [17, 18] to assess pancolonic motility; other, less invasive, methods to assess colonic contractility and transit will soon be available [19]. Furthermore, the association between cerebral activity and bowel function can now also be studied, and carefully constructed protocols employing techniques such as functional magnetic resonance imaging (f-MRI), the assessment of cortical evoked potential, etc. [20–24], will provide essential knowledge concerning the brain–gut axis.

Development and use of these physiological tools has confirmed the importance of suprasphincteric components to continence and defecation. Nevertheless, the pelvic floor and anal sphincters are "the final common path", and, certainly in the surgical setting, represent a frequent source of disturbed function. There is no doubt that anal sphincteric disruption is the main pathogenic mechanism in acquired faecal incontinence, but levator ani failure, including that of the puborectalis, is increasingly recognised to be of aetiological importance [2, 25, 26]. Nevertheless, failure to study and address those other components fundamental to continence will, not surprisingly, lead to poor outcomes following intervention directed solely at sphincteric dysfunction. We recently demonstrated how assessment of rectal sensorimotor function can direct surgery for both incontinence (rectal "augmentation" with or without electrically stimulated gracilis neosphincter for urgency, associated with rectal hypersensitivity, low rectal compliance and exaggerated motor activity [4]) and constipation (vertical rectal reduction for megarectum associated with hyposensitivity and excessive compliance [27]), with functional success associated with normalisation of pathophysiology. It remains unclear exactly how sacral nerve stimulation (SNS) may improve both colonic motility (in cases of inertia [28]) and continence (in incontinence [29]), but it is apparent that the primary effect is certainly not on sphincteric function [30, 31]. Effects on rectal sensorimotor activity are not consistent [30–32], and it may be that we simply do not have the right tools to measure the physiologically significant effects of SNS (possibly central or spinal [21]) and, ultimately, to predict in whom the technique has a good chance of positive effect [29].

Intuitively, anal sensation must be integral to normal continence. It was first systematically assessed by Duthie and Gairns in 1960 [33], since when its measurement and significance has been somewhat questioned [34]. It may be, however, that it is the methodology with which we are currently assessing anal sensation (usually electrostimulation) that is imperfect, as the multitude and density of nerve endings subserving different sensations within the anal transitional zone beg a more influential role. Equally, one may argue that the key to normal anal motor function is the conjoined longitudinal muscle of the anal canal. In the foetus, this structure is thicker than the internal sphincter. As it descends between the internal sphincter and the true intersphincteric space (medial to the external sphincter), it sends extensions medially across the internal sphincter to help support the submucosa of the anal canal (notably the anal cushions), laterally and variably across the external sphincter into the ischiorectal fossa and pelvic side wall fascia, and caudally to insert into the perianal skin [35]. It is, indeed, the anatomy of these lateral and distal extensions that define the components of the external sphincter. Not only does such an arrangement provide a supporting meshwork for the other sphincter components, but the differential responses to neurotransmitters compared with the internal sphincter [36] begs a more active functional role, its contraction flattening the anal cushions, shortening and widening the anal canal, and everting the anal orifice during defecation [37]. Thinning, loss of muscle and fragmentation associated with ageing [38], and perhaps in a more accelerated way, in subjects with pelvic floor weakness and prolapse, are undoubtedly of significance. Another important consideration was highlighted by the discovery of nonadrenergic, noncholinergic (NANC) fibres subserving internal anal sphincter contraction, mediated through the neurotransmitter nitric oxide [36, 39, 40]. This heralded both the acknowledgement of the superspecialised function of this distal continuation of the gut circular muscle and the advent of "reversible chemical sphincterotomy" [41] to reduce resting tone, as well as (less successful) attempts at augmenting sphincter tone with topical sympathomimetic agents [42].

Further study is merited concerning the role of coordinated colorectoanal activity in normal continence and defecation. It is clear that entry of stool or gas into the rectum initiates a series of events (including elicitation of reflexes), the consequences of which may or may not be consciously perceived. Investigation of these reflexes may shed further light on our understanding of the pathophysiology of incontinence. For example, several parameters of the rectoanal inhibitory reflex (RAIR) may be quantified, and the RAIR has been shown to be attenuated in patients with faecal leakage [43–45]. The significance of the rectoanal contractile reflex requires further research, particularly its relation to conscious perception of anorectal distension [3, 46–48].

Although the gross anatomy of the musculature of the anal canal is well known, the same cannot be said of innervation of the pelvic floor and anorectum. Readers will be already highly familiar with the debate concerning the influence of pudendal neuropathy on continence and defecation, its measurement, and usefulness in directing therapy or advising on prognosis following (especially surgical) intervention. Cadaveric studies have demonstrated three variations in pudendal nerve anatomy [49, 50], and its innervation of the levator ani group of muscles remains controversial. In addition, how much variability and asymmetry there is in external anal sphincter innervation has not been explored until recently [51]. There is now, however, growing awareness that the concept of lateral dominance—asymmetry in the neural contribution of a bilaterally innervated midline structure—applies to pudendal nerve innervation [52–54]. This may be particularly important in that damage to the dominant nerve, sustained through whatever injurious mechanism (e.g. traction injury), may leave the individual more susceptible to dysfunction of those structures innervated by the pudendal nerve with resultant incontinence. In a similar vein, *autonomic* innervation to the pelvic viscera remains poorly studied, particularly with reference to the exact neuroanatomy of afferent pathways. Consequently, there remains considerable inconsistency in the literature when describing the correct neurological nomenclature of afferent neurones and pathways to the rectum. However, significant advances are being made: Drs. Bharucha and Blandon have highlighted the finding of rectal intraganglionic laminar endings (rIGLEs) in the guinea pig rectum that serve as slowly adapting mechanoreceptors [55], and other molecular mechanisms involved in mechanosensory transduction have also been identified. For example, rectal sensory nerve fibres expressing the transient receptor potential vanilloid 1 (TRPV1) receptor, which is believed to be involved in neuronal signalling, have been found to be increased in patients with urge faecal incontinence associated with rectal hypersensitivity [56]. The results of further study of both somatic and autonomic innervation may go some way to help resolve recurrent angst and sometimes anger at clinical and research meetings!

One other point that deserves consideration is that faecal incontinence and "constipation" frequently coexist. This perhaps underscores the importance of "normal" defecation to the preservation of continence, in that passive (overflow) faecal leakage, or postdefecation incontinence, may occur as a consequence of incomplete rectal emptying secondary to a "mechanical" (i.e. anatomical, such as large rectocele, intussusception, megarectum etc.) or "functional" outlet obstruction (e.g. pelvic floor dyssynergia, poor defecatory dynamics, nonrelaxing pelvic floor etc.). As such, a comprehension of the normal process of defecation should be considered fundamental to the clinical management of patients with faecal incontinence.

Finally, the complexity of these two biological functions (continence and defecation), which we all take for granted until something goes wrong, means that the risk factors contributing towards disturbed function are often multifactorial and that interventions, especially surgical, that aim to restore primarily anatomy and thus, hopefully, function, are not associated with outcomes that are always satisfactory to the patient. As professionals involved in health delivery, emphasis on research must continue and expand as the basis for effective, targeted and individualised treatment.

References

1. Salvioli B, Bharucha AE, Rath-Harvey D et al (2001) Rectal compliance, capacity, and rectoanal sensation in fecal incontinence. Am J Gastroenterol 96:2158–2168
2. Bharucha AE, Fletcher JG, Harper CM et al (2005) Relationship between symptoms and disordered continence mechanisms in women with idiopathic faecal incontinence. Gut 54:546–555
3. Andrews C, Bharucha AE, Seide B et al (2007) Rectal sensorimotor dysfunction in women with fecal incontinence. Am J Physiol Gastrointest Liver Physiol 292:G282–G289
4. Williams NS, Ogunbiyi OA, Scott SM et al (2001) Rectal augmentation and stimulated gracilis anal neosphincter: a new approach in the management of fecal urgency and incontinence. Dis Colon Rectum 44:192–198
5. Chan CL, Scott SM, Williams NS et al (2005) Rectal hypersensitivity worsens stool frequency, urgency, and lifestyle in patients with urge fecal incontinence. Dis Colon Rectum 48:134–140
6. Chan CL, Lunniss PJ, Wang D (2005) Rectal sensorimotor dysfunction in patients with urge faecal incontinence: evidence from prolonged manometric studies. Gut 54:1263–1272
7. Sun WM, Donnelly TC, Read NW (1992) Utility of a combined test of anorectal manometry, electromyography, and sensation in determining the mechanism of idiopathic faecal incontinence. Gut 33:807–813
8. Siproudhis L, El Abkari M, El Alaoui M et al (2005) Low rectal volumes in patients suffering from fecal incontinence: what does it mean? Aliment Pharmacol Ther 22:989–996
9. Hoffmann BA, Timmcke AE, Gathright JB Jr et al (1995) Fecal seepage and soiling: a problem of rectal sensation. Dis Colon Rectum; 38:746–748
10. Siproudhis L, Bellissant E, Juguet F et al (1999) Perception of and adaptation to rectal isobaric distension in patients with faecal incontinence. Gut 44:687–692
11. Gladman MA, Scott SM, Chan CL et al (2003) Rectal hyposensitivity: prevalence and clinical impact in patients with intractable constipation and fecal incontinence. Dis Colon Rectum 46:238–246
12. Rao SS, Ozturk R, Stessman M (2004) Investigation of the pathophysiology of fecal seepage. Am J Gastroenterol 99:2204–2209
13. Gladman MA, Dvorkin LS, Lunniss PJ et al (2005) Rectal hyposensitivity: a disorder of the rectal wall or the afferent pathway? An assessment using the barostat. Am J Gastroenterol 100:106–114
14. Gladman MA, Lunniss PJ, Scott SM et al (2006) Rectal hyposensitivity. Am J Gastroenterol 101:1140–1151
15. Bampton PA, Dinning PG, Kennedy ML et al (2001) Prolonged multi-point recording of colonic manometry in the unprepared human colon: providing insight into potentially relevant pressure wave parameters. Am J Gastroenterol 96:1838–1848
16. Scott SM (2003) Manometric techniques for the evaluation of colonic motor activity: current status. Neurogastroenterol Motil 15:483–513
17. Herbst F, Kamm MA, Morris GP et al (1997) Gastrointestinal transit and prolonged ambulatory colonic motility in health and faecal incontinence. Gut 41:381–389
18. Rao SS, Sadeghi P, Beaty J et al (2001) Ambulatory 24-h colonic manometry in healthy humans. Am J Physiol Gastrointest Liver Physiol 280:G629–G639
19. Sarosiek I, Majewski M, The SmartPill Trial Group et al (2006) Non-digestible capsule (SmartPill) as a novel diagnostic tool for detecting motility impairment within the gut. Neurogastroenterol Motil 18:786 (Abstract)
20. Turnbull GK, Hamdy S, Aziz Q et al (1999) The cortical topography of human anorectal musculature. Gastroenterology 117:32–39
21. Sheldon R, Kiff ES, Clarke A et al (2005) Sacral nerve stimulation reduces corticoanal excitability in patients with faecal incontinence. Br J Surg 92:1423–1431
22. Harris ML, Hobson AR, Hamdy S et al (2006) Neurophysiological evaluation of healthy human anorectal sensation. Am J Physiol Gastrointest Liver Physiol 291:G950–G958
23. Thompson DG (2006) Neurogastroenterology: imaging of the sensory and motor control of the GI tract. J Psychosom Res 61:301–304
24. Mayer EA, Naliboff BD, Craig AD et al (2006) Neuroimaging of the brain-gut axis: from basic understanding to treatment of functional GI disorders. Gastroenterology 131:1925–1942
25. Fernandez-Fraga X, Azpiroz F, Malagelada JR (2002) Significance of pelvic floor muscles in anal incontinence. Gastroenterology 123:1441–1450
26. Eguare EI, Neary P, Crosbie J et al (2004) Dynamic magnetic resonance imaging of the pelvic floor in patients with idiopathic combined fecal and urinary incontinence. J Gastrointest Surg 8:73–82
27. Gladman MA, Williams NS, Scott SM et al (2005) Medium-term results of vertical reduction rectoplasty and sigmoid colectomy for idiopathic megarectum. Br J Surg 92:624–630
28. Dinning PG, Fuentealba SE, Kennedy ML et al (2007) Sacral nerve stimulation induces pan-colonic propa-

gating pressure waves and increases defecation frequency in patients with slow-transit constipation. Colorectal Dis 9:123–132
29. Gourcerol G, Gallas S, Michot F et al (2007) Sacral nerve stimulation in fecal incontinence: are there factors associated with success? Dis Colon Rectum 50:3–12
30. Michelsen HB, Buntzen S, Krogh K et al (2006) Rectal volume tolerability and anal pressures in patients with fecal incontinence treated with sacral nerve stimulation. Dis Colon Rectum 49:1039–1044
31. Jarrett ME, Mowatt G, Glazener CM et al (2004) Systematic review of sacral nerve stimulation for faecal incontinence and constipation. Br J Surg 91:1559–1569
32. Uludag O, Morren GL, Dejong CH et al (2005) Effect of sacral neuromodulation on the rectum. Br J Surg 92:1017–1023
33. Duthie HL, Gairns FW (1960) Sensory nerve endings and sensation in the anal region of man. Br J Surg 47:585–595
34. Felt-Bersma RJ, Poen AC, Cuesta MA et al (1997) Anal sensitivity test: what does it measure and do we need it? Cause or derivative of anorectal complaints. Dis Colon Rectum 40:811–816
35. Lunniss PJ, Phillips RK (1992) Anatomy and function of the anal longitudinal muscle. Br J Surg 79:882–884
36. O'Kelly TJ, Brading A, Mortensen NJ (1993) In vitro response of the human anal canal longitudinal muscle layer to cholinergic and adrenergic stimulation: evidence of sphincter specialization. Br J Surg 80:1337–1341
37. Shafik A (1976) A new concept of the anatomy of the anal sphincter mechanism and the physiology of defecation. III. The longitudinal anal muscle: anatomy and role in anal sphincter mechanism. Invest Urol 13:271–277
38. Haas PA, Fox TA Jr, Haas GP (1984) The pathogenesis of hemorrhoids. Dis Colon Rectum 27:442–450
39. Burleigh DE (1983) Non-cholinergic, non-adrenergic inhibitory neurons in human internal anal sphincter muscle. J Pharm Pharmacol 35:258–260
40. Cook TA, Brading AF, Mortensen NJMcC (1999) Differences in contractile properties of anorectal smooth muscle and the effects of calcium channel blockade. Br J Surg 86:70–75
41. Loder PB, Kamm MA, Nicholls RJ et al (1994) 'Reversible chemical sphincterotomy' by local application of glyceryl trinitrate. Br J Surg 81:1386–1389
42. Carapeti EA, Kamm MA, Phillips RK (2000) Randomized controlled trial of topical phenylephrine in the treatment of faecal incontinence. Br J Surg 2000 87:38–42
43. Sangwan YP, Coller JA, Schoetz DJ et al (1996) Spectrum of abnormal rectoanal reflex patterns in patients with fecal incontinence. Dis Colon Rectum 39:59–65
44. Zbar AP, Aslam M, Gold DM et al (1998) Parameters of the rectoanal inhibitory reflex in patients with idiopathic fecal incontinence and chronic constipation. Dis Colon Rectum 41:200–208
45. Kaur G, Gardiner A, Duthie GS (2002) Rectoanal reflex parameters in incontinence and constipation. Dis Colon Rectum 45:928–933
46. Akervall S, Fasth S, Nordgren S et al (1989) Rectal reservoir and sensory function studied by graded isobaric distension in normal man. Gut 30:496–502
47. Sun WM, Read NW, Prior A et al (1990) Sensory and motor responses to rectal distention vary according to rate and pattern of balloon inflation. Gastroenterology 99:1008–1015
48. Corsetti M, Cesana B, Bhoori S (2004) Rectal hyperreactivity to distention in patients with irritable bowel syndrome: role of distention rate. Clin Gastroenterol Hepatol 2:49–56
49. Shafik A, el Sherif M, Youssef A et al (1995) Surgical anatomy of the pudendal nerve and its clinical implications. Clin Anat 8:110–115
50. Schraffordt SE, Tjandra JJ, Eizenberg N et al (2004) Anatomy of the pudendal nerve and its terminal branches: a cadaver study. ANZ J Surg 74:23–26
51. Enck P, Hinninghofen H, Wietek B et al (2004) Functional asymmetry of pelvic floor innervation and its role in the pathogenesis of fecal incontinence. Digestion 69:102–111
52. Hamdy S, Enck P, Aziz Q et al (1999) Laterality effects of human pudendal nerve stimulation on corticoanal pathways: evidence for functional asymmetry. Gut 45:58–63
53. Enck P, Hinninghofen H, Merletti R et al (2005) The external anal sphincter and the role of surface electromyography. Neurogastroenterol Motil 17(Suppl 1): 60–67
54. Gooneratne ML, Scott SM, Lunniss PJ (2007) Unilateral pudendal neuropathy is common in patients with fecal incontinence. Dis Colon Rectum *(in press)*
55. Lynn PA, Olsson C, Zagorodnyuk V et al (2003) Rectal intraganglionic laminar endings are transduction sites of extrinsic mechanoreceptors in the guinea pig rectum. Gastroenterology 125:786–794
56. Chan CL, Facer P, Davis JB et al (2003) Sensory fibres expressing capsaicin receptor TRPV1 in patients with rectal hypersensitivity and faecal urgency. Lancet 361:385–391

Epidemiology of Faecal Incontinence

2

Alexandra K. Macmillan, Arend E.H. Merrie

Introduction

This chapter focuses on the prevalence and incidence rate of faecal incontinence in the general population and specific subgroups, including the elderly and children. Epidemiological definitions are described, and problems with measuring faecal incontinence are discussed. Descriptive studies of prevalence and incidence rates are reviewed, including demographic determinants and the reliability of the prevalence estimates. A thorough discussion of risk factors for the development of faecal incontinence is covered elsewhere in this volume. Having highlighted the need for valid, reliable measurement tools, an example of such a tool is given for use in epidemiologic studies.

Definitions

The following epidemiologic definitions are used in this chapter:

Prevalence: the proportion of a population with a disease at a specific point in time. This is also called the "point" prevalence. Prevalence measures are given as proportions, percentages or cases per population.

Incidence Rate: a measure of how rapidly people are newly developing a disease or health status, represented by the number of new cases in a time period divided by the average population in that time period. Although commonly called the "incidence", this is a true rate, as it measures the number of new diagnoses per population *per time period.*

Epidemiological Bias: systematic deviation of study results from the true results because of the way in which the study is conducted. This is usually divided into three types of bias: selection bias, information bias and confounding. Table 1 demonstrates the common causes of bias in prevalence studies of faecal incontinence and their likely effect on the prevalence estimate.

Problems with Measurement

Measuring faecal incontinence has long proved difficult for those wishing to study its epidemiology. When measuring the frequency of faecal incontinence in a population, it is necessary to have a clear idea of both the definition and the criteria for diagnosis. A consistent case definition is vital for data about prevalence and incidence rate to be meaning-

Table 1. Sources of bias in prevalence studies of faecal incontinence and their likely effect on the prevalence rate [1]

Source of bias	Likely effect
Selection bias	
Sample frame	Sampling an older population may overestimate prevalence Sampling healthy workers may underestimate prevalence Sampling general practice or hospital patients may overestimate prevalence
Response rate	Low response rate is likely to result in an overestimate of prevalence by self-selection of those with incontinence and a higher proportion of older participants
Information bias	
Outcome definition	Use of an insensitive definition will underestimate the prevalence, and an oversensitive definition may overestimate it
Data collection method	Face-to-face or telephone interviewing is likely to underestimate the prevalence, and use of anonymous postal questionnaires may overestimate the prevalence

ful and comparable. While faecal incontinence is commonly defined as a loss of voluntary control of the passage of liquid or stool, it is usual for clinicians to use this term to include incontinence of flatus. The term "anal incontinence" has also been used to include the uncontrolled passage of flatus and liquid or solid stool. These two definitions can therefore be confusing, and we recommend the continued use of the term "faecal incontinence" to include the incontinence of flatus as part of a continuum. Some qualification of these definitions with regard to quantity, frequency and impact on quality of life is also required in any assessment of prevalence or incidence rate, particularly if such an assessment is to be useful for planning to meet a community need for assessment and treatment services. Rather than a single disease, faecal incontinence represents a clinical spectrum with diverse manifestations that are closely related to its varied aetiology. This makes classification within the case definition important. The Rome committees [2–4] have provided useful case definitions for functional faecal incontinence that can easily be converted for also defining faecal incontinence with an organic origin.

Some work around definition and classification has been done in the paediatric population in which there is again confusing terminology. There have been several attempts to standardise the definition of functional faecal incontinence in childhood, which accounts for more than 90% of cases [5, 6] The term "encopresis" is commonly used for paediatric faecal incontinence; however, there is variability about its definition in the literature. In 1994, a "classic" set of criteria was defined for encopresis (with or without symptoms of constipation) [7]. The criteria included two or more faecal incontinence episodes per week in children older than 4 years. The Rome II consensus group also defined criteria for nonretentive faecal incontinence of once per week or more for at least 3 months in a child older than 4 years [6, 8]. However, these two definitions exclude faecal incontinence secondary to constipation and faecal retention, which account for a significant proportion of cases [5, 6, 9]. In 2004, a consensus conference on faecal incontinence defined encopresis as the repeated incontinence of a normal bowel movement in inappropriate places by a child aged 4 years or older [9]. Soiling was defined as the involuntary leakage of small amounts of stool, and both encopresis and soiling were encompassed in the term faecal incontinence. No criteria related to frequency were included in this definition. These definitions are summarised in Table 2.

In addition to the inconsistencies in definition and classification noted above, data relating to morbidity from faecal incontinence is not included in routinely collected data sets (such as emergency hospital admissions or deaths). This lack of routine data results in a reliance on self-reported assessments for accurate epidemiologic measurement. A number of methods can be used to collect such data about the prevalence of faecal incontinence, most commonly by telephone or face-to-face interviews or by postal surveys. These methods can either be anonymous or named. Comparison of data collection methods for faecal incontinence has not been undertaken. However, for other socially sensitive behaviours, the validity of data collected via face-to-face or telephone interviews compared with self-administered surveys has been tested. From this testing, anonymous questionnaires are recommended, as they provide a greater degree of validity than either interview method. These measurement challenges are compounded by sufferers' social stigmatisation and community members' reluctance to discuss bowel habits in general [10, 11].

In summary, definitions and survey methods significantly affect the outcomes of studies measuring the frequency of faecal incontinence in the population. We recommend the use of the term "faecal

Table 2. Definitions of functional paediatric faecal incontinence [1]

Authors	Definition	Age criterion	Frequency criterion
Benninga et al. 1994 [6]	Encopresis: voluntary/ involuntary passage of normal bowel movement in the underwear (or other unorthodox locations)	Older than 4 years	On a regular basis
Rome II consensus group 1999 [1]	Nonretentive faecal soiling	Older than 4 years	Once per week for more than 12 weeks
Di Lorenzo and Benninga 2004 [8]	Encopresis: repeated expulsion of normal bowel movement in inappropriate places	Older than 4 years	None given

incontinence" that includes incontinence of flatus for both adults and children. Furthermore, anonymous, self-administered questionnaires are the recommended survey method for cross-sectional studies of faecal incontinence.

Studies Measuring Disease Frequency

Prevalence in the Adult Population

Several cross-sectional prevalence studies have been undertaken; however, they all used different definitions of faecal incontinence, few used anonymous questionnaires and they included different age groups and sample populations. In addition, many of the studies have been hampered by poor response rates. Together, these factors contribute to significant epidemiological bias within studies, limiting estimate interpretation and making prevalence estimates difficult to compare.

This likely explains why the prevalence of faecal incontinence for adults in the community reported in cross-sectional studies varies more than ten-fold. Thomas et al. [12] reported a prevalence of 0.43% among general practice patients in the UK but defined faecal incontinence as "faecal soiling twice or more per month" and relied on face-to-face confirmation of answers to a postal survey. Using a more sensitive definition and an anonymous self-administered questionnaire, Giebel et al. surveyed hospital patients, employees and their families and found a prevalence of any loss of control of stool, "winds" or frequent faecal soiling of almost 20% [13]. The full range of results found in prevalence studies of community adults is demonstrated in Figure 1.

Four studies that minimised epidemiological bias by using anonymous, self-administered questionnaires sampling randomly from the general adult population and achieving a good response rate found a prevalence rate of faecal incontinence ranging from 11% to 17% [14–16]. These studies are summarised in Table 3.

In keeping with a commonly held belief, these studies (Table 3) demonstrated an increasing prevalence of faecal incontinence with increasing age: up to 25% in those aged over 70 years [14]. However, the studies also examined gender differences in preva-

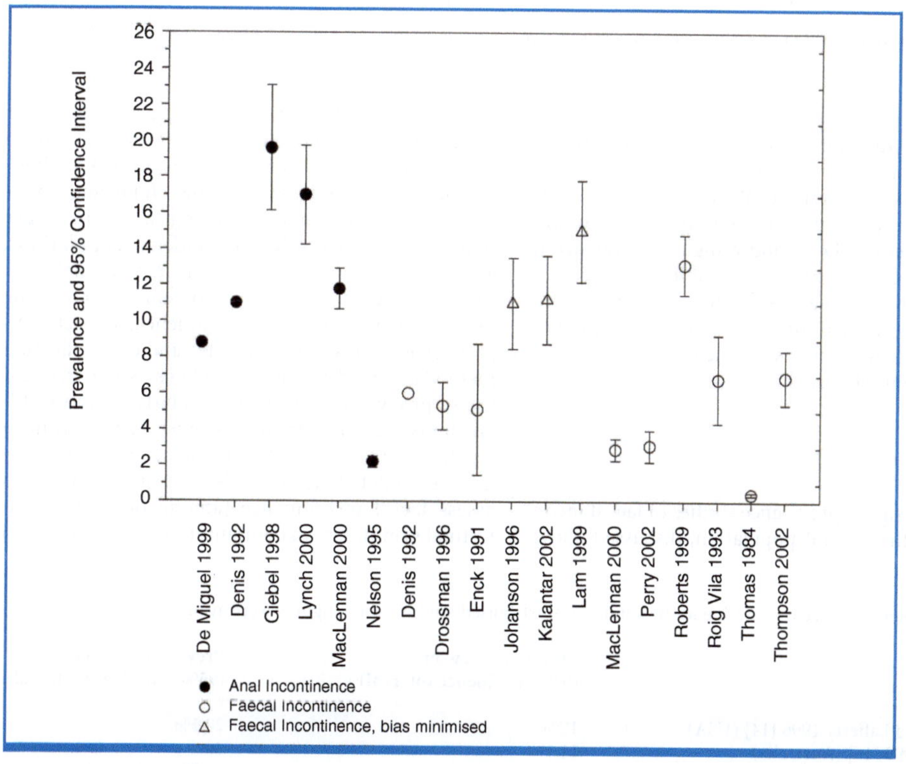

Fig. 1. Variation in prevalence of faecal incontinence in studies of community-dwelling adults. Reprinted with permission from [1]

Table 3. Prevalence of faecal incontinence in studies that minimised sources of epidemiological bias

Study	Population	Sample size (response rate)	Data collection method	Outcome definition	Prevalence (95% confidence interval)
Johanson and Lafferty 1996 [14](USA)	Convenience sample of general-practice patients aged 18–92	586	Anonymous self-administered questionnaire	Any involuntary leakage of stool or soiling of undergarments	Approximately 11% (8.5, 13.5)[a]
Lam et al. 1999 [16] (Australia)	Random sample of Sydney electoral roll, aged over 18	955 (71%)	Anonymous postal questionnaire, core questions validated	At least two of: stool leakage, pad for faecal soiling, incontinence of flatus >25% of the time	15% (12.2, 17.8)[a]
Kalantar et al. 2002 [15] (Australia)	Gender-stratified random sample of Sydney electoral roll, aged over 18	990 (66%)	Anonymous self-administered questionnaire	Unwanted release of liquid or solid faeces at an inappropriate time or place	11.2% (8.8, 13.7)
Siproudhis et al. 2006 [17] (France)	Random stratified cluster sample of noninstitutionalized adults aged over 15	7196 (72%)	Anonymous self-administered postal questionnaire	Uncontrolled anal leakage of stool ever in past 12 months	16.8% (15.9, 17.6)[a]

[a]Estimated from sample size and response rates stated using a simple random sample assumption of design effect

lence, and contrary to popular belief, there was no clear gender difference. Johanson and Lafferty [14] and Lam et al. [16] found a higher prevalence in men than in women, Kalantar et al. [15] found no significant difference between men and women and Siproudhis et al. [17] found a higher prevalence in women (Table 4). Further investigation is required to establish whether there are differences in the frequency of faecal incontinence related to other demographic factors, such as ethnicity, occupation or socioeconomic status.

Prevalence in Older Adults

The best-designed prevalence studies of faecal incontinence in the general population, discussed above, have demonstrated an increasing prevalence with increasing age. Indeed, it has previously been assumed that faecal incontinence is limited to elderly populations and some women following childbirth. A number of epidemiological studies have therefore focused solely on elderly populations, either community dwelling or in institutional care. These studies have similar problems with varying definitions of significant incontinence, subject sampling, age groups, response rates and data collection methods. Added to these problems is the frequent use of proxy respondents, particularly for those elders in institutions. Perhaps the most reliable estimate results from a study by Talley et al. in 1992 [18]. They used a validated self-administered questionnaire to assess faecal incontinence (among other gastrointestinal symptoms) in community-dwelling adults 65

Table 4. Prevalence of faecal incontinence by gender in least-biased studies where figures were available

Study	Prevalence in women (95% confidence interval)	Prevalence in men (95% confidence interval)
Johanson and Lafferty 1996 [14] (USA)	17%	20.5%
Lam et al. 1999 [16] (Australia)	11.1%	20%
Kalantar et al. 2002 [15] (Australia)	11.6% (8.3, 15.0)	10.8% (7.2–14.4)

years and older and found an age-adjusted prevalence of more than once per week of 3.7%, with 6.1% of the same population wearing a pad. There was no difference between men and women and no significant increase in prevalence with age within elders. This prevalence estimate is somewhat lower than that reported for the oldest subjects in the general population studies described above. This is likely to be related to a less sensitive definition of incontinence.

Prevalence in the Paediatric Population

There have been very few prevalence studies of childhood faecal incontinence, and no formal systematic review of epidemiological studies has been undertaken. Bellman's seminal epidemiological studies in the 1960s provided a strong basis for more recent work [19]. As with studies of adult faecal incontinence, these prevalence studies used variable definitions of incontinence, soiling and encopresis, as discussed previously. Issues of low response rate and difficulties with data collection are made more problematic in children because of the need for parental permission and assistance to take part in research. Faecal incontinence is very distressing for children, and they will often attempt to hide their incontinence from their parents [9]. Parents are often also embarrassed and distressed by their child's incontinence, leading to under-reporting [19]. This is likely to result in underestimation of the problem by prevalence studies. Although the accuracy of parental information about bowel habit has been tested [20], no study has investigated the accuracy of information from the child alone. All these factors affect the prevalence found by these studies.

Anonymously collected data from a random questionnaire sample of more than 1,000 6- to 9-year-old Danish school children [21] recently suggested a prevalence higher than that commonly quoted, with a prevalence of 5.6% in girls and 8.3% in boys. However, no definition of faecal incontinence was given. A more recent population-based study of school children (aged 5–6 and 11–12 years) defining encopresis as the involuntary loss of faeces in the underwear once a month or more was reported [22]. Parents were asked about the presence of encopresis on behalf of the child in a face-to-face interview with a doctor while the child was present. The authors reported a prevalence of 4.1% in 5- to 6-year-old children and 1.6% in the 11- to 12-year-old children, with a significantly greater prevalence in boys than in girls. Further demographic associations were identified in the study. In particular, the prevalence of encopresis was significantly higher in children of lower socioeconomic status. These studies demonstrate potential information bias, with the lack of definition in one and method of data collection in the other being likely to underestimate the prevalence.

Incidence-rate Studies

There are no true incidence-rate studies of faecal incontinence in the general population. This dearth of research is a result of the difficulties with measurement discussed above. The incidence rate of faecal incontinence is therefore not known. As a result, the natural history of faecal incontinence in the general population is likewise unclear, in particular with regard to rates of spontaneous remission.

Conclusion

In conclusion, the prevalence of faecal incontinence in the general population is poorly understood. From the available studies, it is likely that the prevalence is between 11% and 17%, which is higher than usually quoted. This appears similar for both genders and increases with age. There is some indication that the prevalence of faecal incontinence also varies by socioeconomic status and ethnicity. In children, there have been too few well-designed studies to estimate a prevalence range; however, it is likely to be higher than that normally quoted for the reasons discussed above.

For future epidemiologic studies, a consensus definition of faecal incontinence is recommended that includes any incontinence of flatus, liquid stool or solid stool that impacts on quality of life in adults and children [1]. Any further prevalence studies should ideally be undertaken using anonymous self-administered questionnaires to aid with minimising bias. Widespread use of a standardised questionnaire would assist with achieving consistency and comparability between further studies. An example of a standardised, valid and reliable self-administered questionnaire [23] is included (Appendix). This questionnaire was constructed and validated in New Zealand, and incorporates with permission the Bristol Stool Form Scale [24–26], Faecal Incontinence Severity Index (with patient weighted scoring) [27] and Faecal Incontinence Quality of Life Index (scored as per Rockwood et al. [28]).

Continued

Appendix

THE UNIVERSITY OF AUCKLAND
FACULTY OF MEDICAL AND HEALTH SCIENCES

BOWEL CONTROL QUESTIONNAIRE

The first section relates to general information, and will help with our data analysis.

1. What is your gender? (*Please tick one*)

Female ☐
Male ☐

2. What is your age in years?

☐

3. Which of these ethnic groups do you identify with most? (*Please tick the box or boxes that apply to you*)

NZ European ☐
Maori ☐
Samoan ☐
Tongan ☐
Cook Island Maori ☐
Niuean ☐
Chinese ☐
Indian ☐

Other ☐
(such as Tokelauan, Japanese)
Please state:

☐

➔ **Go to next page**

4. What is your highest level of education? (*Please tick one*)

No formal qualification ☐
School Certificate ☐
University Entrance (e.g. Bursary) ☐

Trade/Professional Diploma of Certificate ☐
Bachelor's Degree ☐
Postgraduate Degree ☐

5. What is your occupation?

(*e.g. primary school teacher, homemaker/caregiver, motel manager, clothing machinist*)

If retired or currently unemployed, please ***also*** *state most recent occupation*

➔ **Go to next page**

The following questions relate to your usual bowel habit **<u>in the last 3 months</u>**.

6. On average, how often did you pass a bowel motion **<u>in the past 3 months</u>**?
(*Please tick one*)

More than 3 times per day ☐
2 to 3 times per day ☐
Once per day ☐
2 to 3 times per week ☐
Once per week ☐
Less than once per week ☐

7. What has been the usual consistency of your bowel motions **<u>in the past 3 months</u>**?

(*Please circle the ONE type that applies to you USUALLY*)

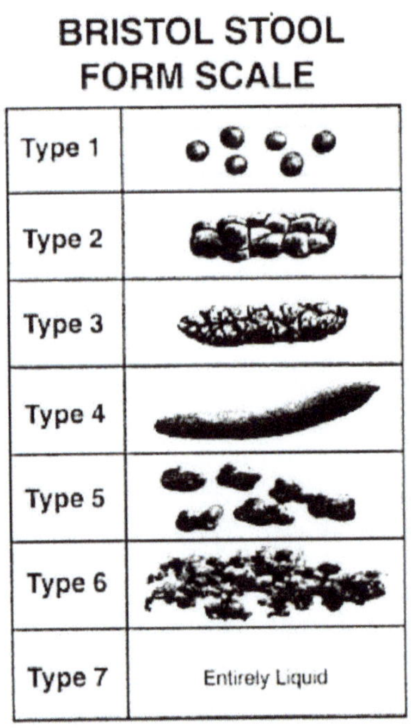

Type	Description
1	Separate hard lumps like nuts (difficult to pass)
2	Sausage shaped but lumpy
3	Like a sausage but with cracks on its surface
4	Like a sausage or snake, smooth and soft
5	Soft blobs with clear-cut edges (passed easily)
6	Fluffy pieces with ragged edges, a mushy stool
7	Water, no solid pieces, ENTIRELY LIQUID

➔ **Go to next page**

The next question relates to any difficulty you may have had passing a bowel motion **in the past 3 months**.

8. **In the past 3 months** have you experienced any of the following? (*Please tick all that apply to you*)

Straining on more than 1 out every 4 bowel motions	☐
Feeling that your bowel motion is incomplete more than a quarter of the time	☐
Feeling of blockage during bowel motions more than a quarter of the time	☐
Need to use fingers or hands to help with passing a bowel motion more than a quarter of the time	☐
None of the above statements apply to me	☐

9. **In the past 3 months** have you used medications regularly, including laxatives or antidiarrhoeal medication, to help you pass a bowel motion?

Yes	☐
No	☐

➔ **Go to next page**

The following section relates to any amount of bowel leakage (accidental loss of gas, mucus or stool/faeces) you may have had in the last month.

10. For each of the following, please mark on average how often **in the past month** you experienced **any amount of bowel leakage**.

(*Ngati Whatua translations are given in brackets*)

PLEASE TICK ONE BOX IN EACH ROW

	Never	**1 to 3 times a month**	**Once a week**	**2 or more times a week**	**Once a day**	**2 or more times a day**
A. LEAKAGE OF GAS (*tete*)	☐	☐	☐	☐	☐	☐
B. LEAKAGE OF MUCUS (*para tutae*)	☐	☐	☐	☐	☐	☐
C. LEAKAGE OF LIQUID STOOL (*tikotiko*)	☐	☐	☐	☐	☐	☐
D. LEAKAGE OF SOLID STOOL (*puru tutae*)	☐	☐	☐	☐	☐	☐

11. How often **in the past month** did you wear a pad because of **bowel leakage**?

2 or more times a day	☐
Once a day	☐
2 or more times a week	☐
Once a week	☐
1 to 3 times a month	☐
Never	☐

➔ **Go to next page**

12. **In the past month**, did you have any warning or feeling when you needed to pass a bowel motion?

Yes ☐
No ☐ (Go to question 13)

If **Yes**, did you have to rush/hurry to reach the toilet as soon as you felt the need to pass a bowel motion?

Yes ☐
No ☐

13. **In the past month**, did you ever have bowel leakage shortly after emptying your bowels or passing a bowel motion?

Yes ☐
No ☐

The following question relates to your bladder control **in the past month**.

14. **In the past month** have you experienced loss of control of your bladder

(a) on coughing, laughing, sneezing or other physical activity?

Yes ☐
No ☐

(b) when feeling an urgent need to pass water (urinate), but not making it to the toilet in time?

Yes ☐
No ☐

➔ Go to next page

The next questions are only for women. **If you are male** ➔ **Go to Question 22 on the next page.**

15. How many children have you given birth to? ☐

If you have had no children ➔ **Go to Question 21.**

16. Thinking back on these births, how many were vaginal deliveries? ☐

17. In your longest labour, how long did you push for (second stage)? (*Please tick one*)

Less than 1 hour ☐
1 to 2 hours ☐
More than 2 hours ☐

18. Thinking back on all your labours, were forceps or instruments ever used?

Yes ☐
No ☐

19. Thinking back on all your labours, did you ever have a tear or episiotomy involving the muscles of your anus (back passage)?

Yes ☐
No ☐

20. Thinking back on all your labours, what was the weight of your largest baby?

☐ **kg** **OR** ☐ **lbs**

21. Have you ever had a hysterectomy (operation to remove your womb)?

Yes ☐
No ☐

If yes, was it............ **Vaginal** ☐
Abdominal ☐

➔ **Go to next page**

The following questions are for everyone.

22. Have you ever had any of the following types of surgery to your bowels or anus (back passage)? (*Please tick all that apply to you*)

Removal and rejoining of party of your bowel ☐
Anal fistula surgery ☐
Operation on anal muscles ☐
Operation for haemorrhoids or piles ☐
Major prostate operation ☐

None of the above ☐

23. Do you have a stoma (bag) for emptying your bowels?

Yes ☐
No ☐

24. Have you ever injured your anus (back passage), not including during labour?

Yes ☐
No ☐

25. Do you suffer from any of the following medical problems? (*Please tick all that apply to you*)

Inflammatory bowel disease ☐
(*Eg Crohn's disease or ulcerative colitis*) ☐

Irritable bowel syndrome ☐
Rectal prolapse ☐
Diabetes ☐
Stroke ☐
Other neurological condition ☐
Decreased mobility ☐

None of the above apply ☐

➔ Go to next page

The following section relates to how your bowel habit may be affecting your lifestyle.

26. In general, would you say your health is:

- Excellent ☐
- Very Good ☐
- Good ☐
- Fair ☐
- Poor ☐

27. For each of the items below, please indicate by circling the appropriate number, how much of the time the item is a concern for you **due to any accidental bowel leakage** (gas, liquid, solid or mucus). If it is a concern for you for another reason (not accidental bowel leakage), then please circle "None of the time".

PLEASE CIRCLE ONE NUMBER IN EACH ROW

Because of accidental bowel leakage:	Most of the time	Some of the time	A little of the time	None of the time	Not Applicable
I am afraid to go out	1	2	3	4	N/A
I avoid visiting my friends	1	2	3	4	N/A
I avoid staying overnight away from home	1	2	3	4	N/A
It is difficult for me to get out and do things like going to a movie or to church	1	2	3	4	N/A
I cut down on how much I eat before I go out	1	2	3	4	N/A
Whenever I am away from home, I try and stay near a toilet as much as possible	1	2	3	4	N/A
It is important to plan my daily activities around my bowel habit	1	2	3	4	N/A
I avoid travelling	1	2	3	4	N/A
I worry about not being able to get to the toilet in time	1	2	3	4	N/A
I feel I have no control over my bowels	1	2	3	4	N/A
I can't hold on to my bowel motion long enough to get to the bathroom	1	2	3	4	N/A
I try to prevent bowel accidents by staying very near a bathroom	1	2	3	4	N/A

➔ **Go to next page**

28. **Because of any accidental bowel leakage**, please indicate, by circling one number in each row, how much you agree or disagree with each of the following statements.

If it is a concern for you for another reason, or not a concern at all, please circle **N/A**.

PLEASE CIRCLE ONE ANSWER IN EACH ROW

Due to accidental bowel leakage:	**Strongly agree**	**Somewhat agree**	**Somewhat disagree**	**Strongly disagree**	**Not Applicable**
I feel ashamed	1	2	3	4	N/A
I cannot do many things I want to do	1	2	3	4	N/A
I worry about bowel accidents	1	2	3	4	N/A
I feel depressed	1	2	3	4	N/A
I worry about the smell	1	2	3	4	N/A
I feel unhealthy	1	2	3	4	N/A
I enjoy life less	1	2	3	4	N/A
I have sex less often than I would like	1	2	3	4	N/A
I feel different from other people	1	2	3	4	N/A
The possibility of bowel accidents is always on my mind	1	2	3	4	N/A
I enjoy life less	1	2	3	4	N/A
I am afraid to have sex	1	2	3	4	N/A
I avoid travelling by plane or public transport	1	2	3	4	N/A
I avoid going out to eat	1	2	3	4	N/A
Whenever I go somewhere new, I make sure I know where the toilets are	1	2	3	4	N/A

➔ **Go to next page**

29. During the past month, have you felt so sad, discouraged, hopeless, or had so many problems that you wondered if anything was worthwhile?

Extremely so- to the point where I have just about given up ☐
Very much so ☐
Quite a bit ☐
Some- Enough to bother me ☐
A little bit ☐
Not at all ☐

30. Have you ever discussed loss of bowel control with anyone? (*Please tick all that apply to you*)

YES Family ☐
Family Doctor ☐
Specialist ☐

Other health professional ☐

Please say what kind of health professional . . . .

NO ☐

31. Have you been referred to any other service for loss of bowel control?

Yes ☐ **Please say where** . . . .
No ☐

This is the end of the questionnaire.

Thank you for your time and assistance.

References

1. Macmillan AK, Merrie AEH, Marshall RJ, Parry BR (2004) The prevalence of fecal incontinence in community-dwelling adults: a systematic review of the literature. Dis Colon Rectum 47:1341–1349
2. Drossman DA (1999) The functional gastrointestinal disorders and the Rome II process. Gut 45:1–5
3. Drossman DA, Corazziare E, Talley NJ et al (eds) Rome II. The functional gastrointestinal disorders. Allen, Lawrence
4. Whitehead WE, Wald A, Diamant NE et al (1999) Functional disorders of the anus and rectum. Gut 45:55–59
5. Loening-Baucke V (1997) Fecal incontinence in children. Am Fam Physician 55:2229–2235
6. Voskuijl WP, Heijmans J, Heijmans HSA et al (2004) Use of Rome II criteria in childhood defecation disorders: Applicability in clinical and research practice. J Pediatr 145:213–217
7. Benninga MA, Buller HA, Heymans HSA et al (1994) Is encopresis always the result of constipation? Arch Dis Child 71:186–193
8. Rasquin-Weber A, Hyman PE, Cucchiara S et al (1999) Childhood functional gastrointestinal disorders. Gut 45(Suppl 2):II60–II68
9. Di Lorenzo C, Benninga MA (2004) Pathophysiology of pediatric fecal incontinence. Gastroenterology 126:S33–S40
10. Dare OO, Cleland JG (1994) Reliability and validity of survey data on sexual behaviour. Health Transit Rev 4:93–110
11. Rossi PH, Wright JD, Anderson AB (eds) (1983) Handbook of survey research. Academic Press, Orlando
12. Thomas TM, Egan M, Walgrove A, Meade TW (1984) The prevalence of faecal and double incontinence. Community Med 6:216–220
13. Giebel GD, Lefering R, Troidl H, Blochl H (1998) Prevalence of fecal incontinence: what can be expected? Int J Colorectal Dis 13:73–77
14. Johanson JF, Lafferty J (1996) Epidemiology of fecal incontinence: the silent affliction. Am J Gastroenterol 91:33–36
15. Kalantar JS, Howell S, Talley NJ (2002) Prevalence of faecal incontinence and associated risk factors; an underdiagnosed problem in the Australian community? Med J Aust 176:54–57
16. Lam TCF, Kennedy ML, Chen FC et al (1999) Prevalence of faecal incontinence: obstetric and constipation-related risk factors; a population-based study. Colorectal Disease 1:197–203
17. Siproudhis L, Pigot F, Godeberge P et al (2006) Defecation disorders: A French population survey. Dis Colon and Rectum 49:219–227
18. Talley NJ, O'Keefe EA, Zinsmeister AR, Melton LJ 3rd (1992) Prevalence of gastrointestinal symptoms in the elderly: A population-based study. Gastroenterology 102:895–901
19. Bellman M (1966) Studies on encopresis. Acta Paediatr Scand 170(Suppl):3–151
20. van der Plas RN, Benninga MA, Redekop WK et al (1997) How accurate is the recall of bowel habits in children with defaecation disorders? Eur J Pediatr 156:178–181
21. Hansen A, Hansen B, Dahm T (1997) Urinary tract infection, day wetting and other voiding symptoms in seven- to eight-year-old Danish children. Acta Paediatr 86:1345–1349
22. van der Wal MF, Benninga MA, Hirasing RA (2005) The prevalence of encopresis in a multicultural population. J Paediatr Gastroenter Nutr 40:345–348
23. Macmillan AK (2004) Design and validation of the New Zealand Faecal Incontinence Questionnaire. Masters thesis, University of Auckland
24. O'Donnell LJD, Virjee J, Heaton KW (1990) Detection of pseudodiarrhoea by simple clinical assessment of intestinal transit rate. BMJ 300:439:440
25. Heaton KW, Ghosh S, Braddon FEM (1991) How bad are the symptoms and bowel dysfunction of patients with the irritable bowel syndrome? A prospective, controlled study with emphasis on stool form. Gut 32:73–79
26. Heaton KW, Radvan J, Cripps H et al (1992) Defecation frequency and timing, and stool form in the general population: a prospective study. Gut 33:818–824
27. Rockwood TH, Church JM, Fleshman JW et al (1999) Patient and surgeon ranking of the severity of symptoms associated with fecal incontinence: the fecal incontinence severitry index. Dis Colon Rectum 42(12):1525–1531
28. Rockwood TH, Church JM, Fleshman JW et al (2000) Fecal incontinence quality of life scale: quality of life instrument for patients with fecal incontinence. Dis Colon Rectum 43:9–17

Pathophysiology of Faecal Incontinence

3

Luigi Zorcolo, David C.C. Bartolo

Introduction

The ability to control evacuation, as discussed in Chapter 1, is guaranteed by many factors. These include intact anal sphincter mechanism, compliant reservoir, efficient evacuation, stool volume and consistency, intestinal motility, pelvic floor structural integrity, cortical awareness, cognitive function, mobility and access to facilities. Normal defecation is a process of integrated somatovisceral responses, which involve coordinated colo-recto-anal function [1]. Incontinence occurs when one or more of these mechanisms are impaired and the remaining mechanisms are unable to compensate. Although integrity of the sphincteric mechanism plays a major part, there are other important aspects, such as stool volume and consistency, colonic transit, rectal compliance and sensation, anorectal sensation and anorectal reflexes [2]. In this chapter, all these aspects are discussed separately, but in the majority of cases (80% according to Rao et al. [3]), the cause of faecal incontinence (FI) is multifactorial [4, 5].

Suprasphincteric Dysfunction

Stool Consistency/Volume and Gastrointestinal Transit

The consistency of the faeces and the rate at which they are introduced into the rectum may play a role in determining incontinence. Liquid stools rapidly delivered to the rectum are able to determine urgency and incontinence even in normal subjects [6]. Many patients with idiopathic FI have chronic diarrhoea, often secondary to irritable bowel syndrome (IBS). In these subjects, sigmoid pressures and sigmoid motility index are usually higher than in the normal population.

Rectal Compliance and Motility

The rectum is a muscular tube composed of a continuous layer of longitudinal muscle that interlaces with the underlying circular muscle. This unique muscle arrangement enables the rectum to serve both as a reservoir and as a pump for emptying stools [7]. A normally distensible rectum is able to maintain low intraluminal pressures despite large volume [8]. If this capacity deteriorates, a smaller quantity of faeces will result in higher pressure, causing urgency and eventually incontinence. This mechanism is clearly evident in patients with ulcerative colitis [9, 10], radiation proctitis [11] or after sphincter-saving operations [12, 13]. Decreased compliance has been noted in many patients with FI [14–17]. However, it is not clear whether this fact always represents a cause or whether it may be a consequence of incontinence itself. Rasmussen et al. [16], having found no differences in rectal compliance between patients with idiopathic or traumatic incontinence, postulated that decreased rectal compliance is likely a consequence of an incompetent anal sphincter and not the cause of incontinence itself.

Rectoanal Inhibitory Reflex

Rectoanal inhibitory reflex (RAIR) enables rectal contents to come into contact with the epithelium of the upper anal canal, where there is a high concentration of free and organised sensory nerve endings [18]. The mechanism is guaranteed by concomitant rectal contraction and internal anal sphincter (IAS) relaxation. At the same time, there is a reflex external anal sphincter (EAS) contraction that prevents accidents. This sampling mechanism occurs several times per hour [19] and allows an accurate distinction between flatus, liquid and solid faces, and for these reasons it has a role in the fine adjustment of continence, allowing the individual to choose whether to retain or discharge their rectal contents. It is likely that minor degrees of sensory impairment are not by themselves causative of incontinence in patients with otherwise normal anorectal function [20]. However, if the sampling mechanism is defective and sphincter function is poor, the patient may be completely unaware of impending incontinence, especially if anal sensation is also reduced [21, 22]. In one of our studies [23], it was noticed that sampling, considered as the moment in which rectal and upper anal pressure are equal, occurred spontaneously in only 33% of incontinent patients compared with 89% of controls ($p<0.05$). These findings confirmed that an impaired sampling mechanism plays an important role in incontinent patients.

Rectal Sensation

The contribution of altered rectal sensation, either in terms of hyposensitivity or hypersensitivity, to disorders of defecation is becoming increasingly recognised [24, 25]. The rectum itself does not have proprioceptors; these are located in the levators, puborectalis (PR) and anal sphincters [26] and subserve the sensation of distension and stretch of the rectal wall. These sensations travel along the pudendal nerve to S_2, S_3 and S_4 roots [27]. The pudendal nerve is a mixed nerve that is the main nerve responsible of innervation of the anorectal wall and sphincteric complex. Its course through the pelvic floor makes it vulnerable to stretch injury, especially during vaginal delivery. Many cases of FI in the presence of a morphologically intact sphincter are related to impaired evacuation and disturbed sensation of the rectum due to intrinsic neuropathy [28–30].

The aetiology of rectal hyposensitivity is unclear, although there is limited evidence to support the role of pelvic nerve injury and abnormal toilet behaviour [25]. More frequently, it is associated with diseases such as altered mental conditions (i.e. dementia; stroke; encephalopathy) and sensory neuropathy (i.e. diabetes; spina bifida; meningocele) [31–34]. Rectal hyposensitivity is more often related to constipation, but it can also be the cause of passive incontinence. Despite a normal or borderline sphincter function, blunted anorectal sensation with impaired EAS contraction during the sampling reflex may result in soiling [35]. This is what typically happens in institutionalised elderly people in whom reduced rectal sensation and poor rectal motility often determine faecal impaction with overflow incontinence secondary to continuous elicitation of the anorectal reflex. Overall, high conscious rectal sensory threshold is probably the primary cause of incontinence in about one third of patients [36].

Rectal hypersensitivity is also a frequent manometric finding in patients with FI and acts as an independent trigger of urgency [1, 37, 38]. Chan et al. [1] found this anomaly in 44% of their patients with urge incontinence. They noticed that when sphincteric dysfunction was associated with rectal hypersensitivity, patients had a significantly increased stool frequency and urgency, a greater use of pads and more lifestyle restrictions compared with patients with isolated sphincter dysfunction. The same authors, utilising a prolonged rectosigmoid manometry, investigated rectosigmoid motor function, demonstrating that rectal hypersensitivity is often associated with an exaggerated rectosigmoid contractile activity [24]. Rectal hypersensitivity is generally the effect of impaired relaxation properties of the rectum [16, 39, 40]. Other mechanisms have been advocated, such as sensitisation of the extrinsic peripheral pathways [41] or central afferent mechanisms [42], low-grade inflammation [43] and abnormalities in perceptual and behavioural processes causing a state of heightened vigilance and focused selective attention [44, 45].

Sphincteric Dysfunction

Internal Anal Sphincter Integrity

The IAS is a circular smooth muscle that is responsible for 50–85% of the resting tone [46–48]. Its continuous maximum contraction is due to both intrinsic myogenic and extrinsic autonomic neurogenic properties [48, 49]. With age, resting pressure progressively decreases because of gradual degeneration of the muscular fibres [50]. Primary degeneration of IAS with atrophy was identified by Vaizey et al. in a group of 45 patients (ten men), and this was the only demonstrable cause of passive incontinence [51]. Structural damage of this muscle is often secondary to anorectal trauma or anal surgery. Several studies have shown that IAS injuries occur in up to 35% of women during childbirth, but in these cases, there is usually an associated damage of the EAS [52].

In these conditions resting tone is low, and EAS contraction may not be sufficient to avoid involuntary loss of gas or liquid stools, and passive incontinence may occur.

More frequently, the IAS appears to be anatomically intact but still unable to maintain a continuous contraction. This has been noticed in about 25% of patients with idiopathic incontinence [53]. With manometric and electromyographic (EMG) studies, we previously noticed that in 92% of patients with neurogenic incontinence, there was a median of four episodes of IAS EMG silence per hour, each lasting a median of 90 s, not associated with sampling mechanism. This phenomenon was not recorded in the control group [54]. These findings have no clear interpretation, but they probably reflect the functional and histological disturbances of the IAS related to neurogenic damage.

Puborectalis, Anorectal Angle, External Anal Sphincter Integrity

Despite the fact that the PR and EAS have somewhat different innervations (see Chapter 1), they act as an indivisible unit, and for this reason, the PR is now considered as the deepest part of external sphincter. These muscles form together the triple loop system described by Shafik [55]. Unlike the other skeletal muscles, which are usually inactive at rest, these muscles maintain a continuous unconscious resting tone [56]. This can be explained by the fact that they are also rich in type I fibres, which are responsible for tonic contractile activity [57, 58].

The PR and the anorectal angle (ARA) due to its U-shaped sling contribute to maintaining gross faecal continence. It has been postulated that this result is guaranteed by a flap-valve mechanism in which the anterior rectal wall occludes the upper anal canal [59, 60]. However, a study performed by us questioned this theory and suggested that, rather, the PR functions by sphincteric occlusion of the anal canal [61]. To demonstrate this, anal and rectal pressures were measured simultaneously together with EAS and PR EMG and synchronously superimposed on an image intensifier displaying the rectum outlined by barium. In this way, we studied 13 subjects at rest and during a Valsalva manoeuvre, and we noticed that there was a significant rise in rectal and sphincter pressures and EAS and PR EMG. In a further 13 patients, Valsalva manoeuvres were performed during proctography alone. In all subjects, the anterior rectal wall was always clearly separated from the upper sphincter despite a maximal effort and a rectum filled with sufficient liquid to produce a desire to defecate.

The involvement of a flap-valve mechanism has also been hypothesised by Bannister et al. [62]. In fact, they noticed that in the normal population, the pressure gradient between rectum and anus is the reverse of that which would be found if an anterior rectal flap valve maintained continence. Instead, they suggested that continence is normally maintained by a reflex contraction of the EAS.

The EAS response to stimuli (such as increased intra-abdominal pressure, rectal distension or anal dilatation) is contraction. In normal conditions, this can be voluntarily sustained for 40–60 s, a period of time which is generally sufficient for the rectum to accommodate [63]. Inability to voluntary activate the EAS for a sufficient period, as happens when the sphincter has been injured during a vaginal delivery, is the commonest cause of urge incontinence in the Western world. Cumulative injuries may occur and often are associated with a decline in pudendal nerve conduction [64]. Such damage has also been noticed after late caesarean deliveries [65]. Less frequently, the sphincter appears morphologically intact but still is unable to provide good contraction because of isolated neurological impairment [66].

Conclusions

FI is a complex problem, and its pathophysiology is often multifactorial, involving both suprasphincteric and sphincteric dysfunction. Many aspects are still unclear and require further studies. Hopefully, a better understanding of neurophysiological mechanisms will be the key to correctly assessing these difficult patients and to choosing the right treatment.

References

1. Chan CL, Scott SM, Williams NS, Lunniss PJ (2005) Rectal hypersensitivity worsens stool frequency, urgency, and lifestyle in patients with urge fecal incontinence. Dis Colon Rectum 48:134–140
2. Kiff ES, Swash M (1984) Slowed conduction in the pudendal nerves in idiopathic faecal incontinence. Br J Surg 71:614–616
3. Rao SSC, Patel RS (1997) How useful are manometric tests of anorectal function in the management of defecation disorders. Am J Gastroenterol 92:469–475
4. Sun WM, Donnelly TC, Read NW (1992) Utility of a combined test of anorectal manometry, electromyography and sensation in determining the mechanism of idiopathic faecal incontinence. Gut 33:807–813
5. Rao SSC (1999) Faecal incontinence. Clinical perspective in gastroenterology 2:277–288
6. Schiller LR (1986) Faecal incontinence. Clin Gastroenterol 15:687–674
7. Rao SSC (2004) Diagnosis and management of faecal incontinence. Am J Gastroenterol 99:1585–1604
8. Arhan P, Faverdin C, Persoz B et al (1976) Relationship between viscoelastic properties of the rectum and anal pressure in man. J Appl Physiol 41:677–682
9. Suzuki H, Fujoka M (1982) Rectal pressure and rectal compliance in ulcerative colitis. Jpn J Surg 12:79–81
10. Denis PH, Colin R, Galmiche JP et al (1979) Elastic properties of the rectal wall in normal adults and in patients with ulcerative colitis. Gastroenterology 77:45–48
11. Varma JS, Smith AN, Busuttil A (1985) Correlation of clinical and manometric abnormalities of rectal function following chronic radiation injury. Br J Surg 72:875–878
12. Nasmyth DG, Johnston D, Godwin PG et al (1986) Factors influencing bowel function after pouch anal anastomosis. Br J Surg 73:469–473
13. Batignani G, Monaci I, Ficari F, Tonelli F (1991) What affects continence after anterior resection of the rectum? Dis Colon Rectum 34:329 335
14. Ihre T (1974) Studies on anal function in continent and incontinent patients. Scand J Gastroenterol 9:1–80
15. Read NW, Harford WV, Schmulen AC et al (1979) A clinical study of patients with faecal incontinence and

diarrhoea. Gastroenterology 76:747–756
16. Rasmussen O, Christensen B, Sorensen M et al (1990) Rectal compliance in the assessment of patients with fecal incontinence. Dis Colon Rectum 33:650–653
17. Womack NR, Morrison JF, Williams NS (1986) The role of pelvic floor denervation in the etiology of idiopathic faecal incontinence. Br J Surg 73:404–407
18. Duthie HL, Gairns FW (1960) Sensory nerve endings and sensation in the anal region in man. Br J Surg 47:585–595
19. Miller R, Lewis GT, Bartolo DCC et al (1988) Sensory discrimination and dynamic activity in the anorectum: evidence using a new ambulatory technique. Br J Surg 75:1003–1007
20. Giordano P, Wexner SD (2001) The assessment of fecal incontinence in women. J Am Coll Surg 193:397–406
21. Roe AM, Bartolo DC, Mortensen NJ (1986) New method for assessment of anal sensation in various anorectal disorders. Br J Surg 73:310–312
22. Bielefeldt K, Enck P, Erckenbrecht JF (1990) Sensory and motor function in the maintenance of anal continence. Dis Colon Rectum 33:674–678
23. Miller R, Bartolo DC, Cervero F, Mortensen NJ (1988) Anorectal sampling: a comparison of normal and incontinent patients. Br J Surg 75:44–47
24. Chan CL, Lunniss PJ, Wang D et al (2005) Rectal sensorimotor dysfunction in patients with urge faecal incontinence: evidence from prolonged manometric studies. Gut 54:1263–1272
25. Gladman MA, Lunniss PJ, Scott SM, Swash M (2006) Rectal hyposensitivity. Am J Gastroenterol 101: 1140–1151
26. Parks AG (1975) Anorectal incontinence. J R Soc Med 68:681–690
27. Goligher JC, Huges ESR (1951) Sensibility of the rectum and colon. Its role in the mechanism of anal continence. Lancet 1:543–547
28. Hancke E, Schurholz M (1987) Impaired rectal sensation in idiopathic faecal incontinence. Int J Colorectal Dis 2:146–148
29. Nagashima M, Iwai N et al (1992) Motility and sensation of the rectosigmoid and the rectum in patients with anorectal malformations. J Pediat Surg 27:1273–1277
30. Lubowski DZ, Nicholls RJ (1988) Faecal incontinence associated with reduced pelvic sensation. Br J Surg 75:1086–1088
31. Wald A, Tunuguntla AK (1984) Anorectal sensorimotor dysfunction in faecal incontinence and diabetes mellitus. Modification with biofeedback therapy. N Engl J Med 310:1282–1287
32. Caruana BJ, Wald A, Hinds JP, Eidelman BH (1991) Anorectal sensory and motor function in neurogenic fecal incontinence. Comparison between multiple sclerosis and diabetes mellitus. Gastroenterology 100:465–470
33. Sun WM, Read NW, Donnelly TC (1990) Anorectal function in incontinent patients with cerebrospinal disease. Gastroenterology 99:1372–1379
34. Sun WM, Read NW, Prior A et al (1990) Sensory and motor responses to rectal distention vary according to rate and pattern of balloon inflation. Gastroenterology 99:1008–1015
35. Sun WM, Read NW, Miner PB (1990) Relationship between rectal sensation and anal function in normal subjects and patients with faecal incontinence. Gut 31:1056–1061
36. Buser WD, Miner PB Jr (1986) Delayed rectal sensation with fecal incontinence. Gastroenterology 91:1186–1191
37. Felt-Bersma RJ, Sloots CE, Poen AC et al (2000) Rectal compliance as a routine measurement: estreme volumes have direct clinical impact and normal volumes exclude rectum as a problem. Dis Colon Rectum 43:1732–1738
38. Santoro GA, Eitan BZ, Pryde A, Bartolo DC (2000) Open study of low-dose amitriptyline in the treatment of patients with idiopathic fecal incontinence. Dis Colon Rectum 43:1676–1681
39. Salvioli B, Bharucha AE, Rath-Harvey D et al (2001) Rectal compliance, capacity and rectoanal sensation in faecal incontinence. Am J Gastroenterol 96:2158–2168
40. Malcom A, Phillips SF, Camileeri M, Hanson RB (1997) Pharmacological modulation of rectal tone alters perception of distention in humans. Am J Gastroenterol 92:2073–2079
41. Lembo T, Munakata J, Mertz H et al (1994) Evidence for hypersensitivity of lumbar splanchnic afferents in irritable bowel syndrome. Gastroenterology 107:1686–1696
42. Mayer EA, Gebhart GF (1994) Basic and clinical aspects of visceral hyperalgesia. Gastroenterology 107:271–293
43. Spiller RC, Jenkins D, Thornley JP et al (2000) Increased rectal mucosal enteroendocrine cells, T lymphocytes, and increased gut permeability following acute Campylobacter enteritis and in post-dysenteric irritable bowel syndrome. Gut 47:804–811
44. Accarino AM, Azpiroz F, Malagelada JR (1997) Attention and distraction: effects on gut perception. Gastroenterology 113:415–422
45. Withehead WE, Palsson OS (1998) Is rectal pain sensitivity a biological marker for irritable bowel syndrome: psychological influences on pain perception. Gastroenterology 115:1263–1271
46. Duthie HL, Watts JM (1965) Contribution of the external anal sphincter to the pressure zone in the anal canal. Gut 6:64–68
47. Schweiger M (1979) Method for determining individual contributions of voluntary and involuntary anal sphincters to resting tone. Dis Colon Rectum 22:415–416
48. Lestar B, Penninckx F, Kerremans R (1989) The composition of anal basal pressure. An in vivo and in vitro study in man. Int J Colorectal Dis 4:118–122
49. Ustach TJ, Tobon F, Hambrecht T et al (1970) Electrophysiological aspects of human sphincter function. J Clin Invest 49:41–48
50. Eckadt VF, Elmer T (1991) Reliability of anal pressure measurements. Dis Colon Rectum 34:72–77
51. Vaizey CJ, Kamm MA, Bartram CI (1997) Primary degeneration of the internal anal sphincter as a cause of passive faecal incontinence. Lancet 349:612–115
52. Sultan AH, Kamm MA, Hudson CN et al (1993) Anal-sphincter disruption during vaginal delivery. N Eng J Med 329:1905–1911

53. Sun WM, Read NW, Donnelly TC (1989) Impaired internal anal sphincter in a subgroup of patients with idiopathic fecal incontinence. Gastroenterology 97:130–135
54. Farouk R, Duthie GS, MacGregor AB, Bartolo DCC (1994) Evidence of electromechanical dissociation of the internal anal sphincter in idiopathic fecal incontinence. Dis Colon Rectum 37:595–601
55. Shafik A (1975) A new concept of the anatomy of the anal sphincter mechanism and the physiology of defecation. II. Anatomy of the levator ani muscle with special reference to puborectalis. Invest Urol 13:175–182
56. Floyd WF, Walls EW (1953) Electromyography of the sphincter ani externus in man. J Physiol 122:599–609
57. Johnston MA, Polgar J, Weightman D, Appleton D (1973) Data on the distribution of the fibers types in thirty-six human muscles: an autopsy study. J Neurol Sci 18:111–129
58. Parks AG, Swash M (1979) Denervation of the anal sphincter causing idiopathic ano-rectal incontinence. J R Coll Surg Edinb 24:94–96
59. Phillips SF, Edwards DA (1965) Some aspects of anal continence and defecation. Gut 6:396–406
60. Parks AG, Porter NH, Hardcastle J (1966) The syndrome of the descending perineum. J R Soc Med 59:477–482
61. Bartolo DC, Roe AM, Locke-Edmunds JC et al (1986) Flap-valve theory of anorectal continence. Br J Surg 73:1012–1014
62. Bannister JJ, Gibbons C, Read NW (1987) Preservation of faecal continence during rises in intra-abdominal pressure: is there a role for the flap valve? Gut 28:1242–1245
63. Schuster MM, Hookman P, Hendrix TR, Mendeloff AI (1965) Simultaneous manometric recording to intenal and external anal sphincter reflexes. Bull Johns Hopkins Hosp 116:79–88
64. Fynes M, Donnelly V, Behan M et al (1999) Effect of second vaginal delivery on anorectal physiology and faecal continence: a prospective study. Lancet 354:983–986
65. Donnelly V, Fynes M, Campbell D et al (1998) Obstetric events leading to anal sphincter damage. Obstet Gynecol 92:955–961
66. Mavrantonis C, Wexner SD (1998) A clinical approach to faecal incontinence. J Clin Gastroenterol 27:108–121

Invited Commentary

Anne-Marie Leroi

Although this chapter by Drs. Zorcolo and Bartolo on the pathophysiology of anal incontinence is quite thorough, I would like to emphasize several points that affect the management of incontinent patients. The role of transit disorders, which is explained in this chapter, is particularly important in the pathophysiology of anal incontinence. Whereas we are used to having patients consult for diarrhea who, in fact, have anal incontinence (unvoiced symptom), we now frequently receive patients consulting for anal incontinence associated with unrecognized diarrhea. This "clinical impression" is confirmed by objective data. We recently published an article on the frequency of transit disorders (diarrhea or constipation) in anal incontinence in 287 consecutive patients in a tertiary care center [1]. One hundred and thirty-four patients (47%) had a transit disorder associated with anal incontinence: 70 patients (24%) had constipation and 64 (22%) had diarrhea. Even if transit orders were not the only cause of anal incontinence, treating this disorder cured or improved incontinence in 62% of cases [1]. When managing an incontinent patient, transit disorders must first be investigated before any specific tests are performed for incontinence. Treatment of transit disorders improves incontinence in more than half the patients, and no further investigations are required. Indeed, if specific treatment for anal incontinence is proposed (sacral nerve stimulation or artificial bowel sphincter, for example) without first taking into account transit disorders, the risk of failure is high.

The active or passive nature of anal incontinence is valuable clinical information that should be systematically determined in incontinent patients. As the authors mentioned, active anal incontinence suggests external anal sphincter defects and/or altered colorectal function (noncompliant, hypersensitive rectum, increased rectosigmoid contractility). Although passive anal incontinence may suggest internal anal sphincter defects, as mentioned by Zorcolo and Bartolo, in our experience, it is more frequently due to incomplete rectal emptying, which should be managed by suggesting medical treatment to improve emptying at the first intention.

Finally, it is also important to add some information about the neurological control of continence because of (1) the frequency of neurological lesions causing anal incontinence, and (2) the development of treatments such as sacral nerve stimulation that may improve rectosphincter function by modulating its neurological control. As with vesicoureteral function, neurological control of anorectal function has a specific segmentary spinal organization. This organization results in the automatic emission of stools in paraplegic patients. However, in healthy subjects, anal continence and defecation seem to be, as with urinary continence and micturition, controlled by the cerebral cortex. Different studies based on registered somatosensory evoked potentials or functional imaging have shown that primary and secondary somesthetic areas responsible for spatial discrimination are activated after anal and rectal stimulation [2, 3]. Other areas involved in affect and attention, such as the insula, anterior cingular cortex, and prefrontal cortex, are also activated, especially after rectal stimulation. Chronic sacral nerve stimulation seems to modify certain cerebral areas involved in consciousness and attention to the feeling of needing to evacuate [4]. As with micturition, there seems to be a supraspinal command center located in the brainstem, probably in a pontic structure near the center for micturition (M center). Thus, a real command center, capable of modifying sphincter tone, has been located in the locus coeruleus [5]. In humans, patients with brainstem lesions have been found to have modified anorectal motricity [6]. This suggests that center(s) in the brainstem (locus coeruleus?) could be similar to that for micturition, responsible for coordination of the sympathetic, parasympathetic, and somatic systems innervating the anorectal nerve apparatus. Thus, the(se) center(s) would coordinate "harmonious" defecation (rectal contraction, relaxation of the internal and external sphincters resulting in opening of the anal canal). The brainstem center of micturition could be controlled by cortical areas in the frontal lobe. Indeed, anorectal functional anomalies have been described in patients with frontal lobe lesions [7].

References

1. Demirci S, Gallas S, Bertot-Sassigneux P et al (2006) Anal incontinence: the role of medical management. Gastroenterol Clin Biol 30:954–960
2. Collet L, Meunier P, Duclaux R et al (1988) Cerebral evoked potentials after endorectal mechanical stimulation in humans. Am J Physiol 254:G477–G482
3. Hobday DI, Aziz Q, Thacker N et al (2001) A study of the cortical processing of ano-rectal sensation using functional MRI. Brain 124:361–368
4. Blok BF, Groen J, Bosch JL et al (2006) Different brain effects during chronic and acute sacral neuromodulation in urge incontinent patients with implanted neurostimulators. BJU Int 98:1238–1243
5. Abysique A, Orsoni P, Bouvier M (1998) Evidence for supraspinal nervous control of external anal sphincter motility in the cat. Brain Res795:147–156
6. Weber J, Denis P, Mihout B et al (1985) Effect of brainstem lesion on colonic and anorectal motility. Study of three patients. Dig Dis Sci 30:419–425
7. Andrew J, Nathan PW (1964) Lesions on the anterior frontal lobes and disturbances of micturition and defaecation. Brain 87:233–262

Risk Factors in Faecal Incontinence

4

S. Mark Scott, Peter J. Lunniss

Introduction

Continence is a highly complex physiological function requiring coordinated activity of brain and central nervous system (CNS), autonomic and enteric nervous systems; a gastrointestinal tract of adequate length and biomechanical properties; and a competent anal sphincter complex, many components of which remain incompletely understood. In a minority of cases, for example incontinence immediately following fistulotomy for a high anal fistula in an otherwise "normal" individual, the cause-effect relationship is clear. For the majority, however, temporal relationships are not so evident, e.g. onset of symptoms several decades following a clinically uneventful vaginal delivery but one in which covert sphincter damage occurred, in which association between event and symptoms is less clear, and in which the event may be just one component of a multifactorial aetiology. Structural sphincteric causes of incontinence are relatively easy to investigate; at the most simplistic level, faecal continence depends upon anal pressure being higher than rectal pressure, and that this situation may be maintained predominantly by internal anal sphincter function, augmented at times of increased rectal pressure by voluntary anal muscle contraction, reflex or conscious, and orchestrated by intact sensation. In the population as a whole, faecal incontinence may, in fact, most commonly occur as "overflow" secondary to faecal impaction, particularly in institutionalised older patients, but incontinence in the form of postdefaecation soiling may result in younger people from one of the many pathophysiologies grouped under the term "rectal evacuatory disorder". The numerous and diverse structural, functional and neurological components to continence are summarised in Table 1, and a list of risk factors together with their probable pathophysiologies are presented in Table 2.

A risk factor is a definable entity that places one individual at greater risk of developing a condition than another individual who has not been exposed to that same factor. For conditions such as lung cancer and ischaemic heart disease, risk factors have been clearly identified and to which odds ratios (ORs) may be ascribed. In contrast, there are few epidemiological studies that have systematically reviewed all potential risk factors for faecal incontinence, although data for obstetric-related symptoms (the most common cause in women) are becoming well recognised. For other risk factors, there is a paucity of prospective data, perhaps not surprising in view of the difficulties related to the carrying out of appropriate methodology, and most evidence comes from retrospective observation. Many specific (diabetes mellitus, multiple sclerosis, Parkinson's disease etc.) and nonspecific (ageing) conditions may be associated with their effect on continence through their effects on mobility, ability to carry out activities of daily living etc., which make cause-effect associations even harder to determine.

The situation is further complicated by the disparities in prevalence of anal incontinence within the female parous population, for example, as reported from epidemiological studies (perhaps approaching 10%) [1–6] and increasing in the elderly [2, 5, 7] and the rates at which women seek help for their symptoms [6, 8–10]. This may be partly explained by differences in the definition of faecal incontinence (the nature and severity of faecal incontinence is variable, ranging from loss of whole motions in relation to incapacitating urgency, to minor staining of the underwear, or rare involuntary leakage of flatus). Nevertheless, a recent study from Norway showed that only three (10%) of 29 patients who felt "disabled" by symptoms of incontinence acquired following obstetric injury had sought medical help [10]. Help seeking is highly complex, involving the nature and severity of symptoms and their impact on quality of life, with primary factors such as neurological, behavioural and environmental impacts upon the condition itself, and with secondary factors such as socioeconomic, psychological and religious impacting on attitudes to seeking help, which must also include coping mechanisms, which presumably ultimately fail.

Table 1. Factors contributing to the maintenance of continence

	Component
Sphincteric	
Structural	
	Internal anal sphincter
	External anal sphincter
	Conjoined longitudinal muscle
	Vascular anal cushions and secondary mucosal folds
Functional	
	Anal resting tone
	Anal canal/high-pressure zone length
	Resting anal pressure gradient
	Voluntary anal squeeze pressure
	Anal sensation
	Anal plasticity and motility
	Rectoanal inhibitory (sampling) reflex
	Rectoanal contractile reflex
Neurological	
	Pudendal nerve
	Sympathetic (hypogastric) nerves
	Parasympathetic (pelvic) nerves
Pelvic	
Structural	
	Levator ani, especially puborectalis
	Perineal resting position/level of descent
	Rectal capacity
	Curvatures/transverse folds
	Flap-valve effect of the anterior wall
	Endopelvic musculofascial support
Functional	
	Tonic levator ani contraction
	Anorectal angle
	Postural pelvic floor reflex
	Rectal sensation
	Rectal tone
	Rectal compliance
	Rectosigmoid motility
	Anorectal pressure gradient
	Rectosigmoid sphincter
Neurological	
	Sacral somatic nerves
	Sympathetic nerves
	Parasympathetic nerves
	Spinal afferent nerves
	Intrinsic (enteric) nerves
Intestinal	
Structural	
	Intestinal length
Functional	
	Stool consistency
	Stool volume
	Gastrointestinal/colonic motility
Neurological	
	Autonomic nerves
	Afferent nerves
	Intrinsic (enteric) nerves
Other	
	Central neurological integrity (brain, spinal cord)
	Psychobehavioural factors
	Normal rectal evacuation (overflow)
	Youth

Table 2. Risk factors for faecal incontinence and pathophysiological mechanisms

Onset/risk factors	Pathophysiology of faecal incontinence
Congenital/childhood	
Anorectal anomalies	Congenital and iatrogenic bowel dysmotility; rectal irritability; sphincteric dysfunction
Spina bifida	Congenital sphincter and neuropathic bowel dysfunction; overflow
Hirschsprung's	Residual primary bowel dysmotility; congenital sphincter dysfunction; overflow; iatrogenic IAS sphincter injury
Behavioural	Wilful soiling; overflow secondary to voluntary faecal retention
Acquired/adulthood	
Diabetes mellitus	Primarily relates to neuropathy: disturbances to bowel motility and sphincteric function; steatorrhoea
CVA	Disruption of cerebrointestinal pathways; cognitive/language deficit; concurrent neuropathy; drugs (secondary effects); overflow
Parkinson's	Disturbances to bowel motility (decreased GI transit); overflow; sphincteric dysfunction
Multiple sclerosis	Conal/supraconal involvement; loss of rectal reservoir function/rectal irritability; sphincteric dysfunction
Spinal cord injury	Depends on site of lesion; disturbances to bowel motility (increased/decreased GI transit); loss of visceral perception; loss of rectoanal coordination; rectal hyperreactivity; sphincteric dysfunction
Other neurological conditions	
	Striated muscle degeneration–sphincteric dysfunction
	Multiple autonomic system atrophy; intestinal myopathy; overflow; sphincteric dysfunction
	Primarily relates to neuropathy: disturbances to bowel motility (increased/decreased GI transit); steatorrhoea
GI infection	Decreased GI transit; colorectal irritability (overwhelmed sphincter); ?secondary enteric neuropathy
Irritable bowel syndrome (IBS)	Heightened visceral perception; disturbed colorectal sensorimotor function; ?enteric neuropathy
Metabolic bowel disease	Steatorrhoea
Irritable bowel disease	Decreased GI transit; loss of rectal reservoir function; rectal irritability/hyper-reactivity; sphincteric dysfunction
Megacolon/megarectum	Loss of visceral perception; secondary decrease in colonic transit; overflow
Anal trauma	Sphincteric injury; pudendal nerve injury
	Decreased GI transit; altered visceral reflexes?
	Decreased GI transit; altered visceral reflexes?
Pelvic surgery	Loss of anatomic supporting structures; autonomic neuropathy; loss of visceral perception
Pelvic malignancy	Loss of reservoir function; altered visceral reflexes?
	Loss of rectal reservoir function; sphincteric dysfunction
Pelvic radiotherapy	Loss of rectal reservoir function; rectal irritability/hyper-reactivity; sphincteric dysfunction
Rectal prolapse	Loss of rectal reservoir function; rectal irritability/hyper-reactivity; sphincteric dysfunction
Rectal evacuatory disorder	Overflow
Anal surgery	Sphincteric injury (primarily IAS and vascular cushions); loss of rectal reservoir function
	Sphincteric injury
	Sphincteric injury (primarily IAS)
	Sphincteric injury (primarily EAS)

CVA cerebrovascular accident, *GI* gastrointestinal, *IAS* internal anal sphincter, *EAS* external anal sphincter

(continued)

Table 2. *(continued)*

Obstetric events	Sphincteric injury; pudendal nerve injury; secondary rectal sensorimotor dysfunction
General	
Ageing	Loss of mobility; overflow; sphincteric dysfunction secondary to degenerative neuropathy and myopathy
Dependence of nursing care	Loss of mobility; overflow; physical restraint; diarrhoea; dementia
Obesity	Overflow; drug-induced steatorrhoea
Psychobehavioural factors	Overflow
Intellectual incapacity	Cognitive contribution to continence; overflow
Drugs	Overflow; diarrhoea
	Anal and colorectal sensorimotor dysfunction; overflow; diarrhoea

CVA cerebrovascular accident, *GI* gastrointestinal, *IAS* internal anal sphincter, *EAS* external anal sphincter

Congenital Risk Factors

Anorectal Anomalies

Anorectal anomalies affect 1:3–5,000 newborn babies [11], most frequently associated with rectourethral fistula in boys and rectovestibular fistula in girls, but which range from low (covered anus) to complex malformations, including persistent cloaca in girls, associated with varying degrees of sacral dysgenesis [12]. The more complex the malformation, the more poorly developed are the levators and external sphincter. Irrespective of adequacy of surgical treatment in terms of anatomical correction, all those born with anorectal anomalies have an abnormal continence mechanism, which in addition to underdeveloped striated musculature includes loss of anal canal sensitivity (and thus faecal continence) and disturbed hindgut motility resulting in a dilated rectum and overflow incontinence [13–15]. Thus, up to 30% of all those born with low defects suffer faecal incontinence, constipation and inability to control flatus, and up to 85% of those with high malformations report social disability relating to incontinence [14].

Spina Bifida

Incontinence is one of the major stigmas affecting patients born with spina bifida, which occurs in about 1:1,000 live births. A cross-sectional nationwide Dutch study [16] has reported a 31% frequency of faecal incontinence among 179 young adults with spina bifida, with symptoms associated with spina bifida aperta, hydrocephalus and a lesion level of L5 or above. Voluntary control of defecation requires rectal sensation, peristalsis and adequate anorectal sphincter function. Neurological defects in patients with spinal lesions may affect one or more of these components, resulting in different types of defecation disorders: faecal incontinence, chronic constipation or both [17]. The external sphincter is often paralysed, so that upon internal sphincter relaxation, soiling is inevitable [18], and delayed colonic transit together with lack of rectal contraction in response to distension compound the problem.

Isolated Sacral Agenesis

This condition, resulting in abnormal parasympathetic innervation, renders all sufferers faecally incontinent [19]. Physiologically, rectal sensitivity is blunted, anal resting pressure is normal, but the rectoanal inhibitory reflex (RAIR) is more pronounced and longer lasting, and squeeze pressures are attenuated.

Hirschsprung's Disease

Up to 50% of children following surgical treatment of Hirschsprung's disease (which affects 1:5,000 live births) suffer constipation or faecal incontinence [20], although by adulthood, most have reasonable function [21, 22]. Physiologically, such disturbances may reside in loss of colonic length, a dysmotile residual colon with increased high-amplitude propagating contractile activity (HAPCs) resulting in rapid stool delivery to the neorectum, and rectal pressures exceeding external anal sphincter pressure, compounded by surgical interventions to relax the internal sphincter and disimpact the rectum, whereas loss of normal urge rectal sensation and failure of internal sphincter relaxation facilitate persistent constipation.

Functional Incontinence in Childhood

Functional faecal retention, commonly occurring at the time of toilet training or around the time of beginning school, is common [23]. Increasing difficulty in evacuation leads to stool withholding behaviour, and over time, the rectum dilates and loses its sensory and motor functions [24], and overflow soiling ensues. This situation appears to be reversible in that the majority are successfully treated by a variety of medical and behavioural strategies, but in a minority of patients, the problem persists into adulthood [25] and may result in megarectum.

Central Nervous System

Cerebrovascular Accidents

Faecal incontinence may affect up to 40% of subjects immediately following a stroke, with a frequency of up to 15% of those who survive 3 years. It is associated with a higher mortality and greater likelihood of need for long-term (institutional) care (exceeding dementia as a reason for requesting nursing home placement). In the immediate poststroke period, incontinence has been shown to be associated with female gender, a history of previous stroke, and comorbidity of other disabling diseases, especially diabetes mellitus and hypertension. The cerebral lesions in those with incontinence are significantly more often a haemorrhage, larger in size, and more often involved the cerebral cortex than those without faecal incontinence [26]. The pathophysiology of urinary incontinence following a stroke has been categorised into three main mechanisms: disruption of neuromicturition pathways, stroke-related cognitive and language deficits and concurrent neuropathy and medication use. Presumably, similar mechanisms may be involved in faecal incontinence, although constipation with overflow may predominate, especially after the acute cerebral event. Although incontinence may resolve during recuperation, in some it may arise as a new problem. At 3 months following the event, stroke-related factors do not appear to independently affect continence but, rather, exert influence through associations with clinical and functional factors, of which the strongest has been reported as needing help to use the toilet [27], a complex factor involving mobility, dexterity, vision, sensation, communication, cognition and affect.

A small physiological study comparing various parameters between subjects with primary idiopathic constipation and those with constipation following a stroke has reported delay in colonic transit to be more generalised in the stroke group–rather than residing in a rectal evacuatory disorder–and rectal sensation to be normal in the stroke group [28]. Risk factors for constipation (and presumably overflow) include decreased mobility, dehydration, dietary factors and the use of drugs, which exert anticholinergic actions on the gut.

Parkinson's Disease

The loss of dopaminergic neurones in Parkinson's disease occurs both in the CNS and enteric nervous system, leading to constipation and slow colonic transit [29]. Voluntary muscle dystonia, including the external sphincter, results in paradoxical contraction and obstructed defecation, whereas reduced anal resting and squeeze pressures increase the risk of faecal incontinence [30–32].

Multiple Sclerosis

Up to 68% of patients with multiple sclerosis have colorectal problems, with 30% suffering episodes of incontinence at least weekly [33, 34]. Incontinence may reside in reduced anal resting and squeeze pressure, reduced anorectal sensitivity, and reduced rectal compliance with rectal hyperirritability [35].

Spinal Cord Injury

The influence of spinal cord injury on continence is complex, being dependent upon the level and completeness of the injury as well as time since the event. The majority of patients suffer with constipation, but faecal incontinence is experienced by 75%, with up to one third having accidents at least monthly [36]. In the acute phase (spinal shock), complete cord severance leads to permanent loss of all voluntary and sensory function and a temporary loss of reflex functions in all segments below the lesion. There is loss of facilitation from above and loss of inhibitory reflexes from below the lesion. The termination of spinal shock, up to 4 weeks following injury, is heralded by a return and then exaggeration of reflex activity. Supraconal lesions are associated with delayed proximal colonic transit (loss of sympathetic activity compounded by muscle weakness and being bedridden), but with exaggerated rectal contractions and anal relaxation in response to relatively low rectal distension volumes, impaired rectal sensitivity and impaired conscious control over the external anal sphincter [37]. Although the rectoanal excitatory reflex may be exaggerated, a lack of temporal association with rectal sensation or contraction suggests that the reflex may not occur at times when continence is threatened. Thus, incontinence may arise through rectal contraction and loss of sensation, or, if the perception of urge arises, this cannot be counteracted by adequate voluntary sphincter contraction.

Conal or cauda equina lesions have a relatively greater impact on rectosigmoid than on the more proximal colonic transit, and an insensitive flaccid rectum, together with attenuated resting pressure and external sphincter function (reflex and voluntary contractions), all contribute to incontinence.

Autonomic Nervous System

Diabetes Mellitus

It is well recognised that lower gastrointestinal symptoms, including diarrhoea and incontinence, are frequently reported by patients with diabetes, more so than in the general population, although the pathogenesis is unclear. A prevalence of 7% among a cohort of 540 diabetics has been reported [38], with some degree of symptom fluctuation (improvement in some, new onset in others) over time. Abnormal gastrointestinal sensorimotor function (including internal sphincter dysfunction [39] and blunted rectal sensitivity) secondary to autonomic neuropathy, glycaemic control and psychological and sociodemographic factors all contribute. However, within the limitations of those studies performed, symptoms suggestive of peripheral (and by inference, autonomic and enteric) neuropathy appear to be the strongest independent risk factors. Pudendal neuropathy may be found, associated with external sphincter weakness, and rapid transit of loose stool to the rectum may occur secondary to bacterial overgrowth (steatorrhoea) or disturbed small-bowel motor activity [40].

Ageing

Faecal incontinence is an underreported symptom in the general population but is especially common in the elderly residing either in the community or within residential/nursing homes [41]. Indeed, it is the second most common reason for request for residential long-term care provision. Faecal incontinence occurs in up to 10% of people older than 65 years in the community and approximately 50% of nursing home residents [41]. A systematic review and metaregression analysis interestingly demonstrated rates of faecal incontinence to be higher in women than in men, but that the difference did not reach statistical significance [42]. Among the elderly, faecal incontinence can be broadly categorised as overflow incontinence, reservoir incontinence and rectosphincteric incontinence. Faecal incontinence among nursing home residents is associated with multiple factors: urinary incontinence, impaired ability to perform activities of daily living, tube feeding, the use of physical restraints, diarrhoea, poor vision and constipation/impaction.

There are relatively little data in the literature relating to specific age-related physiological changes to continence. Given that we know that ageing is associated with changes in the enteric nervous systems of the small bowel and colon, it is not surprising that degenerative changes may occur to components of the continence mechanism. Bannister et al. [43] noted lower anal pressures in the elderly compared with younger subjects, and importantly, in whom lower rectal distension volumes were required to inhibit anal sphincter tone as well as lower rectal urge and maximum toleration volumes–such differences rendering the elderly more susceptible to incontinence. Internal sphincter dysfunction may relate to age-specific thickening and sclerosis of the internal anal sphincter [44], perhaps compounded by age-related autonomic innervation dysfunction [45]. Evidence for reduced squeeze pressures with age is conflicting, and although pudendal nerve conduction slows with age, it is unclear whether slowing occurs in middle age or later life [45–47]. Irrespective of mechanism, Bharucha et al. [48] have recently shown that the risk of faecal incontinence indeed increases with age, with an OR of 1.3 per decade [95% confidence interval (CI): 1.2–1.4).

Intestinal Disorders

It is evident that any acute diarrhoeal state, if sufficiently extreme, will result in temporary incontinence through an otherwise normal anal sphincter mechanism, and more so if the sphincter is compromised from any other causes. Such overwhelming of the sphincters may arise through intestinal inflammation, hypersecretory states, malabsorption, intestinal hypersensitivity and heightened contractility, which result in the rapid delivery of liquid stool to a possibly irritable rectum. Chronic conditions affecting gastrointestinal function in the same way will obviously impact on continence in the long term, with lasting effects on quality of life.

Inflammatory Bowel Disease

Increased frequencies of defecation (>80%), urgency (>80%), the sensation of incomplete evacuation (75%) and tenesmus (63%) were the most common symptoms reported in patients with active ulcerative colitis by Rao et al. [49] and more common in active rather than in quiescent disease but irrespective of proximal colonic involvement, suggesting that such symptoms related to an inflamed, irritable distal colon and rectum. In 1978, Farthing and Lennard-Jones reported lower rectal thresholds to balloon distension in patients with ulcerative colitis compared with controls, the difference being greater in those with active rather than inactive disease [50]. Rao et al. [51] confirmed these findings but also demonstrated lower rectal compliance in active disease and lower rectal volumes required to induce sustained internal sphincter relaxation.

By contrast, in a study of patients with Crohn's disease and faecal urgency, anorectal behaviour appeared to be less important in symptom pathogenesis than did small bowel involvement, with secondary rapid rectal filling [52]. With regard to colonic motility, Bassotti et al. [53] demonstrated greater frequency of HAPCs (but not their amplitude) and low APCs (LAPCs) in patients with moderately active ulcerative colitis compared with irritable bowel syndrome (IBS) sufferers and healthy controls. Such increased propulsive activity (including loss of normal retarding segmental contractions) were suggested to arise through increased gut secretory functions and mucosal inflammation [54].

Irritable Bowel Syndrome

Diarrhoea is a component of several of the functional gastrointestinal disorders defined by Rome III criteria, including idiopathic functional diarrhoea and IBS [55]. The frequencies of urgency and accidental faecal incontinence have been reported in several studies as greater amongst IBS sufferers than in the general population [56–59]. IBS appears to be prevalent in many parts of the world–in those countries where intestinal infections are not common, the adoption of diagnostic criteria means that reported prevalences are perhaps fairly accurate. The limited symptom repertoire of the gut, however, means that in less developed countries, prevalence may be overestimated, although the roles of past infection and inflammation in the possible pathoaetiology of IBS further confuses the issue. Visceral hypersensitivity, whose origin may lie at varying sites along the brain–gut axis, together with disturbed motility, are probably central to symptom generation and influenced by other factors (psychosocial, etc.) [60]. Abnormal motility has been demonstrated in the small bowel [61–63], whole gut [64], proximal colon [65] and rectosigmoid [66–68]. Although intestinal dysmotility is considered a major pathophysiological factor, the specificity of many of the reported abnormal motor patterns at various sites along the gastrointestinal tract is unclear [69]. More frequent and higher-amplitude HAPCs may account for accelerated colonic transit and bowel frequency, and the rapid arrival of more liquid stool to the rectum combined with heightened rectal sensitivity and high rectal pressures may lead to the sphincters, on occasions, being overwhelmed, resulting in accidental defecation [68].

Pelvic Nonintestinal Surgery

Women often ascribe bowel symptoms to gynaecological intervention, especially hysterectomy, the most commonly performed gynaecological procedure. However, functional gut and gynaecological symptoms often coexist [70, 71], and referral to a gynaecologist may prompt hysterectomy. There are four possible factors that may result in bowel dysfunction following uterine excision. The close proximity of the pelvic (sympathetic and parasympathetic) plexus to the bladder, cervix and vagina renders the autonomic innervation to the hindgut at risk of injury, and the more radical the procedure, the greater the risk of such damage [72–74]. Anatomical studies suggest that such risk is reduced if the cardinal ligaments are preserved and less vaginal cuff removed [75]. Secondly, loss of anatomical and functional pelvic supporting structures following hysterectomy may lead to vault prolapse, enterocoele, rectocele and perineal descent [76, 77]. Loss of ovarian function results in reduced serum oestrogen, and the uterus is a potential source of prostaglandins, of which PGF2· has a stimulatory effect on colonic motility. Lastly, the complex issue of psychological influences may contribute to symptomatology.

The fact is, however, that there is a paucity of prospectively accrued data to support an association between gynaecological surgery and bowel disturbance, which has usually been reported from retrospective study as constipatory in nature (straining, ineffective evacuation, loss of urge), and which may be related to increased rectal compliance, blunted rectal sensitivity and reduced motility [78, 79]. Interestingly, a prospective questionnaire study of 121 consecutive patients undergoing hysterectomy found no increase in constipatory symptoms following surgery but that concomitant bilateral salpingo-oophorectomy (but not simple vaginal hysterectomy) resulted in a significantly increased risk of faecal incontinence that persisted at 12 months [80]. The relative ubiquity of hysterectomy in the West and conflicting evidence in respect to effects on hindgut function begs large-scale prospective study of function and physiology.

Rectal Resection

Rectal resection results in loss of the rectal reservoir (the lower the level of resection, the greater the reservoir loss), one of the fundamental components to normal continence, and may be associated also with inadvertent (iatrogenic) sphincter damage [81]. As a result of the observed functional consequences of a low straight coloanal anastomosis, attempts have been made at restoring reservoir function by construction of a short colonic pouch [82], by coloplasty [83] or by end-to-side anastomosis [84]. Such reservoir construction improves (over the first 2 years) but does not abolish the functional consequences of the "conventional" technique, such as urgency, frequency and incontinence, the aetiology of which may also reside in changes in hindgut motility [85, 86].

Pelvic Radiotherapy

Putta and Andreyev published a review of the literature relating to faecal incontinence following pelvic radiotherapy for prostate, gynaecological, bladder, rectal and anal malignancies [87]. They suggested that data reliability was poor because of patient reluctance to admit to incontinence and a lack of prospective studies; nevertheless, rates of late new-onset faecal incontinence ranged from 3% to 53%. The rectal contribution to urgency and incontinence may reside in a stiffer, less compliant rectum [88] and mucosal irritability (proctitis), whilst at the sphincter level, radiotherapy has been associated with reduced resting and squeeze pressures, sphincter scarring on ultrasound and prolonged pudendal nerve terminal motor latencies [89, 90]. The additive effects on continence of high-dose, short-course radiotherapy given before anterior resection for rectal carcinoma have been able to be assessed as a result of the randomised trials designed primarily to determine oncological end points. From the Dutch [91] and Swedish [89] studies, irradiated patients reported significantly greater rates of faecal incontinence than did nonirradiated patients (57–62% vs 26–38%, respectively) and greater rates of soiling, pad usage and bowel frequency than in those undergoing surgery alone.

Sphincteric Risk Factors

Obstetric Events

With respect to acquired faecal incontinence in women, we have recently reported the results of a (necessarily) retrospective cohort analysis of 475 women referred to our Gastrointestinal Physiology Unit for investigation of their symptoms of faecal incontinence [92]. The pertinent findings of that study can be summarised as follows:

The median age of symptom onset was 47 years and symptom duration 26 (range 2–502) months, with symptomatology usually being combined passive and urge incontinence.

Only 1% had histories that contained no volunteered potential risk factor.

The overwhelming risk factor was childbirth (91%), with at least one vaginal delivery reported as complicated (notably perineal trauma, and the use of forceps) in 78%.

Among the 150 women in whom only one risk factor was identifiable, obstetric risk factors were reported in 82%.

Forty percent of women ascribed their symptoms directly to a particular event in their medical histories, including 48 of the 124 women in whom obstetric factors were the only risk.

The median age of onset of symptoms in those women who ascribed their symptoms to childbirth was 26 years less than that of those in whom obstetric factors were the only risk but in whom no association had been made with subsequent symptoms and in whom the median time lag before symptom onset was 18.5 (range 2–55) years, although there was no difference in symptom duration before presentation between the ascribers and nonascribers.

Results of physiological testing were abnormal in all but 4%, and in 64%, there was more than one pathophysiology identified (anal morphology, anal pressures, pudendal nerve function and rectal sensation).

Notwithstanding the limitations of retrospective study (the practicalities of a prospective long-term study, given the time lag to symptom onset amongst many factors, means that such a study has never been performed), there is now clear recognition, supported by a considerable body of evidence, that obstetric trauma is, by far, the major risk factor for the development of acquired faecal incontinence in women [93–96]. Table 3 summarises the prevalence of symptoms of faecal incontinence postpartum in studies involving >130 subjects and shows that greater than 10% of women will complain of bowel symptoms in the first few months following childbirth [1, 2, 4, 5, 97–108]. Although in the majority this

Table 3. Prevalence of incontinence symptoms following childbirth

Author	Date	Vaginal deliveries	Parity P/M	Follow-up (months)	Prevalence of new postpartum symptoms (%)		
					Urgency	Flatus	Faecal
Continence status before delivery known							
Sultan et al. [97]	1993	127	79 P/48 M	1.5	7.1	3.9	0.8
Donnelly et al. [98]	1998	168	168 P	1.5	13.7	13.1	4.2
Chaliha et al. [2]	1999	413	413 P	3	7.3	5.1	[e]1.9
Zetterström et al. [99]	1999	278	278 P	5	-	19.0	1.1
Zetterström et al. [99]	1999	278	278 P	9	-	18.3	0.4
MacArthur et al. [1]	1997	877	363 P/514 M	10	2.2	-	1.9
Summary data: median (range)					7.2 (2.2–13.7)	13.1 (3.9–19.0)	1.5 (0.4–4.2)
Continence status before delivery unknown							
Donnelly et al. [100]	1998	312	312 P	1.5	16.0	15.4	10.3
Abramowitz et al. [101]	2000	202	[e]103 P/100 M	2	-	~6.4	~2.9
Pregazzi et al. [102]	2002	218	218 P	2	-	0.9	1.8
Groutz et al. [103]	1999	300	-	3	-	6.3	0.7
Signorello et al. [104]	2000	612	612 P	3	-	24.3	5.2
MacArthur et al. [4]	2001	6135[a]	2698 P/3316 M	3	-	26.6	4.2
Chaliha et al. [105]	2001	130	130 P	3	16.9	12.3[b]	-
Hannah et al. [106]	2002	404[c]	~202 P/200 M	3	-	9.2	1.0
Eason et al. [5]	2002	834	~515 P/319 M	3	-	25.9	3.2
Sartore et al. [107]	2004	519	519 P	3	-	2.3[b]	
Signorello et al. [104]	2000	612	612 P	6	-	15.2	2.3
Chiarelli et al. [108]	2003	568[d]	298 P/270 M	12	14.8	24.4	6.9
Summary data: median (range)					16.0 (14.8–16.9)	14.3 (0.9–26.6)	3.1 (0.7–10.3)

P primiparous, *M* multiparous
[a]Parity not known in 121 cases
[b]Includes flatus and faecal incontinence
[c]Breech presentation
[d]High-risk delivery (instrumental delivery, or birthweight >4,000 g)
[e]Accurate data not presented; best estimate made

will be restricted to urgency of defecation or "minor" incontinence (i.e. flatus or soiling), approximately 1.5–3% of women [1, 2, 4, 5, 97–108] will suffer "major" or frank stool incontinence. Prevalence rates as high as 10% for major incontinence have been reported by Donnelly et al. [100], although the continence status of patients prior to delivery was not described in this study, and this therefore likely represents an overestimate with regard to new-onset symptoms. However, given that the prevalence of major faecal incontinence in the community as a whole has been reported as 2–4.3% [41, 42], these data indicate that in the vast majority of women, obstetric trauma is indeed the primary aetiological factor.

Several studies have looked at which particular obstetric variables may predispose to the development of incontinence. The predominant independent risk factor appears to be a clinically apparent anal sphincter tear at the time of delivery, with median ORs of between 1.7 and 9.1 reported [5, 99, 101, 102, 110–112]. Other major risk factors are increasing maternal age [99, 108]; multiparity [108, 110, 113]; instrumental delivery [1, 98, 103], particularly involving forceps [1, 4, 5, 101, 114], and a prolonged second stage of labour [98, 101, 103, 114].

Third-degree perineal rupture, which, by definition, involves an anal sphincter tear, has been reported to occur in 0.6–5.9% of vaginal deliveries [115–122]. Nevertheless, it is important to appreciate that occult (i.e. not clinically evident) disruption of the anal sphincter complex occurs in approximately 30% of women during childbirth and is only identifiable on endoanal ultrasound [97, 101, 105, 123–128] (Table 4). This high incidence of covert sphincter damage as a result of vaginal delivery provides the background for the development of symptoms later in life [92, 129–132], when other risk factors (specific

Table 4. Incidence of anal sphincter damage following vaginal delivery: studies utilising endo anal ultrasonography

Author	Date	Number		New sphincter defect %		Newly symptomatic (new defect) %	Newly symptomatic (no defect) %
		P	M	P	M		
Sultan et al. [97]	1993	79	48	35	8	41	1.3
Fynes et al.[a] [123]	1999	59	59	34[b]	5	68	0
Abramowitz et al. [101]	2000	96	106	26	13	23	6.7
Faltin et al. [124]	2000	150	0	28	-	37	6.8
Chaliha et al. [105]	2001	130	0	~45[b‡]	-	-	-
Belmonte-Montes et al. [125]	2001	98	0	29	-	75	0
Nazir et al. [126]	2002	80	0	26		-	-
Pinta et al. [127]	2004	75	0	23	-	47	-
Damon et al. [128]	2005	197	0	34[b]	-	71	4.5
Summary data: median (range)		96 (35–197)		29 (20–45)		44 (0–75)	1.3 (0–6.8)

P primiparous, *M* multiparous
[a]Same cohort studied through first two vaginal deliveries
[b]No pre natal assessment performed, therefore defects may have preexisted, i.e. possible overestimate
[c]Accurate denominator not documented: 58 defects in 125–130 patients (i.e. 44–46%)

and nonspecific) impact (see above).

Numerous studies have attempted to determine which obstetric variables are associated with the risk of sustaining third- and fourth-degree perineal tears [109, 133] (Table 5): first vaginal birth [5, 116, 118–120, 122, 134, 135]; instrumental delivery [98, 121, 136], notably forceps-assisted [5, 115–117, 119–122, 134, 135, 137–139] and by vacuum extraction [5, 118, 119,

Table 5. Multivariate analyses from selected series showing the adjusted odds ratio/relative risk of developing a third- or fourth-degree perineal tear during an instrumental vaginal delivery

	Author	Year	Odds ratio	(95% CI)
Forceps	Poen et al. [115]	1997	3.3	(1.6–6.9)
	de Leeuw et al. [117]	2001	3.3	(3.0–3.7)
	Handa et al. [119]	2001	1.5	(1.4–1.5)
	Eason et al. [5]	2002	12.3[a]	(3.0–50.4)
	Fenner et al. [138]	2003	4.8	(3.4–6.6)
	Christianson et al. [120]	2003	11.9	(4.7–30.4)
	Andrews et al. [140]	2006	6.0	(1.2–19.5)
	Fitzgerald et al. [139]	2007	13.6	(7.9–23.2)
Vacuum extraction	Handa et al. [119]	2001	2.3	(2.2–2.4)
	Eason et al. [5]	2002	7.4[a]	(1.9–28.5)
	Fenner et al. [138]	2003	3.5	(2.6–4.7)
	Fornell et al. [112]	2004	4.2	(1.7–10.4)
Midline episiotomy	Helwig et al. [142]	1993	2.4[a]	(1.7–3.5)
	Signorello et al. [104]	2000	5.5	(1.8–16.2)
	Eason et al. [5]	2002	9.6[a]	(3.2–28.5)
	Fenner et al. [138]	2003	2.2	(1.8–2.8)
	Christianson et al. [120]	2003	2.5	(1.0–6.0)
Mediolateral episiotomy	Poen et a.l [115]	1997	0.5	(0.3–0.9)
	de Leeuw et al. [117]	2001	0.2	(0.2–0.2)
	Fenner et al. [138]	2003	0.7	(0.4–1.2)
	Andrews et al. [140]	2006	4.0	(1.7–9.6)

CI confidence interval
[a]Relative risk (RR)

135, 138]; macrosomia (>4,000 g) [115–121, 135–138, 140]; prolonged second-stage labour [115–117, 134]; and epidural anaesthesia [115, 121] are all reported as principal factors. Other, perhaps less appreciated, factors include maternal age [118, 138], induction of labour [115, 118, 121], shoulder dystocia [135] and Asian race [4, 119, 134, 141].

Two areas of controversy that remain are whether either episiotomy or Caesarean section are protective of anal sphincter rupture or the development of incontinence. Episiotomy may be carried out routinely in the belief that it reduces the severity of perineal trauma; however, there is now strong evidence that median or midline episiotomy is associated with an increased incidence of anal sphincter tears [5, 104, 118, 120, 134, 136–138, 142] and symptoms of altered continence [104]. Data regarding mediolateral episiotomy are conflicting. Shiono et al. [137] reported that the risk of severe perineal laceration was reduced 2.5-fold in primiparous women who received a mediolateral episiotomy; similarly, Poen et al. [115] and de Leeuw et al. [117] have shown ORs of 0.5 and 0.2, respectively, with episiotomy performed mediolaterally, indicating a protective effect. By contrast, others have shown no difference in the rates of incontinence [107] or sphincter tears [138] in women with or without mediolateral episiotomy or, indeed, that mediolateral episiotomy may be an independent risk factor for sphincter rupture [122, 140]. One explanation relates to operative technique in that mediolateral episiotomies are not truly mediolateral but angled towards the midline [140]. What is apparent is that episiotomy performed towards or in the midline increases rather than minimises the risk of incontinence, and comparative studies have shown midline episiotomy to be three times more likely than mediolateral episiotomy to cause anal sphincter laceration [138].

With regard to Caesarean section, many studies have reported that symptoms of incontinence are absent in women who have undergone either an elective or prelabour emergency procedure [4, 97–101, 106, 123]. Both MacArthur et al. [4] and Goldberg et al. [7] have shown a negative association between C-section and faecal incontinence, reporting ORs of 0.6 (95% CI: 0.4–0.97) and 0.4 (95% CI: 0.2–0.9), respectively. Nevertheless, others have shown that emergency section may be associated with altered faecal continence [1, 143], and it was concluded by Fynes et al. [123] that recourse to Caesarean delivery late in labour may not avoid neurological injury. More recently, however, Lal et al. reported that incontinence can occur following both elective and prelabour emergency section [143], and a systematic review of the literature by Nelson et al. [144], covering 15 studies encompassing 3,010 Caesarean sections and 11,440 vaginal deliveries showed no difference between the rates of either faecal or flatus incontinence between the two different modes of delivery. They concluded that Caesarean section does not prevent incontinence. The implication of both of these studies is that it is pregnancy itself, perhaps in relation to connective tissue properties or perhaps an inherited susceptibility [133], that can lead to pelvic floor disorders. Further clinical studies are required to clear up these conflicting results and to elucidate the role of C-section in the prevention of incontinence.

In terms of the pathophysiology of incontinence following obstetric trauma, anal sphincter dysfunction is recognised as the main pathogenic mechanism in the majority [145–147]. A consistent manometric finding is that anal squeeze pressures are significantly decreased following spontaneous and instrumental vaginal delivery, irrespective of postpartum continence status or sphincter integrity [97, 105, 123, 127, 148–154]. For anal resting tone, published findings are more contradictory. Although some prospective studies show significantly decreased resting pressures postpartum compared with antepartum [97, 98, 151, 155], others show no change in resting tone [127, 149, 150] or report that a decrease is confined to those in whom structural defects are found at ultrasound [148], those who have had an instrumental delivery [105] or only those who become incontinent [128]. Caesarean section appears, from the results of most studies, to afford protection against anal structural damage and sphincter dysfunction, as both resting and squeeze pressures are unchanged [97, 98, 105, 123, 156]. However, when performed as an emergency in late labour, Caesarean section may be associated with significantly reduced squeeze pressures (in the absence of anal structural defects), which indicates neurological injury to the anal sphincter mechanism [123, 156].

Structural sphincter damage is best assessed by ultrasonography; the seminal study of Sultan et al. [97] showed that 35% of primiparous and 4% of multiparous women had defects resulting from vaginal delivery (with only two of 150 women having recognised tears of the anal sphincter at the time of delivery), and a strong association was demonstrated between presence of a defect and development of symptoms [97]. The incidence of anal sphincter tears is shown in Table 4. It has been calculated that for a woman presenting with faecal incontinence postpartum, the probability of her having a sphincter defect is ~80% [132].

The external anal sphincter is the structure most threatened during vaginal delivery, and disruption may result, of course, from extension of perineal trauma (either tear or episiotomy). Table 6 clearly

Table 6. Type of anal sphincter disruption identified on endoanal ultrasound

Author	Date	Number of defects	Isolated IAS defects %	Isolated EAS defects %	Combined IAS/EAS defects %	All EAS defects %
Sultan et al. [97]	1993	28	46	18	36	56
Abramowitz et al. [101]	2000	39	10	85	590	
Faltin et al. [124]	2000	42	5	71	24	95
Chaliha et al. 105]	2001	59	17	59	24	83
Belmonte-Montes et al. [125]	2001	28	0	66	34	100
Nazir et al. [126]	2002	14	7	79	14	93
Pinta et al. [127]	2004	17	12	65	23	88
Damon et al. [128]	2005	66	0	74	26	100
Summary data: median (range)		33.5 (14–66)	8.5 (0–46)	68.5 (18–85)	24 (5–36)	91.5 (56–100)

IAS internal anal sphincter, *EAS* external anal sphincter

demonstrates that in women with ultrasonographic confirmation of sphincter defects, approximately 90% involve the external anal sphincter [101, 124–128], either in isolation or combined with rupture of the internal anal sphincter. Isolated internal anal sphincter defects are much less common, accounting for 10% or less of all defects in the majority of studies [101, 124–128]. In the absence of an overt tear (i.e. an intact perineum), it is presumed that such isolated defects in the internal anal sphincter result from shearing forces imposed during delivery [97].

Aside from sphincter damage, the branches of the pudendal nerve, which contains both motor and sensory fibres, are vulnerable to stretch or compression injury, which may occur during childbirth [157–163] when pelvic floor descent and progression of the foetal head towards the pelvic outlet may stretch the nerve as it emerges from Alcock's canal, where its course is relatively fixed along the pelvic sidewall [95]. Multiparity, instrumental delivery (notably forceps), protracted second stage of labour, anal sphincter tears and high birthweight are identified risk factors [97, 123, 148, 157, 160]. In respect to parity, first vaginal delivery appears, from the results of prospective studies, to be the most injurious to sphincter [5, 120, 123, 135] and neural [123, 160] integrity alike, with damage to the pudendal nerves being cumulative with successive deliveries [110, 123, 153, 158, 159, 163]. Importantly, studies assessing pudendal nerve function in patients undergoing emergency versus elective Caesarean have shown that a section performed after the onset of labour (especially during the later stages) does not protect against neural damage [97, 156, 164], especially on the left side [97, 156, 160], although the significance of this is unclear. Association between pudendal neuropathy and symptoms of incontinence acquired following childbirth has been shown in some [98, 154, 159, 161, 165] but not all [97] studies. Prolonged nerve terminal motor latencies are a surrogate marker of pudendal neuropathy and are used as a measure of demyelination (and also axonal injury), and have been demonstrated in 16–30% of primiparous women at around 6 weeks following childbirth [97, 98, 123, 156, 165]. Although latencies may recover with time [97, 152, 157, 160] (i.e. suggesting that the nerve may recover from initial injury), it is feasible that with multiparity [110, 123, 153, 158, 159, 163]–perhaps chronic straining at stool [163, 166, 167] and, indeed, ageing [45]–neuropathy may be cumulative and thence become an independent risk factor resulting in symptoms [153]. It may certainly constitute one of the multiple aetiologies contributing to incontinence in parous women presenting in later life [92, 94, 129–131].

Anal Surgery

After obstetric trauma, the most common aetiological factor associated with the development of acquired faecal incontinence is anal surgery [145]. This is particularly the case in men; a recent retrospective review of 154 incontinent male patients revealed that previous anal surgery was reported by 50% [92]. Of the 76 men in this cohort in whom only a *single* risk factor was evident in their histories, anal surgery was reported by 59%. In such procedures, it is primarily the internal (rather than external) anal sphincter that is susceptible to disruption, either deliberately (e.g. lateral sphincterotomy) or as a complication (e.g. haemorrhoidectomy) [92, 168]. In both genders, the relative incidence of anal surgical procedures has been reported to be almost identical [92], with haemorrhoidectomy the most frequent procedure reported, followed by fistula surgery and sphincterotomy for anal fissure.

Lateral Internal Anal Sphincterotomy

Internal sphincterotomy was introduced into surgical practice more than 50 years ago [169], with the lateral subcutaneous sphincterotomy becoming the procedure of choice after it was first reported by Notaras in 1969 [170]. This represents a "controlled" division of the internal anal sphincter in its caudal part, usually to the dentate line. Although lateral internal sphincterotomy remains the surgical treatment of choice for chronic anal fissures unresponsive to medical therapy, with healing rates of up to 97% reported [171–174], it carries a well-recognised and significant risk of disturbance of anal continence.

Several large studies (>200 patients) have shown that between 23% and 45% of patients will suffer some degree of incontinence in the postoperative period [171, 175, 176]. In the largest of these studies, by Khubchandani et al. [171], the reported incidence of flatus incontinence, soiling and solid stool incontinence in 829 patients responding to a postoperative questionnaire was 35%, 22% and 5%, respectively. Others, however, reported a much lower incidence of incontinence (only 1.4% with loss of control of flatus) following "tailored" surgery, aimed to preserve more sphincter by selecting the height of sphincter to be divided [177]. Long-term studies show that problems with continence may be transient in the majority; for example, Mentefl et al. [174] reported a reduction in incontinence from 7.4% in the immediate postoperative period to 2.9% at 12 months. However, several reports show an incidence of 8–18% of "any" anal incontinence at follow-up ranging from 4.3–5.6 years [172, 178, 179]. Although for solid stool incontinence the incidence may be low in the long term (0–3% [175–177, 180]), flatus incontinence may remain a common problem, with published rates of up to 30% [180].

With regard to pathophysiology, in the majority of cases, this is due to extended division of the internal anal sphincter beyond the therapeutic intention of the surgery [175, 181]. This is consistent with the predominance of passive faecal incontinence observed in the majority [92]. Using ultrasound, Lindsey et al. [181] demonstrated overextension of the sphincterotomy in 15/17 patients with incontinence; in four patients, division of the internal anal sphincter was evident throughout the length of the anal canal. Sultan et al. [182] similarly showed complete division of the internal anal sphincter in nine of ten women though in none of the four men; they suggested this was related to a shorter anal canal length in women. Iatrogenic external anal sphincter injury has also been reported in patients having undergone internal sphincterotomy [181, 183]. Furthermore, a high incidence of coexisting (occult) sphincter defects are present in patients who develop incontinence after sphincterotomy, even in those in whom the procedure has been performed satisfactorily [184]. Indeed, Casillas et al. [181] have reported a higher risk of incontinence following sphincterotomy in women who have had two or more vaginal deliveries, supporting the concept that occult injury contributes to the pathophysiology of disturbed continence in this group [180]. Manometrically, there may be a reversal of the pressure gradient within the anal canal; Zbar et al. [185] suggested that pathophysiology is more complex still, with disturbances to the rectoanal inhibitory reflex, a shorter high-pressure zone and more anal sphincter asymmetry.

Anal Dilatation

Although first described almost two centuries ago, anal dilatation became the primary treatment for anal hypertonia associated with chronic fissure-in-ano and haemorrhoids after the introduction of the now-infamous Lord's procedure [originally an eight-finger (!) anal stretch] in 1968 [186]. The concept was that forceful dilatation would loosen the sphincter muscle and increase blood flow to the anoderm [187]. Despite reported success rates with respect to pain relief of 55–80% [188–190], it is now well documented that this procedure is frequently associated with compromised continence. Furthermore, symptom recurrence may be high over the long term [189, 191].

In prospective studies, minor incontinence (soiling and flatus) rates of 13–27% have been reported immediately following dilatation [189, 192–194]. However, a study by Konsten and Baeten with median follow-up of 17 years in 39 patients who had undergone dilatation and haemorrhoidectomy and 44 patients who had undergone dilatation alone showed a long-term incontinence rate of 52% [191]. Comparative studies have shown that anal dilatation is associated with a greater incidence of postintervention incontinence than is sphincterotomy [192, 195, 196].

Compatible with primarily passive incontinence noted after dilatation, impairment of internal anal sphincter function has been shown manometrically [197], and in symptomatic patients, internal anal sphincter disruption, or indeed fragmentation, appears to be an almost invariable finding. Speakman et al. [198], using ultrasonography, showed that 11 of 12 patients with incontinence following anal stretch had internal anal sphincter defects and the internal anal sphincter was extensively fragmented in ten of these 11. Similarly, Lindsey et al. [181] demonstrated that in 27 patients with incontinence after dilatation, 100% had internal anal sphincter injury; the smooth muscle ring was thinned posteriorly in ten, disrupted posteriorly in 12 and fragmented in five. Of note, they also reported external anal sphincter injury in eight the 27 patients. Occult injury may also be significant, with the potential to impact later in life. Nielsen et al. [193] showed that 11 of 18 *continent* patients had sphincteric damage (nine internal anal sphincter, one external anal sphincter and one combined sphincters) following dilatation and concluded that sphincter injury may occur in more that 50% of patients undergoing this procedure, although relatively few develop symptoms immediately.

As long ago as 1992, the use of anal dilatation was questioned because of the risk of developing incontinence [189], and there is now consensus opinion that this is an outmoded procedure that should be abandoned [145, 187, 191, 196].

Fistula Surgery

Treatment for fistula-in-ano is diverse, with no single technique being universally effective. The major approach is surgical, with the aim of abolishing the primary track and draining any secondary tracks. Although sphincter-preserving techniques are preferable, surgical division of sphincteric musculature is unavoidable in many cases, and this carries with it the risk of iatrogenic incontinence; indeed, the development of incontinence may be almost inescapable after complex anal fistula surgery [145]. Fistulotomy is the classic operation for anal fistulas, in which the track is laid open; however, this involves division of those muscle fibres enclosed by the track. Alternatively, fistulectomy involves excision of the track. Seton threads may also be used, often as part of a staged fistulotomy procedure, either as a long-term loose draining seton or as a tight or "snug" cutting seton [199], which provides slower division of the enclosed muscle.

Overall, irrespective of surgical technique, retrospective studies in large patient series' (200–700), often with long-term follow-up, have shown postoperative incontinence rates ranging from, at best, 4–7% [200, 201] to 26–45% [202–204]. More specifically, impairment of continence following fistulotomy has been reported in up to 54% of patients, whether by lay-open technique [202, 205, 206] or through a cutting seton (see review by Hammond et al. [199]) [205, 207–209]. Certainly, the higher the fistula, the greater the potential for impaired function after fistulotomy. However, even in patients where the consequences of sphincter division would be anticipated to result in minimal functional disturbance (i.e. with low fistulas), incontinence may still occur due to the additive effects of other risk factors, such as previous obstetric injury in women [181]. Importantly, postoperative incontinence is more common than fistula recurrence, and rates of dissatisfaction with surgery may thus be attributable to such disturbances in continence [204].

Mechanistically, various studies have shown that patients who are incontinent following fistula surgery have reduced resting tone in the distal 1 or 2 cm of the anal canal [206, 210–212] and perhaps attenuated anal squeeze pressures also [208, 210, 211], especially following treatment for transsphincteric fistulas.

Haemorrhoidectomy

In terms of structures contributing to continence, the sphincter muscles alone cannot entirely close the anal lumen [213], and approximately 15% of the basal anal canal resting tone is generated by the expansile vascular anal cushions [214], which, along with secondary anal mucosal folds [215], provide a hermetic seal. The importance of these structures becomes evident in patients with prolapsing haemorrhoids, where the mucocutaneous junction, which provides a barrier against mucus and liquid faecal leakage, may be displaced beyond the anal verge [216]. Faecal soiling is not uncommon in such patients [217] and may indeed be cured by haemorrhoidectomy [218, 219]. Contrarily, however, in continent patients with symptomatic haemorrhoids, surgery is now clearly recognised as carrying a risk for the development of incontinence.

There are essentially four varieties of haemorrhoidectomy: the open technique, now referred to as the Milligan–Morgan operation [220]; the closed technique, as popularised by Ferguson [221]; the Parks submucosal technique [222]; and the more recently introduced stapling method, as originally described by Longo in 1998 [223]. Overall, several large series (>380 patients) have shown that the incidence of "severe" and persistent postoperative incontinence is rare, ranging from 0.2–1%, irrespective of surgical technique [224–227]. In addition, transient soiling affecting 35–50% of patients may completely resolve by 6 months [228, 229]. However, minor (flatus) and moderate (soiling) incontinence has been reported in the long term in a significant proportion of patients. Johannsson et al. [230] showed that 33% of patients suffered from disturbed continence up to 7 years following open haemorrhoidectomy; 29% of these patients directly attributed onset of their incontinence to the surgery. Guenin et al. [226] reported a similar incidence of persistent soiling (27%) in 514 patients following closed haemorrhoidectomy. A randomised trial comparing the Milligan-Morgan procedure (109 patients) to the Ferguson technique (102 patients) favoured the latter with regard to development of incontinence, with 13% in both groups suffering from mild incontinence at 1 year. However, only 1% had moderate incontinence following the closed operation compared with 7% after the open procedure [219].

Endoanal ultrasonography, performed in patients complaining of incontinence following haemorrhoidectomy, has shown injury to the internal anal sphincter in the majority. Abbasakoor et al. [231] demonstrated an isolated internal anal sphincter injury in 5/10 patients, a combined internal/external anal sphincter in two and an isolated external anal sphincter defect in one. Two patients had a normal ultrasound [231]. Similarly, Lindsey et al. [181] showed internal anal sphincter injury in 26 of 29 patients with incontinence following Milligan-Morgan haemorrhoidectomy; the internal anal sphincter was thin in 12 and disrupted in 14 at the pedicle excision sites. Furthermore, an adjacent external anal sphincter injury was seen in 24% of patients. It has also been suggested that loss of the endovascular mucosal cushions contributes to the development of incontinence [181, 231, 232].

Rectal Evacuatory Disorder

Faecal impaction is an important risk factor for incontinence and predominantly affects older people, especially those living in institutions [41, 95], but also children [25, 41, 145]. In the elderly, approximately 50% of nursing home residents will suffer from faecal incontinence [41, 233, 234]; prolonged retention of stool in the rectum, perhaps secondary to incomplete evacuation during defecation but also as a consequence of other factors, such as physical immobility, inadequate diet and water intake, depression, dementia, associated metabolic disorders (e.g. hypothyroidism) and use of constipating drugs (e.g. narcotics, antipsychotics and antidepressants), can lead to faecal impaction [95]. This may result in overflow incontinence, which can be exacerbated by laxative use [235], which causes liquid stool to seep around the faecal bolus [236]. The presence of an impacted mass will also stimulate the secretion of large volumes of mucus, which will further aggravate the problem. Such overflow leakage has been attributed to a combination of decreased anorectal sensation and reduced anal pressures, possibly secondary to persistent reflex inhibition of internal anal sphincter tone (although this concept has been challenged [237]), which allows liquid stool to escape through the anal canal [238]. Decreased rectal sensitivity and increased rectal compliance may also contribute to faecal retention by decreasing the frequency and intensity of the desire (and hence the motivation) to defecate [96].

Childhood constipation is a common problem, affecting around 9% of children under 18 years [239]. In children without anorectal anomalies, functional faecal retention, because of fear of painful defecation or other reasons, may also result in faecal impaction and encopresis or overflow soiling [25, 145]. Treatment requires disimpaction, and education focused on alleviating phobias and feelings of guilt by reinforcing self-esteem and incorporating disciplined toileting behaviour [25]. Failure to "retrain" such children may result in progressive dilatation of the rectum (megarectum), leading to chronic impaction, and in a proportion, symptoms may progress into adulthood [240, 241].

Although a considerable body of literature is available regarding impaction-related incontinence at both ends of the age spectrum (i.e. paediatrics/adolescents and geriatrics), there is a relative paucity of information in adults that addresses the concept that rectal evacuatory dysfunction may be an independent risk factor for the involuntary loss of bowel contents [59, 242–245] in spite of the fact that faecal incontinence and "constipation" frequently coexist. Passive (overflow) incontinence, or postdefecation leakage, may occur as a consequence of incomplete rectal emptying following defecation, secondary to a "mechanical" (i.e. anatomical, such as large rectocele, intussusception, megarectum etc.) or "functional" (e.g. pelvic floor dyssynergia, poor defecatory dynamics, nonrelaxing pelvic floor etc.) outlet obstruction. As such, comprehension of the normal process of defecation should be considered fundamental to the clinical management of patients with incontinence, utilising techniques such as balloon expulsion or barium or magnetic resonance (MR) proctography.

Contemporary studies of the pathophysiology of faecal seepage in adults also implicate impaired (blunted) rectal sensation (i.e. *hypo*sensitivity [246]) or increased compliance (i.e. a *hypo*tonic rectum [247, 248]), as seen in conditions of megarectum. This results in the loss of a sense of urgency, faecal impaction and overflow incontinence [249] in the absence of an appropriate "compensatory" sphincteric response [250–254]. In normal subjects, conscious contraction of the external anal sphincter occurs in response to rectal distension, thus preventing incontinence of stool during reflex relaxation of the internal anal sphincter (RAIR) [238]. This is crucially dependent on perception of rectal distension [255, 256]. However, the presence of diminished perception of rectal distension will allow faecal material to enter the rectum without conscious recognition, and thus conscious contraction of the external anal sphincter during reflex internal anal sphincter relaxation cannot occur [255, 257]. This results in a reduction in anal canal pressure and allows stool to enter the anal canal, with the potential for passive leakage [250, 258]. Rectal hyposensitivity may also underlie dyssynergic defecation, exacerbating the retention of faeces in the rectum [243, 254].

Furthermore, impaired perception of rectal distension may also leads to a shorter “warning” between entry of stool into the rectum and impending defecation. This “late” recognition of a large faecal bolus in the rectum, or the passage of stool into the upper anal canal, may account for the sudden, and apparently paradoxical, sense of extreme urgency experienced by some patients with rectal hyposensitivity [250, 259].

Rectal Prolapse

Faecal incontinence occurs in approximately two thirds of patients with overt rectal prolapse [145, 260–263] and 30–40% of patients with symptomatic rectal intussusception (covert or internal prolapse) [264–266].

The pathophysiological basis for this incontinence is unclear and likely to be multifactorial. Repeated dilatation of the anal sphincter mechanism, which may occur as a result of the descending prolapse, may contribute to a dysfunctional internal anal sphincter, resulting in reduced anal pressures [264, 267–269]. Commonly, the internal anal sphincter is thickened, distorted or even fragmented on endoanal ultrasound [270]. A reduction in thickness following rectopexy suggests a partially reversible process [271], and this is consistent with the finding that surgical correction of prolapse/intussusception, which decreases trauma to the internal anal sphincter, improves continence, although often without a rise in sphincter pressures [272–274]. Conversely, continued straining at stool over many years may lead to perineal descent and has been proposed as a major aetiological factor for the development of rectal intussusception and prolapse [269, 275]. This may further stretch and damage the pudendal nerves, increasing the chances of faecal incontinence [276–278]. Pudendal neuropathy has been found in both continent and incontinent patients with bowel-wall prolapse [269, 276, 279, 280], but it is less common and less severe in the continent group [279, 280]. However, the exact relationship between bowel-wall descent, pudendal neuropathy and subsequent faecal incontinence remains unclear. Prolapse may also lead to chronic activation of the rectoanal inhibitory function, with the descending bowel wall acting as a space-occupying lesion in the rectal lumen [268, 281, 282]. Other possible mechanisms include reduced rectal capacity and compliance [274], altered rectal sensorimotor function [269], reversal of the anorectal pressure gradient [269] and a decrease in rectosigmoid transit time [283], whereby the presentation of a greater volume of stool to the (possibly dysfunctional) rectum may stress the continence mechanism and contribute to incontinence.

References

1. MacArthur C, Bick DE, Keighley MR (1997) Faecal incontinence after childbirth. Br J Obstet Gynaecol 104:46–50
2. Chaliha C, Kalia V, Stanton SL et al (1999) Antenatal prediction of postpartum urinary and fecal incontinence. Obstet Gynecol 94:689–694
3. MacLennan AH, Taylor AW, Wilson DH et al (2000) The prevalence of pelvic floor disorders and their relationship to gender, age, parity and mode of delivery. BJOG 107:1460–1470
4. MacArthur C, Glazener CM, Wilson PD, et al (2001) Obstetric practice and faecal incontinence three months after delivery. BJOG 108: 678–683
5. Eason E, Labrecque M, Marcoux S et al (2002) Anal incontinence after childbirth. CMAJ 166: 326–330
6. Thorson AG (2002) Anorectal physiology. Surg Clin North Am 82:1115–1123
7. Goldberg RP, Kwon C, Gandhi S et al (1992) Prevalence of anal incontinence among mothers of multiples and analysis of risk factors. Am J Obstet Gynecol 189:1627–1630
8. Kok AL, Voorhorst FJ, Burger CW et al (1992) Urinary and faecal incontinence in community-residing elderly women. Age Ageing 21:211–215
9. Leigh RJ, Turnberg LA (1982) Faecal incontinence: the unvoiced symptom. Lancet 1:1349–1351
10. Norderval S, Nsubuga D, Bjelke C et al (2004) Anal incontinence after obstetric sphincter tears: incidence in a Norwegian county. Acta Obstet Gynecol Scand 83:989–994
11. Davies MC, Creighton SM, Wilcox DT (2004) Long-term outcomes of anorectal malformations. Pediatr Surg Int 20:567–572
12. Levitt MA, Pena A (2005) Outcomes from the correction of anorectal malformations. Curr Opin Pediatr 17:394–401
13. Ong NT, Beasley SW (1991) Long-term continence in patients with high and intermediate anorectal anomalies treated by sacroperineal (Stephens) rectoplasty. J Pediatr Surg 26:44–48

14. Rintala R, Mildh L, Lindahl H (1994) Fecal continence and quality of life for adult patients with an operated high or intermediate anorectal malformation. J Pediatr Surg 29:777–780
15. Rintala RJ, Lindahl H (1995) Is normal bowel function possible after repair of intermediate and high anorectal malformations? J Pediatr Surg 30:491–494
16. Verhoef M, Lurvink M, Barf HA et al (2005) High prevalence of incontinence among young adults with spina bifida: description, prediction and problem perception. Spinal Cord 43:331–340
17. Lemelle JL, Guillemin F, Aubert D et al (2006) A multicentre study of the management of disorders of defecation in patients with spina bifida. Neurogastroenterol Motil 18:123–128
18. Di Lorenzo C (1997) Chronic constipation and fecal incontinence in children with neurological and neuromuscular handicap. J Pediatr Gastroenterol 25(Suppl 1):S37–S39
19. Morera C, Nurko S (2003) Rectal manometry in patients with isolated sacral agenesis. J Pediatr Gastroenterol Nutr 37:47–52
20. Catto-Smith AG, Coffey CM, Nolan TM et al (1995) Fecal incontinence after the surgical treatment of Hirschsprung's disease. J Pediatr 127:954–957
21. Fortuna RS, Weber TS, Trace JF Jr et al (1996) Critical analysis of the operative treatment of Hirschsprung's disease. Arch Surg 131:520–524
22. Heikkenen M, Rintala RJ, Louhima I (1995) Bowel function and quality of life in adult patients with operated Hirschsprung's disease. Pediatr Surg Int 10:342–324
23. Loening-Baucke V (1998) Constipation in children. N Engl J Med 339:1155–1156
24. Baker SS, Liptak GS, Colletti RB et al (1999) Constipation in infants and children: evaluation and treatment. A medical position statement of the North American Society for Pediatric Gastroenterology and Nutrition. J Pediatr Gastroenterol Nutr 29:612–626
25. Di Lorenzo C, Benninga MA (2004) Pathophysiology of pediatric fecal incontinence. Gastroenterology 126(Suppl 1):S33–S40
26. Nakayama H, Jorgensen HS, Pedersen PM et al (1997) Prevalence and risk factors of incontinence after stroke. The Copenhagen Stroke study. Stroke 28:58–62
27. Harari D, Coshall C, Rudd AG et al (2003) New-onset fecal incontinence after stroke: prevalence, natural history, risk factors, and impact. Stroke 34:144–150
28. Ho YH, Goh HS (1995) Anorectal physiological parameters in chronic constipation of unknown aetiology (primary) and of cerebrovascular accidents–a preliminary report. Ann Acad Med 24:367–368
29. Edwards LL, Pfiffer RF, Quigley EM et al (1991) Gastrointestinal symptoms in Parkinson's disease. Mov Disord 6:151–156
30. Mathers SE, Kempster PA, Law PJ et al (1989) Anal sphincter dysfunction in Parkinson's disease. Arch Neurol 46:1061–1064
31. Edwards LL, Quigley EM, Harned RK et al (1994) Characterization of swallowing and defecation in Parkinson's disease. Am J Gastroenterol 89:15–25
32. Ashraf W, Pfeiffer RF, Quigley EM (1994) Anorectal manometry in the assessment of anorectal function in Parkinson's disease: a comparison with chronic idiopathic constipation. Mov Disord 9:655–663
33. Hinds JP, Eidelmann BH, Wald A (1990) Prevalence of bowel dysfunction in multiple sclerosis. A population study. Gastroenterology 98:1538–1542
34. Chia YM, Fowler CJ, Kamm MA et al (1995) Prevalence of bowel dysfunction in patients with multiple sclerosis and bladder dysfunction. J Neurol 242:105–110
35. Haldeman S, Glick M, Bhatia HH et al (1982) Colometry, cystometry, and evoked potentials in multiple sclerosis. Arch Neurol 39:698–701
36. Krogh K, Christensen P, Laurberg S (2001) Colorectal symptoms in patients with neurological disease. Acta Neurol Scand 103:335–343
37. Sun WM, Read NW, Donnelly TC (1990) Anorectal function in incontinent patients with cerebrospinal disease. Gastroenterology 99:1372–1379
38. Talley NJ, Howell S, Jones MP et al (2002) Predictors of turnover of lower gastrointestinal symptoms in diabetes mellitus. Am J Gastroenterol 97:3087–3094
39. Schiller LR, Santa Ana CA, Schmulen AC et al (1982) Pathogenesis of fecal incontinence in diabetes mellitus: evidence of internal-anal-sphincter dysfunction. N Engl J Med 307:1666–1671
40. Camilleri M, Bharucha AE (1996) Gastrointestinal function in neurologic disease. Sem Neurol 16:203–216
41. Nelson RL (2004) Epidemiology of fecal incontinence. Gastroenterology 126:S3–S7
42. Pretlove SJ, Radley S, Toozs-Hobson PM et al (2006) Prevalence of anal incontinence according to age and gender: a systematic review and meta-regression analysis. Int Urogynecol J Pelvic Floor Dysfunct 17:407–417
43. Bannister JJ, Abouzekry L, Read NW (1987) Effect of aging on anorectal function. Gut 28:353–357
44. Swash M, Gray A, Lubowski DZ et al (1988) Ultrastructural changes in internal anal sphincter in neurogenic faecal incontinence. Gut 29:1692–1698
45. Jameson JS, Chia YW, Kamm MA et al (1994) Effect of age, sex and parity on anorectal function. Br J Surg 81:1689–1692
46. Laurberg S, Swash M (1989) Effects of aging on the anorectal sphincters and their innervation. Dis Colon Rectum 32:737–742
47. Ryhammer AM, Laurberg S, Sorensen FH (1997) Effects of age on anal function in normal women. Int J Colorect Dis 12:225–229
48. Bharucha AE, Zinsmeister AR, Locke GR et al (2006) Risk factors for fecal incontinence: a population-based study in women. Am J Gastroenterol 101:1305–1312
49. Rao SS, Holdsworth CD, Read NW (1988) Symptoms and stool patterns in patients with ulcerative colitis. Gut 29:342–345
50. Farthing MJ, Lennard-Jones JE (1978) Sensibility of the rectum to distension and the anorectal distension reflex in ulcerative colitis. Gut 19:64–69
51. Rao SS, Read NW, Davison PA et al (1987) Anorectal sensitivity and responses to rectal distention in patients with ulcerative colitis. Gastroenterology 93:1270–1275
52. Buchmann P, Kolb E, Alexander-Williams J (1981) Pathogenesis of urgency in defaecation in Crohn's disease. Digestion 22:310–316
53. Bassotti G, de Roberto G, Chistolini F et al (2004) Twenty-four-hour manometric study of colonic

propulsive activity in patients with diarrhea due to inflammatory (ulcerative colitis) and non-inflammatory (irritable bowel syndrome) conditions. Int J Colorect Dis 19:493–497
54. Loening-Baucke V, Metcalf AM, Shirazi S (1989) Rectosigmoid motility in patients with quiescent and active ulcerative colitis. Am J Gastroenterol 84:34–39
55. Longstreth GF, Thompson WG, Chey WD et al (2006) Functional bowel disorders. Gastroenterology 130:1480–1491
56. Drossman DA, Sandler RS, Broom CM et al (1986) Urgency and fecal soiling in people with bowel dysfunction. Dig Dis Sci 31:1221–1225
57. Talley NJ, Zinsmeister AR Van Dyke C et al (1991) Epidemiology of colonic symptoms and the irritable bowel syndrome. Gastroenterology 101:927–934
58. Kwan AC, Hu WH, Chan YK et al (2002) Prevalence of irritable bowel syndrome in Hong Kong. J Gastroenterol Hepatol 17:1180–1186
59. Kalantar JS, Howell S, Talley NJ (2002) Prevalence of faecal incontinence and associated risk factors; an underdiagnosed problem in the Australian community? Med J Aust 176:54–57
60. Kellow JE, Azpiroz F, Delvaux M et al (2006) Applied principles of neurogastroenterology: physiology/motility sensation. Gastroenterology 130:1412–1420
61. Horowitz L, Farrar JT (1962) Intraluminal small intestinal pressure in normal patients and in patients with functional gastrointestinal disorders. Gastroenterology 42:455–464
62. Kellow JE, Phillips SF (1987) Altered small bowel motility in irritable bowel syndrome is correlated with symptoms. Gastroenterology 92:1885–1893
63. Stivland T, Camilleri M, Vassallo M et al (1991) Scintigraphic measurement of regional gut transit in idiopathic constipation. Gastroenterology 101:107–115
64. Cann PA, Read NW, Brown C et al (1983) Irritable bowel syndrome. Relationship of disorders in the transit of a single solid meal to symptom patterns. Gut 24:405–411
65. Vassallo M, Camilleri M, Phillips SF et al (1992) Transit through the proximal colon influences stool weight in the irritable bowel syndrome. Gastroenterology 102:102–108
66. Ritchie J (1973) Pain from distension of the pelvic colon by inflating a balloon in the irritable bowel syndrome. Gut 14:125–132
67. Whitehead WE, Engel BT, Schuster MM (1980) Irritable bowel syndrome: physiological and psychological differences between diarrhea-predominant and constipation-predominant patients. Dig Dis Sci 25:404–413
68. Chey WY, Jin HO, Lee MH et al (2001) Colonic motor abnormality in patients with irritable bowel syndrome exhibiting pain and diarrhea. Am J Gastroenterol 96:1499–1505
69. Quigley EMM (2006) Changing face of irritable bowel syndrome. World J Gastroenterol 12:1–5
70. Hogston P (1987) Irritable bowel syndrome as a cause of chronic pain in women attending a gynaecology clinic. Br Med J 294:934–935
71. Prior A, Whorwell PJ (1989) Gynaecological consultation in patients with the irritable bowel syndrome. Gut 30:996–998
72. Parys BT, Haylen B, Hutton JL et al (1989) The effect of simple hysterectomy on vesicourethral function. Br J Urol 64:594–599
73. Taylor T, Smith AN, Fulton PM (1989) Effect of hysterectomy on bowel function. Br Med J 299:300–301
74. Butler-Manuel SA, Buttery LD, A'Hern RP et al (2000) Pelvic nerve plexus trauma at radical hysterectomy and simple hysterectomy: the nerve content of the uterine supporting ligaments. Cancer 89:834–841
75. Mundy AR (1982) An anatomical explanation for bladder dysfunction following rectal and uterine surgery. Br J Urol 54:501–504
76. Symmonds RE, Williams TJ, Lee RA et al (1981) Posthysterectomy enterocele and vaginal vault prolapse. Am J Obstet Gynecol 140:852–859
77. Karasick S, Spettell CM (1997) The role of parity and hysterectomy on the development of pelvic floor abnormalities revealed by defecography. AJR Am J Roentgenol 169:1555–1558
78. Smith AN, Varma JS, Binnie NR et al (1990) Disordered colorectal motility in intractable constipation following hysterectomy. Br J Surg 77:1361–1365
79. Varma JS (1992) Autonomic influences on colorectal motility and pelvic surgery. World J Surg 16:811–819
80. Altman D, Zetterstrom J, Lopez A et al (2004) Effect of hysterectomy on bowel function. Dis Colon Rectum 47:502–509
81. Farouk R, Duthie GS, Lee PW et al (1998) Endosonographic evidence of injury to the internal anal sphincter after low anterior resection: long term follow-up. Dis Colon Rectum 41:888–891
82. Parc R, Tiret E, Frileux P et al (1986) Resection and colo-anal anastomosis with colonic reservoir for rectal carcinoma. Br J Surg 73:139–141
83. Remzi FH, Fazio VW, Gorgun E et al (2005) Quality of life, functional outcome, and complications of coloplasty pouch after anterior resection. Dis Colon Rectum 48:735–743
84. Machado M, Nygren J, Goldman S et al (2005) Functional and physiologic assessment of the colonic reservoir or side-to-end anastomosis after low anterior resection for rectal cancer: a two-year follow-up. Dis Colon Rectum 48:29–36
85. Yo YH, Tan M, Leong AF et al (2000) Ambulatory manometry in patients with colonic J-pouch and straight coloanal anastomoses: randomized, controlled trial. Dis Colon Rectum 43:793–799
86. Furst A, Burghofer K, Hutzel L et al (2002) Neorectal reservoir is not the functional principle of the colonic J-pouch: the volume of a short colonic J-pouch does not differ from a straight coloanal anastomosis. Dis Colon Rectum 45:660–667
87. Putta S, Andreyev HJ (2005) Faecal incontinence: a late side-effect of pelvic radiotherapy. Clin Oncol 17:469–477
88. Varma JS, Smith AN, Busuttil A (1985) Correlation of clinical and manometric abnormalities of rectal function following chronic radiation injury. Br J Surg 72:875–878
89. Pollack J, Holm T, Cedermark B et al (2006) Long-term effect of preoperative radiation therapy on anorectal function. Dis Colon Rectum 49:345–352

90. Lim JF, Tjandra JJ, Hiscocj R et al (2006) Preoperative chemoradiation for rectal cancer caused prolonged pudendal nerve terminal motor latency. Dis Colon Rectum 49:12–19
91. Peeters KC, van de Velde CJ, Leer JW et al (2005) Late side effects of short-course preoperative radiotherapy combined with total mesorectal excision for rectal cancer: increased bowel dysfunction in irradiated patients–a Dutch colorectal cancer group study. J Clin Oncol 23:6199–6206
92. Lunniss PJ, Gladman MA, Hetzer FH et al (2004) Risk factors in acquired faecal incontinence. J R Soc Med 97:111–116
93. Kamm MA (1994) Obstetric damage and faecal incontinence. Lancet 344:730–733
94. Rao SS (2004) Pathophysiology of adult fecal incontinence. Gastroenterology 126(Suppl 1):S14–S22
95. Madoff RD, Parker SC, Varma MG, et al (2004) Faecal incontinence in adults. Lancet 364:621–632
96. Bharucha AE (2003) Fecal incontinence. Gastroenterology 124:1672–1685
97. Sultan AH, Kamm MA, Hudson CN et al (1993) Anal-sphincter disruption during vaginal delivery. N Engl J Med 329:1905–1911
98. Donnelly V, Fynes M, Campbell D et al (1998) Obstetric events leading to anal sphincter damage. Obstet Gynecol 92:955–961
99. Zetterström JP, López A, Anzén B et al (1999) Anal incontinence after vaginal delivery: a prospective study in primiparous women. Br J Obstet Gynaecol 106:324–330
100. Donnelly V, O'Herlihy C, Campbell DM et al (1998) Postpartum fecal incontinence is more common in women with irritable bowel syndrome. Dis Colon Rectum 41:586–589
101. Abramowitz L, Sobhani I, Ganansia R et al (2000) Are sphincter defects the cause of anal incontinence after vaginal delivery? Results of a prospective study. Dis Colon Rectum 43:590–598
102. Pregazzi R, Sartore A, Bortoli P et al (2002) Immediate postpartum perineal examination as a predictor of puerperal pelvic floor dysfunction. Obstet Gynecol 99:581–584
103. Groutz A, Fait G, Lessing JB et al (1999) Incidence and obstetric risk factors of postpartum anal incontinence. Scand J Gastroenterol 34:315–318
104. Signorello LB, Harlow BL, Chekos AK et al (2000) Midline episiotomy and anal incontinence: retrospective cohort study. BMJ 320:86–90
105. Chaliha C, Sultan AH, Bland JM et al (2001) Anal function: effect of pregnancy and delivery. Am J Obstet Gynecol 185:427–432
106. Hannah ME, Hannah WJ, Hodnett ED et al (2002) Outcomes at 3 months after planned cesarean vs planned vaginal delivery for breech presentation at term: the international randomized Term Breech Trial. JAMA 287:1822–1831
107. Sartore A, De Seta F, Maso G et al (2004) The effects of mediolateral episiotomy on pelvic floor function after vaginal delivery. Obstet Gynecol 2004103:669–673
108. Chiarelli P, Murphy B, Cockburn J (2003) Fecal incontinence after high-risk delivery. Obstet Gynecol 102:1299–1305
109. Wang A, Guess M, Connell K et al (2006) Fecal incontinence: a review of prevalence and obstetric risk factors. Int Urogynecol J Pelvic Floor Dysfunct 17:253–260
110. Pollack J, Nordenstam J, Brismar S (2004) Anal incontinence after vaginal delivery: a five-year prospective cohort study. Obstet Gynecol 104:1397–1402
111. Faltin DL, Otero M, Petignat P et al (2006). Women's health 18 years after rupture of the anal sphincter during childbirth: I. Faecal incontinence. Am J Obstet Gynecol 194:1255–1259
112. Fornell EU, Wingren G, Kjolhede P (2004) Factors associated with pelvic floor dysfunction with emphasis on urinary and fecal incontinence and genital prolapse: an epidemiological study. Acta Obstet Gynecol Scand 83:383–389
113. Ryhammer AM, Bek KM, Laurberg S (1995) Multiple vaginal deliveries increase the risk of permanent incontinence of flatus urine in normal premenopausal women. Dis Colon Rectum 38:1206–1209
114. Guise JM, Morris C, Osterweil P et al (2007) Incidence of fecal incontinence after childbirth. Obstet Gynecol 109:281–288
115. Poen AC, Felt-Bersma RJ, Dekker GA et al (1997) Third degree obstetric perineal tears: risk factors and the preventive role of mediolateral episiotomy. Br J Obstet Gynaecol 104:563–566
116. Wood J, Amos L, Rieger N (1999) Third degree anal sphincter tears: risk factors and outcome. Aust N Z J Obstet Gynaecol 38:414–417
117. de Leeuw JW, Struijk PC, Vierhout ME et al (2001) Risk factors for third degree perineal ruptures during delivery. BJOG 108:383–387
118. Jander C, Lyrenas S (2001) Third and fourth degree perineal tears. Predictor factors in a referral hospital. Acta Obstet Gynecol Scand 80:229–234
119. Handa VL, Danielsen BH, Gilbert WM (2001) Obstetric anal sphincter lacerations. Obstet Gynecol 98:225–230
120. Christianson LM, Bovbjerg VE, McDavitt EC (2003) Risk factors for perineal injury during delivery. Am J Obstet Gynecol 189:255–260
121. Gupta N, Kiran TU, Mulik V et al (2003) The incidence, risk factors and obstetric outcome in primigravid women sustaining anal sphincter tears. Acta Obstet Gynecol Scand 82:736–743
122. Williams A (2003) Third-degree perineal tears: risk factors and outcome after primary repair. J Obstet Gynaecol 23:611–614
123. Fynes M, Donnelly V, Behan M et al (1999) Effect of second vaginal delivery on anorectal physiology and faecal continence: a prospective study. Lancet 354:983–986
124. Faltin DL, Boulvain M, Irion O et al (2000) Diagnosis of anal sphincter tears by postpartum endosonography to predict fecal incontinence. Obstet Gynecol 95:643–647
125. Belmonte-Montes C, Hagerman G, Vega-Yepez PA et al (2001) Anal sphincter injury after vaginal delivery in primiparous females. Dis Colon Rectum 44:1244–1248
126. Nazir M, Carlsen E, Nesheim BI (2002) Do occult anal sphincter injuries, vector volume manometry and delivery variables have any predictive value for bowel

symptoms after first time vaginal delivery without third and fourth degree rupture? A prospective study. Acta Obstet Gynecol Scand 81:720–726

127. Pinta TM, Kylanpaa ML, Teramo KA et al (2004) Sphincter rupture and anal incontinence after first vaginal delivery. Acta Obstet Gynecol Scand 83:917–922
128. Damon H, Bretones S, Henry L et al (2005) Long-term consequences of first vaginal delivery-induced anal sphincter defect. Dis Colon Rectum 48:1772–1776
129. Sultan AH, Stanton SL (1997) Occult obstetric trauma and anal incontinence. Eur J Gastroenterol Hepatol 9:423–427
130. Nygaard IE, Rao SS, Dawson JD (1997) Anal incontinence after anal sphincter disruption: a 30-year retrospective cohort study. Obstet Gynecol 89:896–901
131. Fitzpatrick M, O'Herlihy C (2001) The effects of labour and delivery on the pelvic floor. Best Pract Res Clin Obstet Gynaecol 15:63–79
132. Oberwalder M, Dinnewitzer A, Baig MK et al (2004) The association between late-onset fecal incontinence and obstetric anal sphincter defects. Arch Surg 139:429–432
133. Byrd LM, Hobbiss J, Tasker M (2005) Is it possible to predict or prevent third degree tears? Colorectal Dis 7:311–318
134. Combs CA, Robertson PA, Laros RK Jr (1990) Risk factors for third-degree and fourth-degree perineal lacerations in forceps and vacuum deliveries. Am J Obstet Gynecol 163:100–104
135. Richter HE, Brumfield CG, Cliver SP et al (2002) Risk factors associated with anal sphincter tear: a comparison of primiparous patients, vaginal births after cesarean deliveries, and patients with previous vaginal delivery. Am J Obstet Gynecol 187:1194–1198
136. Simhan H, Krohn M, Heine RP (2004) Obstetric rectal injury: risk factors and the role of physician experience. J Matern Fetal Neonatal Med 16:271–274
137. Shiono P, Klebanoff MA, Carey JC (1990) Midline episiotomies: more harm than good? Obstet Gynecol 75:765–770
138. Fenner DE, Genberg B, Brahma P et al (2003) Fecal and urinary incontinence after vaginal delivery with anal sphincter disruption in an obstetrics unit in the United States. Am J Obstet Gynecol 189:1543–1549
139. Fitzgerald MP, Weber AM, Howden N et al (2007) Risk factors for anal sphincter tear during vaginal delivery. Obstet Gynecol 109:29–34
140. Andrews V, Sultan AH, Thakar R et al (2006) Risk factors for obstetric anal sphincter injury: a prospective study. Birth 33:117–122
141. Guendelman S, Thornton D, Gould J et al (2006) Obstetric complications during labor and delivery: assessing ethnic differences in California. Womens Health Issues 16:189–197
142. Helwig JT, Thorp JM Jr, Bowes WA Jr et al (1993) Does midline episiotomy increase the risk of third- and fourth-degree lacerations in operative vaginal deliveries? Obstet Gynecol 82:276–279
143. Lal M, H Mann C, Callender R et al (2003) Does Cesarean delivery prevent anal incontinence? Obstet Gynecol 101:305–312
144. Nelson RL, Westercamp M, Furner SE (2006) A systematic review of the efficacy of Cesarean section in the preservation of anal continence. Dis Colon Rectum 49:1587–1595
145. Kamm MA (1988) Faecal incontinence. BMJ 316: 528–532
146. Law PJ, Kamm MA, Bartram CI (1991) Anal endosonography in the investigation of faecal incontinence. Br J Surg 78:312–314
147. Nielsen MB, Hauge C, Pedersen JF et al (1993) Endosonographic evaluation of patients with anal incontinence: findings and influence on surgical management. AJR Am J Roentgenol 160:771–775
148. Zetterstrom J, Mellgren A, Jensen LL et al (1999) Effect of delivery on anal sphincter morphology and function. Dis Colon Rectum 42:1253–1260
149. Fornell EK, Berg G, Hallbook O et al (1996) Clinical consequences of anal sphincter rupture during vaginal delivery. J Am Coll Surg 183:553–558
150. Rieger N, Schloithe A, Saccone G et al (1997) The effect of a normal vaginal delivery on anal function. Acta Obstet Gynecol Scand 76:769–772
151. Rieger N, Schloithe A, Saccone G et al (1998) A prospective study of anal sphincter injury due to childbirth. Scand J Gastroenterol 33:950–955
152. Lee SJ, Park JW (2000) Follow-up evaluation of the effect of vaginal delivery on the pelvic floor. Dis Colon Rectum 43:1550–1555
153. Willis S, Faridi A, Schelzig S (2002) Childbirth and incontinence: a prospective study on anal sphincter morphology and function before and early after vaginal delivery. Langenbecks Arch Surg 387:101–107
154. Hojberg KE, Hundborg HH, Ryhammer AM (2003) The impact of delivery on anorectal function in women with and women without anal incontinence-a prospective study. Int Urogynecol J Pelvic Floor Dysfunct 14:38–45
155. Fornell EU, Matthiesen L, Sjodahl R (2005) Obstetric anal sphincter injury ten years after: subjective and objective long term effects. BJOG 112:312–316
156. Fynes M, Donnelly VS, O'Connell PR et al (1998) Cesarean delivery and anal sphincter injury. Obstet Gynecol 92:496–500
157. Snooks SJ, Setchell M, Swash M et al (1984) Injury to innervation of pelvic floor sphincter musculature in childbirth. Lancet 2:546–550
158. Snooks SJ, Swash M, Henry MM et al (1986) Risk factors in childbirth causing damage to the pelvic floor innervation. Int J Colorectal Dis 1:20–24
159. Snooks SJ, Swash M, Mathers SE et al (1990) Effect of vaginal delivery on the pelvic floor: a 5-year follow-up. Br J Surg 77:1358–1360
160. Sultan AH, Kamm MA, Hudson CN (1994) Pudendal nerve damage during labour: prospective study before and after childbirth. Br J Obstet Gynaecol 101:22–28
161. Tetzschner T, Sorensen M, Rasmussen OO et al (1995) Pudendal nerve damage increases the risk of fecal incontinence in women with anal sphincter rupture after childbirth. Acta Obstet Gynecol Scand 74:434–440
162. Tetzschner T, Sorensen M, Jonsson L et al (1997) Delivery and pudendal nerve function. Acta Obstet Gynecol Scand 76:324–331
163. Rieger N, Wattchow D (1999) The effect of vaginal

delivery on anal function. Aust N Z J Surg 69:172–177
164. Allen RE, Hosker GL, Smith AR et al (1990) Pelvic floor damage and childbirth: a neurophysiological study. Br J Obstet Gynaecol 97:770–779
165. Zetterstrom J, Lopez A, Holmstrom B et al (2003) Obstetric sphincter tears and anal incontinence: an observational follow-up study. Acta Obstet Gynecol Scand 82:921–928
166. Kiff ES, Barnes PR, Swash M (1984) Evidence of pudendal neuropathy in patients with perineal descent and chronic straining at stool. Gut 25:1279–1282
167. Engel AF, Kamm MA (1994) The acute effect of straining on pelvic floor neurological function. Int J Colorectal Dis 9:8–12
168. Felt-Bersma RJ, van Baren R, Koorevaar M et al (1995) Unsuspected sphincter defects shown by anal endosonography after anorectal surgery. A prospective study. Dis Colon Rectum 38:249–253
169. Eisenhammer S (1951) The surgical correction of chronic internal anal (sphincteric) contracture. S Afr Med J 25:486–489
170. Notaras MJ (1969) Lateral subcutaneous sphincterotomy for anal fissure–a new technique. Proc R Soc Med 62:713
171. Khubchandani IT, Reed JF (1989) Sequelae of internal sphincterotomy for chronic fissure in ano. Br J Surg 76:431–434
172. Pernikoff BJ, Eisenstat TE, Rubin RJ et al (1994) Reappraisal of partial lateral internal sphincterotomy. Dis Colon Rectum 37:1291–1295
173. Richard CS, Gregoire R, Plewes EA et al (2000). Internal sphincterotomy is superior to topical nitroglycerin in the treatment of chronic anal fissure: results of a randomized, controlled trial by the Canadian Colorectal Surgical Trials Group. Dis Colon Rectum 43:1048–1057
174. Menteﬂ BB, Tezcaner T, Yilmaz U et al (2006) Results of lateral internal sphincterotomy for chronic anal fissure with particular reference to quality of life. Dis Colon Rectum 49:1045–1051
175. Garcia-Aguilar J, Belmonte C, Wong WD et al (1996) Open vs closed sphincterotomy for chronic anal fissure: long-term results. Dis Colon Rectum 39:440–443
176. Nyam DC, Pemberton JH (1999) Long-term results of lateral internal sphincterotomy for chronic anal fissure with particular reference to incidence of fecal incontinence. Dis Colon Rectum 42:1306–1310
177. Littlejohn DR, Newstead GL (1997) Tailored lateral sphincterotomy for anal fissure. Dis Colon Rectum 40:1439–1442
178. Usatoff V, Polglase AL (1995) The longer term results of internal anal sphincterotomy for anal fissure. Aust N Z J Surg 65:576–578
179. Rotholtz NA, Bun M, Mauri MV et al (2005) Long-term assessment of fecal incontinence after lateral internal sphincterotomy. Tech Coloproctol 9:115–118
180. Casillas S, Hull TL, Zutshi M et al (2005) Incontinence after a lateral internal sphincterotomy: are we underestimating it? Dis Colon Rectum 48:1193–1199
181. Lindsey I, Jones OM, Smilgin-Humphreys MM et al (2004) Patterns of fecal incontinence after anal surgery. Dis Colon Rectum 47:1643–1649
182. Sultan AH, Kamm MA, Nicholls RJ et al (1994) Prospective study of the extent of internal anal sphincter division during lateral sphincterotomy. Dis Colon Rectum 37:1031–1033
183. Farouk R, Monson JR, Duthie GS (1997) Technical failure of lateral sphincterotomy for the treatment of chronic anal fissure: a study using endoanal ultrasonography. Br J Surg 84:84–85
184. Tjandra JJ, Han WR, Ooi BS et al (2001) Faecal incontinence after lateral internal sphincterotomy is often associated with coexisting occult sphincter defects: a study using endoanal ultrasonography. ANZ J Surg 71:598–602
185. Zbar AP, Beer-Gabel M, Chiappa AC et al (2001) Fecal incontinence after minor anorectal surgery. Dis Colon Rectum 44:1610–1619
186. Lord PH (1968) A new regime for the treatment of haemorrhoids. Proc R Soc Med 61:935–936
187. Steele SR, Madoff RD (2006) Systematic review: the treatment of anal fissure. Aliment Pharmacol Ther 24:247–257
188. McCaffrey J (1975) Lord treatment of haemorrhoids. Four-year follow-up of fifty patients. Lancet 1:133–134
189. MacDonald A, Smith A, McNeill AD et al (1992) Manual dilatation of the anus. Br J Surg 79:1381–1382
190. Oliver DW, Booth MW, Kernick VF et al (1998) Patient satisfaction and symptom relief after anal dilatation. Int J Colorectal Dis 13:228–231
191. Konsten J, Baeten CG (2000) Hemorrhoidectomy vs. Lord's method: 17-year follow-up of a prospective, randomized trial. Dis Colon Rectum 43:503–536
192. Saad AM, Omer A (1992) Surgical treatment of chronic fissure-in-ano: a prospective randomised study. East Afr Med J 69:613–615
193. Nielsen MB, Rasmussen OO, Pedersen JF et al (1993) Risk of sphincter damage and anal incontinence after anal dilatation for fissure-in-ano. An endosonographic study. Dis Colon Rectum 36:677–680
194. Lindsey I, Jones OM, Cunningham C et al (2004) Chronic anal fissure. Br J Surg 91:270–279
195. Jensen SL, Lund F, Nielsen OV et al (1984) Lateral subcutaneous sphincterotomy versus anal dilatation in the treatment of fissure in ano in outpatients: a prospective randomised study. Br Med J 289:528–530
196. Nelson R (2002) Operative procedures for fissure in ano. Cochrane Database Syst Rev 2:CD002199
197. Snooks S, Henry MM, Swash M (1984) Faecal incontinence after anal dilatation. Br J Surg 71:617–618
198. Speakman CT, Burnett SJ, Kamm MA et al (1991) Sphincter injury after anal dilatation demonstrated by anal endosonography. Br J Surg 78:1429–1430
199. Hammond TM, Knowles CH, Porrett T et al (2006) The Snug Seton: short and medium term results of slow fistulotomy for idiopathic anal fistulae. Colorectal Dis 8:328–337
200. Rosa G, Lolli P, Piccinelli D et al (2006) Fistula in ano: anatomoclinical aspects, surgical therapy and results in 844 patients. Tech Coloproctol 10:215–221
201. Sygut A, Zajdel R, Kedzia-Budziewska R et al (2007) Late results of treatment of anal fistulas. Colorectal Dis 9:151–158
202. Sainio P, Husa A (1985) Fistula-in-ano. Clinical features and long-term results of surgery in 199 adults. Acta Chir Scand 151:169–176

203. van Tets WF, Kuijpers HC (1994) Continence disorders after anal fistulotomy. Dis Colon Rectum 37:1194–1197
204. Garcia-Aguilar J, Belmonte C, Wong WD et al (1996) Anal fistula surgery. Factors associated with recurrence and incontinence. Dis Colon Rectum 39:723–729
205. Williams JG, MacLeod CA, Rothenberger DA et al (1991) Seton treatment of high anal fistulae. Br J Surg 78:1159–1161
206. Lunniss PJ, Kamm MA, Phillips RK (1994) Factors affecting continence after surgery for anal fistula. Br J Surg 81:1382–1385
207. Graf W, Pahlman L, Ejerblad S (1995) Functional results after seton treatment of high transsphincteric anal fistulas. Eur J Surg 161:289–291
208. Hamalainen KP, Sainio AP (1997) Cutting seton for anal fistulas: high risk of minor control defects. Dis Colon Rectum 40:1443–1446
209. Pescatori M, Ayabaca S, Caputo D (2004) Can anal manometry predict anal incontinence after fistulectomy in males? Colorectal Dis 6:97–102
210. Belliveau P, Thomson JP, Parks AG. Fistula-in-ano (1983) A manometric study. Dis Colon Rectum 26:152–154
211. Sainio P (1985) A manometric study of anorectal function after surgery for anal fistula, with special reference to incontinence. Acta Chir Scand 151:695–700
212. Chang SC, Lin JK (2003) Change in anal continence after surgery for intersphincteral anal fistula: a functional and manometric study. Int J Colorectal Dis 18:111–115
213. Gibbons CP, Trowbridge EA, Bannister JJ et al (1986) Role of anal cushions in maintaining continence. Lancet 1:886–888
214. Lestar B, Penninckx F, Kerrimans R (1989) The composition of the anal basal pressure. An in vivo and in vitro study in man. Int J Colorect Dis 4:118–122
215. Rao SS (2004) Diagnosis and management of fecal incontinence. Am J Gastroenterol 99:1585–1604
216. Rasmussen OØ (1994) Anorectal function. Dis Colon Rectum 37:386–403
217. Read MG, Read NW, Haynes WG et al (1982) A prospective study of the effect of haemorrhoidectomy on sphincter function and faecal continence. Br J Surg 69:396–398
218. Murie JA, Sim AJ, Mackenzie I (1982) Rubber band ligation versus haemorrhoidectomy for prolapsing haemorrhoids: a long term prospective clinical trial. Br J Surg 69:536–538
219. Johannsson HO, Pahlman L, Graf W (2006) Randomized clinical trial of the effects on anal function of Milligan-Morgan versus Ferguson haemorrhoidectomy. Br J Surg 93:1208–1214
220. Milligan ETC, Morgan CN, Jones LE et al (1937) Surgical anatomy of the anal canal and operative treatment of hemorrhoids. Lancet 2:1119–1124
221. Ferguson JA, Heaton JR (1959) Closed hemorrhoidectomy. Dis Colon Rectum 2:176–179
222. Parks AG (1956) The surgical treatment of haemorrhoids. Br J Surg 43:337–351
223. Longo A (1998) Treatment of haemorrhoids disease by reduction of mucosa and haemorrhoidal prolapse with circular suturing device: a new procedure. In: Proceedings of the 6th World Congress of Endoscopic Surgery, Rome, pp 777–784
224. McConnell JC, Khubchandani IT (1983) Long-term follow-up of closed hemorrhoidectomy. Dis Colon Rectum 26:797–799
225. Ravo B, Amato A, Bianco V et al (2002) Complications after stapled hemorrhoidectomy: can they be prevented? Tech Coloproctol 6:83–88
226. Guenin MO, Rosenthal R, Kern B et al (2005) Ferguson hemorrhoidectomy: long-term results and patient satisfaction after Ferguson's hemorrhoidectomy. Dis Colon Rectum 48:1523–1527
227. Lan P, Wu X, Zhou X et al (2006) The safety and efficacy of stapled hemorrhoidectomy in the treatment of hemorrhoids: a systematic review and meta-analysis of ten randomized control trials. Int J Colorectal Dis 21:172–178
228. Roe AM, Bartolo DC, Vellacott KD et al (1987) Submucosal versus ligation excision haemorrhoidectomy: a comparison of anal sensation, anal sphincter manometry and postoperative pain and function. Br J Surg 74:948–951
229. Altomare DF, Rinaldi M, Sallustio PL et al (2001) Long-term effects of stapled haemorrhoidectomy on internal anal function and sensitivity. Br J Surg 88:1487–1491
230. Johannsson HO, Graf W, Pahlman L (2002) Long-term results of haemorrhoidectomy. Eur J Surg 168:485–489
231. Abbasakoor F, Nelson M, Beynon J et al (1998) Anal endosonography in patients with anorectal symptoms after haemorrhoidectomy. Br J Surg 85:1522–1524
232. Jorge JM, Wexner SD (1993) Etiology and management of fecal incontinence. Dis Colon Rectum 36:77–97
233. Tobin GW, Brocklehurst JC (1986) Faecal incontinence in residential homes for the elderly: prevalence, aetiology and management. Age Ageing 15:41–46
234. Wald A (2005) Faecal incontinence in the elderly: epidemiology and management. Drugs Aging 22:131–139
235. Cooper ZR, Rose S (2000) Fecal incontinence: a clinical approach. Mt Sinai J Med 67:96–105
236. Read NW, Abouzekry L, Read MG et al (1985) Anorectal function in elderly patients with fecal impaction. Gastroenterology 89:959–966
237. Read NW, Abouzekry L (1986) Why do patients with faecal impaction have faecal incontinence. Gut 27:283–287
238. Loening-Baucke VA, Cruikshank BM (1986) Abnormal defecation dynamics in chronically constipated children with encopresis. J Pediatr 108:562–566
239. van den Berg MM, Benninga MA et al (2006) Epidemiology of childhood constipation: a systematic review. Am J Gastroenterol 101:2401–2409
240. van Ginkel R, Reitsma JB, Buller HA et al (2003) Childhood constipation: longitudinal follow-up beyond puberty. Gastroenterology 125:357–363
241. Voskuijl WP, Reitsma JB, van Ginkel R et al (2006) Longitudinal follow-up of children with functional nonretentive fecal incontinence. Clin Gastroenterol Hepatol 4:67–72
242. Rex DK, Lappas JC (1992) Combined anorectal manometry and defecography in 50 consecutive adults with fecal incontinence. Dis Colon Rectum 35:1040–1045
243. Rao SS, Ozturk R, Stessman M (2004) Investigation of

the pathophysiology of fecal seepage. Am J Gastroenterol 99:2204–2209
244. Scarlett Y (2004) Medical management of fecal incontinence. Gastroenterology 126(Suppl 1):S55–S63
245. Shatari T, Hayes J, Pretlove S et al (2005) Importance of evacuatory disturbance in evaluation of faecal incontinence after third degree obstetric tear. Colorectal Dis 7:18–21
246. Gladman MA, Lunniss PJ, Scott SM et al (2006) Rectal hyposensitivity. Am J Gastroenterol 101:1140–1151
247. Siproudhis L, Bellissant E, Juguet F et al (1999) Perception of and adaptation to rectal isobaric distension in patients with faecal incontinence. Gut 44:687–692
248. Felt-Bersma RJ, Sloots CE, Poen AC et al (2000) Rectal compliance as a routine measurement: extreme volumes have direct clinical impact and normal volumes exclude rectum as a problem. Dis Colon Rectum 43:1732–1738
249. Crowell MD (2004) Pathogenesis of slow transit and pelvic floor dysfunction: from bench to bedside. Rev Gastroenterol Disord 4(Suppl 2):S17–S27
250. Buser WD, Miner PB Jr (1986) Delayed rectal sensation with fecal incontinence. Successful treatment using anorectal manometry. Gastroenterology 91:1186–1191
251. Lubowski DZ, Nicholls RJ (1988) Faecal incontinence associated with reduced pelvic sensation. Br J Surg 75:1086–1088
252. Hoffmann BA, Timmcke AE, Gathright JB Jr et al (1995) Fecal seepage and soiling: a problem of rectal sensation. Dis Colon Rectum 38:746–748
253. Gladman MA, Scott SM, Chan CL et al (2003) Rectal hyposensitivity: prevalence and clinical impact in patients with intractable constipation and fecal incontinence. Dis Colon Rectum 46:238–246
254. Crowell MD, Lacy BE, Schettler VA et al (2004) Subtypes of anal incontinence associated with bowel dysfunction: clinical, physiologic, and psychosocial characterization. Dis Colon Rectum 47:1627–1635
255. Sun WM, Read NW, Miner PB (1990) Relation between rectal sensation and anal function in normal subjects and patients with faecal incontinence. Gut 31:1056–1061
256. Diamant NE, Kamm MA, Wald A et al (1999) AGA technical review on anorectal testing techniques. Gastroenterology 116:735–760
257. Wald A, Tunuguntla AK (1984) Anorectal sensorimotor dysfunction in fecal incontinence and diabetes mellitus. Modification with biofeedback therapy. N Engl J Med 310:1282–1287
258. Sun WM, Donnelly TC, Read NW (1992) Utility of a combined test of anorectal manometry, electromyography, and sensation in determining the mechanism of 'idiopathic' faecal incontinence. Gut 33:807–813
259. Smith AN, Binnie NR (1991) Neurological disorders. In: Kumar D, Waldron DJ, Williams NS, eds. Clinical measurement in coloproctology. Springer-Verlag, London, pp 124–139
260. Broden G, Dolk A, Holmstrom B (1988) Recovery of the internal anal sphincter following rectopexy: a possible explanation for continence improvement. Int J Colorectal Dis 3:23–28
261. Williams JG, Wong WD, Jensen L et al (1991) Incontinence and rectal prolapse: a prospective manometric study. Dis Colon Rectum 34:209–216
262. Farouk R, Duthie GS (1998) Rectal prolapse and rectal invagination. Eur J Surg 164:323–332
263. Kairaluoma MV, Kellokumpu IH (2005) Epidemiologic aspects of complete rectal prolapse. Scand J Surg 94:207–210
264. Ihre T, Seligson U (1975) Intussusception of the rectum-internal procidentia: treatment and results in 90 patients. Dis Colon Rectum 18:391–396
265. Johansson C, Ihrs T, Ahlback SO (1985) Disturbances in the defecation mechanism with special reference to intussusception of the rectum (internal procidentia). Dis Colon Rectum 27:435–441
266. Felt-Bersma RJ, Cuesta MA (2001) Rectal prolapse, rectal intussusception, rectocele, and solitary rectal ulcer syndrome. Gastroenterol Clin North Am 30:199–222
267. Frenckner B, Ihre T (1976) Function of the anal sphincters in patients with intussusception of the rectum. Gut 17:147–151
268. Mackle EJ, Parks TG (1986) The pathogenesis and pathophysiology of rectal prolapse and solitary rectal ulcer syndrome. Clin Gastroenterol 15:985–1002
269. Sun WM, Read NW, Donnelly TC et al (1989) A common pathophysiology for full thickness rectal prolapse, anterior mucosal prolapse and solitary rectal ulcer. Br J Surg 76:290–295
270. Dvorkin LS, Chan CL, Knowles CH et al (2004) Anal sphincter morphology in patients with full-thickness rectal prolapse. Dis Colon Rectum 47:198–203
271. Poen AC, de Brauw M, Felt-Bersma RJ et al (1996) Laparoscopic rectopexy for complete rectal prolapse. Clinical outcome and anorectal function tests. Surg Endosc 10:904–908
272. Scaglia M, Fasth S, Hallgren T et al (1994) Abdominal rectopexy for rectal prolapse. Influence of surgical technique on functional outcome. Dis Colon Rectum 37:805–813
273. Schultz I, Mellgren A, Dolk A et al (1996) Continence is improved after the Ripstein rectopexy. Different mechanisms in rectal prolapse and rectal intussusception? Dis Colon Rectum 39:300–306
274. Lazorthes F, Gamagami R, Cabarrot P et al (1998) Is rectal intussusception a cause of idiopathic incontinence? Dis Colon Rectum 41:602–605
275. Porter NH (1962) A physiological study of the pelvic floor in rectal prolapse. Ann R Coll Surg Engl 31:379–404
276. Parks AG, Swash M, Urich H (1977) Sphincter denervation in anorectal incontinence and rectal prolapse. Gut 18:656–665
277. Jones PN, Lubowski DZ, Swash M et al (1987) Relation between perineal descent and pudendal nerve damage in idiopathic faecal incontinence. Int J Colorectal Dis 2:93–95
278. Lubowski DZ, Swash M, Nicholls RJ et al (1988) Increase in pudendal nerve terminal motor latency with defaecation straining. Br J Surg 75:1095–1097
279. Neill ME, Parks AG, Swash M (1981) Physiological studies of the anal sphincter musculature in faecal incontinence and rectal prolapse. Br J Surg 68:531–536
280. Roig JV, Buch E, Alos R et al (1998) Anorectal function

in patients with complete rectal prolapse. Differences between continent and incontinent individuals. Rev Esp Enferm Dig 90:794–805

281. Duthie GS, Bartolo DC (1992) Abdominal rectopexy for rectal prolapse: a comparison of techniques. Br J Surg 79:107–113

282. Farouk R, Duthie GS, MacGregor AB et al (1994) Rectoanal inhibition and incontinence in patients with rectal prolapse. Br J Surg 81:743–746

283. Prokesch RW, Breitenseher MJ, Kettenbach J et al (1999) Assessment of chronic constipation: colon transit time versus defecography. Eur J Radiol 32:197–203

Psychological Aspects of Faecal Incontinence

5

Julian M. Stern

Introduction: the Individual Behind the Diagnosis

There are many routes to becoming a patient with faecal incontinence (FI), many aetiologies of the disorder, and many personal histories. The "meaning" of the FI will be different for each patient, and his or her way of managing it will depend not only on aetiology but also on a number of personal, social and medical factors. Is the FI secondary to a medical or surgical mishap, or is it the by product of a life-saving surgical resection, an "act of God", or an "act of man"? Has the FI been with the patient since childhood, and has he or she developed coping strategies; or is it of recent onset and as yet "new", foreign and unmanageable? What medical support is available to the patient? What emotional support–from family, partner, friends and work associates–is available? Is the partner supportive, or resentful and disgusted? What habitual defence mechanisms do, the patient use in order to deal with adversity, and are these mechanisms overall successful or counterproductive?

These are but a few questions we need to ask each time a patient with FI presents in the clinic. In other words, beyond the generalisations applying to "patients" with FI lie individual men and women, boys and girls, each with his or her own personal, family, medical, psychological and social histories. What applies to one patient or what works for a particular patient may not apply to or work for another.

Development of Bladder and Bowel Continence

Development of bladder and bowel continence is intimately tied up with the development of the child and his or her role as a competent human being. Freud wrote about the power, pride and control of the little prince on the potty: "His Majesty the Child" [1]. The development of continence in a child is an important developmental step and is praised and rewarded throughout cultures. A crucial part of the child's development is the development of a sense of self and the boundaries between "me" and "not me". Children learn that defecating in the wrong place (pants), at the wrong time or in public is punished or is the cause of humiliation or mockery, and that there is pervasive disapproval of incontinence. Even the word incontinence is linked with loss or lack of control, with phrases in common parlance such as "emotional incontinence" or "verbal incontinence". Very seldom, or perhaps never, is incontinence of any sort seen as having any positive connotations. As we grow older, the pleasurable sensations of defecation are increasingly kept private [2–4]. Both in the personal realm and in the social realm, defecation and faeces have become private and imbued with shame and embarrassment [5–9]. Incontinence is associated with negative images–of the mentally unwell, the learning disabled, or demented elderly patients.

We also know that secondary enuresis or encopresis, i.e. the development of enuresis or encopresis after the achievement of continence, is often associated with emotional or physical trauma in childhood. So it should not surprise us that even when there is an obvious physical aetiology for FI, this is sometimes exacerbated by psychological factors and can be (at least partially) ameliorated by treatments that address the patient's psychology.

Stigma and Quality of Life

People with FI have been found to live in a restricted world, often describing it as being similar to imprisonment. The limits to their world are often dictated by access to toilets, the need to carry a change of clothing with them at all times, and attempts to conceal the problem from family and friends alike.

There are few studies of people's experiences of living with FI, but one study of teenagers with FI [10] found that the powerful social rules associated with this area of life mean that families of teenagers with FI faced public distaste, embarrassment, ridicule, general ignorance and little opportunity for discussion. A community-based research programme [11] explored the feelings of exclusion secondary to FI. This study ran over the course of 5 years and involved a group of women suffering from multiple sclerosis (MS). Some of the main concerns in this group were in managing double incontinence, the effects of MS on sexuality and sexual relationships, and trying to live well despite their chronic illness. The shared group experience gave them the freedom to talk openly about sex and incontinence, subjects about which they had previously felt compelled to be silent. Norton and Chelvanayagam [12] ran two focus groups at St. Mark's Hospital in the UK to develop a research questionnaire titled "Effects of Bowel Leakage". For many participants, this was the first time they had ever spoken openly about their FI, and it was found to be mutually supportive to be able to speak openly to peers about the ever-present stress and risk of potential humiliation. As with Australian women [11], access to toilets and sexual relationships were cited as issues of concern. However, what came through was evidence of the extent to which all aspects of life were affected–skin care, shopping, food, employment, travel, appearance and socialising, to name a few. Additional groups have been conducted at St. Mark's for patients with FI [13]. These groups have shown that common themes include "symptom checking" within the group; envying people with normal continence; sporadic anger towards the medical profession (as well as gratitude); problems with body image, sexuality and sexual functioning; as well as more complex intragroup dynamics, such as envy, rivalry and resentment.

The relationship between FI and its impact on quality of life (QOL) had been studied in the clinic but not in the community until the study by Bharucha et al. [14]. In that study, 23% of the subjects with FI reported that the symptom had a moderate to severe impact on one or more domains of QOL. This figure is similar to the proportion of subjects (32%) who reported that FI had "a lot of impact" on QOL in a UK-based study [15]. The impact on QOL was clearly related to severity of FI. Thus, 35% of patients with moderate FI and 82% with severe FI reported a moderate to severe impact on QOL [14].

The stigma involved accounts for the startling finding that only 10% of women with FI had discussed the symptom with a physician in the past year. Whitehead [16], in an editorial accompanying the study by Bharucha et al. [14], described this finding as "astonishing", especially as the patients with milder symptoms who are least likely to present to their physicians are most likely to be helped by conservative measures. Whitehead wrote: "There is... speculation that patients may be too embarrassed or they may be too sceptical that anything can be done about it" (p. 6). He suggested that researchers need to investigate why patients with FI do not report this symptom to their physicians and that there is a need for the development of public education methods to address this issue.

Sexuality

Little research has been performed on the effects of bowel problems and FI on psychosexual functioning in women. Trachter et al. [17] wrote whilst describing irritable bowel syndrome (IBS): "While there is an abundance of research addressing the medical aspects of irritable bowel disease, the psychosexual impact of these diseases is usually not targeted for investigation" (p. 413). In recognition of this, Collings and Norton [18] conducted a study to explore the psychosocial and psychosexual aspects of women living with FI. This was a small, exploratory study using a semistructured interview format. The participants reported a range of psychosexual issues, including current lack of arousal or desire and abstinence. Unexpectedly to the researchers, this was not a uniform problem, and seven of the 20 participants said it was not really a problem unless FI occurred during sexual contact.

Depression, Shame and Isolation

In the study by Collings and Norton [18], shame and embarrassment were common, and depression, stress, isolation, secrecy, poor self-image and sexual avoidance or aversion were also reported. These narrative-based findings tie in well with results from other studies.

Amongst adolescents with FI, psychosocial impairment was significant on the Child Assessment Schedule, the Child Behaviour Checklist and the Youth Self Report [19]. In a study of community-dwelling adults, FI was found to have a marked negative effect on sexuality and job function and in some cases led to near total social isolation as a result of embarrassment.

Fisher et al. [20] used the Hospital Anxiety and Depression Scale (HADS) on patients with FI. They found that patients who had unsuccessful surgical intervention had significantly higher scores than did subjects with FI who had successful surgical outcomes. This finding mirrors several investigations in the urinary incontinence literature in which patients showed elevated levels of distress when treatment for incontinence was unsuccessful and no longer showed such elevations when treatment was successful

[21–25]. Additional associations exist between FI and anxiety, a fear of going out (which needs to be distinguished from the more traditional psychiatric syndromes of agoraphobia/panic in the absence of FI), poor sleep (especially in those patients who suffer from nocturnal FI) and in some cases, the use of alcohol, and drugs such as hypnotics or illicit drugs.

Coping mechanisms identified by 20 patients with FI in the study by Collings and Norton [18] included practical and psychological measures, such as: restricting activity (five), knowing the location of toilets when out (five), care of diet or fasting (three), separate bedrooms (three), wearing pads (five), denial (five), counselling (five) and turning to religion (one).

Psychological Assessment of the Patient with FI

Psychological assessment of the patient with FI requires a confidential setting that gives the patient a sense of being respected, carefully attended to and not rushed. In our experience at St. Mark's Hospital, it is helpful if the patient recognises he or she is being seen by a mental health professional associated with a gastroenterology team who has an interest in and empathy for such problems and is aware of the shame, embarrassment and fear experienced by many patients with FI. Patients are very sensitive to the reactions of others to their FI and may (correctly in some cases) fear that the mental health professional will be disgusted by the FI, just as other members of the public may be (in fantasy or reality).

The initial moments in the assessment may involve understanding something of the FI–its origins, its aetiology and the impact on the various spheres of the patient's life (family, friends, work associates, occupation, sex, leisure, travel etc.). Usually, the patient is relieved to be able to talk about it and sometimes will become tearful or very angry, especially when there is a grievance (justified or unjustified) against a surgeon, physician, nurse or hospital. It is always important from the beginning to look for features of depressed mood as well as resentment, anger or the inability to express anger. In some cases, there is a manic attitude, which incorporates denial of the anguish involved, denial of the losses as well as pain and stigma.

It is important to take a full personal and family history, understanding something of the main relationships and attachment figures in the patient's past and present, as well as an educational and occupational history. It is crucial to understand aspects of the patient's social and psychosexual functioning, both pre- and post-FI [25, 26]. A medical, psychiatric and drug and/or alcohol history as well as some understanding of the patient's present circumstances are also required. The patient's own personality structure and habitual way of coping and dealing with difficulties and interpersonal relationships will crucially colour his or her "relationship" to and mode of coping with the FI.

In order to fully understand the impact of the FI and its meaning to the individual patient, one must also look for issues of shame, guilt and stigma. Is there any sense that the patient feels he or she is to blame for the FI? Does he or she "deserve it"? Is there any secondary gain involved? Are there any symptoms or behaviours that might worsen the FI, such as an unhelpful diet or any self-destructive behaviour? (For a similar approach to patients, see Stern 2003a and b [27, 28], and with particular reference to parenteral nutrition, see Stern 2006 [29]).

Other features of the assessment will include a brief assessment of the patient's cognitive functioning and a mental-state examination to assess the presence of a formal psychiatric condition. This assessment requires expertise, patience, empathy and time.

Management

Following the assessment described above, management strategies can be devised. This depends not only on the patient's psychological state but also on the availability of treatments in each particular case. For some patients, formal psychiatric management is required, especially if there is severe depression (or an anxiety disorder) that might benefit from pharmacotherapy. Whether or not pharmacotherapy is indicated, it is almost invariably helpful for the patient if there is also some psychological treatment available. Psychological treatment can take many forms, ranging from supportive counselling to cognitive behavioural therapy (CBT) or in-depth psychoanalytic psychotherapy [30, 31]. Treatment may be individual or in a group setting, and we recently described both group therapy and psychoeducational groups for patients with FI [13]. As shown below, some of the main themes from a brief psychotherapy group for women with FI are similar to the main themes from a psychoeducational group for women with FI:

Main themes from psychotherapy group meetings for women with FI

- Symptom checking
- Disclosure of bowel and physical symptoms
- Experiences of health services
- Litigation
- Loss
- Sexual functioning
- Disability and hidden disability
- Employment

Main themes from psychoeducational group meetings for women with FI

- Disclosure of bowel symptoms
- Seeking help and treatment
- Availability of and access to toilets
- Hidden disability
- Psychological aspects

Our experience in these group settings was that not only do patients feel more empowered following group treatment, they also on occasion report a lessening of the severity of their symptoms, indicating a super-added psychogenic component to at least some of the severity of the symptomatology.

Biofeedback has also been proven to have a beneficial effect on patients with FI [32, 33] and is discussed elsewhere in this volume. One should not underemphasise the beneficial effects of the nurse–patient relationship in the biofeedback therapy, one that provides the patient not only with the specific techniques taught in the biofeedback sessions, but crucially, a safe place in which to talk to an empathetic confidante. The similarities between this and the importance of the so-called "non-specific factors" in psychotherapy are obvious [34].

Whilst the main focus so far in this chapter has been on the patients' psychological needs, we should not forget the needs of two other groups–family members, and professionals looking after these patients. The impact on the family, spouse and children can be immense, and support–be it through a social worker, family therapist or groups for family members–should be considered and made available where appropriate. Professionals–for example, specialist nurses on the wards or in the community–caring for these patients have their own needs, too. The impact of dealing with the incontinent patient cannot be underestimated, and nurses (as with all of us!) have their own responses to the reality of FI. None of us are immune from emotions ranging from disgust to empathy, irritation to overidentification, and sadness to reparative wishes. With this in mind, at St. Mark's Hospital, we have developed programmes to support specialist coloproctology nurses deal with the impact of their work on their own psyches, addressing issues such as their own feelings (countertransference) [29, 35, 36], as well as providing all members of the multidisciplinary team with a weekly forum in which to discuss problematic patients or patient–staff interactions. This "care of the staff" is crucial in allowing staff members to work productively and empathetically and to minimise the risk of staff "burnout".

Conclusion

What I have proposed in this chapter is a psychological approach to the patient with FI, recognising that, for each patient, his or her FI will have a very individual, unique meaning based on that person's history, relationships and psychological state. Assessment of the patient's psychological needs is a time-consuming but rewarding experience, and patients can be helped by a variety of means to feel less alone, less stigmatised and less disempowered. Medical staff members, too, can benefit from a forum in which these issues can be discussed. If these psychological factors are denied, they may appear to have gone away, but for the patient and for staff members, this disappearance is illusory.

References

1. Freud S (1914) On narcissism: an introduction. In: Strachey J (ed and trans) The standard edition of the complete psychological works of Sigmund Freud, vol. 14. Hogarth Press, London, pp 73–102
2. Abraham K (1920) The narcissistic evaluation of excretory processes in dreams and neuroses. In: Selected papers of Karl Abraham. Hogarth Press, London
3. Abraham K (1921) Contributions to the theory of the anal character. In: Selected papers of Karl Abraham. Hogarth Press, London
4. Freud S (1908) Character and anal erotism. In: Strachey J (ed and trans). The standard edition of the complete psychological works of Sigmund Freud. Hogarth Press, London
5. Elias N (1978) The History of manners: The civilizing process. New York: Pantheon books
6. Garcia JA, Crocker J, Wyman JF (2005) Breaking the cycle of stigmatisation. J Wound Ostomy Continence Nurs 32(1):38–52
7. Joachim G, Acorn S (2000) Stigma of visible and invisible chronic conditions. J Adv Nurs 32(1):243–248
8. White C (1997) Living with a stoma. Sheldon Press, London
9. Whorton JC (2000) Inner hygiene: constipation and the pursuit of health in modern society. Oxford University Press, New York
10. Cavet J (1998) People don't understand: children, young people and their families living with a hidden disability. National Children's Bureau, London
11. Koch T, Selim P, Kralik D (2002) Enhancing lives through the development of a community-based participatory action research program. J Clin Nurs 11 (2):109–117
12. Norton C, Chelvanayagam S (2004) Bowel continence nursing. Beaconsfield Publishers, Beaconsfield
13. Chelvanayagam S, Stern JM (2007) Using therapeutic groups to support women with faecal incontinence? Br J Nurs 16:214–218
14. Bharucha A, Zinsmeister A, Locke R et al (2005) Prevalence and burden of fecal incontinence: a population-based study in women. Gastroenterology 129:42–49
15. Perry S, Shaw C, McGrother C et al (2002) The prevalence of faecal incontinence in adults aged 40 years or more living in the community. Gut 50:480–484

16. Whitehead W (2005) Diagnosing and managing faecal incontinence: if you don't ask, they won't tell. Gastroenterology 129:6
17. Trachter AB, Rogers A, Leblum SR (2002) Inflammatory bowel disease in women: impact on relationship and sexual health. Inflamm Bowel Dis 8(6):413–421
18. Collings S, Norton C (2004) Women's experiences of faecal incontinence: a study. Br J Community Nurs 9(12):520–523
19. Diseth TH, Emblem R (1996) Somatic function, mental health and psychological adjustment of adolescents with anorectal anomalies. J Pediatr Surg 31:638–643
20. Fisher SE, Breckon K, Andrews H, Keighley M (1989) Psychiatric screening for patients with faecal incontinence or chronic constipation referred for surgical treatment. Br J Surg 76:352–355
21. Hagglof B, Andren O, Bergstrom E et al (1998) Self-esteem in children with nocturnal enuresis and urinary incontinence. Eur Urol 33(Suppl 3):16–19
22. Burgio KL, Locher J, Roth D, Goode P (2001) Psychological improvements associated with behavioural and drug treatment of urge incontinence in older women. J Gerontol B Psychol Sci Soc 56:P46–P51
23. Millard RJ, Oldenburg B (1983) The symptomatic, urodynamic and psychodynamic results of bladder re-education programs. J Urol 130:715–719
24. Rosenzweig BA, Hischke D, Thomas S et al (1991) Stress incontinence in women; psychological status before and after treatment. J Reprod Med 36:835–838
25. Heymen S (2004) Psychological and cognitive variables affecting treatment outcomes for urinary and fecal incontinence. Gastroenterology 126:S146–151
26. Fenner DE, Genberg B, Brahama P et al (2003) Fecal and urinary incontinence after vaginal delivery with anal sphincter disruption in an obstetrics unit in the United States. Am J Obstet Gynecol 189(6)1543–1550
27. Stern JM (2003a) Psychiatry, psychotherapy and gastroenterology: bringing it all together. Aliment Pharmacol Ther 17:175–184
28. Stern JM (2003b) Stomas, sorrow and shame. In: Stigma in healthcare: understanding the psychology of the stigma of incontinence. Simon Foundation, Chicago
29. Stern JM (2006) Home parenteral nutrition and the psyche: psychological challenges for patient and family. Proceedings of the Nutrition Society, vol. 65(3). CABI Publishing, Oxfordshire, pp 222–226
30. Montgomery C (2002) Role of dynamic group therapy in psychiatry. Adv Psychiatr Treat 8(1):34–41
31. Vamos M (2006) Psychotherapy in the medically ill: a commentary. Aus N Z J Psychiatry 40(4):295–309
32. Norton C, Kamm MA (1999) Outcome of biofeedback for faecal incontinence. Br J Surg 86:1159–1163
33. Norton C, Chelvanayagam S, Wilson-Barnett, J et al (2003) Randomised controlled trial of biofeedback for fecal incontinence. Gastrtoenterology 125:1320–1329
34. Frank J (1961) Persuasion and healing. Johns Hopkins Press, Baltimore
35. Stern JM (1999) Psychoanalytic psychotherapy in a medical setting. Psychoanal Psychother 13(1):51–68
36. Stern JM (2005) Psychotherapy-individual, family and group. In: Wright P, Stern J, Phelan M. Core psychiatry, 2nd edn. Elsevier Saunders, London, pp 541–564

Impact of Fecal Incontinence on Quality of Life

6

Todd H. Rockwood

Introduction

Given the psychological, social, and functional impacts that fecal incontinence (FI) has on an individual, the assessment of health-related quality of life (HRQoL) is an important consideration when evaluating the efficacy of treatment. An individual with FI faces a serious set of challenges in living life, and as a result, providers are also faced with consideration of these issues in providing treatment. For example, the implantation of an artificial sphincter is about more than technical procedures; it is also about its impact on the individual's ability to live life.

The role of HRQoL continues to grow, and accompanying this growth is an increase in research in the refinement of the assessment of HRQoL. HRQoL assessment in FI is still relatively new, and the process of specifying the range of issues involved as well as the content of many of the areas identified to date is ongoing. This work continues to improve the understanding and knowledge of FI and expands horizons. The following material focuses on two issues associated with HRQoL assessment and FI. First is a brief review of different measures that are available to assess HRQoL for FI. This is followed by a consideration of issues that are associated with evaluating instruments for use in assessment of HRQoL and the development of HRQoL instruments.

Existing Measures for Quality of Life in Fecal Incontinence

The state of HRQoL measurement in FI is still developing and evolving. A number of reviews of issues associated with and instruments available for measuring HRQoL in FI are available [1–3]. What is apparent from the research is that it is possible to assess HRQoL in FI with success, but the field has by no means matured.

There are three basic instrument types available for the study of HRQoL in FI: (1) general HRQoL instruments, (2) specialized instruments, and (3) condition-specific measures. Each instrument signals a different approach and presents unique strengths as well as associated weaknesses.

Instruments such as the SF-36 [4] and European Quality of Life (EuroQol) [5] have been used with success in numerous studies on FI. The primary concern with the use of general HRQoL instruments is the sensitivity of the instrument to specific issues associated with FI as well as the presence of floor and ceiling effects. While mixed, the findings are encouraging. For example, the new version of the SF-36 (v 2.0) appears to demonstrate increased sensitivity to HRQoL in FI compared with the original SF-36 [6]. At a minimum, these instruments can serve as gross indicators of HRQoL in the FI population and provide the opportunity to compare within as well as between populations [e.g., urinary incontinence (UI) vs. FI].

This ability to compare across populations does come with a price–a question about responsiveness exists: Are the instruments sensitive enough to be able to detect change that is meaningful in the FI population? This issue is compounded with the potential for floor effects emerging. When floor effects are present, there is only one direction for possible change to occur: towards improvement. As a result, the measures can lead to a false conclusion-an overestimation of benefit instead? Finally, when considering these measures, the specification of the treatment outcome needs to be determined. Treatment is often directed and specific, and thus gross measures, such as general HRQoL instruments, might not be able to detect meaningful changes relative to intended outcomes.

Specialized Measures

Specialized scales exist for an incredibly large range of issues [7, 8], and research on QoL in FI could benefit from their utilization in many instances. These measures represent an underutilized area of HRQoL assessment in FI. This underutilization detracts from our ability to further the understanding of HRQoL in

FI. If a treatment, surgical or otherwise, is likely to be strongly related to a specific aspect of HRQoL–e.g., stress/anxiety, depression, control–then selection of specialized instruments that measure that domain would best serve patients, providers, and researchers.

Condition-specific QoL (CSQoL) measures are generally designed based on a model of disease/condition causing change to some other construct, e.g., FI causes changes in the amount or intensity of anxiety experienced by an individual. This assumption is viable, and instruments such as the FIQoL scale make the assumption that FI causes anxiety and the intent is to assess anxiety solely associated with FI.

The above model is generally adequate for most outcomes research, but it cannot be assumed to be adequate for all research, nor is it adequate in the long run. An example of this can actually be found in the evaluation of instruments such as the FIQoL in the postpartum population. This work consistently points out that the assessment of core issues such as shame, embarrassment, and stress are not completely adequate [9, 10]. This is due, in part, to the combined presence of FI, the event of childbirth and a newborn, and all the interactions that are not captured with general HRQoL or CSQoL instruments. The use of specialized scales in these instances would provide a more robust assessment and increase our ability to evaluate the relativistic impacts of the different conditions.

Evaluation of specific treatments, such as biofeedback, could benefit greatly from the use of specialized measures. Depression can be used as an example to illustrate this benefit. Biofeedback targets control, and depression is often a response to lack of control. If biofeedback creates a sense of control, then as a secondary effect, biofeedback could impact depression. Instruments designed specifically around depression, such as the Beck Depression Inventory [7] or the Center for Epidemiologic Studies Depression (CESD) scale [7] would be more sensitive and likely to identify and assess such secondary impacts. Evaluation of these secondary impacts would allow us to begin to unravel an as of yet unanswered question: How much does FI contribute to the emergence and manifestation of depression? Specialized scales would allow us to begin to untangle these types of questions by starting with depression and looking at how FI changes it as opposed to the current approach in which we evaluate depression associated with FI. This knowledge could then be used to refine CSQoL instruments.

Condition-specific Measures for Fecal Incontinence

Recent work on CSQoL measures in FI is encouraging. This work is directed at three key issues: (1) evaluating the content of existing measures and pointing out shortcomings, (2) comparing different measures against each other to identify relative strengths and weaknesses, and (3) developing new instruments or refining the content of existing instruments in general or for application in specific populations.

Three instruments have dominated measurement of HRQoL in FI. The Gastrointestinal Quality of Life Index (GIQLI) [11], the Manchester Health Questionnaire [12], and the FIQL scale [13]. Each of these instruments has been used successfully in the assessment of QoL associated with treatment for with FI. A number of other instruments have also been developed, but their utilization has not been as wide spread. This is in part due to the very specific nature of the instrument, e.g., QoL in a Parkinson's disease population [14], clinical/community epidemiology [15, 16], or children [17].

An encouraging trend in QoL measurement in FI is work that is building upon these base instruments. For example, the sensitive and personal nature of FI underscores the importance of how instruments are administered. Kwon and colleagues have done work to adapt the Manchester Health Questionnaire for telephone administration [18]. Although the results are not definitive, this does represent a critical step [19].

Another encouraging area is work that points out the shortcomings in these base tools, both conceptually and in terms of measurement. For example, work has demonstrated the need to expand the content of the FIQoL to better capture the postpartum mother's experiences [9, 10]. Work such as this is absolutely critical to improving our ability to measure QoL in FI.

Also underway is work that assesses QoL more systemically. The GIQLI is the forerunner of work in this area. It looks at FI within the context of the overall GI system. There are distinct benefits to such instruments in that they focus on interrelated aspects of the body so that, for example, function and effects due to X [irritable bowel syndrome (IBS)] are not as likely to be attributed to Y (FI). Recently, there has been an increase of work focusing on measurement associated with the pelvic floor and FI. Measures in this area have a significant contribution to make. FI is often associated with issues beyond the sphincter, e.g., the pelvic floor, and as a result, its occurrence cannot be disassociated from conditions such as UI. Instruments such as the FIQoL might not be able to disentangle QoL issues when both UI and FI are present [9, 20, 21]. Instruments focusing on the pelvic floor would be appropriate when the root cause of FI is due to the pelvic floor but not appropriate for use when FI is due to something other than the pelvic floor (e.g., sphincter tear).

Health-related Quality of Life and Fecal Incontinence

The following material focuses on central issues in the consideration of what instrument(s) to use as well as the development or refinement of existing instruments. The primary question/issue is to determine what is meant by HRQoL relative to the purpose of the research. Core to this is an assessment of the primary and secondary impacts of treatment. HRQoL can range from observable characteristics (functional status) to abstract constructs that are not directly observable (depression). Phenomena in the latter instance are not straightforward when it comes to conceptualization and measurement.

The notion of stress provides a good illustration of the complexities associated with identifying or developing appropriate measures. Stress is a core issue associated with HRQoL and FI, and the conceptual orientation employed relative to stress can determine both its meaning and how it is measured. Stress can be conceptualized as event based or, alternatively, as an internal coping phenomenon. In the event-based model, stress is conceived of as an individual's response to events. An individual has an FI episode, and this event causes stress. Stress is the result of the event occurring; had the event not occurred, stress would not be induced. Such a model is embedded within much of the work in FI. The relativistic impact of solid versus liquid stool loss events is an illustrative example of such an approach. Alternatively, the coping model does not focus on events that occur or environmental conditions; rather, the focus is the individual's perception of their ability to deal with a stress. In these instances, whether or not a stool loss event has occurred is not particularly relevant. It is the individual's felt ability to cope with the event that is important.

Consideration of scope is an oft-ignored issue in the use HRQoL measures. Returning to the above example of stress, consider two alternative studies: In a surgical treatment of FI in which an artificial sphincter is implanted, the focus on outcomes might use a stress-events model. The intent of the artificial sphincter is to reduce the number of events experienced. Given this, in the assessment of HRQoL, logic would argue that treatment reduces events and reduction in events reduces stress. Alternatively, if the research is focused on psychosocial interventions (e.g., counseling to deal with postpartum FI), then a different logic is employed; treatment increases ability to deal with FI occurring, and increased ability to deal with FI reduces stress associated with FI. Recognizing this distinction is important for both instrument development as well as choosing between existing instruments when conducting studies. Concordance between treatment outcomes and what is being measured is essential to conducting good outcomes research.

HRQoL can range from macro measures associated with existential well-being to micro measures around shame and embarrassment associated with FI. No single instrument can adequately represent the full scope of HRQoL; instruments tend to focus more or less on different aspects. This requires thought when selecting an appropriate instrument. FI is not a condition that has a primary effect on cognitive abilities, but it does have a dramatic impact on daily activities that are usually taken for granted (e.g., shopping) or emotional and psychological conditions (e.g., shame). The intent of CSQoL measures such as the adapted Manchester Health Questionnaire [12, 18] or the FIQoL [13] is to focus on issues that have high salience for FI. These instruments tend to focus toward the microlevel measures in the instrument and focus on the impact FI has on day-to-day activities and life. The instruments do not attempt to measure the impact that FI has on the meaning of life.

Another critical issue in FI research is targeting instruments for particular populations and/or situations. FI research is dominated by work in one of two populations, geriatric or postpartum, with a smaller amount of work in cancer, trauma, and adolescent populations. HRQoL in general and CSQoL in particular is not uniform across populations, and consideration of instrument needs to include an assessment of the population. Instruments such as the GIQLI and the FIQoL are designed for the general FI population, and the unique situations faced by populations such as the new mother or the institutionalized individual bring fundamental changes to the conceptualization of QoL. It is important that this aspect of scope be included in the consideration of measures. Instruments that adapt existing tools for use in specific populations, such as the Manchester Health Questionnaire [12] or the work of Cockell et al. [10] for postpartum or Trajanovska and Catto-Smith in children [17], are central to expanding our knowledge and understanding of FI.

One fundamental issue that has yet to be successfully dealt with in FI research is coping. To date, coping behaviors and mechanisms have been treated in one of two ways in FI research. Figure 1a illustrates the initial treatment of coping in FI research. Coping is a response to severity and as a result is an indicator of the severity of the condition. The impact of this can mediate the impact severity has on HRQoL [22]. Alternatively, Figure 1 illustrates a more recent emergence of the conceptualization of coping [3]. Coping is related to severity as shown in the dashed line but can be viewed as a response to severity or as a means

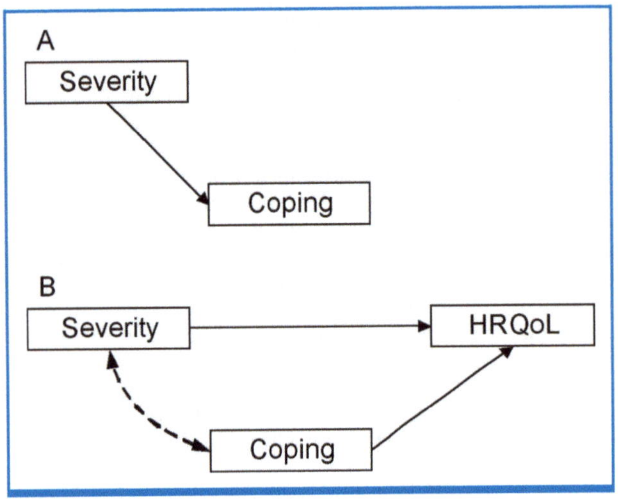

Fig. 1. Conceptualization of coping in fecal incontinence research. *HRQoL* health-related quality of life

of reducing severity. Regardless, it has a direct relationship to HRQoL that has not yet been adequately dealt with.

The final issue associated with conceptual issues has been discussed within the context of the above, but it is the purpose of the assessment of HRQoL. Is the assessment aimed at evaluating the outcome of a particular treatment, an epidemiological evaluation of a population, or general social research evaluating what FI means to life? To date, most instruments in FI research have been developed around the assessment of treatment and outcomes research. This means that instrument content is dominated by issues that should be either directly or indirectly affected by treatment. Moving forward, instruments need to evolve to reflect more of the individual's experience with FI as well as to make the instruments more sensitive to evaluating treatment for FI.

Conclusions

FI is, as conditions go, an incredibly sensitive and difficult issue to deal with relative to QoL assessment. Whereas the condition is not necessarily life threatening physically, it can be seen as life threatening for social and personal life. Because of this, it is important to assess QoL when treating or evaluating treatment for FI.

Research has shown that the basic tools are available to assess HRQoL for individuals with FI and that this assessment is a vital part of the evaluation of treatment of FI. However, there is a need for additional work on QoL measurement in FI to refine the understanding of basic issues, such as coping mechanisms, where they fit in relative to severity on the QoL spectrum, and whether they provide sufficient detail regarding shame and its role in QoL. Going forward, there are several factors that can make work in this area more successful and lead to more rapid development: first is a focus on the development of modules for specific populations that can be appended to existing instruments. Second is building upon the work that has been done to date and pushing it forward, such as the work on QoL postpartum. Finally is to start integrating the patient's perspective into measures at a deeper level.

References

1. Baxter NN, Rothenberger DA, Lowry AC (2003) Measuring fecal incontinence. Dis Colon Rectum 46(12):1591–1605
2. Eton DT, Lepore SJ (2002) Prostate cancer and health-related quality of life: a review of the literature. Psychooncology 11(4):307–326
3. Rockwood TH (2004) Incontinence severity and QOL scales for fecal incontinence. Gastroenterology 126 (1 Suppl 1):S106–S113
4. Ware J et al (1993) SF-36 Health Survey: manual and interpretation guide. The Health Institute, New England Medical Center, Boston
5. Brazier J, Jones N, Kind P (1993) Testing the validity of the EuroQol and comparing it with the SF-36 Health Survey questionnaire. Qual Life Res 2:169–180
6. Bordeianou L et al (2006) Does incontinence severity correlate with quality of life? American Society of Colon and Rectal Surgeons, Seattle, WA, June 2006
7. Robinson JP et al (1991) Measures of personality and social psychological attitudes. In: Measures of social psychological attitudes, vol 1. Academic Press, San Diego

8. McDowell I, Newell C (1996) Measuring health: a guide to rating scales and questionnaires, 2nd edn. Oxford University Press, New York
9. Hatem M, Fraser W, Lepire E (2005) Postpartum urinary and anal incontinence: a population-based study of quality of life of primiparous women in Quebec. J Obstet Gynaecol Can 27(7):682–688
10. Cockell SJ, Oates-Johnson T, Gilmour DT et al (2003) Postpartum flatal and Fecal Incontinence Quality-of-Life Scale: a disease- and population-specific measure. Qual Health Res 13(8):1132–1144
11. Eypasch E, Williams JI, Wood-Dauphinee S et al (1995) Gastrointestinal Quality of Life Index: Development, validation and application of a new instrument. Br J Surg 82:216–222
12. Bug GJ, Kiff ES, Hosker G (2001) A new condition-specific health-related quality-of-life questionnaire for the assessment of women with anal incontinence. BJOG 108(10):1057–1067
13. Rockwood TH, Church JM, Fleshman JW et al (2000) Fecal Incontinence Quality of Life Scale: quality-of-life instrument for patients with fecal incontinence. Dis Colon Rectum 43(1):9–16
14. Sakakibara R, Shinotoh H, Uchiyama T et al (2001) Questionnaire-based assessment of pelvic organ dysfunction in Parkinson's disease. Auton Neurosci 92(1–2):76–85
15. Bharucha AE, Locke GR 3rd, Seide BM, Zinsmeister AR (2004) A new questionnaire for constipation and faecal incontinence. Aliment Pharmacol Ther 20(3):355–364
16. Bharucha AE, Zinsmeister AR, Locke GR et al (2006) Symptoms and quality of life in community women with fecal incontinence. Clin Gastroenterol Hepatol 4(8):1004–1009
17. Trajanovska M, Catto-Smith A-G (2005) Quality of life measures for fecal incontinence and their use in children. J Gastroenterol Hepatol 20(6):919–928
18. Kwon S, Visco AG, Fitzgerald MP et al (2005) Validity and reliability of the Modified Manchester Health Questionnaire in assessing patients with fecal incontinence. Dis Colon Rectum 48(2):323–331
19. Rockwood T (2005) Comment: validity and reliability of the Modified Manchester Health Questionnaire in assessing patients with fecal incontinence. Dis Colon Rectum 48(2):331–334
20. Barber MD, Walters MD, Bump RC (2005) Short forms of two condition-specific quality-of-life questionnaires for women with pelvic floor disorders (PFDI-20 and PFIQ-7). Am J Obstet Gynecol 193(1):103–113
21. Kelly CE (2003) Which questionnaires should be used in female urology practice? Curr Urol Rep 4(5):375–380
22. Jorge JM, Wexner SD (1993) Etiology and management of fecal incontinence. Dis Colon Rectum 36(1):77–97

Social Aspects and Economics of Fecal Incontinence

7

Carlo Ratto, Patrizia Ponzi, Francesca Di Stasi, Angelo Parello, Lorenza Donisi, Giovanni B. Doglietto

Introduction

Health care expenditure in the most economically advanced countries seems to have spiraled out of control over the last few decades. There are three main reasons accounting for this situation: ageing of the population has led to an increase in the numbers requiring health care services, the accelerating pace of technological development has given rise to new techniques that have improved the quality of treatment, and with the introduction of new, increasingly costly, products, patient expectations have changed and patients thus demand better medical treatment. The combination of these three factors has resulted in health care spending becoming increasingly difficult to control.

This means that the available resources must be managed to the best advantage. Clearly, this implies adopting the economic strategy that, according to Samuelson's [1] definition, consists of maximizing the use of very limited resources that could be allocated for other purposes.

The need to control health care expenditure initially prompted decision makers to consider implementing investment cuts, with little regard for the long-term repercussions that these could have. However, it soon became apparent that to optimize the use of resources allocated to health care, expenditure had to be rationalized rather than rationed. Targeted objectives of the health care policy (only the efficacy or only the cost of a service) have, therefore, been superseded by multidimensional objectives, which correlate the efficacy of a program with the costs that it involves. In this light, once clinical efficacy has been established, health care programs must now be assessed in terms of their economic efficiency (technical and allocational) before a new therapeutic approach is introduced.

Economic Assessments in Health Care

An economic assessment is, by definition, "the comparative analysis of alternative courses of action in terms of both their costs and consequences" [2]. The steps to be taken in any assessment are, therefore, to identify, measure, evaluate, and compare the costs and consequences of the alternatives under consideration. These operations apply to all fields, not the least of which is health care services.

As various therapeutic options have to be considered, it is important that the alternatives to be compared are homogeneous. The aim of rationalizing the use of resources requires that costs and effects of a program be compared with costs and effects of programs of the same kind, with a view to ascertaining which is the most advantageous from an economic standpoint. There are, in effect, no set rules governing the choice of the optimal alternative; however, that optimal alternative should always be therapeutically significant (more frequently used and/or more efficacious), readily available, and consistent with the design of the study.

For the economic evaluation to be successful in the field of health care, the purpose of the analysis undertaken must be clarified, primarily to correctly identify the costs and effects under consideration. Cost is a subjective concept. Indeed, a cost must be borne by someone, and assessment of the cost will, therefore, depend on whom that someone is. In the field of health care, an economic assessment can be carried out from various points of view: the third-party payer (insurer), the national health service (NHS), the hospital facility, the patient, or society, the latter comprising all the other categories. The perspective of society is so vast that it embraces all possible costs and effects. To adopt this perspective would be simply too complicated, albeit more interesting. Moreover, society as a whole is unlikely to make direct decisions on the allocation of resources.

Having established the alternatives to be examined and the perspective of the analysis, the problem remains of quantifying costs (Table 1) and effects (Table 2). Both can be subdivided into three categories: direct, indirect, and intangible. Direct costs can be further subdivided into health care and non-health care costs.

Table 1. Classification of costs and examples

Direct	Indirect	Intangible
Drugs		
Hospitalization		
	Loss of work time	Psychological factors
Diagnostics		
	Loss of earnings	Impaired quality of life
Rehabilitation		
Home care		

Table 2. Classification of effects and examples

Direct	Indirect	Intangible
Reduction in costs of personnel and materials		
	Reduction in mortality and morbidity	Alleviation of pain
Reduction in costs due to side-effects		
	Reduction in loss of productivity	Improved quality of life
Improvement in clinical parameters		

Direct Costs

Health Care

Direct health care costs are those that can be directly attributed to the procedures related to the diagnosis, treatment, and rehabilitation involved in the management considered or necessary as a result of the pathological conditions addressed by that management.

Non-health Care

Non-health care costs comprise a range of expenses directly related to the intervention considered but which are not of a health care nature (e.g., the cost of transporting patients).

Indirect Costs

Indirect costs are generally regarded as those due to loss of productivity as a result of a pathological event and the treatment thereof. Estimating these social costs is one of the more difficult aspects encountered in the economic appraisal of health care interventions. Quantifying these costs is useful particularly when the analysis technique is the most complete and the perspective is the broadest, i.e., the perspective of society as a whole. Apart from the difficulty in establishing true productivity losses, estimating these costs often proves critical for various reasons. Thus, with the exception of a few particular cases, these costs are usually ignored.

Intangible Costs

Intangible costs are those borne by the individual as a result of being in a poor state of health. These cannot be assessed directly or evaluated in absolute quantitative terms. Anxiety, stress, and pain are a few examples. Quantifying these costs requires the use of specific techniques and instruments ad hoc.

Direct Effects

These are the effects attributable to the diagnostic, therapeutic, and rehabilitative procedures related to the management of the case. These may manifest as variations in objective clinical parameters, variations in the probability of certain undesirable events such as a heart attack or stroke, or variations in so-called final consequences such as mortality or life expectancy.

Indirect Effects

These are generally interpreted as the effects arising from the loss of productivity caused by the pathological condition and/or by the management adopted.

Intangible Effects

These refer to the effects on the individual due to the impaired state of health. As these are of an intangible nature, they cannot be assessed directly. They concern psychological aspects such as anxiety, stress, and pain that affect the patient's quality of life. To estimate these effects, specific techniques and ad hoc instruments are required, as well as clinical indices (erroneously defined as subjective) capable of estimating the quality of life related to a specific type of treatment or health condition.

Analysis Techniques

Essentially, four different techniques are used to perform the analyses, which, in order of increasing complexity, are: cost minimization analysis (CMA), cost effectiveness/efficacy analysis (CEA), cost utility analysis (CUA), and cost benefit analysis (CBA) [3]. These techniques focus on the pathological condition and its treatment; however, another type of analysis–"not complete" economic evaluation, the cost of illness analysis (CIA)–also focuses on the burden of a pathological condition.

Cost Effectiveness/Efficacy Analysis (CEA)

In a CEA, the costs of the alternatives considered are analyzed in relation to the efficacy of those alternatives as expressed in clinical units. Efficacy may be expressed in terms of intermediate parameters of clinical relevance for a certain pathological condition (blood pressure, cholesterolemia) or as final outcomes (deaths prevented, life-years gained, symptom-free years). The result emerging from this type of analysis provides the ratio in which the numerator is a cost, and therefore expressed in monetary units, and the denominator is an effect, which is expressed in clinical units.

The final result of a CEA is a cost-effectiveness ratio, which may be either pure or incremental. In the latter case, the higher costs resulting from the more efficacious treatment are evaluated in relation to the greater efficacy of that treatment, with a view to establishing its economic efficiency [4]. This type of analysis is undoubtedly the one most commonly used in the economic evaluation of pharmaceutical drugs.

Cost Minimization Analysis (CMA)

CMA is, in essence, a cost-effectiveness analysis. Indeed, if the efficacy of the alternative treatments is identical, a comparison can be made only with regard to costs. The CEA, therefore, becomes a cost minimization analysis, and the alternative chosen will be that generating the lowest costs.

Cost Utility Analysis (CUA)

CUA is a more sophisticated technique than CEA, from which it is derived. In CUA, the results of pharmacological treatment are expressed in utility-weighted years of life saved, or in the equivalent years of good health (Quality Adjusted Life Years or Healthy Years Equivalent). The utility index summarizes and expresses as a number between 0 and 1 the desirability of a healthy condition, also taking into account the intangible aspects, i.e., those concerning quality of life. These assessments have the advantage of also allowing comparisons to be made between heterogeneous types of intervention, as the result is always a ratio, the numerator of which comprises costs (monetary units) and the denominator of which is usually expressed in terms of Quality Adjusted Life Years.

Cost Benefit Analysis (CBA)

In the CBA, health care effects are also expressed, as costs, in monetary terms. This is the most complex of the techniques used. Obviously, it is extremely difficult to convert a life saved into monetary terms and sometimes conceptually controversial. It is achieved by means of highly complex instruments, such as that of "willingness to pay". The result of a CBA is usually expressed in terms of net benefit or cost (the difference between costs and benefits) or as a ratio in which both the numerator (costs) and the denominator (benefits) are translated into monetary units. This technique is rarely applied in pharmacoeconomic studies. Assessments of costs and effects in the various techniques of pharmacoeconomics are summarized in Table 3.

Cost of Illness Analysis (COI)

Studies on the COI highlight the impact of a certain disease on society, focusing on the extra resources required to manage the disease as well as productivity lost as a result of the disease. Where the cost of disease is high, a COI study may help to reveal the need for action to better manage this disease. The COI approach estimates the direct costs associated with an illness, sometimes including the cost to society resulting from lost earnings. It does not account for pain and suffering, the value of lost leisure time, or the costs and benefits of preventive measures. Although COI studies cannot be considered complete economic evaluations, they are still aimed at denoting appropriate choices in resource consequences of health problems in relation to each other.

Very few studies have evaluated the economic impact of fecal incontinence in terms of costs related to the condition itself or the cost of the various treatment options. The studies carried out in various countries using a variety of techniques and mostly focusing on specific interventions and patient groups make it difficult to extrapolate the findings to the entire population with fecal incontinence. Whereas it is difficult to compare economic information related to a pathological condition across countries, it is even more difficult to compare cost-effectiveness information concerning relative treatment options. For this reason, a review is presented herewith concerning findings regarding the costs of the pathological condition, whereas economic aspects related to specific treatment options are not discussed here.

Table 3. Assessment of costs and effects in the various techniques of economic evaluation of pharmaceutical drugs

Type of analysis	Measurement/evaluation of costs for both alternatives	Identification of effects	Measurement/evaluation of effects
Cost effectiveness analysis (CEA)	Monetary units (e.g., euros)	A single target result common to both alternatives but achieved to different degrees	Physical units of measurement (e.g., number of lives saved, years of life gained, reduction in blood pressure, etc.)
Cost minimization analysis (CMA)	Monetary units (e.g., euros)	Identical in all relevant aspects	None
Cost utility analysis (CUA)	Monetary units (e.g., euros)	One or more effects, not necessarily common to both alternatives and achieved to different degrees	Quality Adjusted Life Years: years of life adjusted for quality
Cost benefit analysis (CBA)	Monetary units (e.g., euros)	One or more effects, not necessarily common to both alternatives and achieved to different degrees	Monetary units (e.g., euros)

The Cost of Fecal Incontinence

In a Dutch study [5], published in 2005, the mean annual cost of a patient affected by fecal incontinence was reported to be 2,169 euros, namely 1,051 euros referring to direct costs and 1,118 euros to indirect costs. An Italian investigation [6], conducted in that same year, recorded the direct costs alone as 1,103 euros, an amount almost identical to that reported in the Dutch study (Table 4). The paucity of data available in the literature is, therefore, offset by a certain homogeneity in the results. The individual cost items are examined below, with particular attention being focused on the distinction between the direct costs involved both in health care and non-health care.

Table 4. Cost of fecal incontinence

Costs	Deutekom et al. [5] The Netherlands	Ratto et al. [6] Italy
Type		
Direct	1,051 euros	1,103 euros
Indirect	1,118 euros	
Total	2,169 euros	1,103 euros

Direct Costs

Direct Health Care Costs

Fecal incontinence is a very particular case in that some items of expenditure are not attributable to a single agent. Indeed, the local health care authorities (territorial bodies responsible for financing and providing health care services for the residents in their area) often bear some costs (direct health care costs), which are subsequently borne by the patient (direct non-health care costs). Costs related to diagnostic tests and hospitalization are unequivocally attributable to the NHS.

In the case of fecal incontinence, the costs of instrumental and laboratory tests are not high in absolute terms compared with those related to other common diseases. Indeed, the unit cost of examinations such as manometry and colonoscopy are fairly low, as sophisticated diagnostic technology is not involved. Albeit, costs may rise, as these tests often have to be repeated. Indeed, it is not uncommon for patients to constantly search for a solution to their problem, seeking opinions from different physicians in different places (different hospitals sometimes in different regions) and, therefore, undergo the same instrumental examination several times.

Patients presenting with fecal incontinence are often not hospitalized; for instance, in Italy in 2003, the number of hospitalizations with a diagnosis of fecal incontinence on discharge amounted to 222 [7]. To place this figure in its proper perspective, it should be compared with the number of hospitalizations for two very common disorders with a heavy clinical and social impact, namely, hemorrhoids and urinary incontinence, which accounted for 36,073 and 2,274 hospitalizations, respectively, in 2003 [7].

Two different issues may account for this low frequency of hospitalization. First, these patients face an intricate diagnostic workup and therapeutic procedure. Indeed, the number of patients seeking a solution to the problem of fecal incontinence is far lower than the number actually affected by the disorder. Moreover, of those who consult their general practitioner, not all obtain a diagnosis, whereas others receive no treatment even when a diagnosis is made. This still occurs despite the fact that it has now been demonstrated that the treatment options available are both clinically efficacious and economically efficient and are, therefore, potentially able to offer long-term savings for the NHS.

The second aspect accounting for the low number of hospitalizations for fecal incontinence is related to the nature of the hospitalization itself. Indeed, a patient presenting with this disorder is unlikely to be hospitalized for diagnostic purposes, hospitalization generally being reserved for treatment purposes. In the light of these considerations, clearly, the limited number of cases treated results in a limited number of hospitalizations.

Once diagnosis is made, many patients are not referred for surgery, which could yield a definitive solution to their problem, but undergo lengthy rehabilitation programs, which do not always yield satisfactory results. Considering that in Italy the mean cost to the NHS of a rehabilitation session is 200 euros and that the entire course is usually 10–15 sessions, which are often repeated due to unsatisfactory results, the impact this has on the total cost of the disorder can be readily appreciated.

Direct health care costs also include expenditure on pharmaceutical drugs, which in patients with fecal incontinence are antidiarrheal and laxatives. These drugs do not have a high unit cost, their impact on the total cost of the disorder being <10% (5.4% according to Deutekom et al. [5] and 3.9% according to Ratto et al. [6]).

The items weighing most heavily on the total cost of the disorder undoubtedly concern incontinence materials (disposable diapers and pants, washable nappies, anal tampons, underblankets and waterproof sheets, feces bags, etc.), which account for ~25% of total expenditure [5] and is borne both by the NHS and the patient. In countries with an NHS, the patient receives incontinence materials free of charge and, theoretically at least, does not have to buy them personally. Albeit, what usually happens is that these incontinence materials, due to the need for standardization of products and prices when large quantities of materials are purchased, fail to meet the needs of the individual patient; most patients, therefore, buy the products that they deem most useful. Thus, the expense is incurred twice: once by the NHS (direct health care costs) and once by the patient (direct non-health care costs). This phenomenon, reported by numerous patients and common to all the countries involved, results in a waste of money that could be avoided by more carefully choosing the devices to be supplied to patients. The situation is further aggravated by the fact that those prescribing the devices tend, for convenience, to prescribe the maximum number in order to avoid frequent requests from the patient. In Italy, for example, the maximum number of pads that can be prescribed per patient is 120 per month; the magnitude of the cost can easily be appreciated. A recent Italian study [8] estimated the monthly cost of pads borne by local health care authorities to be 35.79 euros per patient, i.e., an annual expenditure per patient of approximately 500 euros.

Direct Non-health Care Costs

Fecal incontinence compared with other disorders does not appear to have a heavy overall impact on the NHS. Indeed, as already pointed out, the costs related to the disorder are almost entirely borne by the patients themselves or their families. In addition to the cost of pads, other costs have to be borne entirely by the patient. The above-mentioned Dutch study [5] estimated expenditure for antidiarrheal drugs (used by 26% of the patients interviewed), skin care products (11%), special articles of clothing (10%), cleaning products (9%), and special foods (6%).

In terms both of direct and indirect costs, cleaning the incontinent patient accounts for a large proportion of the total costs involved in the disorder. Indeed, taking into account how much time is spent cleaning patients who are permanently in institutions, it has been estimated that the personnel in charge of caring for incontinent patients devote 2 h per day (13.3% of the time available) to this duty. Moreover, the cost is aggravated by the fact that episodes tend to occur more frequently during the night, when fewer staff members are on duty [9]. If 25% of the working hours of a health care worker employed in a residential facility are devoted to cleaning incontinent patients, the same percentage of the salary earned by that person should be regarded as a direct cost generated by fecal incontinence. However, the costs of health care personnel are not limited only to salary; staff members who spend much of their time cleaning incontinent patients are more prone to dissatisfaction and depression as well as to infection than are those engaged in other activities, and they are more likely to give up their jobs [10].

Indirect Costs

The population of incontinent patients is relatively young (33.3% <40 years of age) i.e., of working age [11]. The cost of the disorder in terms of lost work-

Table 5. Cost of fecal incontinence

	Papanicolaou et al. [12]	Papanicolaou et al. [12]	Papanicolaou et al. [12]	Kinchen et al. [13]
Country	UK/Ireland	Germany	Spain	USA
Total costs	359 euros	515 euros	655 euros	$ 800

ing hours is high in that many patients are frequently absent from work or, in the very severe cases, are prompted to take early retirement. Moreover, the indirect costs resulting from reduced working activity are not attributable exclusively to the patients themselves; they may also be generated by absenteeism on the part of those assisting the patient. Indeed, the same considerations made above, with regard to the mean number of hours devoted per day to cleaning institutionalized patients, are also valid with regard to patients who are assisted at home.

The phenomenon of congenital incontinence merits particular attention. This disorder has a heavy impact on parents, who often have to curtail their working activity to take care of their sick children.

Intangible Costs

Intangible costs refer to the cost of a disease in terms of pain, suffering, and discomfort. Whereas these effects cannot be evaluated in monetary terms, they nevertheless contribute to the overall burden of the disorder. In the case of fecal incontinence, the intangible costs primarily concern impaired social activity resulting from the shame and embarrassment that most patients suffer. In other words, fecal incontinence impairs the patient's quality of life.

The issue of intangible costs, which is extremely interesting and important, is discussed in the chapters of this volume concerning specific conditions of FI.

Conclusions

Fecal incontinence has a significant impact on health care expenditure, the burden being comparable to that of better known diseases such as urinary incontinence (with which fecal incontinence is often associated). It accounts, for example, for a mean cost per patient (females) per year of 500 euros in Europe (359 euros in the UK, 515 euros in Germany, and 655 euros in Spain) and US $800 in the USA [12, 13] (Table 5).

Even so, a portion of the total costs of the disease is unknown, as some patients are reluctant to declare they suffer from this disorder. Even when the disease severely affects everyday life, the patient is still reluctant to discuss it with his/her doctor. More than 54% of fecal incontinence patients have never discussed the matter with their doctor [14].

To reduce the financial burden of fecal incontinence, it is important to invest in promoting appropriate treatment of the disorder. As most patients are young when first struck by the disorder, investing money to prevent them from suffering from worsening of the disease or complications should be considered "good value for the money". The few economic studies carried out so far on the different treatment options show a general cost-effectiveness, but more investigations are needed to complete the picture-not only of costs but also benefits-of the different alternatives.

References

1. Samuelson PA (1947) Foundations Of Economic Analysis, Harvard University. Press, Cambridge
2. Drummond MF, O'Brien B, Stoddart GL, Torrance GW (1997) Methods for the economic evaluation of health care programmes. Oxford University Press
3. Attanasio E, Bruzzi P, Capri S et al (1999) Raccomandazioni per la conduzione degli studi di farmacoeconomia: la guida GISF. Mecosan 20:65–72
4. Torrance GW (1986) Measurement of health state utilities for economic appraisal. J Health Econ 5:1–30
5. Deutekom M, Dobben AC, Dijkgraaf MGW et al (2005) Cost of outpatients with fecal incontinence. Scand J Gastroenterol 40:552–558
6. Ratto C, Di Bidino R, Ponzi P et al (2005) Preliminary results from a prospective study protocol on the assessment of costs for faecal incontinence. In: Proceedings of the 2nd annual meeting of Health Technology Assessment International, Rome, Italy 20–22 June 2005. Italian Health Ministry. Ricoveri, diagnosi, interventi effettuati e durata delle degenze di tutti gli ospedali. http://www.ministerosalute.it/programmazione/sdo/ric_informazioni/default.jsp. Cited 16 Mar 2007
8. Cerzani M, Cornago D, Garattini L (2006) I dispositivi per assorbenza: modalità di acquisto e distribuzione in

Italia. Economia & Politica del Farmaco 7:20–26
9. Morris A, Ho MT, Lapsley H et al (2005) Cost of managing urinary and faecal incontinence in a sub-acute care facility: a "bottom-up" approach. Neurourol Urodyn 24:56–62
10. Sells H, McDonagh R (1999) Psychological aspects of incontinence. In: Lucas M, Emery S, Beynon J (eds) Incontinence. Blackwell Science, Oxford, pp 1–11
11. Bharucha AE, Zinmeister AR, Loche GR et al (2005) Prevalence and burden of fecal incontinence: a population-based study in women. Gastroenterology 129:42–49
12. Papanicolaou S, Pons ME, Hampet C et al (2005) Medical resource utilisation and cost of care for women seeking treatment for urinary incontinence in an outpatient setting. Example from three countries participating in the PURE study. Maturitas 52(Suppl 2): S35–S47
13. Kinchen KS, Long S, Chang S et al (2005) The direct cost of stress urinary incontinence among women in Medicaid population. Am J Obstet Gynecol 193: 1936–1944
14. Miner PB (2004) Economic and personal impact of fecal and urinary incontinence. Gastroenterology 126(1 Suppl 1):S8–S13

Section II

Diagnosis of Fecal Incontinence

Clinical Assessment of the Incontinent Patient

8

Héctor Ortiz, Mario De Miguel, Miguel A. Ciga

Introduction

Besides physiologic investigations and radiology imaging, diagnosis of fecal incontinence requires accurate clinical assessment. By means of a structured scheme, clinical assessment aims to evaluate the whole picture: whether the patient is really incontinent, the etiology of the incontinence, and the nature and severity of the problem. Nevertheless, we must keep in mind that when treating an individual patient, these data may not be enough to define the pathophysiology of the symptom and, therefore, we need the investigations we mentioned initially.

The first goal is to determine whether the patient is incontinent. Many patients will not easily admit the symptom. On the one hand, incontinence represents a social stigma and, on the other hand, patients may feel distressed by realizing their physical deterioration reaches the point of not being able to maintain fecal continence. Avoiding the term itself, patients will frequently use other terms, such as diarrhea, fecal urgency, etc. This was shown in a classical study [1] in which data showed how half of the patients referred with chronic diarrhea actually presented incontinence, and less than half of them provided that information to the doctor.

At the same time, we can find continent patients who seem to be incontinent. Physically handicapped patients may find difficulty in entering the bathroom, sitting on the toilet or device for defecation, or even cleaning themselves properly after defecation. Psychiatric patients may feel an inadequate need to defecate even if they are not incontinent. Lastly, we must differentiate between incontinence and soiling due to inadequate hygiene or hemorrhoid prolapse.

Once fecal incontinence has been established, the next step to investigate is the nature of the incontinence: passive or stress incontinence. Passive incontinence deals with patients who are not aware of the leak of gases or feces, while stress incontinence means the impossibility of stopping the leak of gases or feces even if attempting to do so. It also must be ascertained what kind of incontinence (gas, liquid, or solid feces) and the frequency of the episodes.

Physical Examination

Assessment must begin with a general examination to investigate possible underlying systemic illnesses that can cause incontinence. Therefore, it should include a neurologic assessment. Anorectal examination must be undertaken in the most comfortable position for the patient. Different options have been described, but the suitable one is the left lateral position, with flexed thighs and knees and with the buttocks slightly out of the limit of the table. This position usually allows a satisfactory inspection of the perineum. Before the examination starts, it is advisable to inspect the underclothes of the patient to check for soiling and the use of protective pads. Anorectal examination should include inspection, palpation, digital examination, and proctoscopy.

Inspection

Severe incontinence, particularly to liquid feces, can cause erosion and erythema of the perianal skin. Those lesions, as well as scratching erosions that may accompany them, can present signs of infection, frequently due to streptococcus and fungi. In that case, specimen cultures may be taken.

Perineum inspection helps identify scarring from previous trauma, episiotomy, or anal surgery that may indicate the etiology of incontinence. External fistula-in-ano openings or inflammatory areas that can explain the feeling of soiling must also be identified. Multiple external openings lead to the suspicion of inflammatory bowel disease.

It is very important to evaluate the anus by separating the buttocks and checking whether it remains completely closed or becomes patulous and opens easily. In that case, a low resting pressure can be sus-

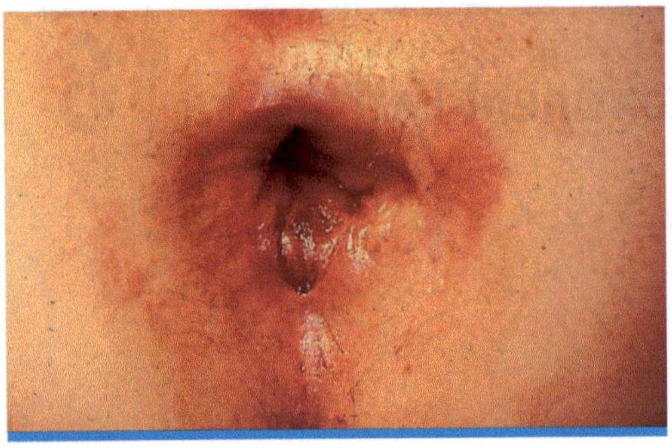

Fig. 1. Patulous anus in a patient with previous anal surgery and neuropathy

pected, suggesting a sphincter gap, occult rectal prolapse, or neuropathy (Fig. 1). Anal deformities, such as key-hole anus, frequently caused after posterior sphincterotomy or fistulotomy, prevent the anus from closing properly and can explain the leak of feces and mucus. The patient should be asked to squeeze so the symmetry and quality of closure can be assessed. Asymmetric collapse of the sphincter ring may reveal a unilateral gap in the sphincter as well as bilateral defects in a different area.

The anus and the perineal area should also be evaluated under the Valsalva maneuver. Under these conditions, rectal prolapse with concentric folds will differ from mucosa prolapse that shows radial folds and is rarely responsible for severe incontinence, although it can explain minor mucus leak. This is also the time to look for third- and fourth-degree hemorrhoids, as well as perineal descent, which is clear when the perineum descends below the level of the ischial tuberosities line. Perineal descent indicates weakness of the pelvic floor and is frequently observed in patients with neuropathic fecal incontinence. Sometimes, the patient's straining permits the observer to see the leak of gas or feces. This maneuver is enhanced by asking the patient to sit in special devices that simulate a toilet and that include a mirror in its inferior plane, allowing a better view of the investigated area with less discomfort for the patient (Fig. 2).

When examining women, the vagina must also be evaluated. Presence of feces in the vagina suggests anovaginal or rectovaginal fistula probably due to obstetric trauma. When large rectoceles are found, it will be observed whether the posterior vaginal wall reaches the vaginal opening during straining.

Palpation

Palpation allows evaluation of sensibility of the perianal area as well as the anal cutaneous reflex. The loss of sensibility in the perianal area suggests a denervation lesion, although it can also be the consequence of surgery. The anal cutaneous reflex (or "wink" reflex) is triggered by stroking the perianal skin (Fig. 3). If present, a sphincter contraction will be observed after stimulation. This spinal reflex finds its afferent and efferent tracts in the pudendal nerves. Its loss suggests pudendal injury.

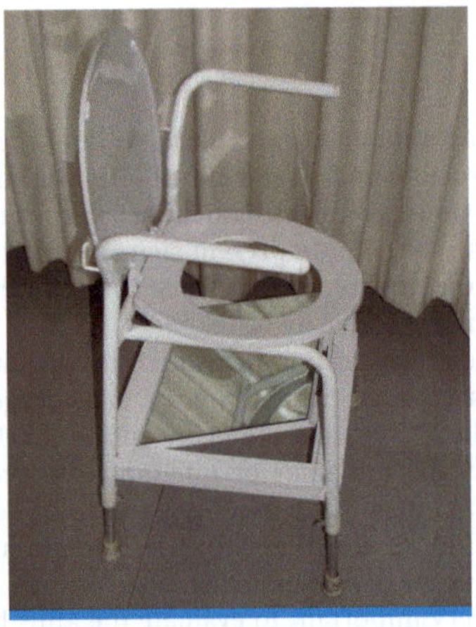

Fig. 2. Special device that simulates a toilet and that includes a mirror in its inferior plane, allowing a better view of the anal and perianal area

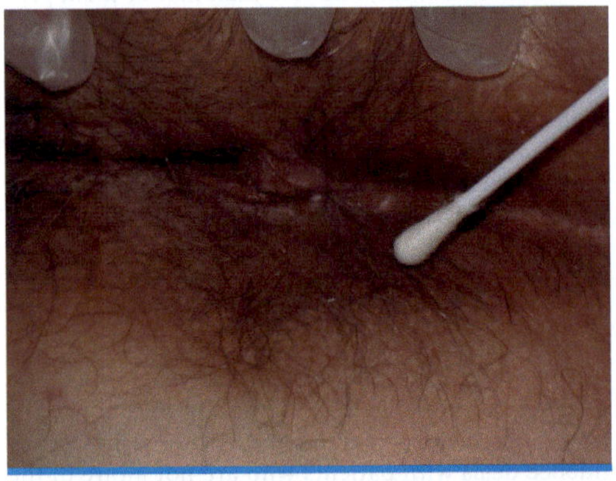

Fig. 3. Anal cutaneous reflex is triggered by stroking the perianal skin. If reflex is present, a sphincter contraction will be observed after stimulation

Digital Examination

When palpating the anal canal in its entire length and circumference, gaps can be observed indicating the presence of sphincter defects. However, the absence of these gaps does not exclude the presence of sphincter defects. Digital examination permits evaluation of the sphincter tone at rest and during squeeze. The positive predictive value of this examination to detect low pressure at rest or during contraction is high [2]. In any case, the perceived tone by digital examination must be considered only as a first approach because it is dependent on multiple factors, including the surgeon's experience, finger measurement of the observer, patient position and cooperation, and coexistence of other illness. As an example, neurologic diseases, even after spinal or cauda equina injuries, may present with an apparently normal sphincter tone, while radial traction at the anal margin or separating the buttocks may show an anal "wink" that normal individuals would not present [3]. Therefore, the assessment of sphincter pressure should rely on anorectal manometry, although this test also has some disadvantages [4].

Digital examination can also evaluate the anal canal length, the integrity of the puborectalis sling, or the anorectal angle by curving the finger above the posterior puborectalis sling at the level of the anorectal junction. Elevation of pelvic floor and perineum can be determined by requesting the patient to provide a voluntary contraction.

The anal canal is most often empty of feces. Finding fecal bolus after digital examination suggests overflow incontinence, which is usually seen in elderly patients or in patients who present a megarectum. Fecal bolus is the most frequent cause of incontinence in the elderly. Nevertheless, in up to 30% of elderly patients who present with large quantity of stool in the upper rectum and sigmoid colon–seen by radiological imaging-feces will not descend to the low rectum and, thus, will not be detected by digital examination [5].

Bimanual examination of the rectovaginal septum helps evaluate the thickness and integrity of the perineal body. This structure is usually involved in obstetric injuries. The Valsalva maneuver during bimanual examination will help detect intussusception, rectocele, cystocele, and enterocele.

Endoscopy

Endoluminal examination is needed to evaluate the lumen and mucosa of the rectum and distal colon and to exclude problems such as proctitis, cancer, and benign secretor tumors, such as villous adenomas, solitary rectal ulcer, or inflammatory bowel disease. It is not necessary to perform a full examination of the colon unless incontinence coexists with diarrhea.

Severity Scores

As opposed to other diseases in which it is possible to establish severity scores from clinical investigation, laboratory tests, or radiology imaging-assessment of severity for incontinent patients depends on the information the patient provides. The aim of severity scores is two fold: they help determine symptom severity and allow comparison of results of the different available treatments. Even if the International Foundation for Functional Gastrointestinal Disorders [6] and the American College of Gastroenterology [7] recommend the use of severity scores, their clinical usefulness has not been demonstrated apart for research purposes.

Two kinds of scores have been proposed to assess severity for incontinence: grading scales and summary scales. Grading scales determine severity by assigning sequential punctuation to incontinent syndromes depending on the type of rectal content the patient is incontinent to, and by considering incontinence to gas; the least important is the latter, and incontinence to solid feces the most important. The most popular grading scale is the Browning and Parks [8] scale (Table 1). This particular score assumes that the more consistent the leaked material is, the greater the damage that can be expected in the sphincter structures. This is the reason that leakage of solid feces is considered more severe than leakage of gas. However, assessment of incontinence severity provided by physicians seems not to be coincident

Table 1. Browing and Parks Scale

Category 1	Category 2	Category 3	Category 4
Normal	Difficult control of flatus & diarrhea	No control of diarrhea	No control of solid stool

Table 2. Cleveland Clinic Florida Fecal Incontinence Score (CCF-FIS)

	Frequency				
Type of incontinence	**Never**	**Rarely**	**Sometimes**	**Usually**	**Always**
Solid	0	1	2	3	4
Liquid	0	1	2	3	4
Gas	0	1	2	3	4
Wears pads	0	1	2	3	4
Lifestyle alteration	0	1	2	3	4

Never 0, *Rarely* <1 month, *Sometimes* <1 week to ≥1 month, *Usually* <1 day to ≥1 week, *Always* ≥1 day

with patients' perceptions [9]. Besides, grading scales have the disadvantage of not taking into consideration the frequency of leakage episodes. These scales are not subtle enough to discriminate among minor differences in incontinence severity and, therefore, to assess slight changes in continence achieved after treatment, which can be of clinical interest. However, grading scales are still used indirectly in studies that review long-term results of incontinence surgery, as such scales assess the kind of rectal content to which the patient is incontinent [10]. Summary scales take into consideration the kind of content and frequency of leakage. Ten scales that consider only clinical data have been proposed. Among them, the Cleveland Clinic Florida Fecal Incontinence Score (CCF-FIS) [11] and those by Pescatori et al. [12], Rockwood et al. [9], and Vaizey et al. [13] have gained greater acceptance. These scales share more similarities than differences. However, the main differences concern the evaluation of quality of life items [11, 13], consideration of constipating treatment, the definition of urgency as the impossibility to defer defecation more than 15 min [13], the fact that it is the patient who punctuates himself or herself [9], and the fact that only the frequency of the most severe type of incontinence is weighted [12]. Even if the scales that use ordinal values seem more perfect, their design presents some weaknesses:

- None of these scales take into consideration defecation frequency, and therefore, in patients with low defecation frequency, incontinence can be underestimated.
- Considering quality of life items may induce errors in the assessment of incontinence severity, as quality of life can depend on the patient's situation totally unrelated to incontinence.
- Considering the use of pads is an error factor, as patients can wear them continuously to prevent soiling in case of leakage, even if leakage is actually not occurring frequently.
- The difference between liquid and solid leakage has not been validated as a factor influencing severity of incontinence.
- The difference between scales where point assignment is made by the physician and those where it is made by the patient has not been assessed. Dis-

Table 3. Vaizey Score: the need to wear a pad or plug, taking constipating medicines, and lack of ability to defer defecation for 15 min

	Frequency				
Type of incontinence	**Never**	**Rarely**	**Sometimes**	**Weekly**	**Daily**
Incontinence for solid stool	0	1	2	3	4
Incontinence for liquid stool	0	1	2	3	4
Incontinence for gas	0	1	2	3	4
Alteration in lifestyle	0	1	2	3	4
Need to wear a pad or plug				0	2
Taking constipating medicines				0	2
Lack of ability to defer defecation for 15 min				0	4

Never no episodes in the past 4 weeks, *Rarely* 1 episode in the past 4 weeks, *Sometimes* >1 episode in the past 4 weeks but <1 a week, *Weekly* 1 or more episodes a week but <1 a day, *Daily* 1 or more episodes a day

tress caused by incontinence can only be reported subjectively, and therefore, it would seem sensible that the patient assign the points. However, this same reason can become a weakness. As refined as the scales can be, they will always be dependent on what the patient reports.

- The attitude of the patient toward incontinence can also alter punctuation if the completely incontinent patient avoids moving far from the toilet.

Another controversial issue concerning the use of scoring systems is the method of data collection. Questionnaires fulfilled in the office and defecation diaries given to the patient can be used. In the first instance, collection depends on the patient's memory. Concerning the usefulness of the second method, which at first seems more consistent, it can be argued that studies evaluating similar diaries for pain [14] show how most patients keep the information without reporting at least for 1 day. In that case, information would not be of better quality than that obtained by questionnaires.

It is difficult to say that summary scales are better than grading scales, because studies evaluating reliability and validity of severity scores are scarce [13]. Finally, the most popular scale is the CCF-FIS [11] (Table 2). However, if assessment of urgency is considered important, then the most suitable scale is that by Vaizey et al. [13] (Table 3). It is also interesting to note that population studies that evaluate the use of scores show how they are rarely used except in referral centers [15].

References

1. Leigh RJ, Turnberg LA (1982) Faecal incontinence: the unvoiced symptom. Lancet 1(8285):1349–1351
2. Hill J, Corson RJ, Brandon H et al (1994) History and examination in the assessment of patients with idiopathic fecal incontinence. Dis Colon Rectum 37:473–477
3. Hardcastle JD, Porter NH (1969) Anal continence. In: Morson BC, ed. Diseases of the colon, rectum and anus. Appleton-Century-Crofts, New York, p 251
4. Eckhardt VF, Kanzler G (1993) How reliable is digital examination for the evaluation of anal sphincter tone? Int J Colorectal Dis 8:95–97
5. Smith RG, Lewis S (1990) The relationship between digital rectal examination and abdominal radiographs in elderly patients. Age Ageing 19:142–143
6. Norton NJ (2004) The perspective of the patient. Gastroenterology 126:S175–S179
7. Rao SSC (2004) Diagnosis and management of fecal incontinence. Practice guidelines. Am J Gastroenterol 99:1585–1604
8. Browning G, Parks A (1983) Postanal repair for neuropathic faecal incontinence: correlation of clinical results and anal canal pressures. Br J Surg 70:101–104
9. Rockwood TH, Church JM, Fleshman JW et al (1999) Patient and surgeon ranking of the severity of symptoms associated with fecal incontinence. The Fecal Incontinence Severity Index. Dis Colon Rectum 42:1525–1532
10. Bravo A, Madoff RD, Lovry AC et al (2004) Long-term results of anterior sphincteroplasty. Dis Colon Rectum 47:727–732
11. Jorge JMN, Wexner SD (1993) Etiology and management of fecal incontinence. Dis Colon Rectum 36:77–97
12. Pescatori M, Anastasio G, Botíni C et al (1992) New grading system and scoring for anal incontinence. Evaluation of 335 patients. Dis Colon Rectum 35:482–487
13. Vaizey CJ, Carapeti E, Cahill JA, Kamm MA (1999) Prospective comparison of faecal incontinence grading systems. Gut 44:77–80
14. Stone AA, Shiffman S, Schwartz JE et al (2002) Patient non-compliance with paper diaries. BMJ 324:1193–1194
15. Dobben AC, Terra MP, Deutekom M et al (2005) Diagnostic work-up for faecal incontinence in daily clinical practice in the Netherlands. Neth J Med 63:265–269

Diagnosis of Fecal Incontinence

9

Satish S. Rao, Junaid Siddiqui

Introduction

Fecal incontinence is a consequence of functional disturbances in the mechanisms that regulate continence and defecation. In this chapter, we review the functional anatomy and physiology of the anorectum, pathogenic mechanisms, and diagnostic approaches for fecal incontinence.

Functional Anatomy and Physiology of the Anorectum

Pelvic Floor

The pelvic floor is a dome-shaped, striated muscular sheet that encloses the bladder, uterus, and rectum. Together with the anal sphincters, it has an important role in the regulation, storage, and evacuation of urine and stool. The neuromuscular integrity of the rectum, anus, and adjoining pelvic floor musculature help to maintain normal continence. The levator ani, which forms the pelvic diaphragm, consist of four contiguous muscles, i.e., pubococcygeus, ileococcygeus, coccygeus, and puborectalis. These muscles are attached peripherally to the pubic body, the ischial spine, and the arcus tendinous, a condensation of obturator fascia in between these areas.

Rectum and Anal Canal

The rectum is a 15- to 20-cm-long hollow muscular tube that extends from the rectosigmoid junction at the level of the third sacral vertebra to the anal orifice (Fig. 1). It is made up of a continuous layer of longitudinal muscle that interlaces with the underlying circular muscle. This unique muscle arrangement enables the rectum to serve both as a reservoir for stool and as a pump for emptying stool. Derived from the embryological hindgut, the upper rectum generally contains feces and can distend toward the peritoneal cavity [1]. The lower part, derived from the cloaca, is surrounded by condensed extraperitoneal connective tissue and is generally empty in normal subjects except during defecation.

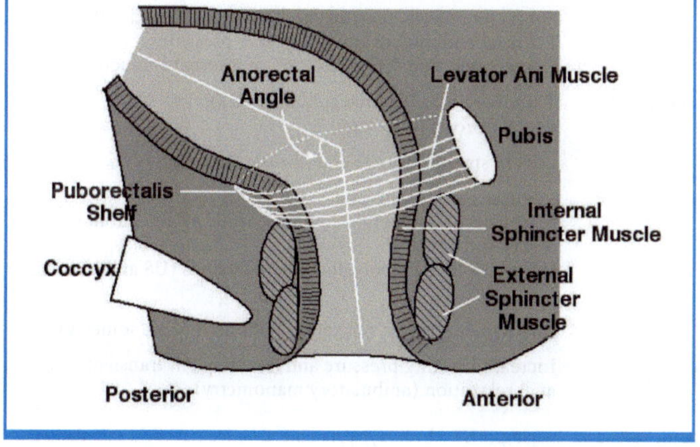

Fig. 1. Diagram of rectum, anal canal, and adjacent structures. The pelvic barrier includes the anal sphincters and pelvic floor muscle

The anal canal is a muscular tube 2- to 4.5-cm long, which at rest forms an angle with the axis of the rectum. At rest, the anorectal angle is approximately 90°. During voluntary squeeze, the angle becomes more acute, approximately 70°, and during defecation, it becomes more obtuse, about 110–130°. The proximal 10 mm of the anal canal is lined by columnar mucosa. The next 15 mm (including the valves) is lined by stratified columnar epithelium. Distal to that is about 10 mm of thick, nonhairy, stratified epithelium called the pecten. The most distal 5–10 mm is lined by hairy skin. The anal sphincter consists of the internal anal sphincter, which is a 0.3- to 0.5-cm-thick expansion of the circular smooth muscle layer of the rectum, and the external anal sphincter, which is a 0.6- to 1-cm-thick expansion of the striated levator ani muscle. Morphologically, both sphincters are separate and heterogeneous [2]. The anus is normally closed by the tonic activity of the internal anal sphincter, and this barrier is reinforced by the voluntary squeeze of the external anal sphincter. The anal mucosal folds together with the expansile, and vascular cushions provide a tight seal. These mechanical barriers are augmented by the puborectalis muscle, which forms a flap-like valve that creates a forward pull and reinforces the anorectal angle to prevent incontinence [2].

The pelvic floor and anorectum are innervated by sympathetic, parasympathetic, and somatic fibers [3]. The nerve supply to the rectum and anal canal is derived from the superior, middle, and inferior rectal plexus. Parasympathetic fibers in the superior and middle rectal plexus synapse with the postganglionic neurons in the myenteric plexus of the rectal wall. The principal somatic innervation to the anorectum is from the pudendal nerve, which arises from the second, third, and fourth sacral nerves (S2, S3, S4), and innervates the external anal sphincter, the anal mucosa, and the rectal wall. This is a mixed nerve and subserves both sensory and motor function [4], and its course through the pelvic floor makes it vulnerable to stretch injury, particularly during vaginal delivery.

The physiological factors that prevent fecal incontinence include the pelvic barrier, rectal compliance and sensation, and other factors such as stool consistency, mobility, etc. In this section, we discuss these factors.

Pelvic Barrier

The internal anal sphincter is responsible for maintaining approximately 70% of the resting anal tone, and this is largely due to tonic sympathetic excitation [5]. The external anal sphincter, which is mostly made up of striated muscle, contributes to the remaining component of the resting tone. The external anal sphincter, the puborectalis, and the levator ani contract further when necessary to preserve continence but relax nearly completely during evacuation. External sphincter contraction may be voluntary or reflexive (e.g., when intra-abdominal pressure increases). Anal resting and/or squeeze pressures are generally reduced in patients with fecal incontinence, suggesting sphincter weakness (Table 1). Inward traction exerted by the puborectalis is reduced in fecal incontinence and is correlated more closely with symptoms than with squeeze pressures, and improves after biofeedback [6].

Common causes of anal sphincter weakness include sphincter damage, neuropathy, or reduced

Table 1. Structural and functional disturbances of the human anal sphincters in disease

Sphincter: condition	Finding (methods)
Internal and external sphincters—FI	Sphincter defects, scarring, and atrophy (US and MRI)? Reduced and resting and/or squeeze pressures Exaggerated transient relaxation of internal sphincter?
Rectum and internal sphincter—scleroderma and FI	Thinning of the internal sphincter (US)? Rectal fibrosis (histology)
Internal sphincter—neurogenic FI	Loss of smooth muscle and fibrosis (histology)?
Internal sphincter—neurogenic FI	Reduced response to pharmacological agents (e.g., catecholaminergic and muscarinic agents but not 5-HT) and EFS?
Internal sphincter—proctalgia Fugax and constipation	Hypertrophy with polyglucosan inclusions (US and histology)?
Internal sphincter—pruritus ani	Abnormal transient relaxation (ambulatory manometry)
Internal sphincter—chronic anal fissure	Increased resting pressure and less frequent transient anal relaxation (ambulatory manometry)

FI fecal incontinence, *US* ultrasound, *MRI* magnetic resonance imaging, *5-HT* 5 hydroxytryptamine, *EFS* electrical field stimulation

input from the cortex or spinal cord. Following is a list of etiologies of fecal incontinence:

- Anal sphincter weakness
- Injury: obstetric trauma related to surgical procedures (e.g., hemorrhoidectomy, internal sphincterotomy, fistulotomy, anorectal infection)
- Nontraumatic: scleroderma, internal sphincter thinning of unknown etiology
- Neuropathy
- Stretch injury, obstetric trauma, diabetes mellitus
- Anatomical disturbances of pelvic floor
- Fistula, rectal prolapse, descending perineum syndrome
- Inflammatory conditions
- Crohn's disease, ulcerative colitis, radiation proctitis
- Central nervous system diseases
- Dementia, stroke, brain tumors, spinal cord lesions, multiple system atrophy (Shy-Drager syndrome), multiple sclerosis
- Diarrhea
- Irritable bowel syndrome, postcholecystectomy diarrhea

Rectal Compliance and Sensation

Distention of the rectum by stool is associated with several processes that serve to preserve continence, or if circumstances are appropriate, to proceed with defecation. Stool is often transferred into the rectum by colonic high-amplitude propagating contractions, which mostly occur after awakening or after meals [7]. It is likely that rectal contents are periodically sensed by the process of "anorectal sampling" [8, 9]. This process may be facilitated by transient relaxation of the internal anal sphincter, which allows the movement of stool or flatus from the rectum into the upper anal canal. Here they may come into contact with the specialized sensory end organs, such as the numerous Krause end-bulbs, Golgi-Mazzoni bodies and genital corpuscles, and the relatively sparse Meissner's corpuscles and pacinian corpuscles [10]. Specialized afferent nerves for touch, cold, tension, and friction subserves these organized nerve endings. An intact sampling reflex allows the individual to choose whether to discharge or retain rectal contents, whereas an impaired sampling reflex may predispose to incontinence. In contrast, the rectal epithelium shows no organized nerve endings [11]. Myelinated and unmyelinated nerve fibers are present adjacent to the rectal mucosa, the submucosa, and the myenteric plexus. These subserve the sensation of distention and stretch. This also mediates the viscerovisceral, the rectoanal inhibitory, and the rectoanal contractile responses [12]. The sensation of rectal distention travels along the parasympathetic system to S2, S3, and S4 [11]. Thus, the sacral nerves are intimately involved with the sensory, motor, and autonomic function of the anorectum and in maintaining continence. Anal sphincter pressure is reduced in most but not all incontinent patients [13]. While most attention has focused on anal sphincter weakness, studies using dynamometer [6] and dynamic magnetic resonance imaging (MRI) [14] have demonstrated weakness of the puborectalis muscle in fecal incontinence.

Other Factors

In addition to normal anorectal function, there are other factors that preserve continence. These include normal stool consistency, intact mental faculties, and adequate physical mobility.

Etiology of Fecal Incontinence

Fecal incontinence occurs when one or more mechanisms that maintain continence are disrupted to an extent that another mechanism(s) is unable to compensate. Thus the cause of fecal incontinence if often multifactorial [13–17]. In a prospective study, 80% of patients had more than one pathogenic abnormality [17]. Following is a list of important information that should be elicited when taking a history in a patient with suspected fecal incontinence:

- Onset and precipitating event(s)
- Duration, severity, and timing
- Stool consistency and urgency
- Coexisting problems/surgery/urinary incontinence/back injury
- Obstetrics: history of forceps delivery, tears, breech presentation, repair
- Drugs, caffeine, diet
- Clinical subtypes: passive or urge incontinence or fecal seepage
- Clinical grading of severity
- History of fecal impaction

The precise role of obstetric trauma and fecal incontinence is unclear, although a clinically overt anal tear occurred in approximately 3.3% of women after vaginal delivery [18]. However, endoanal ultrasound identified anal sphincter defects in 35% of women after their first vaginal delivery [19]. Other important risk factors include forceps delivery, prolonged second stage of labor, large birth weight, and occipitoposterior presentation [20–22]. Perineal tears, even when carefully repaired, can be associated with incontinence, and patients may present with incontinence either immediately following delivery or several years later [19].

Other causes of anatomical disruption include iatrogenic factors such as anorectal surgery for hemorrhoids, fistulae, or fissures and proctitis after radiotherapy for prostate cancer. Postoperative fecal incontinence may affect up to 45% of patients after lateral internal sphincterotomy; 6%, 8%, and 1% reported incontinence to flatus, minor fecal soiling, and loss of solid stool, respectively, 5 years later [23]. Incontinence following lateral internal sphincterotomy does not appear to recover in the long term and appears to be an independent cause of fecal incontinence [24]. Similarly, the risk of fecal incontinence after fistulotomy ranges from 18% to 52% [25]. The internal anal sphincter is occasionally and inadvertently damaged during hemorrhoidectomy [26]. The risk of developing fecal incontinence is about 28.3% in patients receiving "closed" hemorrhoidectomy by Ferguson technique [27], which is now considered a gold standard for hemorrhoidectomy. Pelvic radiotherapy results in chronic anorectal complications, i.e., fistula, stricture, and disabling fecal incontinence, in approximately 5% of patients [28]. In the absence of structural defects, internal anal sphincter dysfunction may occur because of myopathy [29, 30] or internal anal sphincter degeneration [30].

Several neurologic disorders interfere with either sensory perception or motor function or both. Central nervous system disorders that may cause incontinence include multiple sclerosis, dementia, stroke, brain tumors, sedation, and dorsal and spinal cord lesions or injury [31–34]. Peripheral nervous system disorders include diabetic neuropathy, cauda equina lesions, alcohol-induced neuropathy, or traumatic neuropathy [33, 35, 36].

Skeletal muscle disorders such as muscular dystrophy, myasthenia gravis, and other myopathies can affect external anal sphincter and puborectalis function. Reconstructive procedures such as ileoanal or coloanal pouches can increase anorectal capacity and may improve continence [37, 38]. However, up to 40% of patients with an ileoanal pouch experience periodic, often nocturnal, fecal incontinence, possibly related to uncoordinated pouch contractions [39]. Similarly, rectal prolapse may be associated with fecal incontinence in up to 88% of cases [40–42].

Conditions that decrease rectal compliance and accommodation may also cause fecal incontinence. Besides radiation-induced inflammation and fibrosis, other etiologies include ulcerative colitis or Crohn's disease [43–45] and infiltration of the rectum by tumor, ischemia, or following radical hysterectomy [45]. Patients with fecal seepage and/or staining of undergarments often have dyssynergic defecation and incomplete evacuation of stool [46]. Many of these subjects also exhibit impaired rectal sensation [46, 47].

In summary, the origin of fecal incontinence is multifactorial. Hence, it is very important to identify etiologies that may contribute to this condition. . In the following section, we discuss the clinical assessment of fecal incontinence.

Clinical Assessment of Fecal Incontinence

Clinical evaluation, along with the formulation a of diagnostic strategy is essential in for establishing an accurate diagnosis. Many patients who suffer with fecal incontinence inadvertently refer to this condition as "diarrhea" or "urgency" [48]. Thus, the very first step is to establish a rapport with the patient and carefully inquire about the presence of fecal incontinence. Also, it is important to identify whether the patient has passive or urge incontinence or fecal seepage and to grade its severity based on a prospective stool diary. This in combination with physiological testing and imaging will help to determine the underlying pathophysiology and facilitate optimal treatment [49].

Clinical Features

A detailed history is required on the initial visit or contact with the patient. A list of important information that should be elicited when taking history is outlined in under the previous heading: "Etiology of Fecal Incontinence". The temporal relationship between the onset of fecal incontinence and precipitating events should be established. This includes all prior coexisting conditions (diabetes mellitus, etc.), surgeries, spinal injuries, history of physical or sexual abuse, and exposure to radiation. The duration of symptoms should be determined in terms of acute, subacute, or chronic. Incontinence severity is determined by several grading systems. A modified Cleveland Clinic grading system [50] has been validated by investigators at St. Mark's Hospital in the United Kingdom [51]. It provides an objective method of quantifying the degree of incontinence. It can also be used for assessing the efficacy of therapy. The grading system is based on seven parameters that include whether the anal discharge is either solid, liquid, or flatus and whether the problem causes alterations in lifestyle (scores: Never = 0, Always = 5); the need to wear a pad or the need to take antidiarrheal medication, and the ability to defer defecation (scores: No = 0, Yes = 2). Scores range from 0 (continent) to 24 (severe incontinence).

The timing or circumstances under which incontinence occurs should also be determined. This may facilitate identification of the following possible scenarios:

1. Passive incontinence: the involuntary discharge of fecal matter or flatus without any awareness. This suggests a loss of perception and/or impaired rectoanal reflexes either with or without sphincter dysfunction.
2. Urge incontinence: the discharge of fecal matter or flatus in spite of active attempts to retain these contents. This is due to sphincter function or rectal capacity to retain stool.
3. Fecal seepage: the undesired leakage of stool, often after a bowel movement, with otherwise normal continence and evacuation. This condition is mostly due to incomplete evacuation of stool and/or impaired rectal sensation. Here, sphincter function and pudendal nerve function are mostly intact.

There can be an overlap between these three groups, but making a clinical distinction is useful in guiding further investigations and management. One cannot rely on these clinical features alone to establish a diagnosis due to lack of specificity and positive predictive values when compared with more standardized testing (anorectal manometry) [22].

The other important aspect of history is to determine dietary habits (use of coffee, fiber in diet, etc.) and determination of the presence of rectoanal agnosia (inability to differentiate between formed and unformed stools). A prospective stool diary provides an objective assessment of stool habit (Fig. 2).

Physical Exam

A detailed physical exam is essential for establishing an accurate diagnosis and for directing the investigations. The key element of a physical exam in a patient with fecal incontinence is a thorough digital rectal exam (DRE), and a detailed neurological exam especially focused on the testing of sacral nerve dysfunction.

Patient should be examined lying in the left lateral position, with good illumination. The exam begins with an inspection to look for the presence of fecal matter, prolapsed hemorrhoids, dermatitis, scars, skin excoriation, absence of perianal creases, or the presence of a gaping anus. Excessive perianal descent or rectal prolapse can be demonstrated by asking the patient to attempt defecation. An outward bulge that exceeds 3 cm is usually defined as excessive perineal descent [52].

The next step is to check for perianal sensation. The anocutaneous reflex examines the integrity of the connection between sensory nerves and skin; intermediate neurons in the spinal cord segments S2, S3, and S4; and motor innervation of the external anal sphincter. This is assessed by gently stroking the perianal skin with a cotton bud in each of the perianal quadrants. The normal response consists of a brisk contraction of the external anal sphincter. Impaired or absent anocutaneous reflex suggests either afferent or efferent neuronal injury [53].

Stool Diary									
PLEASE RECORD YOUR STOOL HABIT FOR ONE WEEK:							Name: Hosp #:		
Date	Time of Bowel Movement	Incontinence Yes/No	Stool Seepage or Staining Yes/No	Stool Consistency (Type 1-7) See Below	Urgency – unable to postpone BM for more than 15 Minutes Yes/No	Use of Pads Yes/No	Medications	Comments	

Fig. 2. Sample stool diary for assessing patients with fecal incontinence. "Use the following descriptions for describing stool consistency: Type 1: Separate hard lumps. Type 2: Sausage shaped but lumpy. Type 3: Like a sausage but with cracks on its surface. Type 4: Like a sausage or snake, smooth and soft. Type 5: Soft blobs with clear-cut edges (passed easily). Type 6: Fluffy pieces with ragged edges, a mushy stool. Type 7: Watery". Reprinted with permission from [49]

A digital rectal exam is done next to assess resting sphincter tone, length of the anal canal, integrity of the puborectalis sling, acuteness of the anorectal angle, strength of the anal muscle, and elevation of the perineum during voluntary squeeze. Some patients are quite sensitive to a digital exam, and one should exercise considerable gentleness and care. Liberal use of lubrication and use of 2% Xylocaine gel is advisable if the patient experiences discomfort during the exam. Accuracy of the digital rectal exam as an objective tool for assessing anal sphincter pressure has been evaluated in several studies. However, sensitivity, specificity, and positive predictive value of the digital rectal exam is very low [54]. By digital rectal exam, the positive predictive value of detecting low sphincter tone was 67% and low squeeze tone 81% [22]. In another study, agreement between digital exam and resting anal canal pressure was 0.41 and 0.52, respectively [55]. These data suggest that a digital exam is not very reliable and is prone to interobserver differences.

Investigations of Fecal Incontinence

These comprise tests to examine the etiology of diarrhea that accompanies incontinence in many patients.

Endoscopy

Endoscopic evaluation of the rectosigmoid region is recommended in order to exclude colonic mucosal inflammation, a rectal mass, or stricture. This can be achieved by doing a flexible sigmoidoscopy, but a colonoscopy is probably more appropriate, particularly in an older individual.

Stool and Blood Testing

Stool studies, including screening for infection, stool volume, stool osmolality, and electrolytes, may be performed in selected cases with refractory diarrhea. Similarly, blood tests may reveal thyroid dysfunction, diabetes, or other metabolic disorders. Because they are common, breath tests to rule out lactose or fructose intolerance or bacterial overgrowth may also be useful.

Specific Tests to Evaluate Fecal Incontinence

Several specific tests are available for defining the underlying mechanisms of fecal incontinence. These tests are often complementary [53, 56]. A brief description of these tests and their clinical relevance is presented here.

Anorectal Manometry and Sensory Testing

Anorectal manometry with rectal sensory testing is the preferred method of defining functional weakness of the external and internal anal sphincters and for detecting abnormal rectal sensation [49]. Anorectal manometry not only provides an objective assessment of anal sphincter pressures but also assesses rectal sensation, rectoanal reflexes, and rectal compliance [49]. Currently, several types of probes and pressure-recording devices are available, and each system has distinct advantages and drawbacks. A water-perfused probe with multiple closed spaced sensors is a commonly used device. Alternatively, a solid-state probe with microtransducers may be used [53, 57]. This equipment, although more fragile and expensive, is easier to calibrate and more accurate [53, 58]. Anal sphincter pressure can be measured by stationary pull through, but a rapid pull-through technique should be abandoned, as this can give falsely high sphincter pressure readings [53, 59]. Resting anal sphincter pressure predominantly represents internal anal sphincter function, and voluntary-squeeze anal sphincter pressure predominantly measures external anal sphincter function.

Patients with incontinence have low resting and low squeeze sphincter pressures [54, 59–61]. The duration of the sustained squeeze pressure provides an index of sphincter muscle fatigue. The ability of the external anal sphincter to contract in a reflex manner can also be assessed during the abrupt increases of intra-abdominal pressure, such as when coughing [13, 53, 57, 58]. This reflex response causes the anal sphincter pressure to rise above that of the rectal pressure in order to preserve continence. The response may be triggered by receptors in the pelvic floor and mediated through a spinal reflex arc. In patients with spinal cord lesions above the conus medullaris, this reflex response is present but the voluntary squeeze may be absent, whereas in patients with lesions of the cauda equina or sacral plexus, both the reflex response and the voluntary squeeze response are absent [53, 62, 63]. The response may be triggered by receptors on the pelvic floor and mediated through a spinal reflex arc.

Rectal Sensitivity

Rectal hyposensitivity (RH) has been reported in patients with fecal incontinence. This is best documented in patients with diabetes mellitus [64] and multiple sclerosis [32] but has also been seen in patients with "idiopathic" fecal incontinence [65–69]. Rectal balloon distention with either air or water can be used for the assessment of both sensory responses and compliance of the rectal wall. By distending a rectal balloon with incremental volumes, it is possible to assess the thresholds for three common sensations: the first detectable sensation (rectal sensory threshold), the sensation or urgency to defecate, and the sensation of pain (maximum tolerable volume). A higher threshold for sensory perception suggests impaired rectal sensation or RH. Also, the balloon volume required for partial or complete inhibition of anal sphincter tone can be assessed. It has been shown that the volume required to induce reflex anal relaxation is lower in incontinent patients [66, 68].

Quantitative assessment of anal perception using either electrical or thermal stimulation has also been advocated. In a study by Rogers et al. [70] anal mucosal sensation was assessed by recording perception threshold for electrical stimulation of the mid anal canal using a ring electrode, and a combined sensory and motor defect was reported in patients with incontinence. In another study, by Cornes et al. [71] although anal canal perception was impaired immediately after a vaginal delivery, there was no difference at 6 months. The role of thermosensitivity appears controversial [12]. In one study, the ability of healthy anal mucosa to differentiate between small changes in temperature was questioned [72]. Hence, under normal conditions, it is not possible to appreciate the temperature of fecal matter passing from the rectum to the anal canal during sampling [72]. Whether patients have a pure sensory defect of anal perception without coexisting sphincter dysfunction or rectal sensory impairment has not been evaluated.

Rectal compliance is calculated by assessing the changes in rectal pressure during balloon distention with either air or fluids. Rectal compliance is reduced in patients with colitis [43, 44], in patients with low spinal cord lesions, and in diabetic patients with incontinence [32, 35, 73]. In contrast, compliance is increased in high spinal cord lesions [33, 63].

In summary, when performed meticulously, anorectal manometry can provide useful information regarding anorectal function [16, 56, 73–75]. A technical review recommended the use of anorectal manometry for the evaluation of patients with incontinence because it can define the functional weakness of one or both sphincters and helps to perform and evaluate the responses to biofeedback training [56]. Manometric tests of anorectal function may also be useful in assessing objective improvement following drug therapy [76], biofeedback therapy [77], or surgery [78].

Balloon Expulsion Test

A balloon expulsion test can identify impaired evacuation in patients with fecal seepage or in those with fecal impaction and overflow. Most normal subjects can expel a balloon containing 50 ml water [56] or a silicon-filled artificial stool from the rectum in less than a minute [79]. In general, most patients with fecal incontinence have little or no difficulty with evacuation. But patients with fecal seepage [46, 50] and many elderly subjects with fecal incontinence secondary to fecal impaction demonstrate impaired evacuation. In these selected patients, a balloon expulsion test [53, 56, 58] may help to identify dyssynergia and facilitate appropriate therapy.

Pudendal Nerve Terminal Motor Latency

Delayed pudendal nerve terminal motor latency (PNTML) is used as a surrogate marker of pudendal nerve injury and to ascertain whether anal sphincter weakness is attributable to pudendal nerve injury, sphincter defect, or both [56]. PNTML may be useful in assessing patients prior to anal sphincter repair and is particularly helpful in predicting the outcome of surgery. PNTML measures the neuromuscular integrity between the terminal portion of the pudendal nerve and the anal sphincter. An injury to the pudendal nerve leads to denervation of the anal sphincter muscle and muscle weakness. Thus, measurement of nerve latency time can help distinguish a weak sphincter muscle due to muscle injury from that due to nerve injury.

Obstetric Trauma and PNTML

Women who delivered vaginally with a prolonged second stage of labor or had forceps-assisted delivery were found to have a prolonged PNTML compared with women who delivered by caesarian section or spontaneously [80–82]. It has also been shown that women with fecal incontinence after an obstetric injury have both pudendal neuropathy and anal sphincter defects [81, 83, 84]. In a retrospective study of 55 patients with fecal incontinence secondary to obstetric trauma and who underwent surgery, five patients with an intact anal sphincter and six with a nonintact anal sphincter had a poor surgical outcome [85]. Thus, neither anal endosonography nor PNTML could predict surgical outcome. One study showed that surgical repair produced a good to excellent result in 80% of women with fecal incontinence but without pudendal neuropathy compared with 11% of women with neuropathy [81]. Thus, it appears that women with sphincter defects alone fare better following sphincter repair than do women with both sphincter defects and neuropathy. However, two recent reviews of eight uncontrolled studies [80, 86] reported that patients with pudendal neuropathy generally have a poor surgical outcome when compared with those without neuropathy.

A normal PNTML does not exclude pudendal neuropathy. The prognostic value of PNTML will depend to some extent on the degree of each type of injury, the age of the patient, and other coexisting problems [80]. Whether newer tests such as lumboanal or sacroanal motor-evoked potentials provide a more objective and reproducible evaluation of the neuronal innervation of the anorectum remains to be explored [87].

Saline Infusion Test

The saline infusion test can serve as a simple method for evaluating fecal incontinence, in particular for assessing clinical improvement after surgery or biofeedback therapy. This test assesses the overall capacity of the defecation unit to maintain continence during conditions that simulate diarrhea [16, 57, 60, 74, 77, 88].

With the patient lying on the bed, a 2-mm plastic tube is introduced approximately 10 cm into the rectum and taped in position. Next, the patient is transferred to a commode. The tube is connected to an infusion pump, and either 1,500 ml [60, 88] or 800 ml [16, 57, 58] of warm saline (37°C) is infused into the rectum at a rate of 60 ml/min. The patient is instructed to hold the liquid for as long as possible. The volume of saline infused at the onset of the first leak (defined as a leak of at least 15 ml) and the total volume retained at the end of infusion are recorded [16, 57, 60, 88]. Most normal subjects should retain most of this volume without leakage [16, 57], whereas patients with fecal incontinence [54, 60, 77] or patients with impaired rectal compliance, such as ulcerative colitis [88], leak at much lower volumes. The test is also useful in assessing objective improvement of fecal incontinence after biofeedback therapy [77].

Clinical Utility of Tests for Fecal Incontinence

A diagnostic test is useful if it can provide information regarding the patients underlying pathophysiology, confirm a clinical suspicion, or guide clinical management. There are five studies that have evaluated clinical utility of testing patients with incontinence. In one prospective study, history alone could detect an underlying cause in only nine of 80 patients (11%) with fecal incontinence, whereas physiological tests revealed an abnormality in 44 patients (55%) [89]. Undoubtedly, the aforementioned tests help to define the underlying mechanisms, but there is only limited information regarding their clinical utility and their impact on management.

In a large retrospective study of 302 patients with fecal incontinence, an underlying pathophysiological abnormality was identified but only after performing manometry, electromyelogram (EMG), and rectal sensory testing [13]. Most patients had more than one pathophysiologic abnormality. In another large study of 350 patients, incontinent patients had lower resting and squeeze sphincter pressures, a smaller rectal capacity, and leaked earlier following saline infusion in the rectum [74]. However, both a single test or a combination of three different tests (anal manometry, rectal capacity, saline continence test) provided low discriminatory value between continent and incontinent patients. This emphasizes the wide range of normal values and the ability of the body to compensate for the loss of any one mechanism. In a prospective study, anorectal manometry with sensory testing not only confirmed a clinical impression but also provided new information that was not detected clinically [16]. Furthermore, the diagnostic information obtained from these studies influenced both management and outcome of patients with incontinence [16]. A single abnormality was found in 20% of patients, whereas more than one abnormality was found in 80% [16, 17]. In another study, abnormal sphincter pressure was found in 40 patients (71%), whereas altered rectal sensation or poor rectal compliance was present in 42 patients (75%) [88]. These findings have been further confirmed by another study, which showed that physiological tests provided a definitive diagnosis in 66% of patients with incontinence [90].

However, based on these tests alone, it is not possible to predict whether an individual patient is continent or incontinent. Consequently, an abnormal test result must be interpreted along with the patient's symptoms and other complementary tests. Tests of anorectal function provide objective data and define the underlying pathophysiology; most of this information cannot be detected clinically.

Conclusion

Fecal continence is maintained in healthy individuals by various physiological factors, and disruption of these factors may result in fecal incontinence. Fecal incontinence is often multifactorial, and a systematic approach is required to make a correct diagnosis. This includes a thorough history, physical examination, selective laboratory testing, endoscopy, and specific physiological testing. These specific tests are often complementary, and the diagnostic information obtained can influence the management and outcome of patients with fecal incontinence.

References

1. William PL, Warwick R (1980) Splanchnology. In: Grays Anatomy, 36th edn. Churchill Livingston, London, pp 1356–1364
2. Matzel KE, Schmidt RA, Tanagho EA (1990) Neuroanatomy of the striated muscle anal continence mechanism. Implications for the use of neurostimulation. Dis Colon Rectum 33:666–673
3. William PL, Warwick R (1980) Neurology. In: Gray's Anatomy, 36th edn. Churchill Livingston, London, pp 1122–1136
4. Gunterberg B, Kewenter J, Peterson I et al (1976) Anorectal function after major resections of the sacrum with bilateral or unilateral sacrifice of sacral nerves. Br J Surg 63:546–554
5. Frenckner B, Ihre T (1976) Influence of autonomic nerve on the internal anal sphincter in man. Gut 17:306–312
6. Fernandez Fraga X, Azpinoz F, Malagelada JR (2002) Significance of pelvic floor muscles in anal incontinence. Gastroenterology 123:1441–1450
7. Bassotti G, Crowell MD, Whitehead WE (1993) contractile activity of the human colon: lessons from 24 hour studies. Gut 34:129–133
8. Duthie HL, Bennett RC (1963) The relation of sensation in the anal canal to the functional anal sphincter: a possible factor in anal continence. Gut 4:179–182
9. Miller R, Bartolo DC, Cervero F et al (1988) Anorectal sampling: a comparison of normal and incontinent patients. Br J Surg 75:44–47
10. Duthie HL, Gaines FW (1960) Sensory nerve endings and sensation in the anal region of man. Br J Surg 47:585–595
11. Goligher JC, Huges ESR (1951) Sensibility of the rectum and colon. Its role in the mechanism of anal continence. Lancet 1:543–547
12. Rogers J (1992) Anal and rectal sensation. In: Henry MM, ed. Bailliere clinical gastroenterology. Bailliere Tindall, London, pp 179–181
13. Sun WM, Donnelly TC, Read NW (1992) Utility of a combined test of anorectal manometry, electromyography, and sensation in determining the mechanism of 'idiopathic' faecal incontinence. Gut 33:807–813
14. Devroede G, Phillips S, Pemberton J, Shorter R (1991) Functions of the anorectum: defecation and anal continence: the large intestine physiology and disease. Raven, New York, pp 115
15. Bharucha AE, Fletcher JG, Harper CM et al (2005) Relationship between symptoms and disordered continence mechanisms in women with idiopathic fecal incontinence. Gut 54:546–555
16. Rao SSC, Patel RS (1997) How useful are manometric tests of anorectal function in the management of defecation disorders. Am J Gastroenteric 92:469–475
17. Rao SSC (1999) Fecal incontinence. Clinical perspectives in gastroenterology 2:277–288
18. Samuelsson E, Ladfors L, Wennerholm UB et al (2000) Anal sphincter tears: prospective study of obstetric risk factors. BJOG 107:926–931
19. Sultan AH, Kamm MA, Hudson CN et al (1993) Analsphincter disruption during vaginal delivery. N Engl J Med 329:1905–1911
20. Engel AF, Kamm MA, Bartram CI et al (1995) Relationship of symptoms in fecal incontinence to specific sphincter abnormalities. Int J Colorectal Dis 10:152–155
21. Gee AS, Durdey P (1995) Urge incontinence of faeces is a maker of severe external anal sphincter dysfunction. Br J Surg 82:1179–1182
22. Hill J, Corson RJ, Brandon H et al (1994) History and examination in the assessment of patients with idiopathic fecal incontinence. Dis Colon Rectum 37:473–477
23. Nyam DC, Pemberton JH (1999) Long term results of lateral internal sphincterotomy for chronic anal fissure with particular reference to incidence of fecal incontinence. Dis colon rectum 42:1306–1310
24. Rotholtz NA, Bun M et al (2005) Long-term assessment of fecal incontinence after lateral internal sphincterotomy. Tech Coloproctol 9(2):115–118
25. Del Pino A, Nelson RL, Pearl RK, Abcarian H (1996) Island flap anoplasty for treatment of transsphincteric fistula-in-ano. Dis Colon Rectum 39:224–226
26. Abbsakoor F, Nelson M, Beynon J et al (1998) Anal endosonography in patients with anorectal symptoms after hemorrhoidectomy. Br J Surg 85:1522–1524
27. Guenin MO, Rosenthal R, Kern B et al (2005) Ferguson hemorrhoidectomy: long-term results and patient satisfaction after Ferguson's hemorrhoidectomy. Dis Colon Rec 48(8):1523–1527
28. Hayne D, Vaizey CJ, Boulos PB (2001) Anorectal injury following pelvic radiotherapy. Br J Surg 88:1037–1048
29. Engel AF, Kamm MA, Talbot IC (1994) Progressive systemic sclerosis of the internal anal sphincter leading to passive faecal incontinence. Gut 35:857–859
30. Vaizey JS, Kamm MA, Bartram CI (1997) Primary degeneration of the internal anal sphincter as a cause of passive faecal incontinence. Lancet 349:612–615
31. Glickman S, Kamm MA (1996) Bowel dysfunction in spinal cord injury patients. Lancet 347:1651–1653
32. Caruana BJ, Wald A, Hinds J et al (1991) Anorectal sensory and motor function in neurogenic fecal incontinence. Comparison between multiple sclerosis and diabetes mellitus. Gastroenterology 100:465–470
33. Krogh K, Nielson J, Djurhuus JC et al (1997) Colorectal function in patients with spinal cord lesions. Dis Colon Rectum 40:1233–1239
34. Brittain KR, Peet SM, Castleden CM (1998) Stroke and incontinence (review) Stroke 29:524–528
35. Sun WM, Katsinelos P, Horowitz M et al (1996) Disturbances in anorectal function in patients with diabetes mellitus and faecal incontinence. Eur J Gastroenterol Hepatol 8:1007–1012
36. Schiller LR, Santa Ana CA, Schmulen AC et al (1982) Pathogenesis of fecal incontinence in diabetes melli-

tus: evidence for internal-anal-sphincter dysfunction. N Engl J Med 307:1666–1671
37. Parks AG, Nicholls FJ (1978) Proctocolectomy without ileostomy for ulcerative colitis. Br Med J 2:85–88
38. Berger A, Tiret E, Parc R et al (1992) Excision of the rectum with colonic J pouch-anal anastomosis for the adenocarcinoma of the low and mid-rectum. World J Surg 16:470–477
39. Levitt MD, Kamm MA, Van DS Jr et al (1994) Ambulatory pouch and anal motility in patients with ileo-anal reservoirs. Int J Colorectal Dis 9:40–44
40. Farouk R, Duthie GS, MacGregor AB et al (1994) Rectoanal inhibition and incontinence in patients with rectal prolapse. Br J Surg 81:743–746
41. Farouk R, Duthie GS, Bartolo DC et al (1992) Restoration of continence following rectopexy for rectal prolapse and recovery of the internal anal sphincter electromyogram. Br J Surg 79:439–440
42. Felt-Bersma RJF, Cuesta MA (2001) Rectal prolapse, rectal intussusception, rectocele and solitary rectal ulcer syndrome. Gastroenterol Clin North Am 30:199–222
43. Rao SSC, Read NW, Davison P et al (1987) Anorectal sensitivity and responses to rectal distention in patients with ulcerative colitis. Gastroenterology 89:1020–1026
44. Farthing MJG, Lennard-Jones JE (1978) Sensibility of the rectum to distention and the anorectal distention reflex in ulcerative colitis. Gut 19:64–69
45. Herbst F, Kamm MA, Morris GP et al (1997) Gastrointestinal transit and prolonged ambulatory colonic motility in health and feacal incontinence. Gut 41:381–389
46. Rao SSC, Kempf J, Stessman M (1998) Anal seepage: sphincter dysfunction or incomplete evacuation? Gastroenterology 114:A824
47. Rao SSC, Kempf J, Stessman M (1999) Is biofeedback therapy (BT) useful in patients with anal seepage? Gastroenterology 116:G4636
48. Leigh RJ, Turnberg LA (1982) Faecal incontinence: the unvoiced symptom. Lancet 1:1349–1351
49. Rao SSC (2004) Diagnosis and management of fecal incontinence. Practice guidelines: American College of Gastroenterology Practice Parameters Committee. Am J Gastroenterol 99(8):1585–1604
50. Jorge JM, Wexner SD (1993) Etiology and management of fecal incontinence [review]. Dis Colon Rectum 36(1):77–97
51. Vaizey CJ, Carapeti E, Cahill JA et al (1999) Prospective comparison of faecal incontinence grading systems. Gut 44:77–80
52. Harewood GC, Coulie B, Camilleri M et al (1999) Descending perineum syndrome: audit of clinical and laboratory features and outcome of pelvic floor retraining. Am J Gastroenterol 94:126–130
53. Rao SSC, Sun WM (1997) Current techniques of assessing defecation dynamics. Dig Dis 15 (Suppl 1): 64–67
54. Felt-Bersma RJ, Klinkenberg-Knol EC, Meuwissen SGM (1988) Investigation of anorectal function. Br J Surg 75:53–55
55. Eckhardt VF, Kanzler G (1993) How reliable is digital rectal examination for the evaluation of anal sphincter tone? Int J Colorectal Dis 8:95–97
56. Diamant NE, Kamm MA, Wald A et al (1999) AGA technical review on anorectal testing techniques. Gastroenterology 94:735–760
57. Rao SSC (1997) Manometric evaluation of defecation disorders, part II: fecal incontinence. Gastroenterologist 5(2):99–111
58. Rao SSC, Hatfield R, Leistikow J et al (1999) Manometric tests of anorectal function in healthy humans. Am J Gastroenterol 94:773–783
59. McHugh SM, Diamant NE (1987) Effect of age, gender and parity on anal canal pressures. Contribution of impaired anal sphincter function to fecal incontinence. Dig Dis Sci 32:726–736
60. Read NW, Harford WF, Schmulen AC et al (1979) A clinical study of patients with fecal incontinence and diarrhea. Gastroenterology 76:747–756
61. Read NW, Bartollo DC, Read MG (1989) Differences in anal function in patients with incontinence to solids and in patients with incontinence to liquids. Br J Surg 71:39–42
62. Sun W, MacDonagh R, Forster D et al (1995) Anorectal function in patients with complete spinal transection before and after sacral posterior rhizotomy. Gastroenterology 108:990–998
63. MacDonagh R, Sun WM, Thomas DG et al (1992) Anorectal function in patients with complete supraconal spinal cord lesions. Gut 33:1532–1538
64. Wald A, Tunugunta AK (1984) Anorectal sensorimotor dysfunction in fecal incontinence and diabetes mellitus. Modification with biofeedback therapy. N Eng J Med 310:1282–1287
65. Azpiroz F, Enck P, Whitehead WE (2002) Anorectal functional testings: review of collective experience. Am J Gastroenterol 97:232–240
66. Hancke E, Schurholz M (1987) Impaired rectal sensation in idiopathic faecal incontinence. Int J Colorectal Dis 2:146–148
67. Lubowski DZ, Nicholls RJ (1988) Faecal incontinence associated with reduced pelvic sensation. Br J Surg 75:1086–1088
68. Sun WM, Read NW, Miner PB (1990) Relation between rectal sensation and anal function in normal subjects and patients with faecal incontinence. Gut 31:1056–1061
69. Hoffmann BA, Timmcke AE, Gathright JB Jr et al (1995) Fecal seepage and soiling: a problem of rectal sensation. Dis Colon Rectum 38:746–748
70. Rogers J, Henry MM, Misiewicz JJ (1988) Combined motor and sensory deficit in primary neuropathic fecal incontinence. Gut 29:5–9
71. Cornes H, Bartlolo DC, Stirrat GM (1991) Changes in anal canal sensation after child birth. Br J Surg 78(1):74–77
72. Rogers J, Haywood MP, Henry MM et al (1988) Temperature gradient between the rectum and anal canal: evidence against the role of temperature sensation modality in the anal canal or normal subjects. Br J Surg 75:1082–1085
73. Wald A (1994) Colonic and anorectal motility testing in clinical practice. Am J Gastroenterol 89:2109–2115
74. Felt-Bersma RJ, Klinkenberg-Knol EC, Meuwissen SGM (1990) Anorectal function investigations in incontinent and continent patients: differences in discriminatory value. Dis Colon Rectum 33:479–486

75. Rao SSC, Azpiroz F, Diamant N et al (2002) Minimum standards of anorectal manometry. Neurogastroentrol Mot 14:553–559
76. Sun W, Donnelly TC (1996) Effects of loperamide oxide on gastrointestinal transit time and anorectal function in patients with chronic diarrhea and faecal incontinence. Scand J Gastroenterol 32:34–38
77. Rao SSC, Happel J, Welcher K (1996) Can biofeedback therapy improve anorectal function in fecal incontinence? Am J Gastroenterol 91:2360–2366
78. Felt-Bersma RJ, Cuesta MA, Bartram CI (1994) Faecal incontinence 1994: which test and which treatment? Neth J Med 44(5):182–188
79. Pelsang R, Rao SSC, Welcher K (1999) FECOM: a new artificial stool for evaluating defecation. Am J Gastroenterol 94:183–186
80. Olsen AL, Rao SSC (2001) Clinical neurophysiology and electrodiagnostic testing of the pelvic floor. Gastroenterol Clin North Am 30(1):33–54
81. Laurberg S, Swash M, Henry MM (1988) Delayed external sphincter repair for obstetric tear. Br J Surg 75:786–788
82. Snooks SJ, Swash M, Henry MM et al (1986) Risk factors in childbirth causing damage to the pelvic floor innervation. Int J Colorectal Dis 1(1):20–24
83. Donnelly V, Fynes M, Campbell D et al (1998) Obstetric events leading to anal sphincter damage. Obstet Gynecol 92:955–961
84. Tetzschner T, Sorensen M, Lose G et al (1996) Anal and urinary incontinence in women with obstetric anal sphincter rupture. Br J Obstet Gynecol 103:1034–1040
85. Engel AF, Kamm MA, Sultan AH et al (1994) Anterior anal sphincter repair in patients with obstetric trauma. Br J Surg 81:1231–1234
86. Rothholtz NA, Wexner SD (2001) Surgical treatment of constipation and fecal incontinence. Gastroenterol Clin North Am 30(1):131–166
87. Di Lazzaro V, Pilato F et al (2004) Role of motor evoked potential in diagnosis of cauda equina and lumbosacral cord lesions. Neurology 63(12):2266–2271
88. Rao SSC, Read NW, Stobhart JAH et al (1988) Anorectal contractility under basal conditions and during rectal infusion of saline in ulcerative colitis. Gut 29:769–777
89. Wexner SD, Jorge JM (1994) Colorectal physiology tests: use or abuse of technology? Br Jr Surg 160(3):167–174
90. Tjandra JJ, Sharma BR, McKirdy HC et al (1994) Anorectal physiology testing in defecatory disorders: a prospective study. Aus N Z J Surg 64(5):322–326

Imaging of Faecal Incontinence with Endoanal Ultrasound

10

Richelle J.F. Felt-Bersma

Introduction

Endoanal ultrasound (EUS) was introduced 20 years ago by urologists to evaluate the prostate. Later, EUS was extended to other specialists–; first to stage rectal tumors, and next to investigate benign disorders of the anal sphincters and pelvic floor.

EUS has been used for almost every possible disorder in the anal region, and by delineating the anatomy, it has increased insight into anal pathology. Before the introduction of anorectal endosonography (AE), it was believed that pudendal nerve damage was the most common cause of obstetric faecal incontinence [1, 2]. Endosonography has shown that not pudendal nerve damage but obstetric sphincter trauma is the most common cause of faecal incontinence [3–8].

Another important cause of sphincter damage is previous anorectal surgery, i.e., hemorrhoidectomy, lateral sphincterotomy, fistulotomy, and transanal stapling of coloanal or ileoanal anastomoses [9-13]. Other causes of faecal incontinence must be kept in mind: chronic diarrhea or a small rectal compliance should be excluded with medical history and anorectal function tests before making firm decisions concerning surgery for a sphincter defect.

Clinical indications for EUS are faecal incontinence for the detection of defects and atrophy, perianal fistulas and abscesses to demonstrate the fistula tract, and rectal and anal carcinomas for staging and follow-up. There have been some suggestions on the role of endosonography in the prevention of anal incontinence. For example, EUS immediately performed after vaginal delivery allows diagnosis of undetected anal defects that might be associated with subsequent faecal incontinence [14]. Elective cesarean section can be recommended for women at increased risk for anal incontinence [15].

The importance of anal ultrasound in patients with faecal incontinence is detection of a sphincter defect, as this has direct clinical consequences. In a patient with symptomatic faecal incontinence, a significant sphincter defect (exceeding 25% of the circumference) forms an indication to perform sphincter repair. Demonstration of external anal sphincter atrophy is also possible, but as in examination with magnetic resonance imaging (MRI), this remains a difficult issue, which will be discussed elsewhere.

EUS is easy to perform, has a short learning curve, and causes no more discomfort than a routine digital examination. A rotating probe with a 360° radius and a frequency between 5 and 16 MHz is introduced into the rectum. The probe is then slowly withdrawn so that the pelvic floor and subsequently the sphincter complex are seen. With special software, it is also possible to reconstruct three-dimensional (3D) images.

Normal Anatomy and Morphology with Anal Ultrasound

The normal rectum is 11- to 15- cm long and has a maximum diameter of 4 cm. It is generally not empty but is filled with some remainders of faecal material and/or air. This makes it not always easy to obtain an optimal acoustical surrounding for anal ultrasound. On EUS, the normal rectal wall is 2- to 3- cm thick and is composed of a five-layer structure, as is the rest of the digestive tract.

The anal canal is 2- to 4- cm long and is closed in the normal situation. Therefore, excellent images can be obtained with EUS, as the anus lies tight around the probe (Fig. 1). The (inner) circular smooth muscle layer of the rectum continues into the anus where it thickens and becomes the internal anal sphincter (IAS). The (outer) longitudinal component fuses with the external anal sphincter (EAS) along the anal canal. The EAS is a voluntary muscle arising from the levator ani and puborectalis (PR) muscle to form a circular structure around the anal canal. The anatomy of the EAS remains controversial and is usually described as having three parts: a deep part joining with the PR muscle, a superficial part attached to the superficial transverse perinei muscle, and a subcutaneous part continuing below

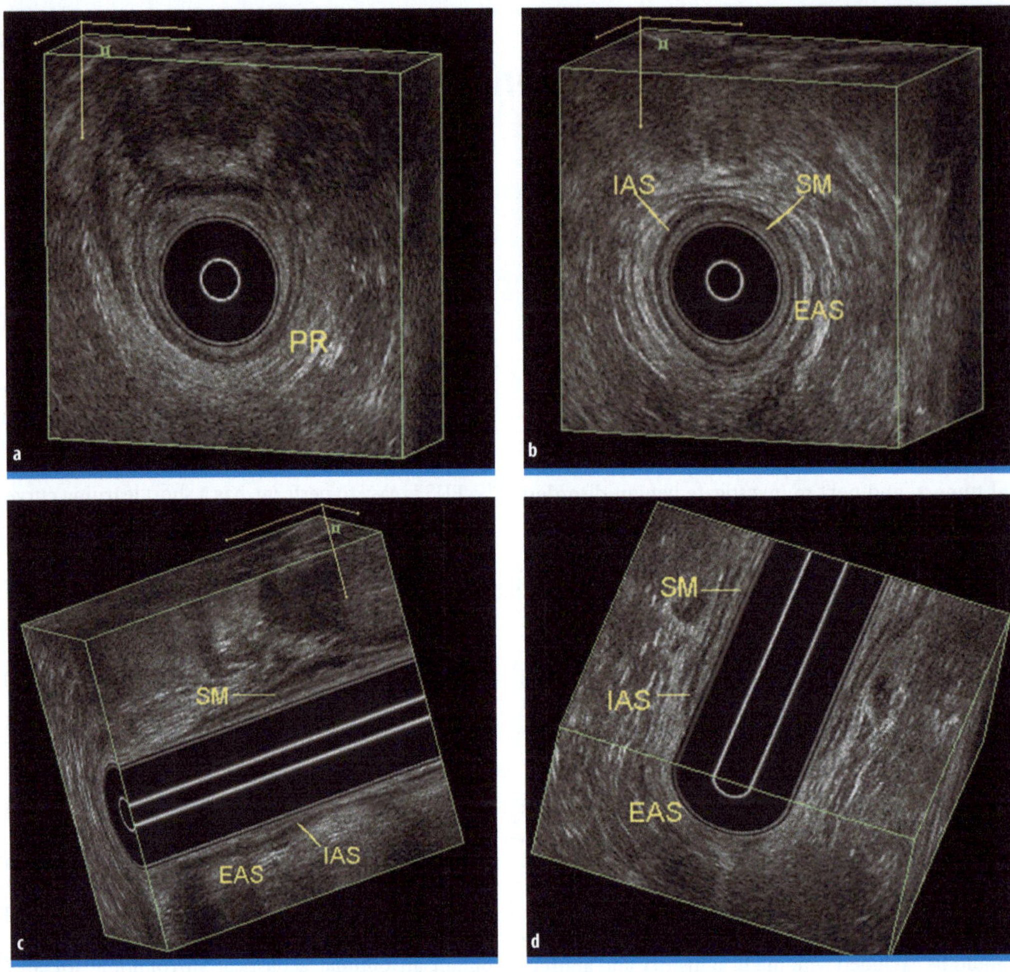

Fig. 1a–d. Anal endosonography. Normal anatomy of the anal sphincter and puborectalis muscle (*PR*) in three-dimensional imaging. **a** Frontal view of the PR; **b** frontal, **c** lateral, and **d** coronal view of the anal sphincters. *SM* submucosa , *IAS* internal anal sphincter, *EAS* external anal sphincter

the IAS. The perineal body is a so-called structure, a junctional zone where fibers from the IAS and EAS converge and fuse with muscles from the anterior urogenital area. Other parts of the pelvic floor are the anococcygeal ligament (posterior), and the levator ani, which consists of three parts: the PR muscle, the iliococcygeal muscle; and the pubococcygeal muscle.

Endosonographic findings in healthy volunteers have been thoroughly investigated [16-26]. Moreover, a number of studies have established basic endosonographic anatomy by making comparisons with anatomical preparations [16, 19, 22, 25]. The PR muscle is almost always easily visualized and can serve as a point of orientation: it appears as a V-shaped echogenic band, which slings dorsally around the rectum (Fig. 1a). When withdrawing the probe, the echogenic band closes anteriorly, thus forming the EAS (Fig. 1b). Figure 1c, d represents the lateral and coronal view, respectively.

Thickness of the EAS is approximately 4–10 mm [18, 20, 23, 24, 26, 27]. In women, it is anteriorly thinner and shorter [17, 23, 26], which makes it more vulnerable to obstetric damage. Besides being related to gender, EAS thickness is also correlated to body weight [23]. There is no clear relationship between EAS thickness and age [26–28].

Inside the EAS lies the IAS, which presents as a

thin, echogenic lucent band of approximately 1–3 mm [18, 20, 21, 23, 24, 26–30]. The IAS increases in thickness and echogenicity with age, both in patients [29, 31] and healthy volunteers [21, 23, 26–28, 30]. These findings are suggestive of sclerosis of the IAS in the elderly, which has been demonstrated histologically [32]. IAS thickness is not related to gender, body weight, or IAS length [21].

The submucosal layer has a mixed echogenic aspect and is partly collapsed by pressure of the endoprobe [25]. Submucosal thickness increases slightly with age [26]. This has also been found to a larger extent in internal haemorrhoids [33] and might be caused by physiological distal displacement or enlargement of the anal cushions [34]. The mucosa cannot be identified separately with the frequencies used.

Other pelvic floor structures around the sphincter complex can also be visualized. There are some reports on visualizing the longitudinal muscle of the EAS, but the importance of this is controversial [17, 20, 22, 25, 35]. The anococcygeal ligament appears as an echo-poor triangle and causes tapering of the EAS or PR muscle [17, 26]. Furthermore, the transverse perineal muscles, the ischiocavernous muscles, the urethra, and pubic bones may be visualized [19, 23, 26].

Vaginal endosonography, to visualize the perianal area and especially the perineum, is an alternative when rectal endosonography is not possible–for instance, when the anus is asymmetrical, causing air artifacts, extreme anal stenosis, or pain [36] (Fig. 2a, b).

Endoanal Imaging

Endoanal Ultrasound Apparatus and Probes

The technique used in this imaging mode is that of the general form of mechanical energy emitted above the frequency of human audibility (20,000 Hz). The operating frequency lies between 2.5 and 16 MHz. The image is formed by reflection at the interfaces of two structures. Part of the signal is transmitted, and part is reflected. Reflections from deeper structures are weaker due to greater signal attenuation. This can be partly corrected by changing the frequency: lower frequencies (2.5 MHz) penetrate better into deeper layers, and superficial structures are better visualized with higher frequencies (16 MHz). Reverberation is an artifact due to a gross mismatch of acoustic impedance at an interface, usually an air-tissue interface. The signal echoes back and forth, giving rise to a series of concentric black and white rings. This is typically a problem in the rectum and in an asymmetrical anus when there is loss of contact with the anal canal.

Several types of ultrasound probes have been developed. The first were single-transducer mechan-

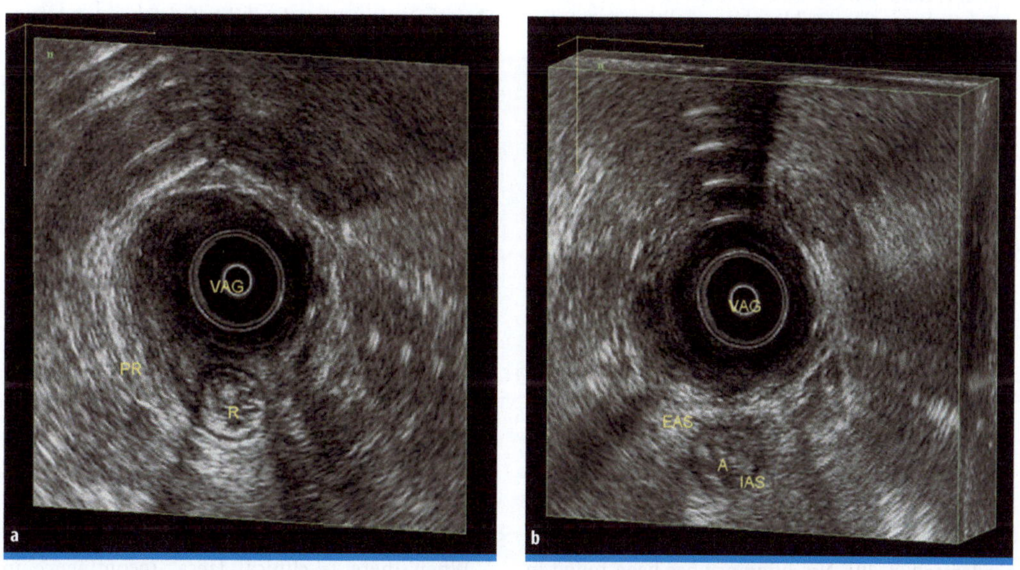

Fig. 2a,b. Vaginal endosonography. Normal image of the pelvic floor. **a** Level of the puborectalis muscle, **b** level of the anal sphincter. *V* vagina, *A* anus, *PR* puborectalis muscle, *R* rectum, *EAS* external anal sphincter, *IAS* internal anal sphincter

ical-sector probes with a limited angle (120–210°) to investigate and puncture the prostate, but they were unsuitable for a sphincter. Later, radial probes were developed with a 360° view. Also, linear and curved array probes with a limited field were developed.

Ultrasound transducers at the tip of an endoscope can be used to evaluate the bowel wall. The advantage is both, an endoscopic and ultrasound image, thus allowing investigation of small abnormalities in the bowel wall. The rubber balloon filled with water is not suitable for the anal canal, as it is compressed and twisted into the rotating probe. A hard, water-filled cone is necessary to image the anal canal.

Several industries provide ultrasound machines. Rigid rotating endoprobes with a 360° view are preferable. Rigid mechanical probes are provided by Bruel & Kjaer Medical (Herlev, Denmark) with a focal range of 5–16 MHz with 360° view, and by Aloka (7.5–12.5 MHz, 270°, Tokyo, Japan). The flexible endoscopic Olympus (Tokyo, Japan) radial scanner (7.5–12 MHz) has a 360° view. Flexible endoscopic sector scanners are by Pentax/Hitachi (sector scanner 100°, 5 and 7.5 MHz) (Tokyo, Japan) and Olympus (180°, 7.5 MHz). Bruel & Kjaer Medical has also developed software to construct a 3D image.

Performance

Generally, the patient is in the left lateral position. A digital rectal examination is mandatory to determine the presence of possible abnormalities (stenosis, painful lesion, tumor). The rigid probes are covered for hygienic reasons with a condom filled with ultrasound gel. Then the probe is covered with a gel on the outside and gently introduced into the rectum, following the anorectal angle. Landmarks are the prostate, vagina, and PR muscle. Then the probe is slowly withdrawn and enters the anal canal, were the anatomy, as described above, can be seen.

EUS Two-Dimensional Versus Three-Dimensional Imaging

With 3D reconstruction, it is not only possible to view the transversal image but also the longitudinal and sagittal images. Subsequently, it is possible to measure the length and volume of the anal sphincters. Men have a longer anterior EAS than do women [37]. Volume measurement has been very disappointing; reproducibility of volume measurement is moderate [38, 39]. No difference has been found in the volume of the EAS of women with faecal incontinence and healthy women [38, 39], and subsequently, this is not a tool to be used to demonstrate sphincter atrophy [40]. Sphincter length and aspect are far more promising markers to show EAS atrophy [41]. Demonstration of sphincter defects may be improved by 3D imaging [42]. The most impressive feature of 3D EUS is the ease of viewing the anal sphincter from all different angles and therefore obtaining a better view and insight into the local pathology.

Accuracy of Demonstrating Anorectal Sphincter Injury with Anal Ultrasound

EUS remains the gold standard in delineating the anatomy of the PR muscle and anal sphincter complex [18, 21, 43–45]. EUS can visualize defects, scarring, thinning and thickening, difference in echogenicity, and other local alterations. The defects should be described, indicating their location (IAS, EAS, PR muscle), their size longitudinally (total, proximal, distal), and their circumference (degrees). Some semantic problems exist concerning the words defect, tear, scar, and fibrosis. Clear disruption of the IAS or EAS are described as defects. Tears are defined by interruption of the fibrillar echo texture; scaring is defined more by loss of normal architecture, with usually low reflectiveness [46]. Endosonography demonstrates sphincter defects with high accuracy [37, 47–52]. Sensitivity and specificity can reach almost 100%. The described defects are confirmed during surgery. There is a good reproducibility for sphincter defects and anal sphincter thickness [37, 53–56]. For the IAS, the agreement is higher than for the EAS. Because of its accuracy and simplicity, endosonography has replaced electromyographical sphincter mapping, which is no more reliable than EUS [50, 52, 57, 58], provides no information about the IAS, and is an invasive, painful, and time-consuming technique [52].

Sphincter defect size correlates with faecal incontinence severity, and postoperative sphincter repair failure correlates with the remaining size of the sphincter defect [59]. Concomitant neuropathy may trouble that relationship [60, 61]. However, finding a sphincter defect does not necessarily mean that it is the cause of faecal incontinence, as many people have sphincter defects without faecal incontinence [62]. On the other hand, patients with faecal incontinence can have intact sphincters, and pudendal or autonomic neuropathy leading to sphincter atrophy is then the cause [2, 13].

When there is clinical faecal incontinence in women with obstetric trauma with low anal pressures and significant sphincter defect, sphincter repair may be considered. When there is no sphincter defect, pudendal neuropathy is the cause of the faecal incontinence, provided that there is no diarrhea or a small rectal capacity [63]. The difficulty comes when there is a small sphincter defect with moderate anal sphincter pressure. Generally, a defect smaller than 25% of the circumference is not considered significant for anal sphincter repair. Another problem is very low sphincter pressures and possible signs of atrophy and a defect of 25%: the very low pressures and signs of atrophy suggest concomitant serious neuropathy, which interferes with successful surgery. Pudendal nerve terminal motor latency (PNTML) measurements are not conclusive either [64], and decisions cannot be made on the results of these measurements.

Internal Anal Sphincter Abnormalities

The majority of lesions of the IAS are due to iatrogenic and obstetric injuries, often in combination with injuries to the EAS, leading to faecal incontinence. Smaller lesions leading to minor faecal incontinence or soiling are due to hemorrhoidectomy or mucosal prolapsectomy. Manual anal dilatation [65] or lateral internal sphincterotomy [66–68] are notorious and have been associated with faecal incontinence in 27% and 50% of patients, respectively. Fistula surgery can cause faecal incontinence in up to 60% of cases [69]. Fortunately, not all traumatic sphincter defects lead to faecal incontinence or soiling. In a study of 50 patients after haemorrhoidectomy (24), fistulectomy (18), and internal sphincterotomy (8), 23 (46%) had a defect of the anal sphincter (13 IAS, one EAS, nine combined defect) three after hemorrhoidectomy, 13 after fistulectomy, and seven after internal sphincterotomy. Seven patients (30%) had symptoms, and they all had a sphincter defect. In the other 16 (70%), the sphincter defect did not produce symptoms [62].

Defects of the IAS are easily recognized due to the prominent appearance of the IAS in the anal canal, as the defects appear as hyperechoic breaks in the hypoechogenic ring. The pattern of disruption is related to the type of surgery or trauma [70]. Manual dilatation will lead to several disruptions or sometimes to a diffuse thinning of the IAS. Patients after a lateral internal sphincterotomy will have a single lateral defect associated with a thickening of the remaining IAS due to retraction of the remaining muscle (Fig. 3a–c) [65, 67]. After hemorrhoidectomy, defects can be seen where the hemorrhoids were removed. Fistula surgery leads to combined defects of IAS and EAS in the fistula tract.

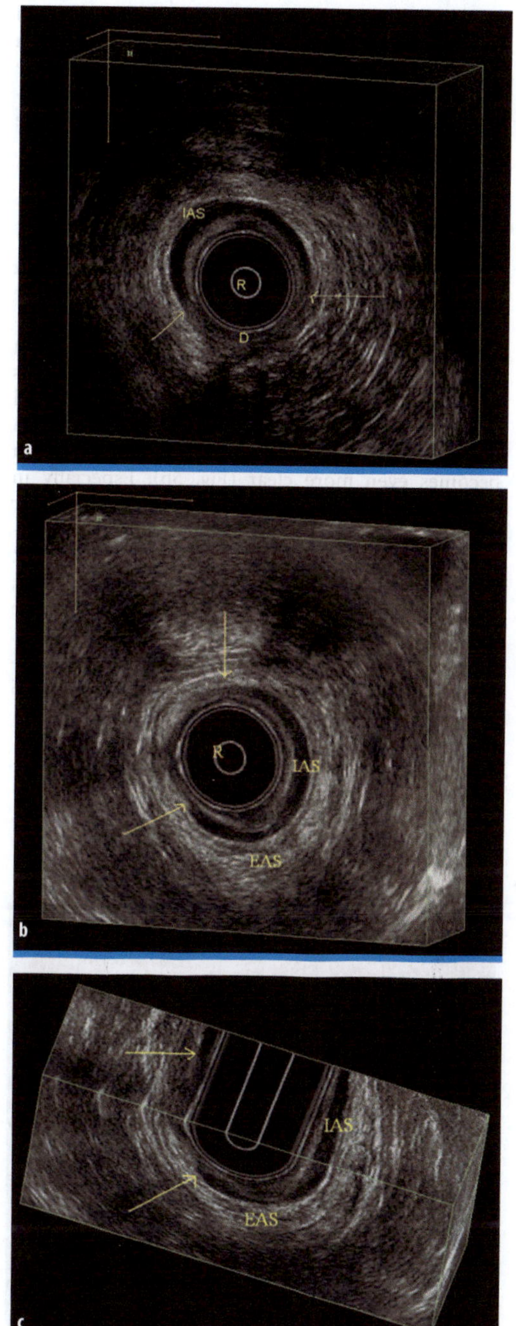

Fig. 3a–c. Internal anal sphincter defect (ISD) due to lateral internal sphincterotomy. **a** Frontal view of a dorsolateral left defect, **b** frontal and **c** coronal view of a right lateral ISD. *R* rectum, *IAS* internal anal sphincter, *EAS* external anal sphincter, *D* defect

Reports have appeared about rare causes of faecal incontinence, such as primary IAS degeneration in passive faecal incontinence [13] and sclerosis of the IAS in mixed connective tissue disease [71] and systemic sclerosis [72]. In these patients, there is diffuse thinning (<0.2 mm) of the IAS.

External Anal Sphincter Abnormalities

The most frequent cause of faecal incontinence is an obstetric injury to the EAS. The typical appearance of this EAS defect is an anterior break in the circumferential integrity of the hyperechogenic band to a more hypoechogenic aspect (Figs. 4a, b; 5a, b). This corresponds to replacement of the normal striated muscle with granulation tissue and fibrosis. With vaginal EUS, the relationship with the vagina becomes even more clear (Fig. 5b). Especially in women, an anterior sphincter defect (irregular mixed echogenic to hypoechogenic) must be well differentiated from the natural gap between the PR muscle in the upper anal canal (hypoechogenic; smooth, regular edges). Surgical defects will be at the location of the surgery.

There is wide variation in the incidence of clinically occult anal sphincter injuries diagnosed by EUS after the first vaginal delivery [3, 7, 73–79]. For primipara, the risk of developing a sphincter tear is 25%, and for subsequent deliveries, it is 4% [3, 80]. Faecal incontinence develops in 25% [80] of such deliveries. Instrumental delivery (forceps more than vacuum extraction), the second stage of labor, and high birth weight are associated with increased risk of anal sphincter injury [73, 80, 81]. In patients with perianal fistula with external fistula openings, the fistula tract can be differentiated from a defect by becoming hyperechogenic after introduction of hydrogen peroxide [82]. EAS atrophy detection with EUS is also possible, but the technique requires more research (see Chapter 28).

Puborectalis Muscle Abnormalities

As with the EAS, the PR muscle is a striated muscle and can also acquire defects or become atrophic. Defects of the PR muscle are rare and are related to dramatic anorectal trauma, such as speedboat or traffic accidents (Fig. 6a). Sometimes with a high anorectal fistula, a defect of the PR muscle can be seen (Fig. 6b, c). A greater shortening of the PR muscle during contraction has been observed in patients with faecal incontinence [83].

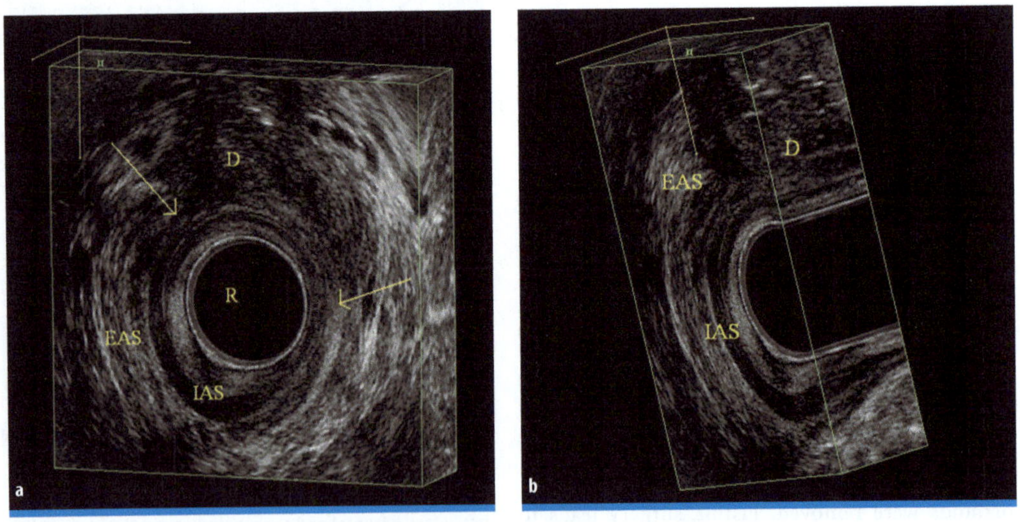

Fig. 4a, b. Combined defect of internal and external anal sphincter. **a** Frontal. **b** Lateral view. *R* rectum, *IAS* internal anal sphincter, *EAS* external anal sphincter, *D* defect

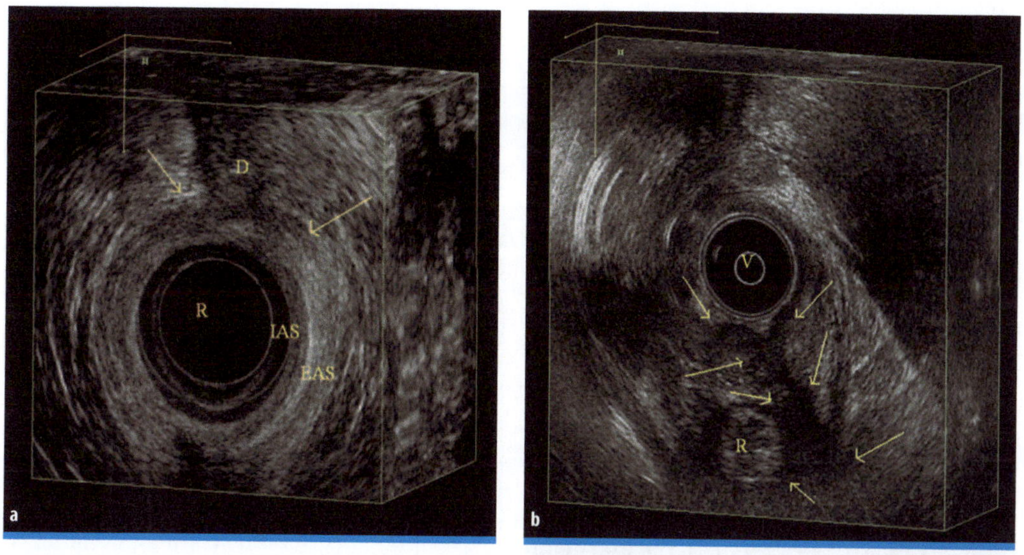

Fig. 5a, b. External anal sphincter defect. **a** Rectal image. **b** Vaginal image. *Arrows* indicate large defect. *V* vagina, *R* rectum, *IAS* internal anal sphincter, *EAS* external anal sphincter, *D* defect

EUS Versus Endoanal MRI

Several studies compared the diagnostic accuracy of EUS and endoanal MRI regarding anal sphincter defects. One report suggests that endosonography is superior to MRI in diagnosing IAS injury but equal in diagnosing EAS defects [84]. Interobserver agreement for sphincter defects in MRI is moderate and less than that reported for EUS [85]. Generally, detection by EUS is equal to that by MRI [40, 41, 86, 87], although some claim MRI is superior in imaging the EAS [88, 89]. In patients with anorectal disorders, EUS provides more information and can be performed during surgery [90]. Some variability can be explained by differences in study design, patient population, physician experience, and interest in the techniques used. Both techniques are very reliable methods and can be used to demonstrate sphincter defects. It has been reported that MRI is the preferred tool to demonstrate sphincter atrophy [91, 92] However, with anal endosonography, it is also possible to detect EAS atrophy, and the technique compares well with MRI findings [41] (see Chapter 28).

EUS and Anal Manometry

Anal manometry selects patients with low pressures in anal incontinence; however, there is an overlap between healthy individuals and patients with incontinence [93]. Anal manometry correlates rather poorly with the presence of sphincter defects [94–98]. This is obvious because anal manometry reflects only the functional result – that is, low anal pressures – but not the cause (sphincter defect or neuropathy). On the other hand, EUS demonstrates a sphincter defect regardless of its functional results on anal pressures. However, it seems logical that a large defect will result in low anal pressures. Both anal manometry and EUS are incapable of predicting clinical outcome in patients with faecal incontinence [99]. However, the indication to perform EUS is demonstration of a sphincter defect. The relationship between anal pressures measured with anal manometry and anal sphincter features measured with EUS is not clear. Sphincter defects of IAS and EAS correlated with maximal basal and squeeze pressure, respectively [100]. A correlation was found between posterior sphincter length measured on 3D EUS and sphincter length measured during manometry in healthy subjects and between IAS volume and resting anal pressure in incontinent women [40].

EUS and Surgery

Patients with a significant sphincter defect without clinically obvious neuropathy and/or atrophy can thus be selected for sphincter repair. Endosonography is also useful in selecting patients with persistent

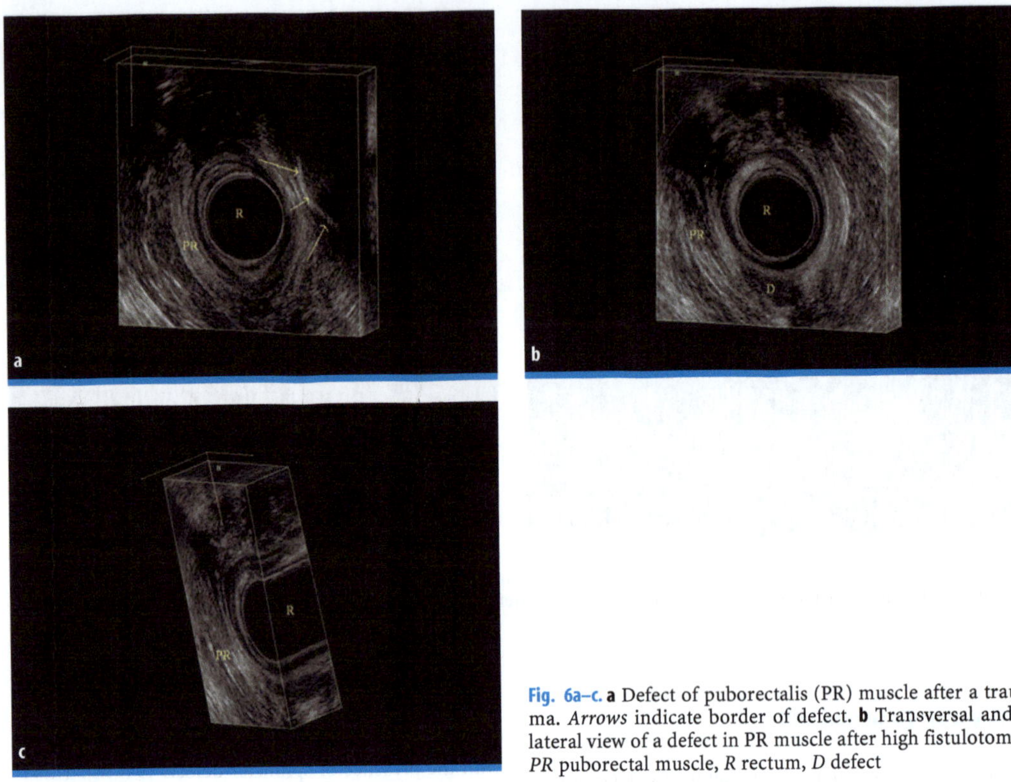

Fig. 6a–c. a Defect of puborectalis (PR) muscle after a trauma. *Arrows* indicate border of defect. **b** Transversal and **c** lateral view of a defect in PR muscle after high fistulotomy. *PR* puborectal muscle, *R* rectum, *D* defect

sphincter defects after failed repair, as the presence of such a rest defect correlates with poor clinical outcome [101–110]. Repeat repair can improve continence score [81]. Sometimes, a typical overlap sign may be observed after sphincter repair [111].

Conclusion

EUS is a very good tool to demonstrate anal sphincter defects of both the EUS and the IAS. The size of the sphincter defect in combination with other anorectal function tests results (low anal pressures, normal rectal, compliance) without diarrhea form an indication to perform an anal sphincter repair. EUS has good reproducibility, compares well with surgery, and has equal results with EAS defects and possibly better results with IAS defects than does MRI. Atrophy detection is also possible but requires more research. Three-dimensional EUS gives more insight into the anatomy and therefore may demonstrate defects better, but it is probably more the ease of viewing the image. Volume measurements for the anal sphincters have no value.

References

1. Parks AG, Swash M, Urich H (1977) Sphincter denervation in anorectal incontinence and rectal prolapse. Gut 18:656–665
2. Snooks SJ, Swash M, Setchell M, Henry MM (1984) Injury to innervation of pelvic floor sphincter musculature in childbirth. Lancet 2(8402):546–550
3. Sultan AH, Kamm MA, Hudson CN et al (1993) Anal-sphincter disruption during vaginal delivery. New Engl J Med 329:1905–1911
4. Kamm MA (1994) Obstetric damage and faecal incontinence. Lancet 344:730–733
5. Oberwalder M, Connor J, Wexner SD (2003) Meta-analysis to determine the incidence of obstetric anal sphincter damage. Br J Surg 90:1333–1337
6. Zetterstrom J, Lopez A, Holmstrom B et al (2003) Obstetric sphincter tears and anal incontinence: an

observational follow-up study. Acta Obstet Gynecol Scand 82:921–928
7. Abramowitz L, Sobhani I, Ganansia R et al (2000) Are sphincter defects the cause of anal incontinence after vaginal delivery? Results of a prospective study. Dis Colon Rectum 43:590–596
8. Benifla JL, Abramowitz L, Sobhani I et al (2000) Post-partum sphincter rupture and anal incontinence: prospective study with 259 patients. Gynecol Obstet Fertil 28:15–22
9. Felt-Bersma RJ, Koorevaar M, Strijers RL, Cuesta MA (1995) Unsuspected sphincter defects shown by anal endosonography after anorectal surgery. A prospective study. Dis Colon Rectum 38:249–253
10. Sultan AH, Kamm MA, Nicholls RJ, Bartram CI (1994) Prospective study of the extent of internal anal sphincter division during lateral sphincterotomy. Dis Colon Rectum 37:1031–1033
11. Farouk R, Drew P, Duthie G et al (1996) Disruption of the internal anal sphincter can occur after transanal stapling. Br J Surg 83:1400
12. Silvis R, van Eekelen JW, Delemarre JB, Gooszen HG (1995) Endosonography of the anal sphincter after ileal pouch-anal anastomosis. Relation with anal manometry and fecal continence. Dis Colon Rectum 38:383–388
13. Vaizey CJ, Kamm MA, Bartram CI (1997) Primary degeneration of the internal anal sphincter as a cause of passive faecal incontinence. Lancet 349:612–615
14. Faltin DL, Boulvain M, Irion O et al (2000) Diagnosis of anal sphincter tears by postpartum endosonography predict fecal incontinence. Obstet Gynecol 95:643–647
15. Faridi A, Willis S, Schelzig P et al (2002) Anal sphincter injury during vaginal delivery - an argument for cesarean section on request? J Perinat Med 30:379–387
16. Eckardt VF, Jung B, Fischer B, Lierse W et al (1994) Anal endosonography in healthy subjects and patients with idiopathic fecal incontinence. Dis Colon Rectum 37:235–242
17. Law PJ, Bartram CI (1989) Anal endosonography. Technique and normal anatomy. Gastrointest Radiol 14:349–353
18. Nielsen MB, Pedersen JF, Hauge C et al (1991) Endosonography of the anal sphincter: Findings in healthy volunteers. AJR Am J Roentgenol 157:1199–1202
19. Tjandra JJ, Milsom JW, Stolfi VM et al (1992) Endoluminal ultrasound defines anatomy of the anal canal and pelvic floor. Dis Colon Rectum 35:465–470
20. Nielsen MB, Hauge C, Rasmussen OO et al (1992) Anal sphincter size measured by endosonography in healthy volunteers. Effect of age, sex and parity. Acta Radiol 33:453–456
21. Burnett SJ, Bartram CI (1991) Endosonographic variations in the normal internal anal sphincter. Int J Colorect Dis 6:2–4
22. Sultan AH, Nicholls RJ, Kamm MA et al (1993) Anal endosonography and correlation with in vitro and in vivo anatomy. Br J Surg 80:508–511
23. Sultan AH, Kamm MA, Hudson CN et al (1994) Endosonography of the anal sphincters: normal anatomy and comparison with manometry. Clin Radiol 49:368–374
24. Papachrysostomou M, Pye SD, Wild SR, Smith AN (1993) Anal endosonography in asymptomatic subjects. Scand J Gastroenterol 28:551–556
25. Gerdes B, Kohler HH, Zielke A et al (1997) The anatomical basis of anal endosonography–a study in postmortem specimens. Surg Endoscopy 11:986–990
26. Poen AC, Felt-Bersma RJF, Cuesta MA, Meuwissen SGM (1997) Normal values and reproducibility of anal endosonographic measurements. Eur J Ultrasound 6:103–110
27. Papachrysostomou M, Pye SD, Wild SR, Smith AN (1994) Significance of the thickness of the anal sphincters with age and its relevance in faecal incontinence. Scand J Gastroenterol 29:710–714
28. Nielsen MB, Pedersen JF (1996) Changes in the anal sphincter with age. An endosonographic study. Acta Radiol 37:357–361
29. Schafer R, Heyer T, Gantke B et al (1997) Anal endosonography and manometry: comparison in patients with defecation problems. Dis Colon Rectum 40:293–297
30. Gantke B, Schafer A, Enck P, Lubke HJ (1993) Sonographic, manometric, and myographic evaluation of the anal sphincters morphology and function. Dis Colon Rectum 36:1037–1041
31. Emblem R, Dhaenens G, Stien R et al (1994) The importance of anal endosonography in the evaluation of idiopathic fecal incontinence. Dis Colon Rectum 37:42–48
32. Klosterhalfen B, Offner F, Topf N et al (1990) Sclerosis of the internal anal sphincter–A process of aging. Dis Colon Rectum 33:606–609
33. Poen AC, Felt-Bersma RJF, Cuesta MA, Meuwissen SGM (1999) Anal endosonography in haemorroidal disease: do anatomical changes have clinical implications? Colorectal Dis 1:146–150
34. Loder PB, Kamm MA, Nicholls RJ et al (1994) Pathology, pathophysiology and aetiology. Br J Surg 81:946–954
35. Lunniss PJ, Phillips R (1992) Anatomy and function of the anal longitudinal muscle. Br J Surg 79:882–884
36. Poen AC, Felt-Bersma RJF, Cuesta MA, Meuwissen SGM (1998) Vaginal endosonography of the anal sphincter complex is important in the diagnosis of faecal incontinence and perianal sepsis. Br J Surg 85:359–363
37. Gold DM, Bartram CI, Halligan S et al (1999) Three-dimensional endoanal sonography in assessing anal canal injury. Br J Surg 86:365–370
38. West RL, Felt-Bersma RJ, Hansen BE et al (2005) Volume measurements of the anal sphincter complex in healthy controls and fecal-incontinent patients with a three-dimensional reconstruction of endoanal ultrasonography images. Dis Colon Rectum 48:540–548
39. Gregory WT, Boyles SH, Simmons K et al (2006) External anal sphincter volume measurements using 3-dimensional endoanal ultrasound. Am J Obstet Gynecol 194:1243–1248
40. West RL, Dwarkasing S, Briel JW et al (2005) Can three-dimensional endoanal ultrasonography detect external anal sphincter atrophy? A comparison with endoanal magnetic resonance imaging. Int J Colorectal Dis 20:328–333

41. Cazemier M, Terra MP, Stoker J et al (2006) Atrophy and defects detection of the external anal sphincter: comparison between three-dimensional anal endosonography and endoanal magnetic resonance imaging. Dis Colon Rectum 49:20–27
42. Christensen AF, Nyhuus B, Nielsen MB, Christensen H (2005) Three-dimensional anal endosonography may improve diagnostic confidence of detecting damage to the anal sphincter complex. Br J Radiol 78:308–311
43. Bartram CI (2003) Ultrasound. In: Bartram CI, deLancy JOL (eds) Imaging pelvic floor disorders. Springer Berlin Heidelberg New York
44. Williams AB, Cheetham MJ, Bartram CI et al (2000) Gender differences in the longitudinal pressure profile of the anal canal related to anatomical structure as demonstrated on three-dimensional anal endosonography. Br J Surg 87:1674–1679
45. Kumar A, Scholefield JH (2000) Endosonography of the anal canal and rectum. World J Surg 24:208–115. Review
46. Rociu E, Stoker J, Zwamborn AW, Lameris JS (1999) Endoanal MR imaging of the anal sphincter in fecal incontinence. Radiographics S171–177
47. Meyenberger C, Bertschinger P, Zala GF, Buchmann P (1996) Anal sphincter defects in fecal incontinence: correlation between endosonography and surgery. Endoscopy 28:217–224
48. Sultan AH, Kamm MA, Talbot IC et al (1994) Anal endosonography for identifying external sphincter defects confirmed histologically. Br J Surg 81:463–465
49. Romano G, Rotondano G, Esposito P et al (1996) External anal sphincter defects: correlation between pre-operative anal endosonography and intraoperative findings. Br J Radiol 69:6–9
50. Burnett SJ, Speakman CT, Kamm MA, Bartram CI (1991) Confirmation of endosonographic detection of external anal sphincter defects by simultaneous electromyographic mapping. Br J Surg 78:448–450
51. Deen KI, Kumar D, Williams JG et al (1993) Anal sphincter defects: Correlation between endoanal ultrasound and surgery. Ann Surg 218:201–205
52. Tjandra JJ, Milsom JW, Schroeder T, Fazio VW (1993) Endoluminal ultrasound is preferable to electromyography in mapping anal sphincteric defects. Dis Colon Rectum 36:689–692
53. Poen AC, Felt-Bersma RJF, Cuesta MA, Meuwissen SGM (1997) Normal values and reproducibility of anal endosonographic measurements. Eur J Ultrasound 6:103–110
54. Falk PM, Blatchford GJ, Cali RL et al (1994) Transanal ultrasound and manometry in the evaluation of fecal incontinence. Dis Colon Rectum 37:468–472
55. Pinta TM, Kylanpaa ML, Salmi TK et al (2004) Primary sphincter repair: are the results of the operation good enough? Dis Colon Rectum 47:18–23
56. Fritsch H, Brenner E, Lienemann A, Ludwikowski B (2002) Anal sphincter complex: reinterpreted morphology and its clinical relevance. Dis Colon Rectum 45:188–194
57. Law PJ, Kamm MA, Bartram CI (1990) A comparison between electromyography and anal endosonography in mapping external anal sphincter defects. Dis Colon Rectum 33:370–373
58. Enck P, von GHJ, Schafer A et al (1996) Comparison of anal sonography with conventional needle electromyography in the evaluation of anal sphincter defects. Am J Gastroenterol 91:2539–2543
59. Felt-Bersma RJ, Cuesta MA, Koorevaar M (1996) Anal sphincter repair improves anorectal function and endosonographic image. A prospective clinical study. Dis Colon Rectum 39:878–885
60. Voyvodic F, Rieger NA, Skinner S et al (2003) Endosonographic imaging of anal sphincter injury: does the size of the tear correlate with the degree of dysfunction? Dis Colon Rectum 46:735–741
61. Felt-Bersma RJ (2004) Comment on Voyvodic et al (2003) Endosonographic imaging of anal sphincter injury. Dis Colon Rectum 47(4):546–547
62. Felt-Bersma RJ, van Baren R,Koorevaar M et al (1995) Unsuspected sphincter defects shown by anal endosonography after anorectal surgery. A prospective study. Dis Colon Rectum 38:249–253
63. Felt-Bersma RJ, Sloots CE, Poen AC et al (2000) Rectal compliance as a routine measurement: extreme volumes have direct clinical impact and normal volumes exclude rectum as a problem. Dis Colon Rectum 43:1732–1738
64. Riccard R, Melgren AF, Madoff RD et al (2006) The utility of pudendal nerve terminal latencies in idiopathic incontinence. Dis Colon Rectum 49(6):852–857
65. Speakman CT, Burnett SJ, Kamm MA, Bartram CI (1991) Sphincter injury after anal dilatation demonstrated by anal endosonography. Br J Surg 78:1429–1430
66. Khubchandani IT, Reed JF (1989) Sequelae of internal sphincterotomy for chronic fissure in ano. Br J Surg 76:431–434
67. Tjandra JJ, Han WR, Ooi BS et al (2001) Faecal incontinence after lateral internal sphincterotomy is often associated with coexisting occult sphincter defects: a study using endoanal ultrasonography. ANZ J Surg 71:598–602
68. Sultan AH, Kamm MA, Nicholls RJ, Bartram CI (1994) Prospective study of the extent of internal anal sphincter division during lateral sphincterotomy. Dis Colon Rectum 37(10):1031–1033
69. Kennedy HL, Zegarra JP (1990) Fistulotomy without external sphincter division for high anal fistulae. Br J Surg 77:898–901
70. Farouk R, Bartolo DC (1994) The use of endoluminal ultrasound in the assessment of patients with faecal incontinence. J R Coll Surg Edinb 39:312–318
71. Engel AF, Kamm MA, Talbot IC (1994) Progressive systemic sclerosis of the internal anal sphincter leading to passive faecal incontinence. Gut 35:857–859
72. Daniel F, De Parades V, Cellier C (2005) Abnormal appearance of the internal anal sphincter at ultrasound: a specific feature of progressive systemic sclerosis? Gastroenterol Clin Biol 29:597–599
73. Handa VL, Danielsen BH, Gilbert WM (2001) Obstetric anal sphincter lacerations. Obstet Gynecol 98:225–230
74. de Parades V, Etienney I, Thabut D et al (2004) Anal sphincter injury after forceps delivery: myth or reality? A prospective ultrasound study of 93 females. Dis Colon Rectum 47:24–34
75. Lee SJ, Park JW (2000) Follow-up evaluation of the

effect of vaginal delivery on the pelvic floor. Dis Colon Rectum 43:1550–1555
76. Snooks SJ, Swash M, Mathers SE, Henry MM (1990) Effect of vaginal delivery on the pelvic floor: a 5-year follow-up. Br J Surg 77:1358–1360
77. Martinez Hernandez Magro P, Villanueva Saenz E, Jaime Zavala M et al (2003) Endoanal sonography in assessment of fecal incontinence following obstetric trauma. Ultrasound Obstet Gynecol 22:616–621
78. Deen KI, Kumar D, Williams JG et al (1993) The prevalence of anal sphincter defects in faecal incontinence: a prospective endosonic study. Gut 34:685–688
79. Williams AB, Bartram CI, Halligan S et al (2001) Anal sphincter damage after vaginal delivery using three-dimensional endosonography. Obstet Gynecol 97:770–775
80. Donnelly V, Fynes M, Campbell D et al (1998) Obstetric events leading to anal sphincter damage. Obstet Gynecol 92:955–961
81. Poen AC, Felt-Bersma RJ, Strijers RL et al (1998) Third-degree obstetric perineal tear: long-term clinical and functional results after primary repair. Br J Surg 85:1433–1438
82. Poen AC, Felt-Bersma RJ, Eijsbouts QA et al (1998) Hydrogen-peroxide-enhanced transanal ultrasound in the assessment of fistula-in-ano. Dis Colon Rectum 41:1147–1152
83. Tankova L, Draganov V, Damyanov N (2001) Endosonography for assessment of anorectal changes in patients with fecal incontinence. Eur J Ultrasound 12:221–225
84. Malouf AJ, Williams AB, Halligan S et al (2000) Prospective assessment of accuracy of endoanal MR imaging and endosonography in patients with fecal incontinence. AJR Am J Roentgenol 175:741–745
85. Malouf AJ, Halligan S, Williams AB et al (2001) Prospective assessment of interobserver agreement for endoanal MRI in fecal Incontinence. Abdom Imaging 26:76–78
86. Pinta T, Kylanpaa ML, Luukkonen P et al (2004) Anal incontinence: diagnosis by endoanal US or endovaginal MRI. Eur Radiol 14:1472–1477
87. Williams AB, Bartram CI, Halligan S et al (2002) Endosonographic anatomy of the normal anal canal compared with endocoil magnetic resonance imaging. Dis Colon Rectum 45:176–183
88. Rociu E, Stoker J, Eijkemans MJ, Lameris JS (2000) Normal anal sphincter anatomy and age- and sex-related variations at high-spatial-resolution endoanal MR imaging. Radiology 217:395–401
89. Beets-Tan RG, Morren GL, Beets GL et al (2001) Measurement of anal sphincter muscles: endoanal US, endoanal MR imaging, or phased-array MR imaging? A study with healthy volunteers. Radiology 220:81–89
90. Jones NM, Humphreys MS, Goodman TR et al (2003) The value of anal endosonography compared with magnetic resonance imaging following the repair of anorectal malformations. Pediatr Radiol 33:183–185
91. Briel JW, Zimmerman DD, Stoker J et al (2000) Relationship between sphincter morphology on endoanal MRI and histopathological aspects of the external anal sphincter. Int J Colorectal Dis 15:87–90
92. Terra MP, Deutekom M, Beets-Tan RG et al (2006) Relationship between external anal sphincter atrophy at endoanal magnetic resonance imaging and clinical, functional, and anatomic characteristics in patients with fecal incontinence. Dis Colon Rectum 49:668–678
93. Felt-Bersma R, Gort G, Meuwissen S (1991) Normal values in anal manometry and rectal sensation: A problem of range. Hepato Gastroenterol 38:444–449
94. Burnett SJ, Spence Jones C, Speakman CT et al (1991) Unsuspected sphincter damage following childbirth revealed by anal endosonography. Br J Radiol 64: 225–227
95. Felt-Bersma RJF, Cuesta MA, Koorevaar M et al (1992) Anal endosonography: Relationship with anal manometry and neurophysiologic tests. Dis Colon Rectum 35:944–949
96. Sultan AH, Kamm MA, Talbot IC et al (1994) Anal endosonography for identifying external sphincter defects confirmed histologically. Br J Surg 81:463–465
97. Nielsen MB, Hauge C, Pedersen JF, Christiansen J (1993) Endosonographic evaluation of patients with anal incontinence: Findings and influence on surgical management. AJR Am J Roentgenol 160:771–775
98. Rieger NA, Sweeney JL, Hoffmann DC et al (1996) Investigation of fecal incontinence with endoanal ultrasound. Dis Colon Rectum 39:860–864
99. Hill K, Fanning S, Fennerty MB, Faigel DO (2006) Endoanal ultrasound compared to anorectal manometry for the evaluation of fecal incontinence: a study of the effect these tests have on clinical outcome. Dig Dis Sci 51:235–240
100. Barthet M, Bellon P, Abou E et al (2002) Anal endosonography for assessment of anal incontinence with a linear probe: relationships with clinical and manometric features. Int J Colorectal Dis 17:123–128
101. Felt-Bersma RJ, Cuesta MA, Koorevaar M (1996) Anal sphincter repair improves anorectal function and endosonographic image. A prospective clinical study. Dis Colon Rectum 39:878–885
102. Nielsen MB, Dammegaard L, Pedersen JF (1994) Endosonographic assessment of the anal sphincter after surgical reconstruction. Dis Colon Rectum 37:434–438
103. Poen AC, Felt-Bersma RJ, Cuesta MA, Meuwissen SGM (1998) Third degree perineal rupture: long term clinical and functional results after primary repair. Br J Surg 85:1433–1438
104. Sitzler PJ, Thomson JP (1996) Overlap repair of damaged anal sphincter. A single surgeon's series. Dis Colon Rectum 39:1356–1360
105. Engel AF, Kamm MA, Sultan AH et al (1994) Anterior anal sphincter repair in patients with obstetric trauma. Br J Surg 81:1231–1234
106. Ternent CA, Shashidharan M, Blatchford GJ et al (1997) Transanal ultrasound and anorectal physiology findings affecting continence after sphincteroplasty. Dis Colon Rectum 40:462–467
107. Starck M, Bohe M, Valentin L (2006) The extent of endosonographic anal sphincter defects after primary repair of obstetric sphincter tears increases over time and is related to anal incontinence. Ultrasound Obstet Gynecol 27:188–197
108. Allgayer H, Dietrich CF, Rohde W et al (2005) Prospec-

tive comparison of short- and long-term effects of pelvic floor exercise/biofeedback training in patients with fecal incontinence after surgery plus irradiation versus surgery alone for colorectal cancer: clinical, functional and endoscopic/endosonographic findings. Scand J Gastroenterol 40:1168–1175
109. Norderval S, Oian P, Revhaug A, Vonen B (2005) Anal incontinence after obstetric sphincter tears: outcome of anatomic primary repairs. Dis Colon Rectum 48:1055–1061
110. Giordano P, Renzi A, Efron J et al (2002) Previous sphincter repair does not affect the outcome of repeat repair. Dis Colon Rectum 45:635–640
111. Savoye-Collet C, Savoye G, Koning E et al (1999) Anal endosonography after sphincter repair: specific patterns related to clinical outcome. Abdom Imaging 24:569–573

Imaging of Fecal Incontinence

11

Andrea Maier

Introduction

Fecal incontinence, the inability to deliberately control the anal sphincter, is a common disease and may affect up to 20% of the age group above 65 years [1]. Fecal incontinence has a substantial impact on quality of life. It is a socially disabling problem that prevents up to one third of patients from seeking medical advice for it. The most common causes include traumatic (obstetric, surgical) sphincter defects, neurogenic dysfunction of the musculature of the pelvic floor, and rectal prolapse. The prevalence of fecal incontinence in women is eight times higher than in men [2]. The most common cause in women is childbirth, during which the sphincter muscles are commonly damaged [3–5]. Traumatic rupture of the anal sphincters may result in immediate-onset fecal incontinence. Pudendal neuropathy, caused by stretching the branches of the pudendal nerve to the sphincter and levator ani as the fetal head pushes down on the pelvic floor to dilate the introitus, leads to delayed-onset incontinence. Following vaginal delivery, the pudendal nerve terminal motor latencies (PNTML) are increased for about 6 months, and there is a fall in squeeze pressure regardless of sphincter damage [6]. Nerve damage appears to be cumulative, whereas direct sphincter damage most likely occurs in the first delivery. An occult sphincter defect may precipitate overt symptoms later as the effects of menopause, neuropathy, and muscle loss accumulate. Indeed, in 80% of affected women, an obstetric trauma is present. Sultan et al. [4] demonstrated that 35% of primiparous and 44% of multiparous women show defects of the internal and/or external sphincter muscles after vaginal delivery. One third of these women also have direct disturbances of anal continence.

Diabetes may be associated with profound autonomic neuropathy, leading to dysfunction of the rectum and the sphincter muscles. Abnormal thinning of the internal sphincter is common and of unknown etiology. Pelvic floor descent is common with advanced age. It may be secondary to prolonged straining, and the condition has been considered to cause primary damage to the pudendal nerves by stretching [7]. Fecal incontinence may be divided into passive, where leakage is the main problem, and urge, where stool cannot be held back. The passive form is more likely to be due to internal damage, while urge incontinence can be attributed to external sphincter damage.

In treating fecal incontinence, the physician can choose from several modalities, depending on localization of the impairment. Isolated external sphincter defects can be treated conservatively by physical therapy, including biofeedback. The pelvic floor may be trained to take on the function of the arbitrary sphincter muscle. In isolated internal sphincter defects, physical therapy alone is unsuccessful because other muscles cannot compensate for the work of this involuntary muscle. Local measures and a dietetic or medicinally triggered increase of fecal consistency are necessary to obtain a good quality of life. Patients with sphincter damage may benefit from surgical repair. To perform optimal surgery, an accurate description of the position, extent, and type of lesion is necessary. Postanal and sphincter repair are the established operative techniques. Long-term results of sphincter repair show success rates of 50–75%, although this technique repairs a circumscribed defect with intact surrounding muscle [8]. Long-term results for postanal repair are not good due to primary diffuse impairment of sphincter function [9]. Total pelvic repair has a success rate of 11% [10].

Choice of an optimal therapy is determined on the basis of proper assessment, especially accurate images of the anal sphincter complex. Imaging methods applied are defecography, endoanal ultrasonography, and magnetic resonance (MR) imaging. Conventional defecography is important for accurate diagnosis of intussusception and rectoceles. Endoanal ultrasound (EUS) is the preferred diagnostic technique and has replaced the invasive method of electromyography. Recently, MR imaging, especially with endorectal coils, has been shown to be accurate in delineating the anatomy of the sphincter complex.

Diagnosis

The four-grade classification after Browning and Parks has been the standard for clinically grading fecal incontinence for many years [11]. Grade I means involuntary loss of gas, grade II is soiling, grade III means loss of solid material, and grade IV refers to complete incontinence. The Jorge and Wexner questionnaire [12], which comprises an estimation of leakage frequency with the need to wear a pad and the overall effect on lifestyle, has become widely used since its implementation in 1993. With this system, a score of 0 indicates perfect continence and a score of 20 indicates complete incontinence.

For assessment of fecal incontinence, digital palpation, manometry (balloon or vector manometry), and measurement of pudendal nerve motor latency are used. In manometry, pressure at rest and pressure at contraction are quantified in a station-pull-through technique. A low pressure at rest is due to functional impairment of the internal sphincter, and a low pressure at contraction is due to impairment of the external sphincter muscle. However, even modern vector manometry cannot provide precise definition of localization and extent of sphincter defects [13]. PNTML is prolonged in patients with idiopathic fecal incontinence. Pudendal latency is increased in patients with long-standing constipation, perineal descent, or, generally, pelvic floor disorders. However, with all of these methods, structural defects cannot be assessed [13]. Diagnosis of sphincter defects is important because patients may be helped by surgery that aims to restore integrity to the sphincter ring. The prime role of anal imaging, whether sonography or MR, is to detect those patients who have an underlying tear and to direct them to surgery. Just as important, imaging can confidently exclude those patients who have no laceration, sparing them an operation that is likely to be unhelpful and instead directing them to more appropriate treatments, such as biofeedback behavioral therapy, sacral nerve stimulation, or sphincter reconstruction using either muscular flaps or implantable devices.

Endoanal Ultrasound

Since its implementation, EUS has been the gold standard in the morphological diagnosis of the anal canal. Muscular discontinuation of anal sphincters can be clearly discriminated from diffuse atony without structural defects [14, 15]. Moreover, EUS is easily available, inexpensive, and patient compliant.

EUS is performed with dedicated equipment including a high-frequency, mechanically rotated transducer for a 360° axial image. For acoustic coupling, the transducer is encased by a hard plastic cone filled with degassed water. The plastic cone is covered with a condom after application of a lubricant to the surfaces of the condom and the cone. The most commonly used system is the type 1850 and 2050 rotating endoprobe (B-K Medical, Herlev, Denmark). Initially, a 7-MHz crystal was used, but image resolution has been greatly improved with the advent of the 10-MHz probe, which has a focal length of 1–4 cm and a beam width of 0.8 mm. Anal endosonography may be performed with the patient in the left lateral, prone, or lithotomy position and then rotated so that the 12 o'clock position is anterior [16]. The probe is inserted through the anus into the lower rectum, where contact is lost between the probe surface and the bowel wall, which leads to characteristic reverberation echo distortion. As the probe is withdrawn further, the first anatomical landmark seen is the sling of the puborectalis muscle. The examination then begins in earnest, and the anal canal distal to this level is carefully examined.

With regard to anal canal anatomy, three layers can be differentiated endosonographically: the highly reflective submucosa, the low-reflective internal sphincter muscle, and the moderately reflective external muscle. The width of the internal sphincter increases with age: normal width for a patient 55 years old or younger is 2.4–2.7 mm, but above this age, the normal range increases to 2.8–3.4 mm. As the width of the sphincter increases, it becomes progressively more reflective and indistinct, which may be due to a relative increase in fibroelastic content of this muscle as a consequence of aging [17, 18]. The external sphincter muscle is of moderate reflectivity, with the longitudinal muscle of a similar reflectivity situated between the two sphincters in the intersphincteric space. The deep part of the external anal sphincter merges with the puborectalis muscle dorsally, with the superficial ends at the caudal extent of the internal sphincter. The anal canal mucosa is not seen because it is lost within the bright reflection from outside of the probe cone (Fig. 1).

Muscle reflectivity depends more on its fibroelastic content and the orientation of these fibers rather than on the type of muscle cells, as these on their own are all of low reflectivity. The internal sphincter has low fibroelastic content and presents as a well-defined ring of low reflectivity. The external sphincter is more variable in fiber content [19]. There is a difference between genders in the appearance of the external sphincter. In men, it is more symmetric, less

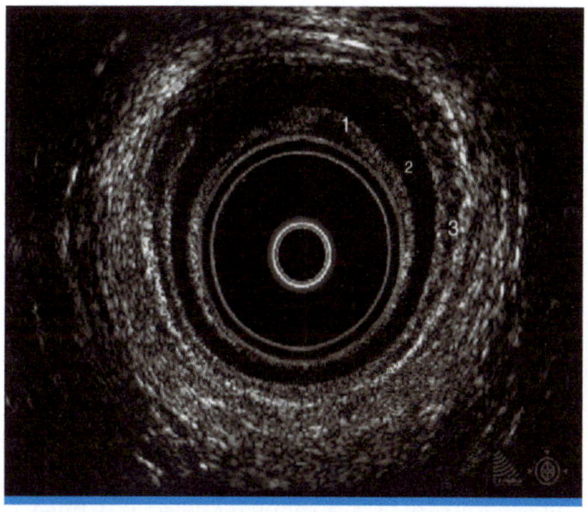

Fig. 1. Normal anal endosonography. Subepithelium (*1*), internal sphincter (*2*), external sphincter (*3*)

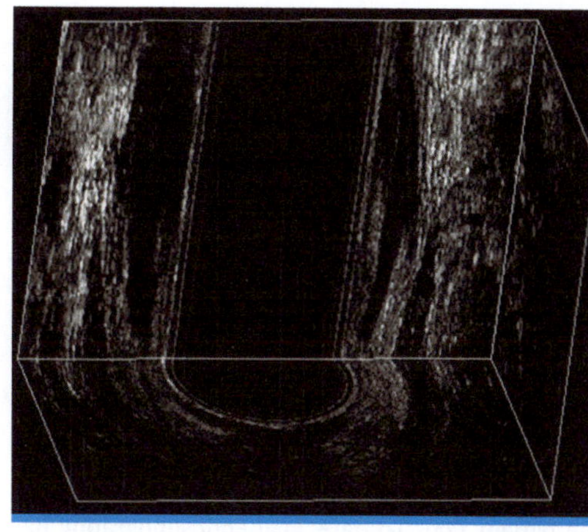

Fig. 2. Three-dimensional endosonography, normal anatomy

reflective, and easier to delineate, while in women, the anterior part of this sphincter is shorter and the perineal body seems void of any structure, as it is mainly fibroelastic in content.

Three-dimensional (3D) ultrasound extends the usefulness of anal endosonography. The same type of probes also facilitates 3D imaging techniques. A 3D reconstruction is based on a high number of parallel transaxial images acquired using an electronic pull-back mover. For endoanal application, the usual setting is 0.2–0.3 mm between adjacent transaxial images over a distance of 60 mm. Data from a series of closely spaced, two-dimensional (2D) images is combined to create a 3D image that can be freely rotated and sliced to allow the operator to get the most information out of the data while not being under the time pressure of the examination itself. Data stored in a file originating from this one acquisition can then be reviewed at any time. After a data set is acquired, it is immediately possible to select coronal anterior–posterior or posterior–anterior as well as sagittal right-left views. These views offer an unsurpassed source of information to use in evaluating the patient. The great advantage of 3D imaging is that once a data set has been obtained, the volume contains all of the data for that examination. Standard 2D anal sonography, as with most ultrasound examinations, is a dynamic process that is observer dependent. In contrast, 3D systems acquire a volume of digital data that can be retrieved for subsequent radiologist review. Three-dimensional reconstruction of anal endosonography is now increasingly available [20, 21], and while its clinical role is uncertain, it does permit multiplanar assessment of sphincter injury for the first time (Fig. 2).

Any break in the continuity of the ring of low reflectiveness representing the internal sphincter muscle is abnormal and is considered to be indicative of direct trauma, particularly from surgical procedures such as anal stretch, lateral internal anal sphincterotomy, fistulotomy for fistula, or part of generalized sphincter trauma from vaginal delivery 3–5, 22] (Fig. 3). A general thinning may be found in internal sphincter degeneration. Tears in the external sphincter muscle are defined by an interruption of the fine parallel fibrillar echo texture. In childbirth,

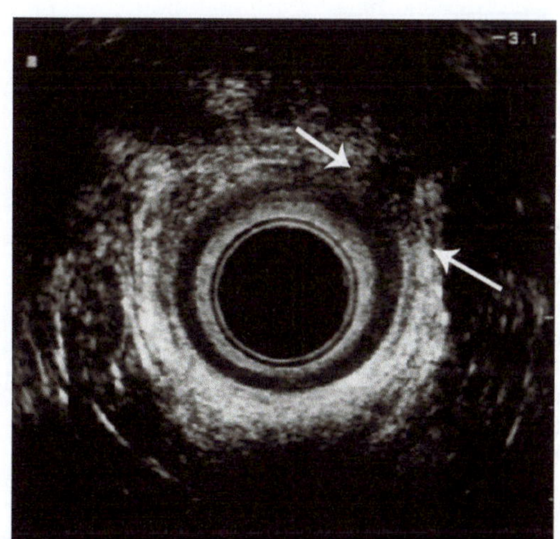

Fig. 3. Anterior external sphincter defect after obstetric injury (*arrows*)

tears result from overstretching or extension from an adjacent rupture or episiotomy. Scars are characterized by loss of normal architecture, with an area of amorphous texture that usually shows low reflectiveness corresponding to fibrosis. Generalized external sphincter atrophy is difficult to appreciate because of the vague contours of the muscle ring. Fat replacement within the atrophied muscle causes loss of the normal muscle/fat interface border at the outer margin of the external sphincter. The outer border of the external sphincter is then not defined, and thickness cannot be accurately measured. MR imaging is the more reliable method for evaluation in this instance.

The main advantage of the use of endosonography is the exact delineation of internal and external sphincter morphology with minimum discomfort for the patient [23]. To date, anal endosonography has almost completely replaced the painful needle-electromyographic mapping in use at the beginning of the last decade and has given a new comprehension of morphological changes of the sphincter muscles in the genesis of fecal incontinence [4, 24]. Operator dependence and common pitfalls, related to aberrant bundles of the external sphincter and gender-related anatomy, are currently the relative limitations of this method [19]. Anal endosonography is more sensitive in the evaluation of fecal incontinence than is anal manometry due to the morphologic depiction of sphincter defects. Endosonography should be mandatory in the assessment of fecal incontinence, even to confirm intact sphincter muscles in suspected neurogenic causes.

MR Imaging

Endoanal MR imaging has the advantages of multiplanar imaging and high soft-tissue contrast, especially for defining the components of the external sphincter muscle [25–28]. MR imaging is performed at 1.0 or 1.5 Tesla units and endoanal surface coils with diameters ranging from 12 to 19 mm and lengths of 50–75 mm. The endoanal coil is covered with a condom and a lubricant and then applied with the patient rotated to the left. External coil holders can be used but may increase patient discomfort. The MR imaging examination is performed in the supine position after application of hyoscine butyl bromide (Buscopan) or glucagon IV to reduce peristaltic bowel movement [27–29].

An optimal imaging protocol for fecal incontinence has not been established to date. However, the use of T2-weighted turbo spin echo (TSE) and 3D gradient echo sequences with a slice thickness of 2–4 mm in the axial, coronal, and sagittal orientation should be performed. On T2-weighted images, the external sphincter and longitudinal muscle return a relatively low signal, whereas the internal sphincter returns a relatively high signal. The subepithelial tissue has a signal intensity value between that of the internal and external sphincters. The lateral border of the external sphincter is well defined, especially when compared with the rather indistinct images of endosonography (Fig. 4). The coronal and the sagittal planes should be oriented perpendicular to the long axis of the endoanal coil. The examination time should not exceed 30 min [30].

Recent literature has evaluated high-resolution MR imaging of the anal sphincter complex using phased-array coils, but its role in fecal incontinence must still be determined. For the visualization of sphincter defects, however, the use of an endoanal coil is necessary [31]. A sphincter defect is defined as a discontinuity of the muscle ring (Fig. 5). Scarring is defined as a hypointense deformation of the normal pattern of the muscle layer due to replacement of muscle cells by fibrous tissue.

MR imaging is comparable with endosonography with regard to characterization of damage to the internal sphincter. With regard to characterization of damage to the external sphincter, however, MR imaging allows good distinction among muscles,

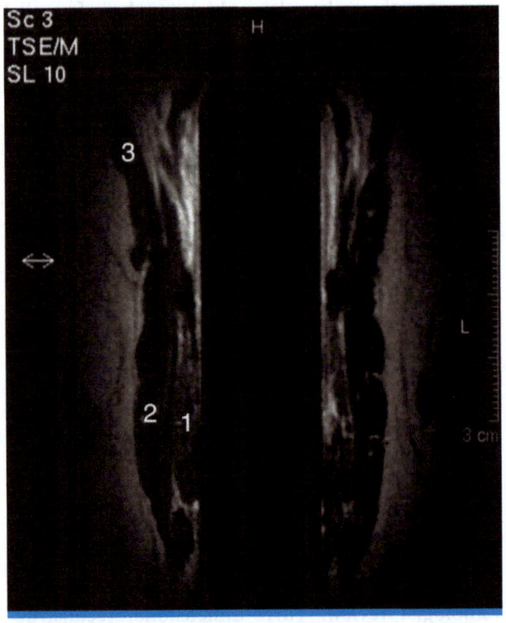

Fig. 4. Coronal T2-weighted magnetic resonance (MR) images of the anal canal with applied endorectal coil. MR image shows normal anatomy internal sphincter (*1*), external sphincter (*2*), and levator plate (*3*)

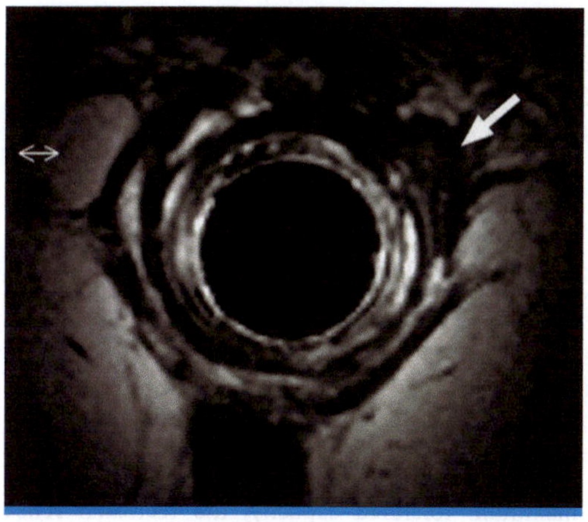

Fig. 5. A 53-year-old woman with fecal incontinence after obstetric trauma. Axial T2-weighted magnetic resonance (MR) image of the anal canal using an endocoil shows discontinuity of the external muscle at 2 o'clock, corresponding to a sphincter tear (*arrow*)

scars, and fat tissue, which facilitates accurate detection of local thinning, which is not possible with endosonography, and gives a more precise description of the extent and structure of complex lesions [32].

Endocoil MR imaging allows accurate assessment of thickness and fat content of the external sphincter. External sphincter atrophy is usually associated with generalized thinning and reduction of the striated muscle with fatty replacement. Endosonography alone is not a reliable modality for this imaging task [33, 34]. MR imaging has been shown to be able to determine the presence or absence of external sphincter atrophy with a sensitivity of 89% and a specificity of 94% [35]. This finding is important because patients who have both an atrophic external sphincter and a coexisting sphincter defect have been found to fare poorly after surgical repair of the defect, presumable because residual muscle is functionally inadequate [35, 36]. The degree of fat replacement may be precisely quantified using MR [37], but the appearances of atrophic muscle are equally well appreciated by simple inspection once the investigator has sufficient experience to recognize the morphology of normal muscle. An atrophic external sphincter has reduced bulk when compared with a normal sphincter, and the quality of that muscle that is present is patchy and indistinct. Sphincter atrophy may also affect the internal sphincter, a phenomenon known as idiopathic internal anal sphincter degeneration [38]. The internal sphincter normally thickens with age, but patients with idiopathic degeneration show progressive thinning, a finding that is probably best assessed using anal ultrasound. Generally, a diagnosis of idiopathic degeneration should be considered in any adult patient with passive incontinence in combination with a thin but intact internal sphincter.

Recently, dynamic MR defecography, with the advantages of a dynamic analysis of pelvic floor organ and soft tissue, decreased invasiveness, and lack of ionizing radiation in anorectal disease, has been introduced [39]. The limitations of MR imaging is the supine position and underestimation of rectal abnormalities. Interest in this modality for pelvic floor imaging has been relatively recent, and validation of the accuracy of MR imaging and optimal technique for the study is still in the process of being determined. When MR imaging has been compared with evacuation proctography, the results have been variable [40–42]. Studies in larger numbers will help to clarify the sensitivity and accuracy of MR imaging compared with proctography, which is the traditional test.

Defecography

Defecography (evacuation proctography) documents the process of rectal evacuation. It provides objective information about rectocele size and emptying and demonstrates coexistent enteroceles. This radiographic technique is a useful method for diagnosis of rectal intussusception, the mechanism by which rectal prolapse occurs.

The rectum is filled with up to 300 ml of a thick barium paste (to approximate the consistency of fecal material). The patient is seated on a radiolucent toilet chair mounted at the footplate of a remote-control stand. A series of lateral images and video films of the rectum and the anal canal are obtained during the process of rectal evacuation. Films are generally obtained at rest, on voluntary contraction of the anal sphincter and pelvic floor muscles, on straining down, and during defecation. The vagina is also opacified. To visualize the loops of the small bowel in the pelvis, barium contrast medium is given orally half an hour prior to examination [43–45].

A large number of incontinent patients have concomitant symptoms of pelvic outlet obstruction. In this group, defecography is useful for demonstrating large, nonemptying rectoceles, a spastic pelvic floor, and intussusception. Intussusception is the mechanism by which rectal prolapse occurs (Fig. 6) [46]. It usually starts as an infolding 6–8 cm inside the rectum, originating from the anterior wall in an annular

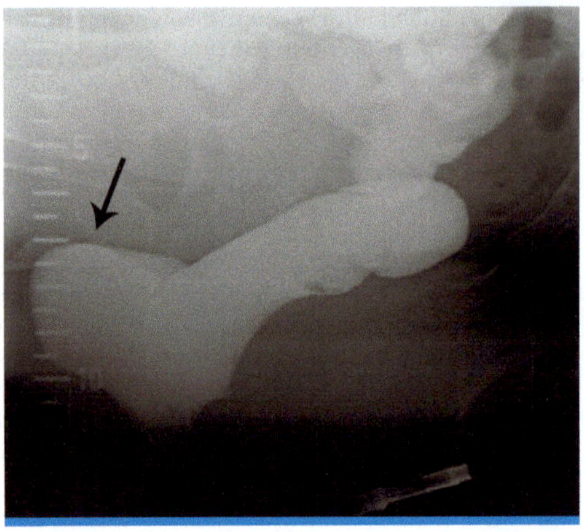

Fig. 6. A 57-year-old woman with fecal incontinence and pelvic outlet obstruction. Lateral view of defecography shows large anterior rectocele with a diameter of 5 cm (*arrow*)

fashion [47]. On continued straining in patients with rectal prolapse, the intussusception advances down into the anal canal and then through the anal orifice, constituting a complete rectal prolapse. Rectoceles are evident at defecography as an outpouching of the anterior rectal wall during evacuation (Fig. 7). Enteroceles are suspected when a separation of the upper vagina from the adjacent rectum by 2 cm or more is present. The definite diagnosis, however, requires the demonstration of herniated loops of small bowel within the widened rectovaginal space [48].

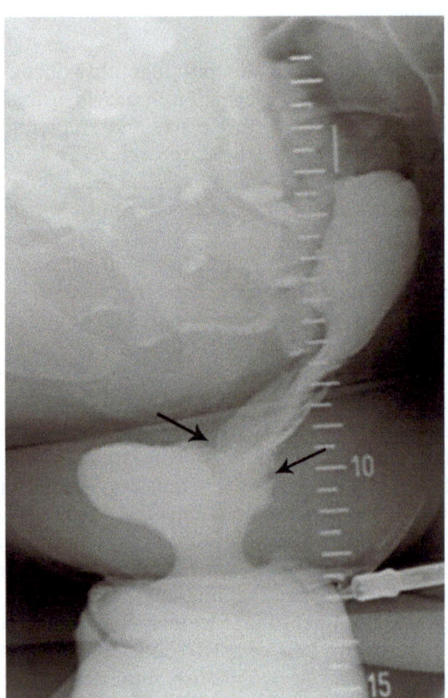

Fig. 7. An 80-year-old woman with fecal incontinence (soiling) and pelvic outlet obstruction. Anteroposterior view of defecography shows circumferential intussusception (*arrows*)

When the patient is seated for defecography, the weight of the abdominal contents stresses the pelvic floor to reveal the abnormal position of the pelvic floor at rest. Leakage of contrast at rest on defecography is also a good indication of sphincter weakness and is found only in patients with overt fecal incontinence [49]. This depends on how much contrast is injected into the rectum. If the rectum is filled to the maximum tolerated capacity, the rectoanal reflex that causes leakage is invoked [6].

Defecography is also used to assess anismus and spastic pelvic floor syndrome. However, overall defecography is of rather limited value in incontinent patients unless they suffer from associated obstructive symptoms [45].

Conclusion

Fecal incontinence is often multifactorial. Clinical examination may not detect the cause in at least 25% of patients. Defecography provides both structural and functional information for rectal voiding and prolapse. Defecography may demonstrate pelvic floor and sphincter weakness by abnormal descent at rest and anal leakage. Anal endosonography and MR imaging are complementary with regard to surgical decision making. The advantages of endosonography are, as stated above, that it is less expensive, more widely available, and faster than MR imaging.

Endosonography is valuable as a screening procedure to detect sphincter tears amenable to surgical treatment and is the method of choice to show damage to the sphincter muscles, either with general thinning as found in degeneration, or from focal discontinuities due to any traumatic cause. MR imaging is a powerful tool with which to investigate weakness of the pelvic floor generally and atrophy of the external sphincter, an important predictive factor for the outcome of sphincter repair.

References

1. Roberts RO, Jacobson SJ, Reilly WT et al (1999) Prevalence of combined fecal and urinary incontinence: a community-based study. J Am Geriatr Soc 47:837–841
2. Keighley MRB, Williams NS (1993) Faecal inconti-

nence. In: Keighley MRB, Williams NS (eds) Surgery of the anus, rectum and colon. Saunders, London, pp 592–700
3. Sultan AH, Kamm MA, Bartram CI, Hudson CN (1993) Anal sphincter trauma during instrumental delivery. Int J Gynecol Obstet 43:263–270
4. Sultan AH, Kamm MA, Hudson CN et al (1993) Anal-sphincter disruption during vaginal delivery. N Engl J Med 329:1905–1911
5. Sultan AH, Kamm MA, Nicholls RJ, Bartram C (1994) Prospective study of the extent of sphincter division during lateral sphincterotomy. Dis Colon Rectum 37:1031–1033
6. Bartram CI (2003) Faecal incontinence. In: Bartram CI, DeLancey JOL (eds) Imaging pelvic floor disorders. Springer, Berlin, Heidelberg, New York, pp 159–164
7. Parks AG, Hardcastle JD (1966) The syndrome of the descending perineum. Proc R Soc Med 59:477–482
8. Felt-Bersma RJF, Cuesta M, Koorevaar M (1996) Anal sphincter repair improves anorectal function and endosonographic image: a prospective clinical study. Dis Colon Rectum 39:878–885
9. Setti Carraro P, Kamm MA, Nicholls RJ (1994) Long-term results of postanal repair for neurogenic faecal incontinence. Br J Surg 81:140–144
10. Pinho M, Ortiz J, Oya M et al (1992) Total pelvic floor repair for the treatment of neuropathic faecal incontinence. Am J Surg 163:340–343
11. Browning GG, Parks AG (1983) Postanal repair for neuropathic faecal incontinence: correlation of clinical results and anal canal pressures. Br J Surg 70:101–104
12. Jorge JM, Wexner SD (1993) Etiology and management of fecal incontinence. Dis Colon Rectum 36:77–97
13. Braun JC, Treutner KH, Drew B et al (1994) Vectormanometry for differential diagnosis of fecal incontinence. Dis Colon Rectum 37:989–996
14. Burnett SJ, Spence-Jones C, Speakman CT et al (1991) Unsuspected sphincter damage following childbirth revealed by anal endosonography. Br J Radiol 64:225–227
15. Law PJ, Kamm MA, Bartram CI (1991) Anal endosonography in the investigation of fecal incontinence. Br J Surg 78:312–314
16. Law PJ, Bartram CI (1989) Anal endosonography; technique and normal anatomy. Gastrointest Radiol 14:349–353
17. Burnett SJ, Bartram CI (1991) Endosonographic variations in the normal internal anal sphincter. Int J Colorectal Dis 6:2–4
18. Sultan AH, Nicholls RJ, Kamm MA et al (1993) Anal endosonography and correlation with in vitro and in vivo anatomy. Br J Surg 80:508–511
19. Bartram CI, Frudinger A (1997) Normal anatomy of the anal canal. In: Handbook of anal endosonography. Wrightson Biomedical Publishing, Petersfield, pp 21–42
20. Gold DM, Bartram CI, Halligan S et al (1999) Three-dimensional endoanal sonography in assessing anal canal injury. Br J Surg 86:365–370
21. Williams AB, Cheetham MJ, Bartram CI et al (2000) Gender differences in the longitudinal pressure profile of the anal canal related to anatomical structure as demonstrated on three-dimensional anal endosonography. Br J Surg 87:1674–1679
22. Nielson MB, Hauge C, Pederson JF, Christiansen J (1993) Endosonographic evaluation of patients with anal incontinence: findings and influence on surgical management. Am J Roentgenol 160:771–775
23. Deen KI, Kumar D, Williams MCH et al (1993) Anal sphincter defects. Correlation between endoanal ultrasound and surgery. Ann Surg 218:201–205
24. Maier A, Fuchsjäger M, Alt J, Herbst F et al (2001) Value of endoanal sonography in the assessment of faecal incontinence. Fortschr Röntgenstr 173: 1104–1108
25. De Souza NM, Puni R, Kmiot WA et al (1995) MRI of the anal sphincter. J Comput Assist Tomogr 19:745–751
26. De Souza NM, Puni R, Zbar A et al (1996) MR imaging of the anal sphincter in multiparous women using an endoanal coil: correlation with in vitro anatomy and appearances in fecal incontinence. AJR Am J Roentgenol 167:1465–1471
27. Maier A, Fuchsjäger M, Funovics M (2000) Endoanal magnetic resonance tomography in fecal incontinence. Radiologe 40:465–468
28. Rociu E, Stoker J, Eijkemans MJC et al (1999) Fecal incontinence: endoanal US versus endoanal MR imaging. Radiology 212:453–458
29. Stoker J, Rociu E (1999) Endoluminal MR imaging of anorectal diseases. J Magn Reson Imaging 9:631–634
30. Stoker J, Bartram CI, Halligan S (2002) Imaging of the posterior pelvic floor. Eur Radiol 12:779–788
31. Hussain SM, Stoker J, Lameris JS (1995) Anal sphincter complex: endoanal MR imaging of normal anatomy. Radiology 197:671–677
32. Briel JW, Zimmerman DD, Stoker J et al (2000) Relationship between sphincter morphology on endoanal MRI and histopathological aspects of the external anal sphincter. Int J Colorectal Dis 15:87–90
33. Gold DM, Halligan S, Kmiot WA, Bartram CI (1999) Intraobserver and interobserver agreement in anal endosonography. Br J Surg 86:371–375
34. Williams AB, Bartram CI, Modhwadia D et al (2001) Endocoil magnetic resonance imaging quantification of external sphincter atrophy. Br J Surg 88:853–859
35. Briel JW, Stoker J, Rociu E et al (1999) External anal sphincter atrophy on endoanal magnetic resonance imaging adversely affects continence after sphincteroplasty. Br J Surg 86:1322–1327
36. Williams AB, Bartram CI, Chelvanayagam S et al (2001) Imaging predicts the results from anterior external anal sphincter repair following obstetric trauma. Colorectal Dis 3:82
37. Williams AB, Malouf AJ, Bartram CI et al (2001) Assessment of external anal sphincter morphology in idiopathic faecal incontinence with endo-coil magnetic resonance imaging. Digest Dis Sci 46:1466–1471
38. Vaizey CJ, Kamm MA, Bartram CI (1997) Primary degeneration of the internal anal sphincter as a cause of passive faecal incontinence. Lancet 346. 612–615
39. Paetzel C, Strotzer M, Fürst A et al (2001) Dynamic magnetic resonance defecography in the diagnosis of

combined pelvic floor disorders in proctology. Fortschr Röntgenstr 173:410–415
40. Delemarre JBVM, Kruyt RH, Doornbos J et al (1994) Anterior rectocele: assessment with radiographic defecography, dynamic magnetic resonance imaging, and physical examination. Dis Colon Rectum 37:249–259
41. Gufler H, Laubenberger J, DeGregorio G et al (1999) Pelvic floor descent: dynamic MR imaging using a half-Fourier RARE sequence. J Mag Reson Imaging 9:378–383
42. Lienemann A, Anthuber C, Baron A et al (1997) Dynamic MR colpocystorectography assessing pelvic-floor descent. Eur Radiol 7:1309–1317
43. Ekberg O, Nylander G, Fork FT (1985) Defecography. Radiology 155:45–48
44. Felt-Bersma RJF, Luth WJ, Janssen JJ, Meuwissen SGM (1990) Defecography in patients with anorectal disorders: which clinical findings are relevant? Dis Colon Rectum 33:277–284
45. Kelvin FM, Maglinte DDT, Benson JT (1994) Evacuation proctography (defecography): an aid to the investigation of pelvic floor disorders. Obstet Gynecol 82:307–314
46. Broden B, Snellman B (1968) Procidentia of the rectum studied with cineradiography: a contribution to the discussion of causative mechanism. Dis Colon Rectum 11:330–347
47. Mahieu P, Pringot J, Bodart P (1984) Defecography: II. Contribution to the diagnosis of defecation disorders. Gastrointest Radiol 9:253–261
48. Kelvin FM, Maglinte DDT, Hornback JA, Benson JT (1992) Pelvic prolapse: assessment with evacuation proctography (defecography). Radiology 184:547–551
49. Rex DK, Lappas JC (1992) Combined anorectal manometry and defecography in 50 consecutive adults with faecal incontinence. Dis Colon Rectum 35: 1040–1045

Invited Commentary

Tracy L. Hull

Anal endosonography has revolutionized the treatment of fecal incontinence. In the early 1990s, research appeared that documented the normal anal sphincter complex and its components [1–3]. Mapping out the normal appearance of the internal and external sphincters allowed actual visualization of defects in the anal sphincter. Prior to this, patients with fecal incontinence (mostly women) were evaluated with physical exam, anal physiology, and needle electromyelogram (EMG) [4–6]. This limited evaluation was not precise, and probably many sphincter defects (usually as a result of childbirth) were missed [7]. Prior to anal endosonography, patients with fecal incontinence that manifested years after the injury were labeled as having "idiopathic" fecal incontinence. Whereas this category still exists, anal endosonography allows precise anatomical delineation in an effort to tailor treatment for the individual patient.

Currently, anal endosonography remains the most popular tool with which to study patients with fecal incontinence. Some patients have obvious defects, which do not require preoperative imaging studies, but many have sphincter defects that are difficult to quantify. Visualization of defects in this group of patients may be beneficial as a guide when planning surgical intervention.

As with any procedure, there are preferences in performing it and a learning curve in becoming proficient at it. The actual number of anal endosonographic exams needed to become skilled enough to identify defects is not clear but is probably low. The most difficult aspect of using the two-dimensional (2D) instrument is learning how to work the different tuning mechanisms, which intensify and manipulate the image. Once this is mastered, seeing defects in the black internal anal sphincter is quite easy. However, the striated external anal sphincter image is sometimes most difficult to visualize. Asking the patient to squeeze his or her anal muscle while the probe is rotating will sometimes delineate the ends of the muscle. Also, the examiner placing a finger in the patient's vagina while the probe is rotating may enhance visualization of the anal sphincters, particularly the external anal sphincter. This is especially true for the inexperienced sonographer or when imaging a patient with a sphincter that is difficult to see.

I prefer to use a balloon around the crystal at the end of the probe rather than the hard plastic cone as discussed in the primary manuscript. I find the cone at times has a diameter that does not allow consistent coupling to the mucosa in patients with decreased tone, and thus shadowing from air distorts the image. The balloon is filled with degassed water and does not need to be overly filled and thus can be controlled to allow just the right amount of fluid to enhance balloon coupling against the anal canal mucosa.

Three-dimensional (3D) anal endosonography is relatively new and the machine expensive enough that many institutions do not have that equipment. The advantage of this modality is that it allows image acquisition and later reconstruction to study the sphincter complex in detail from multiple angles [8]. This can be an advantage, as it allows for intense study of the complex at a later time. However, this can also be a disadvantage, as it takes more time to configure and study the images versus the 2D procedure. The advantage of the degree of improved precision offered by the 3D unit is not clear, and at this point, particularly in light of the added time and expense, the 3D machine is not mandatory for optimal care.

Vaginal endosonography to view the muscle complex "through the rectovaginal septum" is practiced by some caregivers, particularly those from gynecologic backgrounds where transvaginal endosonography is also used to evaluate the ovaries and uterus. This could be considered a natural extension of its use. Without specific experience performing the procedure from this route, I cannot give a fair commentary other than to say that proponents feel they attain equivalent sphincter evaluation.

Other modalities have been examined to study the anal canal anatomy. The only one that provides information close to the endosonography machine is magnetic resonance imaging (MRI) with anal coil [9].

When consideration of time, expense, and degree of visualization is weighed against the MRI with coil, I consider endosonography superior.

At our institution, nearly all patients with fecal incontinence undergo anal endosonography when a surgical intervention is contemplated. We use the 2D machine, and the exam takes about 10 min or less. The exam is done in the office after the patient is given an enema. The enema also is an inexpensive test that crudely assesses the patient's ability to contain liquid in their rectal reservoir. The test is performed in the left lateral position with a 10-MHz probe. The anal endosonography, combined with a careful history and physical exam, guide us in treatment strategy.

As I practice at a teaching institution, anal physiology testing is also done; however, this is less helpful in my opinion. Considering the results from anal physiology testing, I particularly look at the pudendal nerve terminal motor latency (PNTML) and the compliance [10]. If the latency is prolonged, I will generally still repair a defect but explain to the patient that even with defect repair, the results will most likely be suboptimal. However, there is no good method to predict who will or will not be helped with sphincter repair. Therefore, I almost always offer repair to symptomatic patients, even those with a nerve prolongation. The other way I find anal physiology testing useful is to look at rectal compliance. This number reflects the elasticity of the rectum. If the compliance is low, the rectum is stiff and will not optimally store stool. Patients with low compliance can have an element of urgency, which negatively affects their defecation. Nonetheless, I still would repair a defective muscle in a patient with low compliance, as it may provide more time for the patient to reach the toilet. Even a few minutes may be a tremendous advantage.

The most common repair of the sphincter muscle is the overlapping anterior anal sphincteroplasty. This defect is usually a result of injury at the time of childbirth, and the woman's sphincter muscles may compensate for many years after the injury before debilitating symptoms develop. Long-term results of sphincter repair have been disappointing [11, 12], but if symptoms recur after surgery, anal endosonography is useful to verify that the muscle is optimally repaired. If a defect persists, surgical repeat repair is considered. Other novel treatments are being developed, but many will rely on accurate anatomy as outlined by anal endosonography to guide the treatment algorithm.

Other traumatic causes of fecal incontinence include consequences of surgery to address other anorectal disease. Fistulotomy and hemorrhoidectomy can leave various degrees of defects in the muscle or anal topography that lead to leakage. Sometimes these problems can be surgically improved by smoothing the scar ridge or reapproximating the muscle ends. However, internal anal sphincter disruption from stretching or hemorrhoid excisional surgery that includes some muscle fibers may not respond to conventional muscle reapproximation and necessitate consideration of one of the novel approaches to improve fecal leakage. Once again, the ability to detect defects in specific sphincter components and the size and configuration is mandatory.

In conclusion, anal endosonography has emerged over the past 15 years as a primary tool used to evaluate the anal sphincters. Its use has led the way for new and exciting research geared toward improving fecal incontinence by selecting the appropriate patient based on anal anatomy. This evaluation tool continues to evolve, and the 3D unit may prove to be indispensable as treatment options diversify and become targeted for very specific sphincter problems.

References

1. Deen KI, Kumar D, Williams JG et al (1993) Anal sphincter defects. Correlation between endoanal ultrasound and surgery. Ann Surg 218:201–205
2. Law PJ, Bartram CI (1989) Anal endosonography: Technique and normal anatomy. Gastrointest Radiol 14:349–353
3. Sultan AH, Nicholls RJ, Kamm MA et al (1993) Anal endosonography and correlation with in vitro and in vivo anatomy. Br J Surg 80:508–511
4. Wexner SD, Jorge JM (1994) Colorectal physiological tests: Use or abuse of technology? Eur J Surg 160:167–174
5. Cheong DM, Vaccaro CA, Salanga VD et al (1995) Electrodiagnostic evaluation of fecal incontinence. Muscle nerve 18:612–619
6. Tjandra JJ, Milsom JW, Schroeder T et al (1993) Endoluminal ultrasound is preferable to electromyography in mapping and sphincteric defects. Dis Colon Rectum 36:689–692
7. Law PJ, Kamm MA, Bartram CI (1990) A comparison between electromyography and anal endosonography in mapping external anal sphincter defects. Dis Colon Rectum 33:370–373
8. Gold DM, Bartram CI, Halligan S et al (1999) Three-dimensional endoanal sonography in assessing anal canal injury. Br J Surg 86:365–370
9. Malouf AJ, Williams AB, Halligan S et al (2000) Prospective assessment of accuracy of endoanal MR imaging and endosonography in patients with fecal incontinence. AJR Am J Roentgenol 175:741–745
10. Gilliland R, Altomare DF, Moreira H Jr et al (1998) Pudendal neuropathy is predictive of failure following anterior overlapping sphincteroplasty. Dis Colon Rectum 41:1516–1522
11. Halverson AL, Hull TL (2000) Long-term outcome of overlapping sphincter repair. Dis Colon Rectum 43:813–820
12. Gutierrez AB, Madoff RD, Lowry AC et al (2004) Long-term results of anterior sphincteroplasty. Dis Colon Rectum 47:727–732

Invited Commentary

Giulio A. Santoro

Introduction

The preceding chapter highlights the current state of the art for imaging of fecal incontinence. Endoanal ultrasonography (EAUS), endoanal magnetic resonance imaging (MRI), external phased-array MRI, and defecography provide different and possibly complementary information on the anatomy of the pelvic floor and anal sphincters. For the most part, MRI has been of limited clinical use due to cost and access problems. At present, EAUS remains the method of choice to show damage to the sphincter muscles and provides sufficient information for clinical decision making in many cases [1]. However, with the currently available ultrasonographic equipment and techniques, many elements of the image cannot be correctly recognized as components of a three-dimensional (3D) structure–or at least not perceived in their true spatial relationships–and a good deal of relevant information may remain hidden. The advent of high-resolution 3D EAUS and volume render mode (VRM), a technique to analyze information inside a 3D volume by digitally enhancing individual voxels, promise to offer additional information on anatomical structures in the pelvis, bringing improvement for both planning and conduct of surgical procedures [2]. In addition to the techniques described by Andrea Maier, transvaginal (TVUS) and transperineal (TPUS) ultrasonography represent two additional procedures to evaluate dysfunction that can occur in the pelvic floor region in women with fecal incontinence [3]. For these reasons, this commentary focuses on discussing the developments to date of US imaging techniques and suggests areas for future research.

High-resolution Three-dimensional Endoanal Ultrasonography

A 3D model may be constructed from a synthesis of a high number of parallel transaxial two-dimensional (2D) images. Automatic image acquisition is achieved by using a motor action within the transducer itself, allowing acquisition of a multitude of sectional planes. These can be integrated into a volume. Adding the third dimension means that the pixel is transformed in a small 3D picture element called a voxel (the correct term for a pixel that has a defined location in space). Ideally, a voxel should be a cubic structure; however, the dimension in the Z plane is often slightly larger than that in the X and Y planes. Voxel depth is critical to 3D image resolution, and this depth is directly related to the spacing between two adjacent images. High-resolution 3D US acquires four to five transaxial images sampled per 1 mm of acquisition length in the Z plane. This means that an acquisition based upon a sampling of transaxial images over a distance of 60 mm in the human body will result in a data volume block consisting of between 240 and 300 transaxial images. High-resolution data volumes will consist of typical voxel sizes around 0.15×0.15×0.2 mm. Because of this resolution in the longitudinal plane, which is close to the axial and transverse resolution of the 2D image, this technique ensures true dimensions of the 3D data cube in the reconstructed Z plane as well, and provides accurate distance, area, angle, and volume measurement [2].

The ability to visualize information in the 3D image depends critically on the rendering technique. VRM is a special feature that can be applied to high-resolution 3D data volume so information inside the cube is reconstructed to some extent. This technique uses a ray-tracing model as its basic operation. Depending on the various render mode settings of the four different postprocessing display parameters (opacity, luminance, thickness, and filter), data from each voxel may be discarded, it may be used to modify the existing value of the ray, or it may be stored for reference to the next voxel and used in a filtering calculation. All of these calculations result in the current color or intensity of the ray being modified in some way, providing better visualization performance when there are not large differences in the signal levels of pathologic structures compared with surrounding tissues [2].

Transvaginal Ultrasonography

TVUS involves placing the probe inside the vagina. For this application, two different types of probes can be used. To evaluate transaxial projections, a high-frequency (up to 16 MHz), 360° transducer is used. The image plane of this transducer is 90° to the longitudinal axis. For sagittal and conventional transverse imaging of the pelvic floor, including color Doppler, a biplane, high-frequency transducer with a long linear and transverse array is used. Both arrays are placed at 90° to each other and at 90° to the longitudinal axis. The probe can be placed resting on the posterior vaginal wall. With the patient lying on her back on a table or in a gynecological chair, the anterior vaginal wall will softly contact the surface of the US transducer without disturbing the functional anatomy. TVUS allows evaluation of a complex set of anatomical structures of the pelvic floor (Fig. 1) [3]. At the external urethral meatus level, the anal canal will be seen posteriorly in the image, together with the external anal sphincter (EAS), the internal anal sphincter (IAS), and often the superficial transverse perineal muscles within the perineal body in nullipara women. Introducing the transducer further in the cephalad direction (proximal), the ischiopubic rami, the symphysis pubis, the urethra, the pubourethral ligament, and the pubococcygeus muscle can be visualized. The puborectalis muscle (PR) will be seen inferior and lateral to the anal canal, depicting a soft curve upward anterior and lateral to the vagina, forming almost an ellipsoidal structure before attaching itself to the inferior side of the symphysis pubis. Posteriorly to the anal canal, the anococcygeal ligament can be identified as a black triangle in the US image. For transvaginal scanning, 3D US offers significant advantages over conventional techniques, in particular if combined with VRM.

Transperineal Ultrasonography

TPUS is a relatively simple technique for assessing morphologic integrity of both the IAS and EAS [4]. It is performed with a convex 6-MHz probe placed on the perineum. Most often, the patient will lie on her back, with hips flexed and slightly abducted. The left lateral, sitting, and standing positions are seldom used. Examination of the anus is made with the transducer initially applied transversely to the perineal body, identifying the axial view of the anus using the IAS hypoechoic ring as the landmark in an image that is similar to that obtained in the mid anal canal using EAUS. The transducer is then turned 180° to obtain a longitudinal view of the rectum, with extension of the hypoechoic IAS appearing above and below the anal canal in profile. The bright hyperechoic elliptical bundle of the PR sling is well demonstrated.

TPUS offers a dynamic evaluation of the pelvic

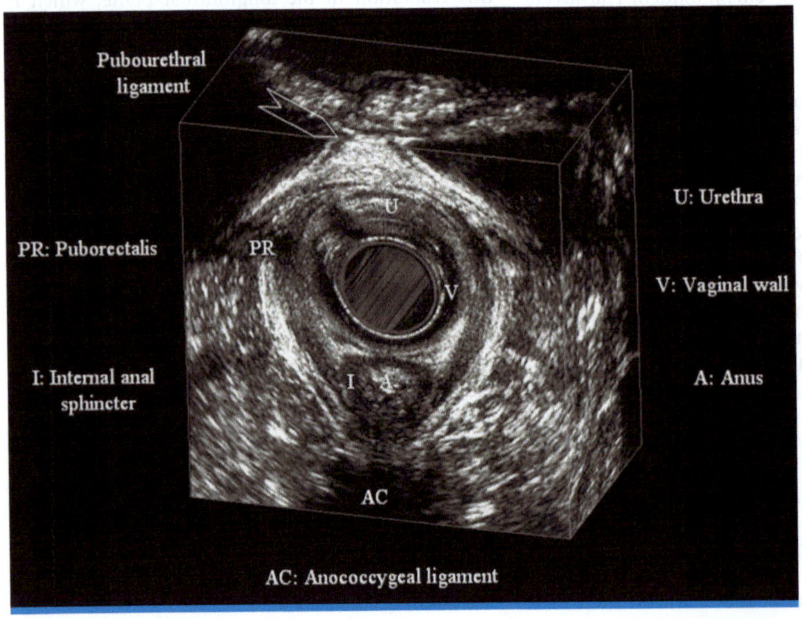

Fig. 1. Transvaginal ultrasonography (TVUS) of the pelvic floor. Reproduced with permission from [5]

floor [6]. After examination performed at rest, the patient can be examined during forcible straining and simulated evacuation so that structures can be evaluated during action. Observation of the levator ani (LA) during contraction and on Valsalva may increase the likelihood of detecting abnormalities of levator morphology [7–10].

Clinical Application

Anal sphincter defects are a major cause of fecal incontinence. These defects are often the result of vaginal delivery [11] or anal surgery (i.e., hemorrhoidectomy, sphincterotomy, fistula surgery). Dr. Maier has provided a comprehensively written and extensively referenced section on the importance of EAUS in distinguishing incontinent patients with intact anal sphincters and those with sphincter lesions. A limitation of EAUS remains scar identification and evaluation of EAS atrophy in patients with idiopathic fecal incontinence [1].

An advantage of high-resolution 3D EAUS is the possibility of measuring EAS length, thickness, area, and volume. The relationship between the radial angle and longitudinal extent of a sphincter tear can be assessed and graded. The length of the remaining intact sphincter muscle can also be evaluated, improving patient selection for surgical repair of the anal sphincter complex and helping the surgeon to judge how far the repair should extend. Volume rendering can be particularly useful in evaluating anal sphincter lesions [2]. Compared with normal mode, setting VRM with high opacity, normal thickness, and high luminance parameters allows better visualization of a rupture of the hyperechoic external sphincter complex in the anal canal. External sphincter tear will appear as a low-intensity defect in the context of the competent, brightest segments of this striated muscle [2]. To better delineate IAS tears, VRM should be used with low opacity and normal thickness setting. It is also possible to detect EAS atrophy by using VRM with normal opacity, high thickness, and high luminance setting to separate color and intensity data of muscular fibers and fatty tissue replacement (Fig. 2) [2].

Dr. Maier concentrated most of her chapter on detecting anal sphincter disruption or atrophy, but it is increasingly well recognized that many incontinent women have intact sphincter muscles. In these cases, LA muscle atrophy or damage is believed to cause the symptoms [12]. Research demonstrates that the LA is critically important in supporting the pelvic organs and maintaining their continence [7–9]. Though regarded as a single muscle, it is composed of two functional components: a supportive component (the iliococcygeus) and a sphincteric component (the pubococcygeus and the PR). The PR is responsible for maintaining anorectal junction angulation and contributes to anal continence. It moves dorsoven-

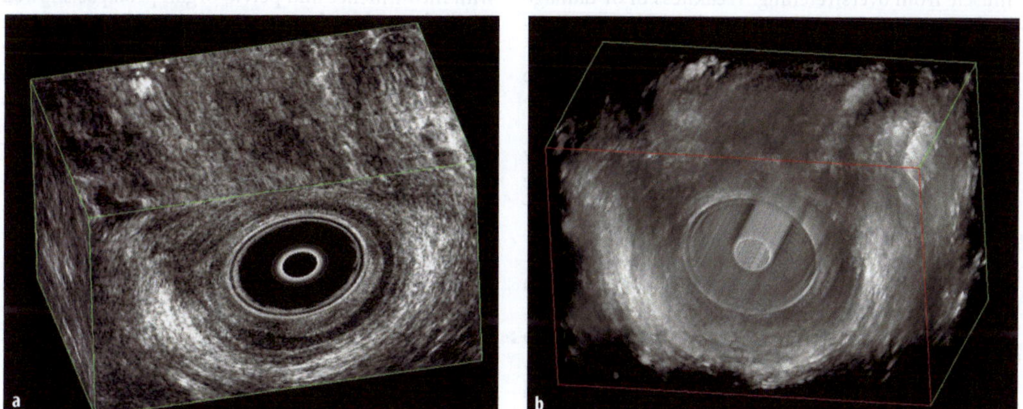

Fig. 2a, b. A 57-year-old woman with a large anterior external anal sphincter (EAS) tear between the 9 and 3 o'clock positions combined with an internal anal sphincter (IAS) defect between the 7 and 11 o'clock positions as consequence of an obstetric trauma. Three-dimensional (3D) endoanal ultrasound (EAUS) with normal mode (**a**). By using volume render mode (VRM) with normal opacity, high thickness, and high luminance setting, it is also possible to detect EAS atrophy of the remaining muscular fibers (**b**). Reproduced with permission from [2]

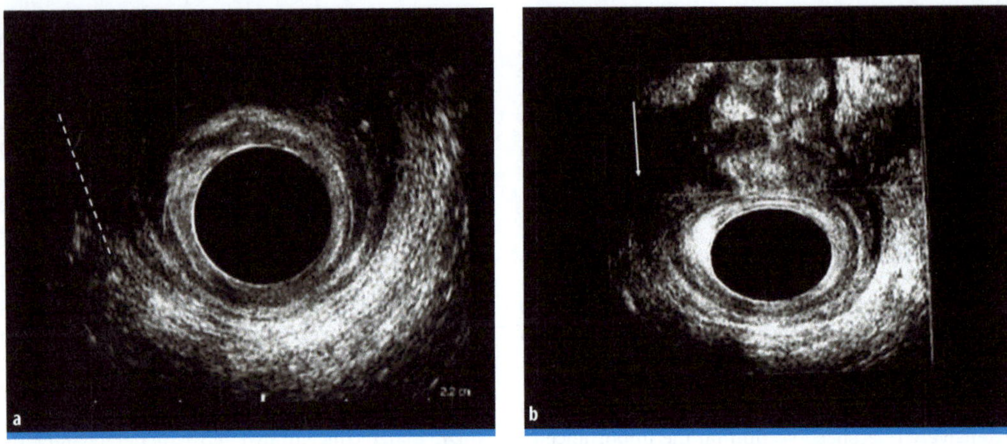

Fig. 3a, b. Example of a major defect of the right arm of the puborectalis muscle. Axial image (**a**). Three-dimensional (3D) reconstruction (**b**)

trally, narrowing the levator hiatus on straining, whereas the iliococcygeus moves craniocaudally. LA damage in women with pelvic floor dysfunction has been documented using MRI [13–17] or TPUS [7–10], and the origin of this damage during vaginal birth has been described [18, 19]. Damage usually appears in localized regions and more often in the pubic portion (pubococcygeal and PR) rather than in the iliococcygeal portion. Lien et al. [20] demonstrated that the pubococcygeal muscle seen to be injured is the part of the LA that undergoes the greatest degree of lengthening during vaginal delivery, suggesting that this injury may be due to rupture of the muscle from overstretching. Weakness of or damage to the LA may result in pelvic organ prolapse and urinary or fecal incontinence.

The complex shape and fiber arrangement of the LA precludes useful measurements of the muscle being made in standard 2D axial plane. The disadvantage of 2D US stems from its inability to easily disclose the 3D relationships, which may be at the root of the defects that lead to clinical pelvic floor pathology. To better understand the specific anatomic defects in women with fecal incontinence, we evaluated LA morphology and integrity by using 3D EAUS and 3D TVUS. Three-dimensional reconstruction and establishing muscle fascicle direction in 3D space provides accurate evaluation of LA morphology. Findings noted in axial sections can be correlated with findings seen in coronal and longitudinal planes to confirm the nature and extent of muscle damage (Fig. 3). In our center, 42 women, 16 with pelvic organ prolapse and fecal incontinence and 26 asymptomatic volunteers were studied using 3D EAUS and 3D TVUS. Axial, coronal, and longitudinal images were obtained and the following parameters measured: levator muscle shape, levator sling arm thickness, levator hiatus width (left-to-right distance), and length (anterior–posterior distance). Abnormalities of the pubovisceral portion were determined on each side and defect severity scored in each muscle from 0 (no defect) to 3 (complete muscle loss). A summed score for the two sides (0–6) was assigned and grouped as minor (1–3) or major (4–6) defects. A summed score of 3 occurring from a unilateral score of 3 was classified in the major group. In the control group, bilaterally intact levator sling arms were observed. In the patient group, ten women (62.5%) with incontinence and pelvic-organ prolapse showed PR defects: four had major defects, involving the right branch in three cases and the left branch in one case; six presented minor defects of the right branch (four cases) or left branch (two cases). Lesion site was more frequently the right branch (seven patients) than the left branch (three patients). Mean values of PR right- and left-branch thickness were significantly higher in controls than in patients (9±0.3 mm vs. 7±0.3 mm and 8±0.6 mm vs. 6±0.2 mm, respectively; $P<0.05$). Posterior PR thickness was similar in both groups (7±0.4 mm vs. 7±0.2 mm). Our 3D data confirm previous reports [13, 14] that levator atrophy and structural integrity loss are major cofactors in female pelvic floor dysfunction.

Conclusions

Ultrasound imaging is becoming the diagnostic standard in fecal incontinence. Several factors are contributing to its increasing acceptance, the most important being the availability of suitable equipment. Recent developments such as high-resolution 3D EAUS with VRM and 3D TVUS and TPUS enhance the clinical usefulness of the method. It is hoped that increasing parameter standardization will make it easier for clinicians and researchers to compare data.

References

1. Santoro GA, Gizzi G (2006) Accuracy and reliability of endoanal ultrasonography in the evaluation of anal sphincter injury. In: Santoro GA, Di Falco G. Benign anorectal diseases. Springer-Verlag Italia, pp 87–98
2. Santoro GA, Fortling B (2007) The advantages of volume rendering in three-dimensional endosonography of the anorectum. Dis Colon Rectum 50:359–368
3. Tunn R, Petri E (2003) Introital and transvaginal ultrasound as the main tool in the assessment of urogenital and pelvic floor dysfunction: an imaging panel and practical approach. Ultrasound Obstet Gynecol 22:205–213
4. Kleinubing H Jr, Jannini JF, Malafaia O et al (2000) Transperineal ultrasonography: new method to image the anorectal region. Dis Colon Rectum 43:1572–1574
5. Santoro GA, Di Falco G (2006) Benign Anorectal Diseases. Springer-Verlag Italia
6. Beer-Gabel M, Teshler M, Barzilai N et al (2002) Dynamic transperineal ultrasound in the diagnosis of pelvic floor disorders. Pilot study. Dis Colon Rectum 45:239–248
7. Dietz HP (2004) Ultrasound imaging of the pelvic floor. Part I: two dimensional aspects. Ultrasound Obstet Gynecol 23:80–92
8. Dietz HP (2004) Ultrasound imaging of the pelvic floor. Part II: three-dimensional or volume imaging. Ultrasound Obstet Gynecol 23:615–625
9. Dietz HP, Steensma AB (2005) Posterior compartment prolapse on two-dimensional and three-dimensional pelvic floor ultrasound: the distinction between true rectocele, perineal hypermobility and enterocele. Ultrasound Obstet Gynecol 26:73–77
10. Dietz HP, Steensma AB, Hastings R (2003) Three-dimensional ultrasound imaging of the pelvic floor: the effect of parturition on paravaginal support structures. Ultrasound Obstet Gynecol 21:589–595
11. Santoro GA, Pellegrini L, Di Falco G (2006) Update in perineal anatomy and its relevance to obstetric trauma. In: Santoro GA, Di Falco G. Benign anorectal diseases. Springer-Verlag Italia, pp 99–113
12. DeLancey JOL (2005) The hidden epidemic of pelvic floor dysfunction: achievable goals for improved prevention and treatment. Am J Obstet Gynecol 192:1488–1495
13. Singh K, Reid WMN, Berger LA (2002) Magnetic resonance imaging of normal levator ani anatomy and function. Obstet Gynecol 99:433–438
14. Singh K, Jakab M, Reid WMN et al (2003) Three-dimensional magnetic resonance imaging assessment of levator ani morphologic features in different grades of prolapse. Am J Obstet Gynecol 188:910–915
15. Hoyte L, Schierlitz L, Zou K et al (2001) Two and 3-dimensional MRI comparison of levator ani structure, volume, and integrity in women with stress incontinence and prolapse. Am J Obstet Gynecol 185:11–19
16. DeLancey JOL, Kearney R, Chou Q et al (2003) The appearance of levator ani muscle abnormalities in magnetic resonance images after vaginal delivery. Obstet Gynecol 101:46–53
17. Chen L, Hsu Y, Ashton-Miller JA, DeLancey JOL (2006) Measurement of the pubic portion of the levator ani muscle in women with unilateral defects in 3D models from MR images. Int J Gynecol Obstet 92:234–241
18. Kearney R, Miller JM, Ashton-Miller JA, DeLancey JOL (2006) Obstetric factors associated with levator ani muscle injury after vaginal birth. Obstet Gynecol 107:144–149
19. Kearney R, Sawhney R, DeLancey JOL (2004) Levator ani muscle anatomy evaluated by origin-insertion pairs. Obstet Gynecol 104:168–173
20. Lien K-C, Mooney B, DeLancey JOL, Ashton-Miller JA (2004) Levator ani muscle stretch induced by simulated vaginal birth. Obstet Gynecol 103:31–40

Diagnostic Workup in Incontinent Patients: An Integrated Approach

12

Carlo Ratto, Angelo Parello, Lorenza Donisi, Francesco Litta, Giovanni B. Doglietto

Introduction

Anal continence is assured by the activity of complex anatomical and physiological structures (anal sphincters, pelvic floor musculature, rectal curvatures, transverse rectal folds, rectal reservoir, rectal sensation). It is dependent also on numerous other factors, such as stool consistency, patient's mental faculties and mobility, and social convenience. Only if there is an effective, coordinated integration between these elements can defecation proceed normally. On the other hand, fecal incontinence (FI) is the result of disruption of one or several of these different entities: frequently, it can be due to a multifactorial pathogenesis, and in many cases, it is not secondary to sphincter tears. The disruption could lie in alterations intrinsic to the anorectal neuromuscular structures of continence control or be extrinsic to them, involving extrapelvic control mechanisms. The primary aim of an effective therapeutic approach must be the improvement-better, the resolution-of this distressing condition. Different forms of therapy are now available so that physicians must select the best option for each patient. Consequently, the diagnostic workup is fundamental to assess, as accurately as possible, the functional condition of every component involved in the continence mechanism and identify presumed causes of incontinence. In this regard, some clinicians are very aggressive in using a variety of tests, whereas others are very minimalist. This is despite evidence that approximately 20% of women with FI report a moderate or severe impact on their quality of life, and 84% of them with poor FI ask for a physician's help [1]. Even if there is full agreement concerning the role played by adequate data collection of patient history and accurate physical examination, the importance of each symptom or sign in the pathophysiologic assessment and in selecting the appropriate management of each individual patient's FI is still debated. On the other hand, related to the progressive improvement of knowledge on continence physiology, several specific instrumental tests have been designed for defining the underlying mechanisms of FI, which are available in a clinical setting or for investigational purposes. However, disagreement remains on the choice of diagnostic procedures and timing.

Clinical Assessment

Investigation of a patient's history is of utmost importance. Considering the embarrassment and reluctance related to FI, it is important to initiate a positive relationship with the patient. A background of psychological and emotional suffering is also characteristic of incontinent patients. Moreover, there is a wide range of personal motivation in searching for a solution. Some patients have looked for specialists in this field, perhaps having overcome the lack of interest or lack of knowledge of general practitioners; some have become convinced that the problem cannot be solved. The task of the specialist is to encourage patients to undergo clinical assessment and then to schedule a possible effective treatment.

Maximum efforts must be made to identify symptoms of pathogenetic significance and define the type of FI (urge incontinence, passive incontinence, fecal soiling, or seepage). However, classification is not always easy, and an in-depth interview of the patient is of pivotal importance. It is important to detail characteristics of normal defecation (occurring without incontinence) and thereafter ascertain the fundamental features of the incontinence: timing, duration, and frequency; type of stool lost; use of pads; rectoanal sensation during normal defecation and FI episodes; and influences on health status and quality of life. These features should be related to possible events in the patient's history, including metabolic and neurological diseases, obstetric and pelvic surgery, neurosurgery, pelvic trauma, chronic inflammatory bowel diseases, pelvic irradiation, psychiatric conditions, and physical and sexual abuse.

The patient interview should effectively address the physical examination, utilizing all exploratory and diagnostic techniques necessary to observe physical alterations of the anus, perineum, and pelvis and to elicit specific reflexes. The checklist shown in Table 1 could be of help.

Patient's symptoms and signs should be considered to classify FI into grades, not only to evaluate the severity but also to assess the effectiveness of the therapeutic approach. A number of scales have been proposed for these purposes, and disagreement exists on their use; grading systems suggested by the Cleveland Clinic [2] and Pescatori et al. [3] are some of the most frequently used.

Another important aspect must be considered: the patient's quality of life. This should be considered in both evaluation of FI severity and treatment assessment. For this parameter also, numerous criteria have been proposed. Some do not specifically addressed FI, whereas others do not evaluate the influence of FI on the general health status of patients [4–6].

Table 1. Physical examination of patients with fecal incontinence (FI)

Examinations	Signs
Perianal inspection	Skin excoriation/infection Perianal/perineal scars Patulous anus Perineal soiling Anal ectropion Hemorrhoidal prolapse Rectal prolapse Sphincter deficit Loss of perineal body Perineal descent Fistula
Palpation	Pinprick touch Resting tone Squeeze tone Puborectalis at rest, squeezing, straining Sphincter deficits Perianal/perineal scars Anal/rectal neoplasms Intussusception Rectocele
Endoscopy	Hemorrhoids Anal/rectal tumors Inflammatory bowel disease Solitary rectal ulcer
Neurological	Perianal sensation Anal reflex Mental status

Physiological Investigations

The primary aims of tests used in FI patients are to better elucidate the pathophysiology and address the treatment. This is particularly complex, not only due to the lack of comprehensive knowledge on pelvic floor morphology and physiology but also because of the wide variety of tests used, not always as standard procedures. This assessment must concern both function [mostly provided by anorectal manometry (ARM), rectal sensations investigation, and anorectal electrophysiology (AREP)] and structure [given by endoanal ultrasound (EAUS) and/or magnetic resonance imaging (MRI)] of all components, pelvic and extrapelvic, involved in the continence mechanisms. Due to the multifactorial nature of FI, no one test alone is sufficient to provide these two types of information, and an integration of investigations is needed. When FI occurs with diarrhea, other possible causes should be explored by endoscopy and stool tests. As well, when clinical examination suggests that FI could be secondary to metabolic, neurological, or neurosurgical disorders; trauma; bowel inflammation; irradiation; or psychiatric disturbances, specific investigations should be programmed.

Anorectal Manometry and Rectal Sensation

These procedures are usually performed in the same setting and include the evaluation of rectoanal reflexes and rectal compliance. Although they are the most frequently used diagnostic procedures in proctology, particularly in FI patients, they are carried out heterogeneously because of wide technical variations in computer software, probes (water perfused or solid state; uni- or multichannel; difference in number, location, and shape of openings; difference in location and material of balloon), acquisition modality of pressures (pull through or stationary), and sensations (inflation of either air or water or using barostat). For these technical differences, it is not possible to standardize either examination or normal values. Therefore, it is advisable to establish procedure and normal values in each laboratory according to age- and gender-matched healthy subjects [7]. In a study by Simpson et al. [8], five different manometric procedures (water-perfused side hole, water-perfused end hole, microtransducer, microballoon, air-filled probe) were compared; no significant variations in anal pressures were found using standard manometry techniques, whereas pressures recorded by the air-filled probe were lower.

In incontinent patients, both resting and squeeze pressures should be calculated (Fig. 1). The investigator should be very careful to evaluate not only the

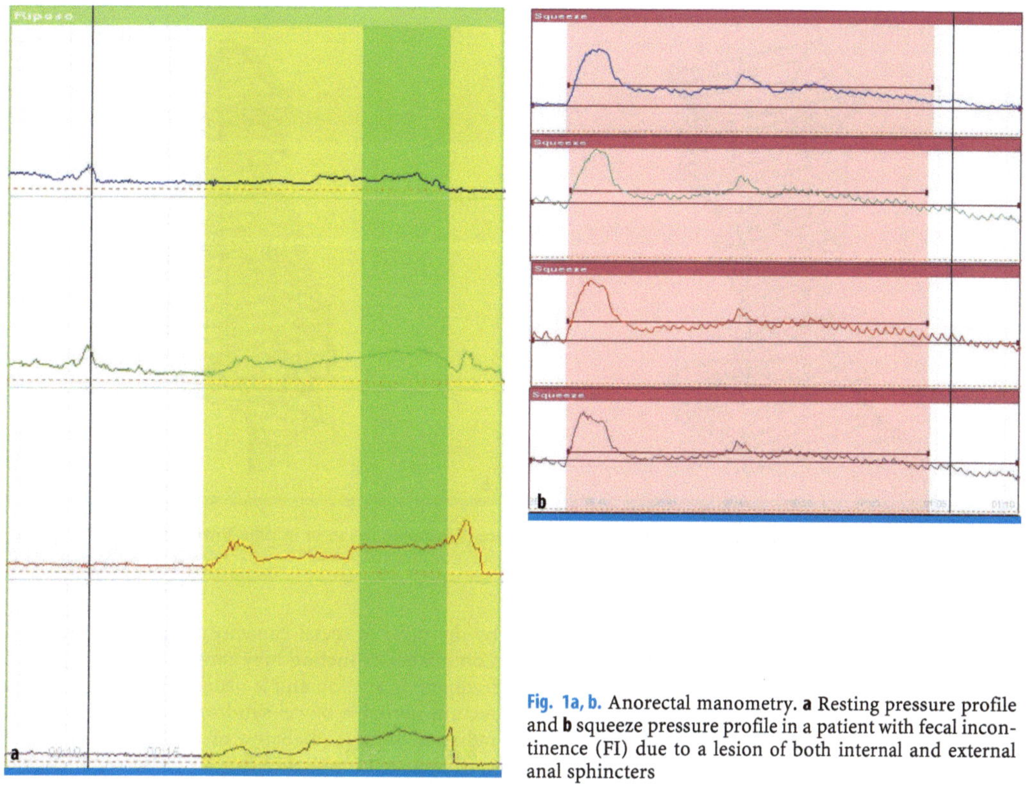

Fig. 1a, b. Anorectal manometry. **a** Resting pressure profile and **b** squeeze pressure profile in a patient with fecal incontinence (FI) due to a lesion of both internal and external anal sphincters

numeric value (i.e., mean or median) but also to consider pressure profiles, providing information on asymmetry in the anal canal [due to a limited lesion of the internal anal sphincter (IAS) or the external anal sphincter (EAS)] or decreased EAS endurance to muscle fatigue during prolonged squeeze. Based on a multichannel acquisition of resting-pressure profile, it is usually possible to visualize a "vector manometry" and identify segments of the anal canal with increased or decreased pressure (Fig. 2). Following the routine use of EAUS, clinical utility of vector manometry has progressively reduced [9], even if, more recently, an inverted vector manometry has been suggested, giving good correlations with EAUS and providing combined functional and anatomic information [10]. On the other hand, in a number of incontinent patients, resting and/or squeeze pressures could be normal, related to a nontraumatic pathophysiology of their incontinence. Although the rectoanal inhibitory reflex (RAIR) is routinely evoked (Fig. 3), its meaning in pathophysiological assessment of FI is not well established. With this test, the threshold of the reflex and the percentage of sphincter relaxation, as well as relaxation time and contraction time, can be calculated. Other reflexes (coughing) should be elicited to investigate the level of possible spinal cord lesions. Very important parameters to be investigated in FI patients are rectal sensations, commonly studied by inflation of air in a rectal balloon to elicit threshold and urge sensations, and maximum tolerated volume. It seems that other modalities using either electrical or thermal stimulation cannot be standardized at this time [9].

Altered values can be found in FI patients with metabolic or neurological diseases or following bowel irradiation, as well as in "idiopathic" FI; however, in other incontinent patients, rectal sensation values could be within normal range. Indeed, either a normosensitive, hypersensitive, or hyposensitive rectum can be found in FI. Despite these different patterns, rectal sensation assessment should be regarded as one of the most useful parameters. In comparison with baseline values, variations in rectal sensation measured under treatment can be of help in the evaluation of therapeutic effectiveness. Rectal compliance is assessed by progressive inflation (with air or water, manually or with barostat) of a rectal balloon and registration of rectal pressure; it is defined

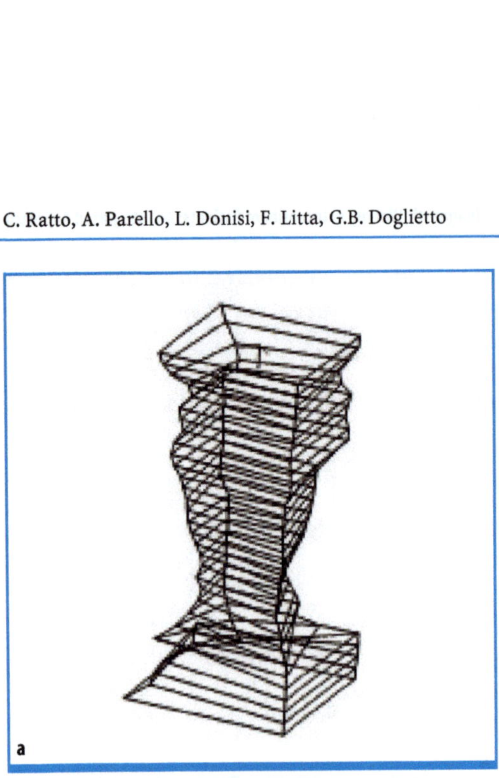

a

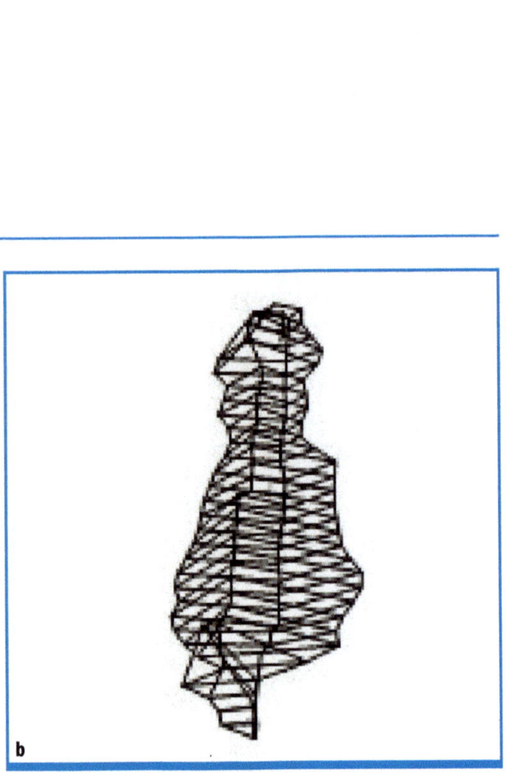

b

Fig. 2a, b. Vector manometry in a patient with fecal incontinence (FI) due to lesion of middle-lower internal anal sphincter, **a** "standard" vector, **b** "inverted" vector

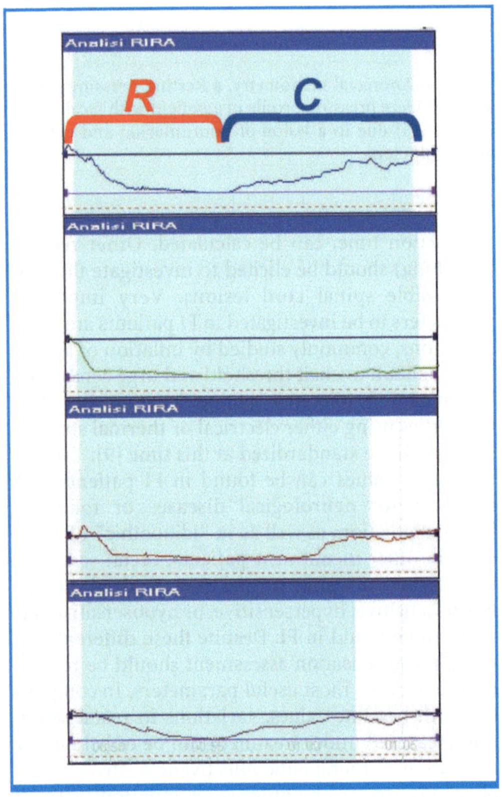

Fig. 3. Rectoanal inhibitory reflex (RAIR). *R* relaxation time, *C* contraction time

by the ratio of rectal capacity to gradient pressure. Compliance reduction may cause rectal urgency and frequent defecation and is usually found in inflamed rectum (irritable bowel syndrome, ulcerative colitis, radiation injury), diabetes, or following low spinal cord lesions. Compliance may be increased in higher spinal cord lesions.

Endoanal Ultrasound

Specifically designed ultrasound probes and software are available to investigate the anal canal and rectum with EAUS. The most useful are those including radial probes with a full 360° field of view and a frequency range between 5 and 16 MHz. The probe outer diameter is 1.7 cm or less to minimize any anatomical distortion. EAUS is usually performed with the patient in left lateral decubitus position. During the examination, the probe is inserted into the anal canal reaching the puborectalis sling showing the U-shaped aspect. From this level, a manual or mechanical pull-through examination is performed evaluating the distinct layers and structures of the anal canal: submucosa, IAS, longitudinal sphincter, EAS, puborectalis, anococcygeal ligament, puboanalis muscle, and perineal body (Fig. 4). By convention, when an axial view is visualized, the anterior edge of the anal canal should be shown on the screen at 12 o'clock, the left lateral at 3 o'clock, the posterior at 6 o'clock, and the right lateral at 9 o'clock. However, a more recent EAUS technique allows three-dimensional imaging (3D-EAUS): the 3D structure

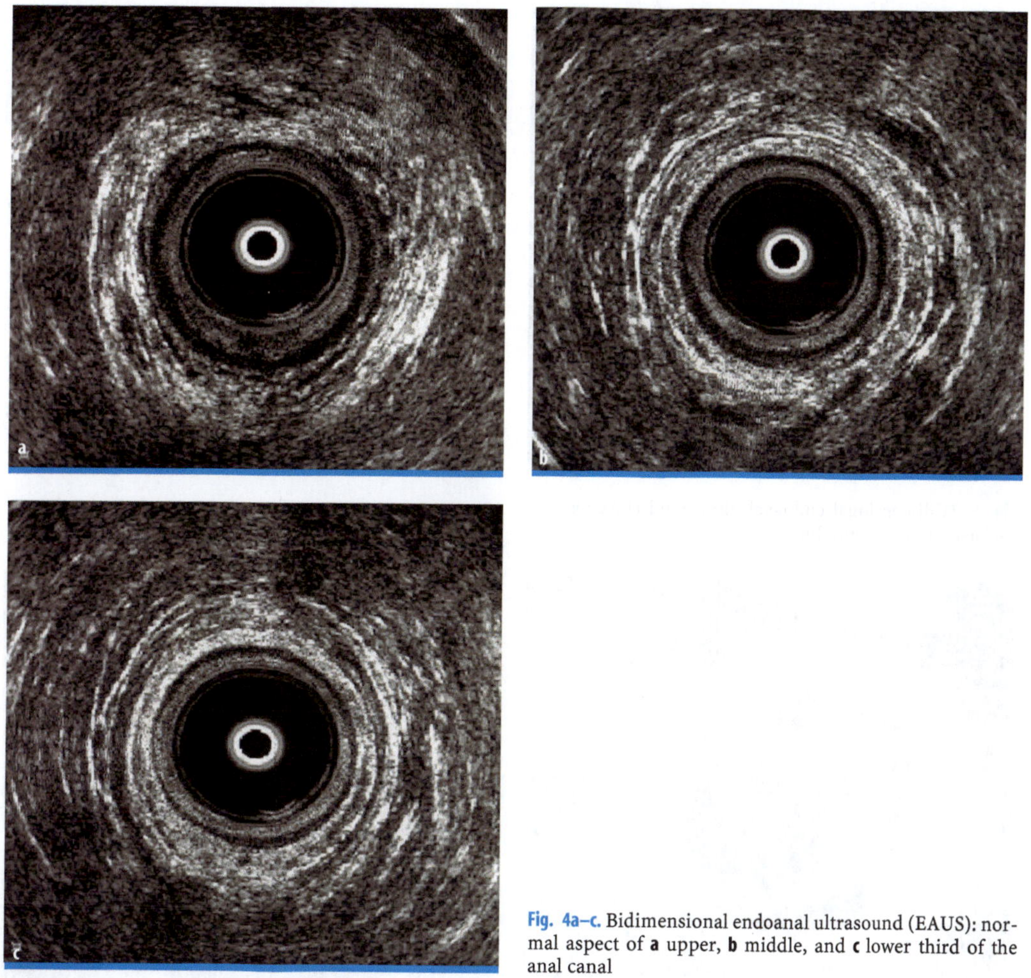

Fig. 4a–c. Bidimensional endoanal ultrasound (EAUS): normal aspect of **a** upper, **b** middle, and **c** lower third of the anal canal

obtained is the result of numerous axial, rapidly acquired, two-dimensional (2D) slices. Immediately after the examination and acquisition of these slices, the operator is able to navigate inside the 3D structure observing the anal canal not only in the axial but also in longitudinal and oblique views (Fig. 5). An area or volume can be calculated if deemed useful. Sphincter lesion appears as an hypoechoic area involving a circumferential segment of the IAS, EAS, or both (Fig. 6). EAUS is also particularly useful in differentiating FI patients with and without sphincter tears. Clinical utility of 3D-EAUS measurement of the anal sphincter complex in FI patients is under investigation [11]. Moreover, a "surface render mode" application is available in the most recently implemented ultrasonographic systems for EAUS (i.e., B-K Medical Hardware, equipped with 2050 endoprobe). This image processing allows changing the depth information of 3D data volume to "see the content inside a box" and offers accuracy in localizing sphincter tears.

Anorectal Electrophysiology

AREP includes a few tests directed to patients already investigated with history and physical assessment and other procedures (mainly ARM and ultrasound) in whom pelvic muscular and/or nervous functions seem to be altered. These tests, used to study the anorectum, have been derived from myographic and nerve conduction examinations performed in other

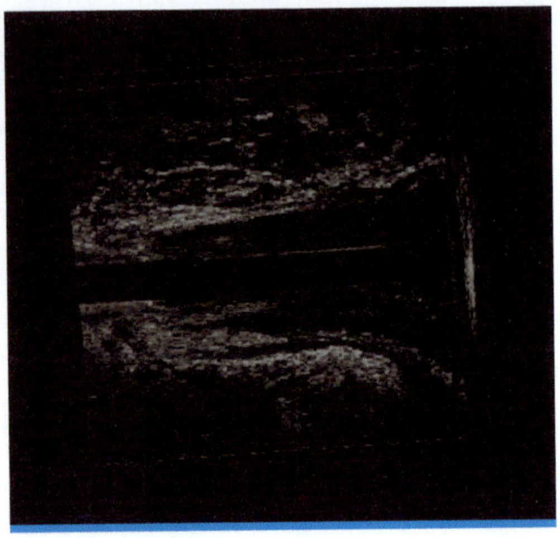

Fig. 5. Tridimensional endoanal ultrasound (EAUS): normal aspect in a longitudinal view

parts of the body. Since the mid-1980s, an evolution of instruments, techniques of examination, and indications has been registered. Electrophysiological studies are usually carried out with a neuromyograph system equipped with software dedicated to anorectal physiology to evaluate electrical muscle activity and nerve functionality. In performing such tests, either a recording function or an electrostimulating function or both can be requested. The neuromyograph instrument has to be connected to dedicated cables and electrodes. A ground electrode soaked in normal saline is placed around the thigh. The most preferred patient position is left lateral.

The purpose of electromyography (EMG) is to investigate the electrical activity of the EAS and the other striated pelvic floor muscles at rest and during squeezing and straining. Muscle denervation or reinnervation could be found in incontinent patients.

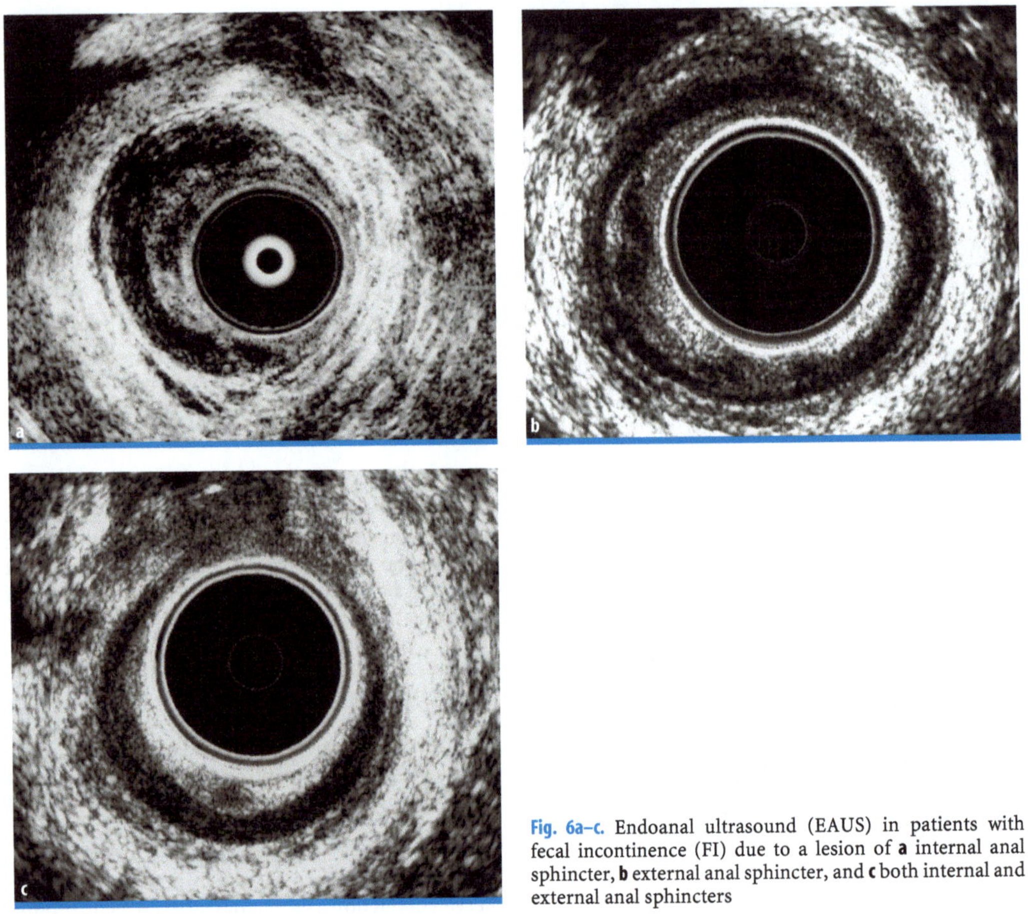

Fig. 6a–c. Endoanal ultrasound (EAUS) in patients with fecal incontinence (FI) due to a lesion of **a** internal anal sphincter, **b** external anal sphincter, and **c** both internal and external anal sphincters

Over time, four different types of electrodes have been developed: concentric needle, monopolar wire, single fiber, and surface. The concentric needle electrode consists of a thin needle (0.1 mm in diameter) covered by an insulating resin, which is able to uptake electrical activity of the small area of the EAS or puborectalis where it has been inserted under the guide of digital exploration. This needle is unable to record single muscle fiber action potentials; recordings from the four anal canal quadrants should be obtained. This procedure is quite uncomfortable for the patient, and even if multiple recording samples are taken, the mapping obtained is considered far from sufficient to delineate accurately the area of normal and abnormal muscle. The monopolar wire should reduce discomfort and avoid the electrode sliding because it is kept in site by a small hook placed at the electrode tip. The single-fiber electrode is thinner than the monopolar wire and is able to record individual motor-unit potentials. An appropriate amplification of the signals recorded is necessary. Also, fiber density can be calculated based on 20 different recordings from each anal hemisphere. Evaluation with single-fiber electrode is more accurate than the two electrodes previously described but remains uncomfortable. Surface electrodes, mounted on an endoanal plug or a small external adhesive plaque, are able to record gross muscle activity but unable to delimit areas of functional deficit. They are more useful to study paradoxical contraction of striated muscles than to evaluate sphincter damage in incontinent patients. Small polyphasic motor unit potentials (MUPs) may be identified when myopathic damage has occurred, whereas large polyphasic MUPs are found in neurogenic damage; also, a mixed pattern can be found. This test should be used when a neurogenic sphincter weakness is suspected and to distinguish selectively disorders of EAS and puborectalis.

Mucosal sensation can be evaluated with electrostimulation not only in the rectum (as with ARM) but also in the anal canal using a bipolar ring electrode (containing two platinum wires 1-cm apart) mounted on a Foley catheter. An appropriate setting of stimulus duration and rate must be done before starting the examination. During this test, the electrode is inserted into the anus first. From zero, the current amplitude is slowly increased until the patient feels a buzzing or tingling sensation in the anus. At least three measurements need to be taken, choosing the lower threshold value for the report. A similar procedure is used for mucosal sensation analysis in the rectum. Rectal ampulla must be reached by the electrode; under slowly increasing current (parameter setting is different compared with that used for anal sensation test), three values should be obtained, taking the lowest as the rectal threshold sensation to be reported.

Pudendal nerve terminal motor latency (PNTML) is measured, allowing evaluation of the pelvic floor neuromuscular integrity (Fig. 7). A disposable St.

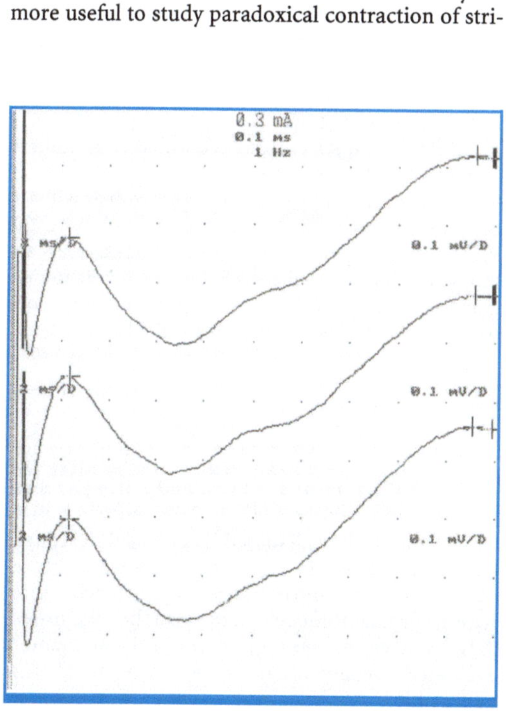

Fig. 7. Normal pudendal nerve terminal motor latency (PNTML)

Mark's pudendal electrode is used, mounted onto the volar side of the examiner's gloved index finger. The index finger is inserted into the rectum, reaching with the fingertip the course of each pudendal nerve and laying with the proximal finger phalanx within the anal canal. During this test, both electrostimulation and recording function have to be activated. Four cables run within the electrode, conveying stimuli (0.1- or 0.2-ms duration, 1-s. interval, not exceeding 15 mA) from the machine to the fingertip (to the anode and cathode) to stimulate the pudendal nerve fibers, and from the fingertip to the machine to record the striated muscle response, which is visualized on the screen. The latency (expressed in milliseconds) from the onset of the stimulus to the first deflection of the response is calculated for each pudendal nerve (n.v.: 2.0±0.2 ms). Because only the fastest conducting fibers are elicited during this test, it is possible to find a normal PNTML value in the presence of pudendal neuropathy, sparing a small amount of conducting fibers. Imprecise reproducibility and uncertain sensitivity and specificity are other limits of PNTML.

Evoked potentials can be obtained by stimulating the cortex or sacral roots to assess the central and peripheral motor (MEPs) and somatosensory (SEPs) pathways. Either electrical or magnetic stimulation can be used, the latter having the advantage of being painless and able to stimulate deep nervous structures. Both MEPs and SEPs allow the evaluation of conduction time of the stimulus (i.e., latency) and excitability of the intracortical circuit. Sacral MEPs have been proposed to replace PNTML [12], although the technical artefacts rate (up to 25%) is relevant [13–15]. These have been attributed also to vicinity of recording electrodes to the magnetic field, and use of an intrarectal ground electrode has been proposed to minimize artefacts [16]. Evaluation of SEPs can be performed by application of stimulus to the rectum, anal canal, anal verge, penis, or clitoris; this test could be helpful in assessing sensory fiber lesions, particularly in cases of perineal deficits. [17–19].

AREP could also include quantification of electrical or thermal sensory thresholds (QSTs) within the anal canal, sacral anal reflex (SAR) latency measurement in response to pudendal nerve or perianal stimulation, and perianal recording of sympathetic skin responses (SSRs) [19]. Integration between different tests can allow a reliable assessment of neuropathy. Lefaucheur [19] suggests that "needle EMG signs of sphincter denervation or prolonged TML give evidence for anal motor nerve lesion; SEP/QST or SSR abnormalities can suggest sensory or autonomic neuropathy; and in the absence of peripheral nerve disorder, MEPs, SEPs, SSRs, and SARs can assist in demonstrating and localizing spinal or supraspinal disease".

As mentioned above, indications for AREP are usually decided on the basis of a patient's history and physical assessment if pelvic muscular and/or nervous disorders are hypothesized; moreover, data from other diagnostic procedures (mainly ARM and ultrasound) should confirm the opportunity to submit the patient to the AREP.

In patients with sphincter lesion, no electrical activity may be found in case of wide, complete replacement of normal muscular tissue with scar, or, more frequently, polyphasic potentials as signs of a reinnervation process. Polyphasic potentials do present multiple spikes of muscle activity, prolonged in duration, and an increased fiber density. In evaluating sphincter injury, EAUS has higher sensitivity and specificity compared with EMG in mapping the lesion; however, only EMG can assess neuromuscular integrity. In this view, these two procedures are complementary to each other.

Evaluation of anal mucosal electrosensitivity could have a clinical relevance in a few clinical conditions. In neurogenic incontinence, a wide spectrum of findings can be observed, probably related to the degree of pudendal neuropathy. Also, rectal sensation measurements by electrophysiological study are meaningful. In incontinent patients with sphincter lesion(s) only, mucosal electrosensitivity could be normal. In those with neurogenic incontinence, there could be a wide variability of findings. As concerning manometric rectal sensation measurement, its meaning has to be intensively interpreted and correlated to results from other tests.

Alterations of PNTML are identified in relation to patient's age, being more frequent in older subjects. In a large number of patients with FI (with or without urinary incontinence) and rectal prolapse, the PNTML is abnormally prolonged. PNTML levels are thought to have a predicting value in patients undergoing treatment, but this assumption remains controversial.

Defecography and Magnetic Resonance

Defecography is able to assess pelvic floor physiology, recording motions at rest and during squeezing, straining, and coughing. The anorectal angle (ARA) should be calculated. A perineal descent is frequently found in incontinent patients. Moreover, rectorectal intussusception, rectocele, enterocele, or sigmoidocele may also be diagnosed; pelvic muscle dyssynergia needs to be adequately evaluated because it can cause continence disturbances [20].

MRI of anal sphincters has been evaluated using phased-array coils, but an endoanal coil has been preferred in studying FI patients [21] because of a superior accuracy in delimitating the EAS and sphincter defect; these should be the major advantages of MRI when compared with EAUS. However, controversy exists about preference toward endoanal coil [22]. EAS atrophy is more adequately visualized by MRI than by EAUS, as sphincter thinning occurs due to a decreased amount of muscle tissue and replacement with fat [23]. However, more recently, it has been reported that external phased-array MRI is comparable with endoanal MRI in depicting EAS atrophy [24]. Endoanal MRI and 3D-EAUS have a comparable accuracy in detecting atrophy and defects of the EAS, even if there is a substantial difference in grading of external anal sphincter atrophy [25]. On the other hand, idiopathic IAS degeneration, or IAS atrophy, is better investigated with EAUS. Terra and Stoker [26], in reviewing imaging techniques in FI, concluded that both external phased-array MRI and 3D-EAUS are "valuable tools in the diagnostic work up of faecal incontinence. Decisions about the preferred technique will mainly be determined by availability and local expertise".

More recently, use of MRI defecography suggested [27] to be included in the diagnostic workup of FI patients to detect previously missed functional alterations of anterior, middle, or posterior pelvic compartments. This examination should improve diagnosis of rectocele and internal prolapse when compared with clinical evaluation and allow the choice of a more adequate treatment.

Critical Choice of an Effective Diagnostic Workup

Every kind of examination should contribute to the diagnosis, offering an interpretation key of the pathophysiology of a certain disease. Diagnostic assessment, provided by a panel of clinical and instrumental tests, should be finalized to plan the treatment, and those tests should legitimate the therapy chosen. There is evidence concerning the usefulness of anorectal testing in the diagnostic workup of FI: it can add diagnostic information in 19–98% of patients, influence the management plan in 75–84% of patients, and alter the management plan in 10–19% of patients compared with clinical assessment alone [28]. Also, a critical evaluation of cost/effectiveness ratio is of interest. Moreover, post-treatment reassessment could provide information on the impact of a particular therapy on the continence mechanisms. From this perspective, clinical evaluation and anorectal tests (including those assessing both structure and function) should be complementary.

However, correct diagnostic workup is still debated [29–31]. There is disagreement concerning the usefulness of instrumental (by ARM) instead of clinical measurement (i.e., digital examination, of anal resting and squeeze pressures, as well as the primary role of EAUS in diagnosing sphincter tears), although there is agreement about the necessity of tests to assess anorectal sensory functions and possible neuropathy [31].

Use of anorectal tests needs to be performed scrupulously, and their results must be related to the entire clinical condition. Of primary importance is the examiner's expertise in order to give adequate indication to a certain test, correct interpretation to test data, and to visualize imaging of true sphincter lesions to be distinguished from anatomical asymmetry of the sphincters. In these conditions, anorectal testing is very well tolerate by most patients with FI, as demonstrated by Deutekom et al. [32] in a study evaluating pain, embarrassment, discomfort, and anxiety in 211 patients with FI undergoing defecography, MRI, and combined anorectal tests (including ARM, PNTML, rectal capacity, and sensation). Those items were classified by Likert scales (ranging from 1 = none to 5 = extreme). The mean scores ranged between 1 and 2 for all four items performing all three tests, being MRI, the procedure with the lowest mean score, and defecography, with the highest score.

A complete anorectal investigation is justified primarily considering the wide range of possible therapeutic options, which include not only regulation of bowel habits, pelvic floor retraining, and traditional surgery (i.e., repair of sphincter tears), but also injection of bulking agents, treatment with sacral nerve stimulation (SNS), and dynamic graciloplasty or artificial sphincter. In particular, correct indications to SNS play a crucial role in obtaining the best results in this innovative and very effective therapy. Potential benefits of this therapy seem to be increasing over the time, covering not only idiopathic neuropathy but also neuropathy secondary to other diseases or nervous trauma and, more recently, sphincter lesions, in the past suitable for sphincteroplasty [33–45].

Hallan et al. [46] found good correlation between digital basal score and maximum basal pressure and digital squeeze score and maximum squeeze pressure, even if there were wide ranges of sphincter function on digital and manometric assessment, with considerable overlap between patient groups. In that report, there were similar sensitivities and specificities of digital scores and ARM in distinguishing continent and incontinent patients. Agreement exists about this assumption [29–31]. However, ARM shows higher accuracy in detecting minor abnormalities in anal pressures and increased pressures in patients with abnormal sphincter relaxation and subsequent fecal seepage [47].

Only minimal attention has been dedicated to RAIR in FI patients: a possible role of relaxation and contraction times needs to be elucidated in cases of mild continence disturbances. Concerning rectal sensations, even if they are frequently found to be altered (reduced or increased) in FI patients, in other cases, they can be normal [48, 49]. The assessment of rectal sensation is preliminary in patients who are possible candidates for sensory retraining. Indeed, preservation of rectal sensation before therapy and its improvement determined by the therapy are suggested as major determinants of biofeedback success [50].

In some incontinent patients, rectal urgency could be associated with a hypersensitive rectum and/or reduced rectal capacity [48, 51] without any sphincter disruption. In fact, cases with intact sphincters but presenting a severe/moderate FI need to be investigated for the presence of other possible causes.

EAUS and MRI represent crucial diagnostic tests in determining which kind of factors plays a major role in pathophysiology of FI. In particular, both techniques may detect sphincter defects following anorectal surgery, even if clinically unsuspected [52]. However, MRI, particularly if dynamic, could give adjunctive information in selected cases of FI suspected to be associated with perineal descent or rectocele [53]: it is superior to clinical examination and barium defecography [7, 54].

Table 2. A proposed schema of an integrated diagnostic workup in patients with fecal incontinence (FI)

	Diagnostic tests: **** mandatory; *** optional; ** on demand; * useless						
Type of FI	**ARM + rectal sensory**	**EAUS**	**AREP**	**MRI**	**Dynamic MRI**	**Barium defecography**	**Others**
Obstetric lesions	****	****	*** (PNTML)	***	**	**	
Iatrogenic lesions	****	****	**** (PNTML)	***	*	*	
Sphincter atrophy	****	**** (only for IAS)	**** (EMG, sensory, PNTML, EP)	**** (Only for EAS)	*	*	
Rectal prolapse	****	****	**** (Sensory, PNTML)	***	***	****	Proctoscopy
Rectal resection	****	****	**** (Sensory, PNTML)	***	*	*	Proctoscopy
Pelvic radiotherapy	****	****	**** (Sensory, PNTML)	*	*	*	Proctoscopy
Peripheral and central neuropathies	****	****	**** (EMG, sensory, PNTML, EP)	*	*	*	MRI of CNS
Diabetes and metabolic diseases	****	****	**** (Sensory, PNTML, EP)	*	*	*	Metabolic assessment
Elderly and institutionalized patients	****	****	**** (EMG, sensory, PNTML, EP)	*	*	*	Psychiatric tests
Congenital	****	****	**** (EMG, PNTML, EP)	*	***	****	Urological evaluation

ARM anorectal manometry, *EAUS* endoanal ultrasound, *AREP* anorectal electrophysiology, *MRI* pelvic magnetic resonance imaging, *EMG* electromyography, *PNTML* pudendal nerve terminal motor latency, *EP* evoked potentials, *CNS* central nervous system

AREP needs to be performed by experts: under these circumstances, patient compliance is higher [48] and results more reliable. Clinical utility of EMG in mapping sphincter lesions has decreased over time because of the significant reliability of EAUS; however, it should have a role in cases due to neurogenic sphincter weakness. PNTML has been a very promising test, but some peculiar indications in selecting patients to specific treatments or to predict therapy outcome have not been supported by recent data [7, 55]. On the contrary, in a retrospective study in FI patients without sphincter lesions, Ricciardi et al. [56] found that only a bilateral (but not unilateral) prolonged PNTML is associated with poorer function and physiology.

Which Tests in Which Condition?

Because there are now numerous therapeutic options, it seems justified to intensively evaluate patients with FI to corroborate the choice. Depending upon diagnostic tests only could cause inaccurate pathophysiological assessment and ineffective treatment. The decision process as to which diagnostic tests should be used in a specific clinical condition is inevitably related to the specific attitude developed in a team involved in a patient's evaluation and cure.

In Table 2, a proposed schema of an integrated diagnostic workup is presented. From a general point of view, ARM and rectal sensation assessment should be considered mandatory in almost every clinical condition, being widely performed in coloproctological laboratories, moderately time consuming, and allowing considerable useful information. However, even if ARM could show a pressure pattern of sphincter asymmetry, it is not enough to diagnose a sphincter lesion; therefore, integration with other diagnostic tests is mandatory. Rectal sensation assessment should be useful to eventually identify alterations due to central or peripheral neuropathy, metabolic diseases (i.e., diabetes), or radiotherapy given for pelvic neoplasms (situated at the anus, rectum, prostate, bladder, or gynecological organs).

Concerning physiological assessment, AREP should play a crucial role, although its use is rather limited because specific experience in electrophysiology is required. EMG performed to map sphincter lesions is no longer frequently used, but it could be of interest to visualize denervation or reinnervation patterns in many clinical conditions (i.e., sphincter atrophy, neuropathies, elderly patients). AREP allows assessment of both anal and rectal threshold sensations, which should be mandatory when investigating FI due to rectal prolapse, after rectal resection or irradiation, in neuropathy and metabolic diseases, and in elderly patients. PNTML assessment could reveal a pudendal neuropathy and, then, be useful in a number of FI cases: in both obstetric and iatrogenic sphincter lesions, being suggested of importance in choosing some therapeutic approach (i.e., sphincteroplasty); in sphincter atrophy; in rectal prolapse or resection; in irradiated patients; in central/peripheral neuropathies; in metabolic diseases; and in FI found in either elderly or pediatric patients. Evoked potentials should complete the AREP evaluation in suspected neuropathies.

In structural assessment of sphincters, there is discussion concerning the preference toward EAUS instead of MR, or vice versa, depending on specific experience in using one test versus the other. In this debate, it should be considered that EAUS can be performed by nonradiologists, and it is usually simpler, more available, and less time consuming and expensive compared with MRI. On the other hand, MRI needs dedicated personnel with specific experience. Therefore, even if both EAUS and MRI should allow similar diagnostic accuracy, in most cases, EAUS is the preferred mandatory test for imaging, with MRI being an optional investigation in the more complex cases. On the contrary, MRI could be used as a first-line imaging, if chosen. Only for specific conditions should clinicians prefer one or the other (i.e., EAUS in suspected IAS atrophy and MRI in suspected EAS atrophy).

Availability of a certain instrumental or diagnostic procedure is a determinant factor in the diagnostic process. In some condition, barium defecography could be the only procedure available to study the functional imaging in the pelvis, whereas in other centers, the availability of dynamic MR could allow a more accurate evaluation. This is the case in FI due to rectal prolapse or when other pelvic disruptions (i.e., rectocele) could have occurred following obstetric sphincter lesions.

Finally, but not negligibly, other procedures could be needed to assess specific problems: proctoscopy in FI due to rectal prolapse (eventual proctitis or solitary ulcer), rectal resection (evaluation of rectal remnant, anastomosis, proctitis), or pelvic irradiation (assessment of proctitis); central nervous system MRI in FI cases of suspected central or peripheral neuropathy; in-depth biochemical assessment in metabolic diseases; psychiatric and psychometric tests in FI elderly; and integration of urologic evaluation in any case of double fecal and urologic incontinence, particularly in pediatric patients.

References

1. Bharucha AE, Zinsmeister AR, Locke GR et al (2005) Prevalence and burden of fecal incontinence: a popu-

lation based study in women. Gastroenterology 129:42–49
2. Jorge JM, Wexner SD (1993) Etiology and management of fecal incontinence. Dis Colon Rectum 36:77–97
3. Pescatori M, Anastasio G, Bottini C (1992) New grading and scoring for anal incontinence. Evaluation of 335 patients. Dis Colon Rectum 35:482–487
4. Ware JE Jr, Sherbourne CD (1992) The MOS 36-Item Short-Form Health Survey (SF-36). I. Conceptual framework and item selection. Med Care 30:473–483
5. Rockwood TH, Church JM, Fleshman JW et al (2000) Fecal Incontinence Quality of Life Scale: quality of life instrument for patients with fecal incontinence. Dis Colon Rectum 43:9–16
6. Donovan J, Bosch R, Gotoh M et al (2005) Symptom and quality of life assessment. In: Abrams P, Cardozo L, Khoury S, Wein AJ (eds), Incontinence, vol. 1. Health Publications, Plymouth, pp 267–316
7. Barnett JL, Hasler WL, Camilleri M (1999) American Gastroenterological Association medical position statement on anorectal testing techniques. American Gastroenterological Association. Gastroenterology 116:732–760
8. Simpson RR, Kennedy ML, Hung Nguyen M et al (2006) Anal manometry: a comparison of techniques. Dis Colon Rectum 49:1033–1038
9. Bharucha AE (2006) Update of tests of colon and rectal structure and function. J Clin Gastroenterol 40:96–103
10. Kaur G, Gardiner A, Duthie GS (2006) A new method of assessing anal sphincter integrity using inverted vectormanometry. Dis Colon Rectum 49:1160–1166
11. West RL, Felt-Bersma RJ, Hansen BE et al (2005) Volume measurements of the anal sphincter complex in healthy controls and fecal-incontinent patients with a three-dimensional reconstruction of endoanal ultrasonography images. Dis Colon Rectum 48:540–548
12. Morren GL, Walter S, Lindehammar H et al (2001) Evaluation of the sacroanal motor pathway by magnetic and electric stimulation in patients with fecal incontinence. Dis Colon Rectum 44:167–172
13. Jost WH, Schimrigk K (1994) A new method to determine pudendal nerve motor latency and central motor conduction time to the external anal sphincter. Electroencephalogr Clin Neurophysiol 93:237–239
14. Loening-Baucke V, Read NW, Yamada T, Barker AT (1994) Evaluation of the motor and sensory components of the pudendal nerve. Electroencephalogr Clin Neurophysiol 93:35–41
15. Sato T, Konishi F, Minakami H et al (2001) Pelvic floor disturbance after childbirth: vaginal delivery damages the upper levels of sphincter innervation. Dis Colon Rectum 44:1155–1161
16. Lefaucheur JP (2005) Intrarectal ground electrode improves the reliability of motor evoked potentials recorded in the anal sphincter. Muscle Nerve 32:110–112
17. Jost WH, Loch EG, Muller-Lobeck H (1998) Electrophysiologic studies of fecal incontinence in the woman. Zentralbl Gynakol 120:153–159
18. Uher EM, Swash M (1998) Sacral reflexes: physiology and clinical application. Dis Colon Rectum 41:1165–1177
19. Lefaucheur JP (2006) Neurophysiological testing in anorectal disorders. Muscle Nerve 33:324–333
20. Rao SS, Ozturk R, Stessman M (2004) Investigation of the pathophysiology of fecal seepage. Am J Gastroenterol 99:2204–2209
21. Hussain SM, Stoker J, Lameris JS (1995) Anal sphincter complex: endoanal MR imaging of normal anatomy. Radiology 197:671–677
22. Terra MP, Beets-Tan RG, van Der Hulst VP et al (2005) Anal sphincter defects in patients with fecal incontinence: endoanal versus external phased-array MR imaging. Radiology 236:886–895
23. Williams AB, Malouf AJ, Bartram CI et al (2001) Assessment of external anal sphincter morphology in idiopathic fecal incontinence with endocoil magnetic resonance imaging. Dig Dis Sci 46:1466–1471
24. Terra MP, Beets-Tan RG, van der Hulst VP et al (2006) MRI in evaluating atrophy of the external anal sphincter in patients with fecal incontinence. AJR Am J Roentgenol 187:991–999
25. Cazemier M, Terra MP, Stoker J et al (2006) Atrophy and defects detection of the external anal sphincter: comparison between three-dimensional anal endosonography and endoanal magnetic resonance imaging. Dis Colon Rectum 49:20–27
26. Terra MP, Stoker J (2006) The current role of imaging techniques in faecal incontinence. Eur Radiol 16:1727–1736
27. Hetzer FH, Andreisek G, Tsagari C et al (2006) MR defecography in patients with fecal incontinence: imaging findings and their effect on surgical management. Radiology 240:449–457
28. Liberman H, Faria J, Ternent CA et al (2001) A prospective evaluation of the value of anorectal physiology in the management of fecal incontinence. Dis Colon Rectum 44:1567–1574
29. Bharucha AE (2006) Pro: Anorectal testing is useful in fecal incontinence. Am J Gastroenterol 101:2679–2681
30. Wald A (2006) Con: Anorectal manometry and imaging are not necessary in patients with fecal incontinence. Am J Gastroenterol 101:2681–2683
31. Rao SS (2006) A balancing view: fecal incontinence: test or treat empirically-which strategy is best? Am J Gastroenterol 101:2683–2684
32. Deutekom M, Terra MP, Dijkgraaf MG et al (2006) Patients' perception of tests in the assessment of faecal incontinence. Br J Radiol 79:94–100
33. Matzel K, Stadelmaier M, Hohenfellner FP (1995) Electrical stimulation of sacral spinal nerves for treatment of faecal incontinence. Lancet 346:1124–1127
34. Ganio E, Realis Luc A, Ratto C et al (2005) Sacral nerve modulation for fecal incontinence: functional results and assessment of the quality of life. http://www.colorep.it/Rivista%20CEC/sacral_nerve_modulation_for_feca.htm. Cited 28 Nov 2005
35. Jarrett ME, Varma JS, Duthie GS et al (2004) Sacral nerve stimulation for faecal incontinence in the UK. Br J Surg 91:755–761
36. Bernstein AJ, Peters KM (2005) Expanding indications for neuromodulation. Urol Clin North Am 32:59–63
37. Jarrett ME, Matzel KE, Christiansen J et al (2005) Sacral nerve stimulation for faecal incontinence in patients with previous partial spinal injury including disc prolapse. Br J Surg 92:734–739
38. Kenefick NJ, Vaizey CJ, Nicholls RJ et al (2002) Sacral nerve stimulation for faecal incontinence due to sys-

temic sclerosis. Gut 51:881–883
39. Matzel K, Stadelmaier U, Hohenfellner M et al (2001) Chronic sacral spinal nerve stimulation for faecal incontinence: long-term results with foramen and cuff electrodes. Dis Colon Rectum 44:59–66
40. Malouf AJ, Vaizey CJ, Nicholls RJ et al (2000) Permanent sacral nerve stimulation for faecal incontinence. Ann. Surg 232:143–148
41. Leroi AM, Michot F, Grise P et al (2001) Effect of sacral nerve stimulation in patients with faecal and urinary incontinence. Dis Colon Rectum 44:779–789
42. Jarrett ME, Matzel KE, Stosser M et al (2005) Sacral nerve stimulation for fecal incontinence following surgery for rectal prolapse repair: a multicenter study. Dis Colon Rectum 48:1243–1248
43. Matzel KE, Stadelmaier U, Bittorf B et al (2002) Bilateral sacral spinal nerve stimulation for fecal incontinence after low anterior rectum resection. Int J Colorectal Dis 17:430–434
44. Ratto C, Grillo E, Parello A et al (2005) Sacral neuromodulation in treatment of fecal incontinence following anterior resection and chemoradiation for rectal cancer. Dis Colon Rectum 48:1027–1036
45. Jarrett ME, Matzel KE, Stosser M et al (2005) Sacral nerve stimulation for faecal incontinence following a rectosigmoid resection for colorectal cancer. Int J Colorectal Dis 20:446–451
46. Hallan RI, Marzouk DE, Waldron DJ et al (1989) Comparison of digital and manometric assessment of anal sphincter function. Br J Surg 76:973–975
47. Rao SS, Ozturk R, Stessman M (2004) Investigation of the pathophysiology of fecal seepage. Am J Gastroenterol 99:2204–2209
48. Bharucha AE, Fletcher JG, Harper CM et al (2005) Relationship between symptoms and disordered continence mechanisms in women with idiopathic fecal incontinence. Gut 54:546–555
49. Sun WM, Donnelly TC, Read NW (1992) Utility of a combined test of anorectal manometry, electromyography, and sensation in determining the mechanism of 'idiopathic' faecal incontinence. Gut 33:807–813
50. Chiarioni G, Bassotti G, Stanganini S et al (2002) Sensory retraining is key to biofeedback therapy for formed stool fecal incontinence. Am J Gastroenterol 97:109–117
51. Siproudhis L, El Abkari M, El Alaoui M et al (2005) Low rectal volumes in patients suffering from fecal incontinence: What does it mean? Aliment Pharmacol Ther 22:989–996
52. Felt-Bersma RJ, van Baren R, Koorevaar M et al (1995) Unsuspected sphincter defects shown by anal endosonography after anorectal surgery. A prospective study. Dis Colon Rectum 38:249–253
53. Stoker J, Halligan S, Bartram CI (2001) Pelvic floor imaging. Radiology 218:621–641
54. Bharucha AE, Fletcher JG, Seide B et al (2005) Phenotypic variation in functional disorders of defecation. Gastroenterology 128:1199–1210
55. Malouf AJ, Norton CS, Engel AF et al (2000) Long-term results of overlapping anterior anal-sphincter repair for obstetric trauma. Lancet 355:260–265
56. Ricciardi R, Mellgren AF, Madoff RD et al (2006) The utility of pudendal nerve terminal motor latencies in idiopathic incontinence. Dis Colon Rectum 49:852–857

Invited Commentary

Scott R. Steele, Ann C. Lowry, Anders F. Mellgren

In this era of evidence-based medicine, it is more important than ever to base clinical decisions on reliable information. The dilemma that clinicians face is how to fully evaluate the patient without performing unnecessary testing. This decision is particularly difficult in patients presenting with fecal incontinence for a number of reasons: the complex nature of continence, the frequency of concomitant conditions contributing to the incontinence, and, in general, a lack of correlation among many of the available tests. The introduction of multiple new treatment options with only limited data about their relative roles makes it even more complicated. The review by Ratto et al. illustrates some important points regarding the need to have a focused diagnostic approach to patients presenting with fecal incontinence.

Normal continence is an intricate process that involves the coordinated interaction between multiple different neuronal pathways and the pelvic and perineal musculature [1]. In addition, multiple other factors, including systemic disease, emotional affect, bowel motility, stool consistency, evacuation efficiency, pelvic floor stability, and sphincter integrity play a role in normal regulation [2]. Failure at any level may result in an impaired ability to control gas or stool.

As pointed out by the authors in Table 1, invaluable information can be gathered from physical examination. At this assessment, it is imperative for the physician to be able to differentiate normal from abnormal findings, a skill that can only be garnered from a complete perineal examination for the many different types of patients seen by the colorectal surgeon, not just those with fecal incontinence. However, even a well-performed physical examination has limitations. Anal inspection and digital rectal examination are poor for detecting sphincter defects, especially those less than 90° [3]. Furthermore, specific questions relating to the overall health and bowel function of the patient need to be ascertained. However, even with the most adept history taking and physical examination, as the authors state, fecal incontinence often demands further workup with ancillary studies.

We are in full agreement with the authors in the value of an integrated approach. The patient presenting with fecal incontinence may have a plethora of concomitant pelvic floor defects that will not only affect their current function but also impact results of therapy. Physicians need to have an organized approach to evaluation to optimally manage these patients and avoid pitfalls that may ultimately lead to failed outcomes. In a retrospective review of 21 patients with full-thickness rectal prolapse, 71% were found to have sphincter defects on ultrasound evaluation, likely contributing to the persistent or recurrent fecal incontinence following successful repair of the rectal prolapse [4]. Similarly, in a study of 28 patients undergoing overlapping sphincteroplasty who underwent thorough physiologic evaluation, all patients were found to have associated pelvic floor disorders, with 57% having more than one abnormality [5]. Further highlighting this point, Hetzer and colleagues used magnetic resonance (MR) defecography to demonstrate concomitant pathology in up to 43% of patients undergoing workup for fecal incontinence, which resulted in a change in the surgical approach in 27 of 33 patients who underwent surgery [6]. Therefore, identification of concomitant pathologies may be a clinically important factor for optimal treatment outcomes, as pointed out by the authors of the current study.

Although questions have been raised recently about the relative contribution of sphincter injuries to incontinence, sphincter defects are still considered to play a significant role in the condition. The most common cause of surgically correctable fecal incontinence is a traumatic injury in the sphincter complex that can be treated by overlapping sphincteroplasty. Combined with the increasing success of sacral nerve stimulation and bulking agents [7–10] for patients with either a normal pelvic floor or abnormal pelvic floor anatomy with neuropathy or dyssynergia, it may be most prudent to first rule out an anatomical defect. Ancillary tests such as endoanal ultrasound, MR imaging (MRI), and/or defecography enable visualization of anatomical abnormalities otherwise not seen by physical examination alone. The authors have provided an excellent discussion of the various modalities of identification of sphincter injuries. We agree with the authors' proposed algorithm that endoanal ultrasound is the most cost-effective, readily available examination for anatomical evaluation.

Despite its frequent use, sphincteroplasty alone leaves many patients with recurrent symptoms when reexamined at extended follow-up intervals [11–13]. In contrast to the recent long-term success reported by Maslekar and colleagues [14] where anterior sphincteroplasty was deemed successful in 80% of patients at a median follow-up of 84 months, we previously reported that only 40% of our 191 patients undergoing overlapping sphincteroplasty had maintenance of continence at long-term follow-up of 10 years [15]. There may be several factors contributing to a suboptimal outcome after sphincteroplasty, including weakening of the muscle with time, technical problems at the original repair, postoperative infection, failure to achieve a lasting circumferential sphincter integrity, or unidentified or uncorrected pelvic floor disorders present at the time of initial surgery. Atrophy of the external sphincter may also play a role; if so, MRI may become a more important part of the preoperative evaluation.

The question remains as to which tests should be performed in patients with fecal incontinence. Per the authors' schema, both anorectal manometry and anorectal electrophysiology are mandatory in almost all incontinent patients. Whereas we feel that each of these procedures provides valuable additional information, they do have some drawbacks, as identified by the authors. Manometry lacks specific correlation with any anatomical defect as well as the wide variations in normal pressures with age and gender [16, 17], and manometry has variable efficacy in correlating with postoperative symptomatic improvement [18]. Anal electromyography has similarly shown variable effects on predicting success following repair, thus limiting its overall use. In a study of 96 patients with fecal incontinence, pudendal neuropathy was only found in 59% [19]. Furthermore, pudendal neuropathy, when present, is highly variable for predicting improvements in continence following repair [20, 21]. We have previously looked at 83 patients with fecal incontinence with intact sphincters on ultrasound and no prolapse on defecography [22]. Only 28% had prolonged pudendal nerve terminal motor latency (PNTML), and unilateral neuropathy did not correlate with manometric or fecal incontinence severity scores, although bilateral neuropathy did correlate with worse scores and decreased mean resting but not squeeze pressures. Thus, results of the PNTML are variable. Unfortunately, the presence of neuropathy may not predict outcome of repair, and normal PNTML does not exclude problems with pelvic dysfunction.

In summary, due to the complex nature of the distal 5–10 cm of the distal alimentary tract and frequency of concomitant conditions, patients with fecal incontinence cannot be accurately assessed by one study alone. Availability may be a determining factor for what studies can be performed. If access is limited, endoanal ultrasound with the goal of identifying a sphincter injury is the most likely examination to affect the treatment recommendation. However, limiting evaluation to one test risks missing other significant factors that could influence treatment outcome. Although our understanding of incontinence and appropriate evaluation has improved, further research is necessary to develop the most effective and efficient algorithm.

References

1. Bannister JJ, Gibbons C, Read NW (1987) Preservation of faecal continence during rises in intra-abdominal pressure: is there a role for the flap-valve? Gut 28:1242–1244
2. Mavrantonis C, Wexner SD (1998) A clinical approach to fecal incontinence. J Clin Gastrol 27(2):108–121
3. Dobben AC, Terra MP, Deutekom M et al (2006) Anal inspection and digital rectal examination compared to anorectal physiology tests and endoanal ultrasonography in evaluating fecal incontinence. Int J Colorectal Dis (Epub ahead of print)
4. Woods R, Voyvodic F, Schloithe AC et al (2003) Anal sphincter tears in patients with rectal prolapse and faecal incontinence. Colorectal Dis 5(6):544–548
5. Steele SR, Lee PY, Mullenix PS et al (2006) Is there a role for concomitant pelvic floor repair in patients with sphincter defects in the treatment of fecal incontinence? Int J Colorectal Dis 21:508–514
6. Hetzer FH, Andreisek G, Tsagari C et al (2006) MR defecography in patients with fecal incontinence: imaging findings and their effect on surgical management. Radiology 240(2):449–457
7. Conaghan P, Farouk R (2005) Sacral nerve stimulation can be successful in patients with ultrasound evidence of external anal sphincter disruption. Dis Colon Rectum 48(8):1610–1614
8. Rasmussen OO, Buntzen S, Sorensen M et al (2004 Sacral nerve stimulation in fecal incontinence. Dis Colon Rectum 47(7):1158–1161
9. Tjandra JJ, Lim JF, Hiscock R, Rajendra P (2004) Injectable silicone biomaterial for fecal incontinence caused by internal anal sphincter dysfunction is effective. Dis Colon Rectum 47(12):2138–2146
10. Malouf AJ, Vaizey CJ, Norton CS, Kamm MA (2001) Internal anal sphincter augmentation for fecal incontinence using injectable silicone biomaterial. Dis Colon Rectum 44(4):595–600
11. Barisic GI, Krivokapic ZV, Markovic VA, Popovic MA (2006) Outcome of overlapping anal sphincter repair after 3 months and after a mean of 80 months. Int J

Colorectal Dis 21(1):52–56
12. Londono-Schimmer EE, Garcia-Guperly R, Nicholls RJ et al (1994) Overlapping anal sphincter repair for faecal incontinence due to sphincter trauma: five-year follow-up of functional results. Int J Colorectal Dis 9:100–103
13. Yoshioka K, Keighley MR (1989) Sphincter repair for fecal incontinence. Dis Colon Rectum 32:39–42
14. Maslekar S, Gardiner AB, Duthie GS (2007) Anterior anal sphincter repair for fecal incontinence: Good long-term results are possible. J Am Coll Surg 204(1):40–46
15. Bravo Gutierrez A, Madoff RD, Lowry AC Et al (2004) Long-term results of anterior sphincteroplasty. Dis Colon Rectum 47(5):727–731; discussion 731–732
16. Cali RL, Blatchfored GJ, Perry RE et al (1992) Normal variation in anorectal manometry. Dis Colon Rectum 35:1161–1164
17. Emblem R, Dhaenens G, Stien R et al (1994) The importance of anal endosonography in the evaluation of idiopathic fecal incontinence. Dis Colon Rectum 37:42–48
18. Hill K, Fanning S, Fennerty MB, Faigel DO (2006) Endoanal ultrasound compared to anorectal manometry for the evaluation of fecal incontinence: a study of the effect these tests have on clinical outcome. Dig Dis Sci 51(2):235–240
19. Roig JV, Villoslada C, Lledo S et al (1995) Prevalence of pudendal neuropathy in fecal incontinence. Results of a prospective study. Dis Colon Rectum 38(9):952–958
20. Chen AS, Luchtefeld MA, Senagore AJ et al (1998) Pudendal nerve latency. Does it predict outcome of anal sphincter repair? Dis Colon Rectum 41(8):1005–1009
21. Osterberg A, Graf W, Edebol Eeg-Olofsson K et al (2000) Results of neurophysiologic evaluation in fecal incontinence. Dis Colon Rectum 43(9):1256–1261
22. Ricciardi R, Mellgren AF, Madoff RD et al (2006) The utility of pudendal nerve terminal motor latencies in idiopathic incontinence. Dis Colon Rectum 49(6) 852–857

SECTION III

Treatment of Fecal Incontinence

Patient Selection and Treatment Evaluation

13

Carlo Ratto, Angelo Parello, Lorenza Donisi, Francesco Litta,
Giovanni B. Doglietto

Introduction

Criteria for patient selection to a certain treatment are of central importance in the management of fecal incontinence (FI). Even though the understanding of continence physiology has improved, there persists a lack of comprehensive knowledge regarding the very complex mechanisms by which various structures contribute to the regulation of continence control. It is now assumed that a continuous modulation of different stimuli is necessary to effectively maintain the various functions involved with continence. On the other hand, the instruments available to measure or analyze parameters associated with continence, albeit numerous and sometimes sophisticated, are not used in a standardized manner, so that data obtained at one center are not comparable with those obtained in another. Also, the entire diagnostic workup is still debatable, being routinely limited to clinical examination in the opinion of some, whereas others recommend extensive evaluation. However, other aspects must be considered in the decision-making process surrounding treatment choice. These aspects include the patient's background and feelings about his or her FI and the clinician's attitude toward proposing a particular treatment. Usually, patients are very frustrated about their FI, and are sometimes convinced that it is ineluctable and incurable. Sometimes they are highly motivated to find the right solution but want to avoid suffering or very complicated solutions that can significantly alter their lifestyle. Sometimes they are so depressed about their FI that they are willing to undergo whichever form of treatment their physician recommends.

Whereas it is necessary for the physician to consider the patient's perspective when making a treatment decision, it is also necessary to consider the consequences of treatment, some possibly ineffective, when deciding upon a first-line approach. For instance, submitting a patient with very poor continence to a prolonged period of rehabilitation during which significant improvement is not seen could increase the patient's skepticism to the point of refusing any other form of therapy. On the other hand, choosing a complex therapy as the first-line approach, for example, dynamic graciloplasty or artificial sphincter, must be based on very strict criteria in order to avoid submitting the patient to excessive treatment. Finally, but fundamental in our opinion, it is unreasonable and irresponsible to offer the patient a stoma as a unique solution for FI without an appropriate diagnosis and a rational therapeutic approach.

Another aspect that influences patient selection to treatment is the evaluation of results from the application of different therapies. These evaluations should help the identification of specific subgroups of patients to be recommended for a specific approach as well as allow assessment of the effectiveness of a particular therapy. However, there are many published reports about treatment of patients inhomogeneously selected to a therapy. Moreover, the rapid evolution of new techniques has determined that in a few years, the same type of patients will be treated with very different methods. Indeed, treatment selection criteria are rapidly changing parallel with technical advances. On the other hand, there remains debate about how to measure the effectiveness of a treatment for FI: reduction of FI episodes; positive impact on quality of life; changing of physiological parameters.

Patient Selection

Baseline evaluation of symptoms described by a patient presenting with FI is fundamental in order to establish severity of continence dysfunction and its impact on the patient's lifestyle. Usually, this can be derived from a clinical assessment (including clinical history and physical examination), as well as from the evaluation of a diary kept by the patient concerning normal bowel movements and episodes of FI, specifying which kind of material has been lost (gas, liquid, solid stool). Frequency, circumstances, and the patient's sensations and attempts to avoid leakage before and during stool passage, are of interest.

Clinical features allow the physician to establish an FI score according to different available scales. Thereafter, more information about the pathophysiology of FI can be gleaned from instrumental examination, including anorectal manometry (ARM) and sensory testing, endoanal ultrasound (EAUS), anorectal electrophysiology (AREP), magnetic resonance (MR), and defecography.

Instrumental assessment is worthwhile because clinical findings alone are not sufficient to correctly plan treatment. Ternent et al. [1] found that using ARM, EAUS, and pudendal nerve terminal motor latency (PNTML) changes the treatment plan in 20% of patients. This tendency was confirmed by the same group of researchers [2] on 90 patients submitted initially to a clinical evaluation from which a pretest therapeutic plan was documented (medical for 45 patients, surgical for 45 patients). Thereafter, ARM, EAUS, and PNTML were performed, and a posttest management consensus was reached. In 10% (nine patients), a change of treatment plan was observed after the physiological tests (from medical to surgical in five patients; from surgical to medical in three patients; change of surgical procedure in one patient). Within patients assigned to a pretest medical treatment, EAUS was the only anorectal test significantly responsible of changing the strategy: among patients indicated for pretest surgical approach, EAUS and PNTML prompted the variation. In a similar study performed at our institution in 2002 involving 63 patients (unpublished data), we found that clinical features alone were unable to indicate treatment in 25 patients (39.7%), whereas after ARM, EAUS, and AREP, these "undefined" patients were assigned to medical treatment in 13 cases and to surgery in 12 cases. For the entire group of patients, including those "undefined," a disagreement between pretest and posttest treatment plan was found in 30 cases (47.6%). In five patients (7.9%), there was a change of pretest approach (from medical to surgical in two; from surgical to medical in three). Numerous other studies have supported the integration of clinical assessment and physiological tests to improve the understanding of FI and patient treatment selection [3–6].

Medical Treatment

Medical treatment includes diet, drugs, supportive measures, rehabilitation, and biofeedback. They are usually chosen for either "elective" reasons or for patients who cannot be treated by a surgical approach. Specifically, poor clinical conditions limiting anesthesia and/or surgery could be valid criteria for a nonoperative approach, whereas a patient's age could be only relatively limiting. On the other hand, psychological problems or disturbances should suggest avoidance of very complex surgical procedures that require patient compliance. Specific bowel diseases (chronic inflammatory diseases; irritable bowel syndrome) with uncontrolled symptoms should contraindicate a major surgical approach. When life-threatening clinical conditions are involved (evolving diseases; chronic diseases; neoplasms not radically treated), the choice of treatment should consider the patient's life expectancy and the possible benefits in quality of life.

"Elective" indication for medical therapy should include minor FI without physiologic or morphologic alterations; in cases with minor abnormalities, a medical approach could be considered as a first-line intervention. Also, individuals with continence dysfunctions related to altered feces quality (i.e., diarrhea) should be expected to gain benefit from a conservative treatment approach. In this area, the patient must be advised to improve perianal hygiene, carefully use absorbent cotton diapers and tampons, and reduce or avoid foods that induce loose stools and increase gastrointestinal transit and gas production (milk derivates; legumes; excess fiber). Diarrhea needs to be fully investigated and, consequently, treated with medication when appropriate. Specific drug treatment has to be initiated in cases of chronic bowel disease. Also, the pathophysiology of soiling should be fully elucidated to determine between operative and nonoperative treatment; when it is minor, occasional, or without either significant physiologic dysfunction or sphincter lesions, a conservative approach can be attempted using postevacuation irrigating water enema or anal plugs as supportive measures.

Pelvic floor rehabilitation, including biofeedback, kinesitherapy, sensory retraining, and electrostimulation, is frequently regarded as a first-line treatment for FI. However, disagreement exists about indications for rehabilitative techniques. Lack of standardized methods makes it difficult to compare results of this approach, even in patients accurately selected. Moreover, in the limited number of well-conducted studies, there is no agreement concerning outcome parameters to measure or predict therapy outcome [7, 8]. A rational modulation of the algorithm for rehabilitation could play a key role for therapy success. Patient compliance and good psychological status are preliminary requirements for rehabilitation, being predictors of therapy success [9, 10]. Selection criteria cannot be based on anal pressures [11–14], whereas altered threshold and rectal urgency sensations have been found to be predictive of a positive treatment response [7, 14–16]. Sensory retraining could be used both in individuals with reduced rectal sensation and in patients with very high sensory levels [16–18]. Although controversies exist about the outcome predictive value of PNTML in individuals undergoing rehabilitation [7, 8, 13], its alteration seems to be regarded as a predictor of negative response [7, 8]. However, an external anal sphincter defect is not an absolute negative predictor of success [7, 8, 19]. Biofeedback, electrostimulation, and kinesitherapy could be scheduled in patients with such a defect.

Surgical Treatment

Until the recent past, in cases of intractable severe FI, criteria for selecting patients to surgical treatment concerned sphincter lesions or pudendal neuropathy with perineal descent and altered anorectal angle. In the former condition, a sphincteroplasty was indicated in cases of limited lesion without PNTML alteration, whereas a sphincter replacement operation (dynamic graciloplasty, artificial sphincter, gluteoplasty) was indicated when a wide lesion, fragmented sphincters, or failure of previous sphincteroplasty occurred. In the latter condition, a postanal repair was indicated. Recently, other therapies have been more widely used, such as injectable bulking agents or the recently introduced radiofrequency. Since 1995, sacral nerve stimulation (SNS) has been introduced into the panorama of treatment options, determining a significant rearrangement of selection criteria.

Sphincteroplasty

Sphincter lesions due to obstetric trauma (third- and fourth-degree tears) have traditionally been submitted electively to sphincteroplasty. This technique can be performed by edge-to-edge approximation or overlapping of the external anal sphincter (Fig. 1). Immediate repair, at the time of delivery or delayed to 24 h, has been suggested to obtain best results. However, sphincteroplasty can frequently be performed a few decades after childbirth, when the patient presents clinically with FI. Manometric parameters (squeeze pressure; resting pressure; anal canal length) seem not to be useful for patient selection to sphincteroplasty, whereas a pudendal neuropathy, measured by a prolonged PNTML (particularly if bilateral), should be considered as a predictor of poor outcome [20–26]. However, conflicting results are also reported [27–31], attributable to correct definition of PNTML normality, adequate evalu-

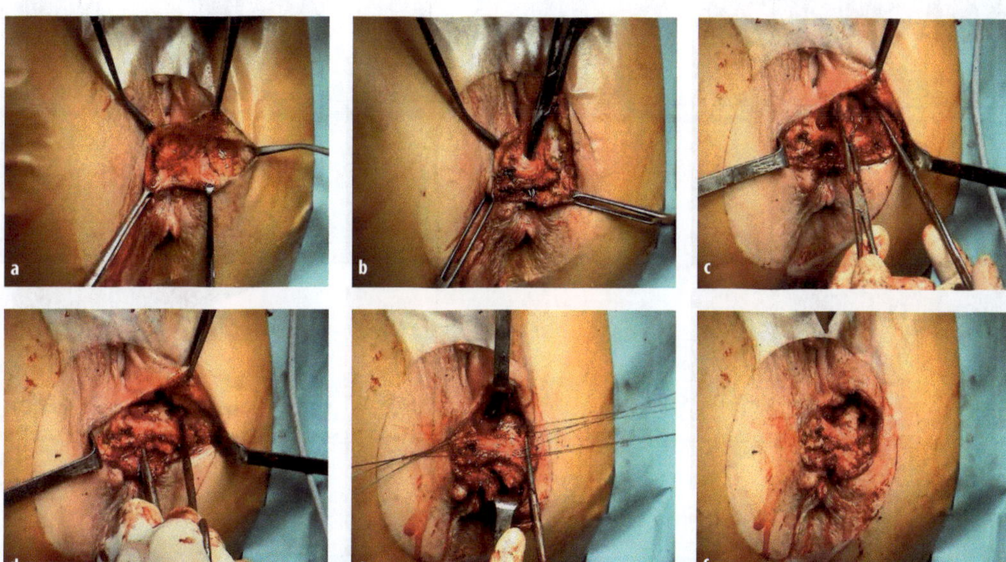

Fig. 1a–f. Sphincteroplasty. **a** Perineal incision. **b** The external anal sphincter is isolated at the level of a scar. **c** The external anal sphincter is incised at the level of the scar. **d** The overlapping sphincteroplasty is prepared. **e** Multiple stitches are placed. **f** The overlapping sphincteroplasty is completed

ation of pudendal neuropathy when assessed by standard PNTML measurement with St. Mark's electrode, and the role of symmetric pudendal innervation [31]. Although EAUS is determinant today in diagnosing a sphincter tear, ultrasonographic aspects are not considered valid criteria to select patients to this procedure. To improve the long-term results displayed by sphincteroplasty alone, which are sometimes limited [32–34], this operation has been performed within a total pelvic floor repair [35] or with anterior levatorplasty [36]. However, again, anorectal physiological parameters were not predictive of symptom improvement.

Postanal Repair

Neuropathic FI associated with perineal descent and without sphincter lesions seems, theoretically, to be the best indication to postanal repair. Unfortunately, no physiological parameters have been found to be indicative for this approach [37–40]. Considering the limited long-term effectiveness of this treatment, patients with these indications could be more effectively approached by other procedures. Indeed, indications for postanal repair have been significantly reduced over time. The procedure has been advocated as part of a total pelvic floor repair in conjunction with anterior levatorplasty.

Dynamic Graciloplasty, Artificial Bowel Sphincter, Gluteoplasty

These procedures must be regarded as major sphincter replacement operations, dedicated only to patients with very severe FI due to a wide sphincter lesion (more than half the circumference) or fragmented sphincters not amenable to neither sphincteroplasty or other surgical approaches (i.e., SNS). In case of failure of previous sphincteroplasty (when there is no indication to redo it), which is not suitable for SNS, these techniques can also be indicated. Moreover, if severe FI is consequent to neuropathy or anorectal malformations, one of these operations could be performed (specifically, in cases of neuropathy when SNS has failed). Usually, patients present a very low or absent squeeze pressure, which is associated with a decreased or absent resting pressure if an internal sphincter lesion/alteration coexists. When pudendal neuropathy occurs, PNTML could be altered. Dysfunctions of rectal sensations should be regarded as negative predictors of success, as reported in different experiences [41–43]. The

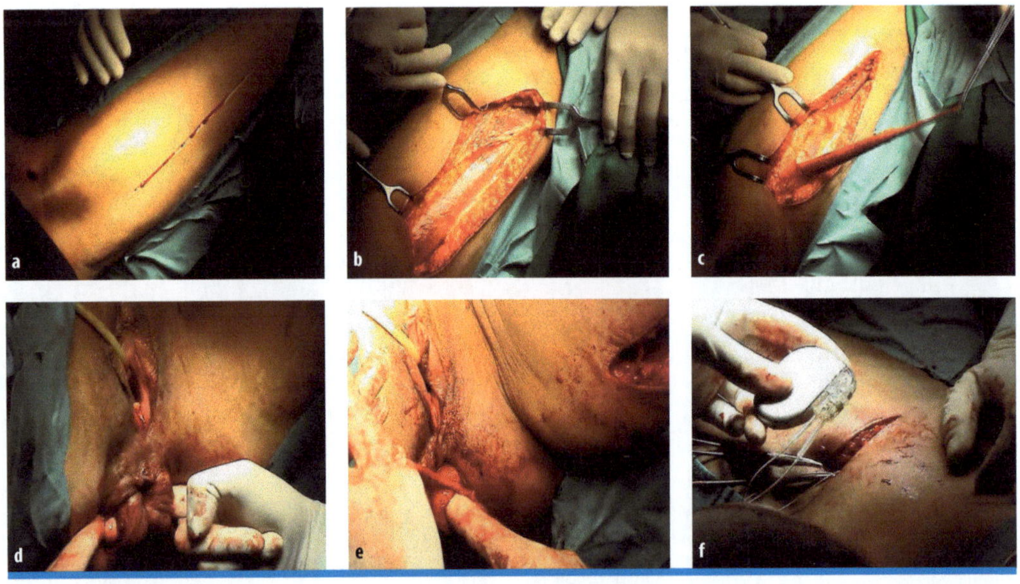

Fig. 2a–f. Dynamic graciloplasty, **a** skin incision, **b** gracilis muscle is exposed and **c** isolated, **d** perianal tunnel is prepared, **e** gracilis muscle has been transposed in perianal space and a "gamma" loop is prepared, **f** the electrostimulator (connected to the electrodes implanted close to the nerve pedicle of the gracilis muscle) is placed in a subfascial pocket at the level of the rectum abdominis muscle

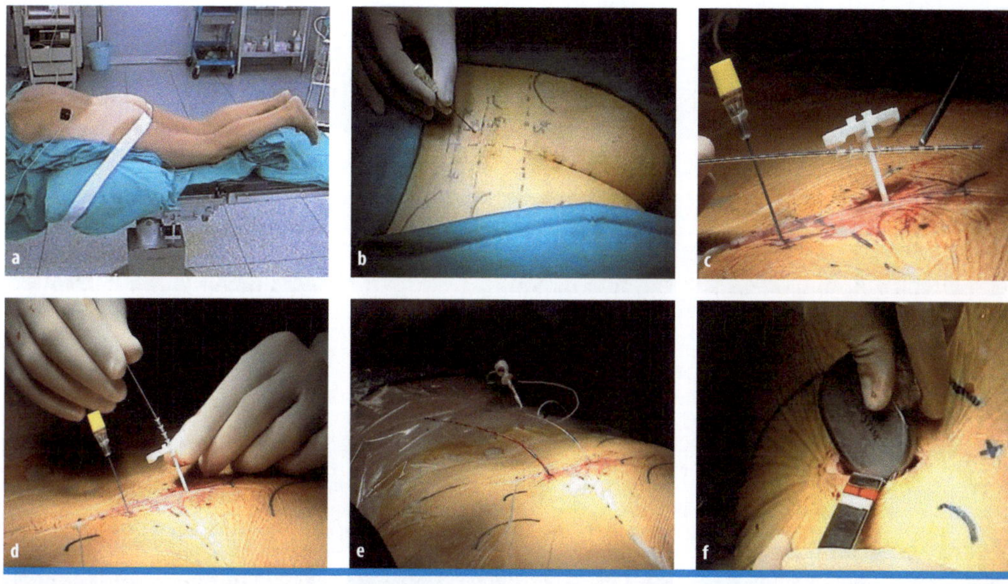

Fig. 3a–f. Sacral nerve stimulation, **a** patient's position in the operating room, **b** following local anesthesia, a needle is inserted through the right third sacral foramen, **c** a needle has been inserted into the left third sacral foramen, and the electrode introducer has been placed through the right third sacral foramen; a permanent quadripolar electrode is shown, **d** insertion of the permanent quadripolar electrode through the introducer, **e** bilateral placement of permanent electrodes into the right and left third sacral foramina, **f** subcutaneous placement of the electrostimulator. Reprinted with permission from [88]

only major contraindications to the sphincter replacement procedures are very severe chronic bowel diseases causing intractable defecation dysfunctions (severe diarrhea as well as severe constipation) and coexistence of rectal prolapse, intussusception, rectocele, or enterocele.

Although indications for dynamic graciloplasty (Fig. 2), artificial bowel sphincter, and gluteoplasty overlap, there are various differences between them concerning surgeon preference and expertise, techniques and materials used, evaluation of perioperative morbidity, and long-term results [44–56]. These aspects are treated in details in other chapters in this book. It must be noted that because all outcome variables can reach very poor or very good levels primarily in relation to correct indications and surgeon expertise, it seems reasonable that these operations must be performed by surgeons dedicated to the management of severe FI.

Sacral Nerve Stimulation

SNS now plays a central role in the algorithm of FI management (Fig. 3). Even if of recent clinical application in anorectal dysfunction [57], this approach has rapidly expanded, and step by step, acceptable indications have been suggested. Initial applications concerned patients with dysfunctions of nonlesioned striated anal muscles, then with a prevalent neurogenic etiology [58–64]. Thereafter, as clinical use and understanding of action mechanisms made progress, SNS expanded to other indications, including idiopathic sphincter degeneration, iatrogenic internal sphincter damage, partial spinal cord injury, scleroderma, limited lesions of internal or external anal sphincters, rectal prolapse repair, and low anterior resection of the rectum [65–78]. Actually, alterations of the sacrum or skin in the implantation area, very wide sphincter tears, pregnancy, and very severe uncontrolled chronic bowel diseases are regarded as the main contraindications for SNS.

A variety of physiological patterns has been observed at patient presentation, and, in most studies, none of these parameters has been elucidated as a prognostic indicator of outcome. Alterations of any one manometric parameter did not contraindicate this therapy. Variations of rectal sensation between baseline to postimplant toward normal range seem to be related to better results, despite whether baseline values were higher or lower than normal [79, 80]; this would demonstrate the "modulation" effect of SNS.

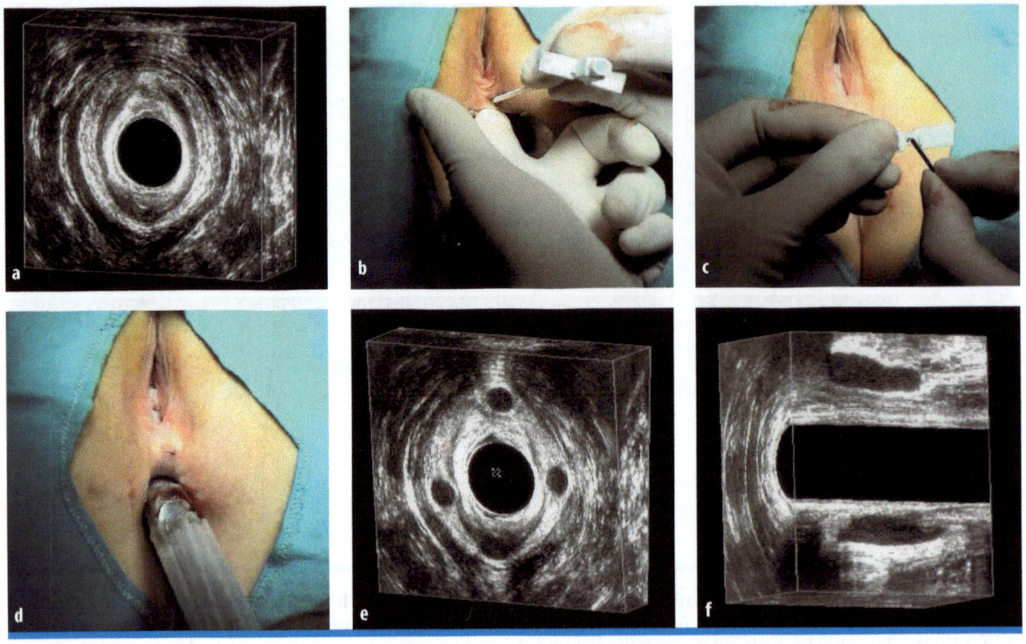

Fig. 4a–f. Implantation of a new bulking agent for fecal incontinence (FI), the Anal Gatekeeper (Medtronic, Inc., Minneapolis, MN, USA), **a** endoanal ultrasound (EAUS) of a patient with FI following rectal prolapse previously repaired with Delorme procedure, **b** following locoregional anesthesia (perineal block), insertion of the introducer through a small skin incision to reach the intersphincteric space; introducer site should be confirmed by EAUS, **c** placement of the thin solid prosthesis through the introducer to reach the intersphincteric space, followed by removal of the introducer, **d** final check by EAUS, **e** coronal and **f** longitudinal views of EAUS 6 months after four prostheses implant; in 24 h, each prosthesis became thicker and very soft

Prolonged PNTML, previously considered a negative prognostic factor for treatment success, now is regarded, per se, as a noninfluencing indicator. Other studies have underlined the influence of SNS on the central nervous system [81, 82], explaining why this approach could be effective in partial spinal cord lesions but ineffective in cases of total lesions. Very recently, Gourcerol et al. [83] investigated prognostic factors associated with SNS success during temporary and definitive stimulation. They found that only patient age was prognostic of outcome during temporary test, whereas bulbocavernosus reflex latency was the only factor influencing success after definitive device implantation. In their opinion, patients with neurogenic FI should be candidates for SNS.

Injectable Bulking Agents

This treatment approach is regarded as attractive because it is not invasive. However, only a very accurate patient selection can allow positive effects of bulking agents on FI. Usually, patients with either limited internal sphincter lesion or a weak anus without tears are indicated to this kind of treatment. Moreover, individuals who cannot be submitted to other major surgical approaches due to their poor general clinical conditions could be amenable to injection of bulking agents. The increasing variety of agents proposed and used (Fig. 4) to create a bulking effect, with different methods of injection (through anal mucosa or transsphincteric), different placement sites (submucosal or intersphincteric), and different check procedures (digital examination or EAUS), have determined criteria incomparable for selecting the most appropriate approach [84].

Radiofrequency

This therapy also seems to be indicated in individuals with weak anal sphincters, but lesions contraindicate its use, as does chronic diarrhea, inflammatory bowel disease, or anal sepsis. Due to the recent clinical application [85–87] and lack of large studies, it is not possible, at this time, to determine stricter selection criteria.

Treatment Evaluation

A variety of aspects can affect evaluation of the effectiveness of a certain therapy for FI. Identification of factors reflecting the treatment impact and methods measuring the improvement obtained is of crucial importance. This should be derived from well-conducted studies with a sufficiently large number of patients selected with strict criteria. However, frequently, the available reports are mostly affected by an inhomogeneous patient selection. Also, criteria used to define response to therapy are not standardized. This could depend on the end point of that treatment: care of symptoms (i.e., reduction of FI episodes; improved control of solid vs. liquid stools vs. gas; ability to postpone defecation), improvement in quality of life, improvement in multifactorial aspects (i.e., scores), or normalization of physiological parameters (i.e., manometric; electrophysiologic; ultrasonographic).

Conceptually, considering a good response as an improvement of at least 50% in FI could be debatable. In fact, in a patient treated for very severe FI, a 50% reduction in FI episodes (for instance, from ten to five episodes per week) probably is not enough to significantly improve that patient's pretreatment quality of life and life style (need to ware pads; living close to the bathroom; constrained to stay at home). Moreover, even if perfect control to solid stools has been regained after treatment, incontinence to liquids or gas could remain very detrimental. Because there is disagreement on clinical parameters to define treatment response, available data from reports must be evaluated thoroughly and critically.

On the other hand, the available scoring systems for FI measurement as well as quality of life questionnaires are not fully shared. They could be too vague and subjective. Patient "satisfaction" would probably be the most comprehensive concept reflecting therapy success, but it is difficult to quantify. Moreover, each score needs to be validated according to the patient's specific social, cultural, and environmental factors.

Physiological parameters are used to demonstrate the objective impact of a treatment. However, very frequently, conflicting data are obtained when a single parameter is considered because of the multifactorial origin of FI. Moreover, the influence of a particular treatment could be different in different subgroups of patients, each with particular physiological features.

All the above-mentioned considerations highlight the difficulty of interpreting data from reports on FI management. In the following chapters, the authors offer a complete panorama of medical, rehabilitative, and surgical methods to cure FI. They discuss techniques and results, as well as the pros and cons of using each approach.

References

1. Ternent CA, Shashidharan M, Blatchford GJ et al (1996) Do anorectal physiology tests result in altered therapy for fecal incontinence? Gastroenterology 110:A43
2. Liberman H, Faria J, Ternent CA et al (2001) A prospective evaluation of the value of anorectal physiology in the management of fecal incontinence. Dis Colon Rectum 44:1567–1574
3. Keating JP, Stewart PJ, Eyers AA et al (1997) Are special investigations of value in the management of patients with fecal incontinence? Dis Colon Rectum 40:896–901
4. Rao SS, Patel RS (1997) How useful are manometric tests of anorectal function in the management of defecation disorders? Am J Gastroenterol 92:469–475
5. Speakman CT, Henry MM (1992) The work of an anorectal physiology laboratory. Baillieres Clin Gastroenterol 6:59–73
6. Wexner SD, Jorge JM (1994) Colorectal physiological tests: use or abuse of technology? Eur J Surg 160:167–174
7. Norton C, Kamm MA (2001) Anal sphincter biofeedback and pelvic floor exercises for faecal incontinence in adults. Aliment Pharmacol Ther 15:1147–1154
8. Whitehead W, Wald A, Norton J (2001) Treatment options for fecal incontinence. Dis Colon Rectum 44: 131–144
9. Cerulli MA, Nikoomanesh P, Schuster MM (1979) Progress in biofeedback conditioning for fecal incontinence. Gastroenterology 76:742–746
10. Wald A (1981) Biofeedback therapy for fecal incontinence. Ann Intern Med 95:146–149
11. Sangwan YP, Coller JA, Barrett RC et al (1995) Can manometric parameters predict response to biofeedback therapy in fecal incontinence? Dis Colon Rectum 38:1021–1025
12. Fernandez-Fraga X, Azpiroz F, Aparici A et al (2003) Predictors of response to biofeedback treatment in anal incontinence. Dis Colon Rectum 46:1218–1225
13. Rieger NA, Wattchow DA, Sarre RG et al (1997) Prospective trial of pelvic floor retraining in patients with fecal incontinence. Dis Colon Rectum 40:821–826
14. Chiarioni G, Bassotti G, Stegagnini S et al (2002) Sensory retraining is key to biofeedback therapy for formed stool fecal incontinence. Am J Gastroenterol 97:109–117
15. Rao SS, Welcher KD, Happel J (1996) Can biofeedback therapy improve anorectal function in fecal incontinence? Am J Gastroenterol 91:2360–2366
16. Bharucha AE (2003) Fecal incontinence. Gastroenterology 124: 1672–1685
17. Buser WD, Miner PB Jr (1986) Delayed rectal sensation with fecal incontinence. Successful treatment

using anorectal manometry. Gastroenterology 91: 1186–1191
18. Sun WM, Read NW, Miner PB (1990) Relation between rectal sensation and anal function in normal subjects and patients with fecal incontinence. Gut 31:807–813
19. Leroi AM, Dorival MP, Lecouturier MF et al (1999) Pudendal neuropathy and severity of incontinence but not presence of an anal sphincter defect may determine the response to biofeedback therapy in fecal incontinence. Dis Colon Rectum 42:762–769
20. Laurberg S, Swash M, Snooks SJ, Henry MM (1988) Neurologic cause of idiopathic incontinence. Arch Neurol 45:1250–1253
21. Wexner SD, Marchetti F, Jagelman DG (1991) The role of sphincteroplasty for fecal incontinence re-evaluated: a prospective physiologic and functional review. Dis Colon Rectum 34:22–30
22. Oliveira L, Pfeifer J, Wexner SD (1996) Physiological and clinical outcome of anterior sphincteroplasty. Br J Surg 83:502–505
23. Gilliland R, Altomare DF, Moreira H Jr et al (1998) Pudendal neuropathy is predictive of failure following anterior overlapping sphincteroplasty. Dis Colon Rectum 41:1516–1522
24. Londono-Schimmer EE, Garcia-Duperly R, Nicholls RJ et al (1994) Overlapping anal sphincter repair for faecal incontinence due to sphincter trauma: five year follow-up functional results. Int J Colorectal Dis 9:110–113
25. Sangwan YP, CollerJA, Barrett RC et al (1996) Unilateral pudendal neuropathy. Impact on outcome of anal sphincter repair. Dis Colon Rectum 39:686–689
26. Sitzler PJ, Thomson JPS (1996) Overlap repair of damaged anal sphincter. A single surgeon's series. Dis Colon Rectum 39:1356–1360
27. Nikiteas N, Korsgen S, Kumar D, Keighley MRB (1996) Audit of sphincter repair. Factors associated with poor outcome. Dis Colon Rectum 39:1164–1170
28. Rasmussen OO, Colstrup H, Lose G, Christiansen J (1990) A technique for the dynamic assessment of anal sphincter function. Int J Colorectal Dis 5:135–141
29. Young CJ, Mathur MN, Eyers AA, Solomon MJ (1998) Successful overlapping anal sphincter repair: relationship to patient age, neuropathy and colostomy formation. Dis Colon Rectum 41:344–349
30. Chen AS, Luchtefeld MA, Senagore AJ et al (1998) Pudendal nerve latency. Does it predict outcome of anal sphincter repair? Dis Colon Rectum 41:1005–1009
31. Buie WD, Lowry AC, Rothenberger DA, Madoff RD (2001) Clinical rather than laboratory assessment predicts continence after anterior sphincteroplasty. Dis Colon Rectum 44:1255–1260
32. Halverson AL, Hull TL (2002) Long-term outcome of overlapping anal sphincter repair. Dis Colon Rectum 45:345–348
33. Bravo Gutierrez A, Madoff RD, Lowry AC et al (2004) Long-term results of anterior sphincteroplasty. Dis Colon Rectum 47:727–731
34. Trowbridge ER, Morgan D, Trowbridge MJ et al (2006) Sexual function, quality of life, and severity of anal incontinence after anal sphincteroplasty. Am J Obstet Gynecol 195:1753–1757
35. Steele SR, Lee P, Mullenix PS et al (2006) Is there a role for concomitant pelvic floor repair in patients with sphincter defects in the treatment of fecal incontinence? Int J Colorectal Dis 21:508–514
36. Evans C, Davis K, Kumar D (2006) Overlapping anal sphincter repair and anterior levatorplasty: effect of patient's age and duration of follow-up. Int J Colorectal Dis 21:795–801
37. Vaizey CJ, Kamm MA, Nicholls RJ (1998) Recent advances in the surgical treatment of faecal incontinence. Br J Surg 85:596–603
38. Athanasiadis S, Sanchez M, Kuprian A (1995) Long - term follow-up of Parks posterior repair. An electromyographic, manometric and radiologic study of 31 patients. Langenbeck Arch Chir 380:22–30
39. Rockwood TH, Church JM, Fleshman S et al (1999) Patient and surgeon ranking of the severity of symptoms associated with fecal incontinence: the fecal incontinence severity index. Dis Colon Rectum 42:1525–1531
40. Rockwood TH, Church JM, Fleshman JW (2000) Fecal incontinence quality of life scale. Dis Colon Rectum 43:10–16
41. Korsgen S, Keighley MRB (1995) Stimulated gracilis neosphincter-not as good as previously thought. Report of four cases. Dis Colon Rectum 38:1331–1333
42. Baeten CG, Geerdes BP, Adang EM et al (1995) Anal dynamic graciloplasty in the treatment of intractable fecal incontinence. N Engl J Med 332:1600–1605
43. Koch SM, Uludag O, Rongen MJ et al (2004) Dynamic graciloplasty in patients born with an anorectal malformation. Dis Colon Rectum 47:1711–1719
44. Geerdes BP, Heineman E, Konsten J et al (1996) Dynamic graciloplasty. Complications and management. Dis Colon Rectum 39:912–917
45. Wexner SD, Gonzalez-Padron A, Rius J et al (1996) Stimulated gracilis neosphincter operation. Initial experience, pitfalls, and complications. Dis Colon Rectum 39(9):957–964
46. Baeten CG, Bailey HR, Bakka A et al (2000) Safety and efficacy of dynamic graciloplasty for fecal incontinence: report of a prospective, multicenter trial Dynamic Graciloplasty Therapy Study Group. Dis Colon Rectum 43:743–751
47. Rongen MJ, Uludag Ö, El Naggar K et al (2003) Long-term follow-up of dynamic graciloplasty for faecal incontinence. Dis Colon Rectum 46:716–721
48. Lehur PA, Michot F, Denis P et al (1996) Results of artificial sphincter in severe anal incontinence. Report of 14 consecutive implantations. Dis Colon Rectum 39:1352–1355
49. Lehur PA, Zerbib F, Glemain P et al (2002) Comparison of quality of life and anorectal function after artificial sphincter implantation. Dis Colon Rectum 45:508–513
50. Parker SC, Spencer MP, Madoff RD (2003) Artificial bowel sphincter: long-term experience at a single institution. Dis Colon Rectum 46:722–729
51. O'Brien PE, Dixon JB, Skinner S et al (2004) A prospective randomised controlled clinical trial of placement of the artificial bowel sphincter (Acticon Neosphincter) for the control of fecal incontinence. Dis Colon Rectum 47(11):1852–1860
52. Mundy L, Merlin TL, Maddern GJ, Hiller JE (2004) Sys-

tematic review of safety and effectiveness of an artificial bowel sphincter for faecal incontinence. Br J Surg 91:665–672
53. Michot F, Costaglioli B, Leroi AM, Denis P (2003) Artificial anal sphincter in severe fecal incontinence: outcome of prospective experience with 37 patients in one institution. Ann Surg 237:52–56
54. Bruining HA, Bos KE, Colthoff EG et al (1981) Creation of an anal sphincter mechanism by bilateral proximally based gluteal muscle transposition. Plast Reconstr Surg 67:70–72
55. Guelinckx PJ, Sinsel NK, Gruwez JA (1996) Anal sphincter reconstruction with the gluteus maximus muscle: anatomic and physiologic considerations concerning conventional and dynamic gluteoplasty. Plast Reconstr Surg 98:293–302
56. Hultman CS, Zenn MR, Agarwal T et al (2006) Restoration of fecal continence after functional gluteoplasty: Long-term results, technical refinements, and donor-site morbidity. Ann Plast Surg 56:65–71
57. Matzel KE, Stadelmaier U, Hohenfellner M et al (1994) Electrical stimulation of sacral spinal nerves for treatment of faecal incontinence. Lancet 346:1124–1127
58. Matzel KE, Stadelmaier U, Hohenfellner M, Gall FP (1995) Electrical stimulation for the treatment of faecal incontinence. Lancet 346:1124–1127
59. Matzel KE (2001) Sacral spinal nerve stimulation in treatment of fecal incontinence. Semin Colon Rectal Surg 12:121–130
60. Leroi AM, Michot F, Grise P, Denis P (2001) Effect of sacral nerve stimulation in patients with fecal and urinary incontinence. Dis Colon Rectum 44:779–789
61. Ganio E, Ratto C, Masin A et al (2001) Neuromodulation for fecal incontinence: outcome in 16 patients with definitive implant. The initial Italian Sacral Neurostimulation Group (GINS) experience. Dis Colon Rectum 44:965–970
62. Matzel KE, Stadelmaier U, Hohenberger W (2004) Innovations in fecal incontinence: Sacral nerve stimulation. Dis Colon Rectum 47:1720–1728
63. Matzel KE, Kamm MA, Stösser M et al MDT 301 Study Group (2004) Sacral nerve stimulation for fecal incontinence: a multicenter study. Lancet 363:1270–1276
64. Tjandra JJ, Lim JF, Matzel KE (2004) Sacral nerve stimulation - an emerging treatment for faecal incontinence. ANZ J Surg 74:1098–1106
65. Rosen HR, Urbarz C, Holzer B et al (2001) Sacral nerve stimulation as a treatment for fecal incontinence. Gastroenterology 121:536–541
66. Malouf AJ, Vaizey CJ, Nicholls RJ, Kamm MA (2000) Permanent sacral nerve stimulation for faecal incontinence. Ann. Surg 232:143–148
67. Ganio E, Realis Luc A, Ratto C et al (2003) Sacral nerve modulation for fecal incontinence: functional results and assessment of the quality of life. http://www.colorep.it/Rivista%20CEC/sacral_nerve_modulation_for_feca.htm. Cited 28 Nov 2005
68. Jarrett ME, Varma JS, Duthie GS et al (2004) Sacral nerve stimulation for faecal incontinence in the UK. Br J Surg 91:755–761
69. Bernstein AJ, Peters KM (2005) Expanding indications for neuromodulation. Urol Clin North Am 32:59–63
70. Jarrett ME, Matzel KE, Christiansen J et al (2005) Sacral nerve stimulation for faecal incontinence in patients with previous partial spinal injury including disc prolapse. Br J Surg 92:734–739
71. Kenefick NJ, Vaizey CJ, Nicholls RJ et al (2002) Sacral nerve stimulation for faecal incontinence due to systemic sclerosis. Gut 51:881–883
72. Leroi AM, Michot F, Grise P, Denis P (2001) Effect of sacral nerve stimulation in patients with faecal and urinary incontinence. Dis Colon Rectum 44:779–789
73. Jarrett ME, Matzel KE, Stosser M et al (2005) Sacral nerve stimulation for fecal incontinence following surgery for rectal prolapse repair: a multicenter study. Dis Colon Rectum 48:1243–1248
74. Matzel KE, Stadelmaier U, Bittorf B et al (2002) Bilateral sacral spinal nerve stimulation for fecal incontinence after low anterior rectum resection. Int J Colorectal Dis 17:430–434
75. Uludag O, Dejong HC (2002) Sacral neuromodulation for faecal incontinence. Dis Colon Rectum 45:34–36
76. Matzel KE, Bittorf B, Stadelmaier U, Hohenberger W (2003) Sacral nerve stimulation in the treatment of faecal incontinence. Chirurg 74:26–32
77. Ratto C, Grillo E, Parello A et al (2005) Sacral neuromodulation in treatment of fecal incontinence following anterior resection and chemoradiation for rectal cancer. Dis Colon Rectum 48:1027–1036
78. Jarrett ME, Matzel KE, Stosser M et al (2005) Sacral nerve stimulation for faecal incontinence following a rectosigmoid resection for colorectal cancer. Int J Colorectal Dis 20:446–451
79. Ratto C, Petrolino M, Altomare DF et al (2004) The effects of sacral neuromodulation on rectal sensation can predict improvement of fecal incontinence. Dis Colon Rectum 47:611
80. Rosen H (2004) SNS-How does it work. Proceedings from Meeting of European Association of Coloproctology, Geneva
81. Braun PM, Baezner H, Seif C et al (2002) Alterations of cortical electrical activity in patients with sacral neuromodulator. Eur Urol 41:562–566
82. Malaguti S, Spinelli M, Giardiello G et al (2003) Neurophysiological evidence may predict the outcome of sacral neuromodulation. J Urol 170:2323–2326
83. Gourcerol G, Gallas S, Michot F et al (2007) Sacral nerve stimulation in fecal incontinence: are there factors associated with success? Dis Colon Rectum 50:3–12
84. Vaizey CJ, Kamm MA (2005) Injectable bulking agents for treating faecal incontinence. Br J Surg 92:521–527
85. Efron JE, Corman ML, Fleshman J et al (2003) Safety and effectiveness of temperature-controlled radio-frequency energy delivery to the anal canal (Secca procedure) for the treatment of fecal incontinence. Dis Colon Rectum 46:1606–1616
86. Takahashi T, Garcia-Osogobio S, Valdovinos MA et al (2003) Extended two-year results of radio-frequency energy delivery for the treatment of fecal incontinence (the Secca procedure). Dis Colon Rectum 46:711–715
87. Efron JE (2004) The SECCA procedure: a new therapy for treatment of fecal incontinence. Surg Technol Int 13:107–110
88. Ratto C, Parello A, Donisi L (2007) Sacral Neuromodulation in the treatment of defecation disorders. Acta Neurochir 97 (Suppl) 341–350

Medical Treatment of Fecal Incontinence

14

Carlo Ratto, Angelo Parello, Lorenza Donisi, Francesco Litta,
Giovanni B. Doglietto

Introduction

Management of fecal incontinence (FI) should be based on a meticulous assessment of pathophysiology through both clinical and physiological diagnostic workup. There are cases with prevalently altered diet and hygiene. Very frequently, diarrhea and constipation can be found involved in the development and maintenance of FI [1–3], both in the presence or absence of other traumatic or nontraumatic causes. Consequently, in those cases, treatment must be directed toward cure of these dysfunctions, either as single-line or combined treatment. Little evidence exists in the available literature about medical therapy for FI; recently, a Cochrane Database Review highlighted that "there is little evidence with which to assess the use of drug therapies for the management of fecal incontinence" [4]. Therefore, medical treatment in FI is debatable and often pragmatic.

Diet and Patient Education

Patients should be educated to avoid excessive straining at defecation to reduce the risk of pudendal nerve damage. Perianal hygiene must be addressed, including delicate soaps specifically for use in the perianal area, to avoid perianal irritation and pruritus. Only in selected cases should absorbents, diapers, and tampons be recommended. Patients must be educated to reduce or avoid foods that induce loose stools, excessive gastrointestinal transit, or increased intestinal gas production (i.e., milk and derivates, excessive legumes and vegetables, chocolate, tomatoes, caffeine, prunes, grapes, figs).

Chronic Diarrhea

Up to 50% of patients with chronic diarrhea can present FI [5]. The most common cause of chronic diarrhea associated with FI is irritable bowel syndrome (IBS) [6]. In these patients, abdominal pain or discomfort, altered stool frequency, altered stool form, and/or relief of discomfort after a bowel movement may coexist [7–9]. FI can also be associated with other causes of chronic diarrhea:

- Lactose intolerance
- Excess of medications (laxatives, antacids, prostaglandins, nonsteroidal anti-inflammatory drugs)
- Hyperthyroidism
- Diabetes
- Nonabsorbable sugars
- Crohn's disease
- Ulcerative colitis
- Benign or malignant rectal tumors
- Small-bowel bacterial overgrowth
- Bile acid malabsorption
- Celiac sprue
- Microscopic colitis
- Chronic pancreatitis

Usually, these causes create excessive water and electrolyte passage into the small/large bowel, loss of protein and fluid, alteration of intestinal peristalsis, and stool transit time.

For FI associated with mild chronic diarrhea or mild chronic constipation, *bulking agents* of either natural (psyllium, gum arabic, methyl cellulose) or synthetic (calcium polycarbophil) fibers should be considered as first-line treatment. Moreover, a daily fiber supplementation for 1 month has been demonstrated to significantly reduce FI [10].

Persistence of diarrhea should be treated with specific *antidiarrheal agents*. Patients should always be warned about the possible constipating effect of these agents. *Loperamide* is a synthetic opioid with both calcium-receptor-antagonist- and calcium-channel-blocking actions. Then, due to this action, augmented water and electrolyte absorption is obtained by reduction of intestinal peristalsis and prolonged gastrointestinal transit time. Moreover, it increases internal anal sphincter tone and reduces urge sensation and bowel-movement frequency by reducing sensitivity to the rectoanal inhibitory reflex (RAIR). Compared with diphenoxylate, loperamide is more effective in reducing urgency, stool frequency, and central nervous system (CNS) adverse events (it does not cross the blood-brain barrier) [11–13]. However, caution must be used in dosage to avoid undesirable constipation. Only a few studies have been directed toward evaluating the benefits of loperamide in FI patients [14–16]. *Diphenoxylate* and *difenoxin* are opioids with antiperistaltic action, but they cross the blood-brain barrier, causing mild euphoria if taken in excess, requiring atropine. No effects on anal pressures have been demonstrated. An overdosage could cause toxic megacolon in an inflamed colon. Clinical studies have tested the effectiveness of *phenylephrine gel* in patients with FI. This is a selective alpha 1 adrenergic agonist, increasing internal anal sphincter tone and resting anal pressure [17, 18]. *Amitriptyline*, a tricyclic antidepressant with anticholinergic, serotonergic, and antimuscarinic actions, has been demonstrated to reduce amplitude and frequency of rectal motor complexes, increase colonic transit time, and improve symptoms in patients with FI or IBS [19–21].

Chronic Constipation

FI can occur in patients affected by chronic constipation as a consequence of stool retention in the rectum, resulting in overflow incontinence. Chronic fecal retention determines a significantly decreased anorectal sensation. On the other hand, constipation can be caused by excessive consumption of drugs, including antidiarrheals, narcotics, calcium-channel blockers, antidepressants, and other psychotropic agents. Finally, particularly in the older subjects, dehydration and insufficient fiber and fluid intake cause chronic constipation. Overflow FI is particularly frequent in institutionalized patients. It can require manual disimpaction, stool softeners, laxatives, enemas, or suppositories [22].

Accurate diagnosis of constipation-FI sequence is determinant to avoid planning incorrect or excessive treatment. Physical examination, anorectal manometry and electrophysiology, endoanal ultrasound, contrast defecography, and radiologic transit time evaluation can contribute to the identification of pathophysiological processes and exclude other causes of both constipation and FI.

The above-mentioned *bulking agents* as well as *laxatives* and *stool softeners* can be used, provided that caution is used to avoid excessively loose feces, thus worsening FI. Dietary manipulation, by improving fiber intake (including wheat bran, psyllium husk, methylcellulose, polycarbophils), can be effective because stool weight is increased and consistency is decreased.

Both lactulose and sorbitol stimulate intestinal peristalsis by a water-transport mechanism into the bowel. Undesirable side effects are abdominal bloating and flatulence, with subsequent patient discomfort. Glycerin, given as an enema, can obtain rectal emptying. Saline laxatives interfere with bowel osmosis and peristalsis, improving intestinal motility. However, administration to patients with cardiac or renal failure or electrolyte anomalies needs special caution.

Some 5-HT mediators display a different mechanism of action. Tegaserod is a 5-HT4 agonist that improves intestinal peristalsis and increases transit time of both the small intestine and the colon; also, it may ameliorate abdominal pain and distention [23, 24].

References

1. Nelson R, Furner S, Jesudason V (1998) Fecal incontinence in Wisconsin nursing homes: prevalence and associations. Dis Colon Rectum 41:1226–1229
2. Chassagne P, Landrin I, Neveu C et al (1999) Fecal incontinence in the institutionalized elderly: incidence, risk factors, and prognosis. Am J Med 106:185–190
3. Levine MD (1975) Children with encopresis: A descriptive analysis. Pediatrics 56:412–416
4. Cheetham M, Brazzelli M, Norton C et al (2003) Drug treatment for fecal incontinence in adults. Cochrane Database Syst Rev 4:1–26
5. Goode PS, Burgio KL, Halli AD et al (2005) Prevalence and correlates of fecal incontinence in community-dwelling older adults. J Am Geriatr Soc 53:629–635
6. Drossman DA (1989) What can be done to control incontinence associated with irritable bowel syndrome? Am J Gastroenterol 84:365–366
7. Olden KW (2002) Diagnosis of irritable bowel syndrome. Gastroenterology 122:1701–1714
8. Lembo TJ, Fink RN (2002) Clinical assessment of irritable bowel syndrome. J Clin Gastroenterol 35: S31–S36
9. Fine KD, Meyer RL, Lee EL (1997) The prevalence and causes of chronic diarrhea in patients with celiac sprue treated with a gluten-free diet Gastroenterology 112:1830–1838
10. Bliss DZ, Jung HJ, Savok K et al (2001) Supplementation with dietary fiber improves fecal incontinence. Nurs Res 50:203–213
11. Palmer KR, Corbett CL, Holdsworth CD (1980) Double-blind cross-over study comparing loperamide, codeine and diphenoxylate in the treatment of chronic diarrhea. Gastroenterology 79:1272–1275
12. Read MG, Read NM, Duthie HL (1979) Effect of loperamide in anal sphincter function in patients with diarrhea. Gut 20:A942
13. Bergman L, Djarv L (1981) A comparative study of loperamide and diphenoxylate in the treatment of chronic diarrhoea caused by intestinal resection. Ann Clin Res 13:402–405

14. Read M, Read NW, Barber DC et al (1982) Effects of loperamide on anal sphincter function in patients complaining of chronic diarrhea with fecal incontinence and urgency. Dig Dis Sci 27:807–814
15. Hallgren T, Fasth S, Delbro DS et al (1994) Loperamide improves anal sphincter function and continence after restorative proctocolectomy. Dig Dis Sci 39:2612–2618
16. Arnbjornsson E, Breland U, Kullendorff CM et al (1986) Effect of loperamide on faecal control after rectoplasty for high imperforate anus. Acta Chir Scand 152:215–216
17. Carapeti EA, Kamm MA, Evans BK et al (1999) Topical phenylephrine increases anal sphincter resting pressure. Br J Surg 86:267–270
18. Cheetham MJ, Kamm MA, Phillips RK (2001) Topical phenylephrine increases anal canal resting pressure in patients with faecal incontinence. Gut 48:356–359
19. Ritchie JA, Truelove SC (1980) Comparison of various treatments for irritable bowel syndrome. Br Med J 281:1317–1319
20. Farrar JT (1982) The effects of drugs on intestinal motility. Clin Gastroenterol 11:673–681
21. Santoro GA, Eitan BZ, Pryde A et al (2000) Open study of low-dose amitriptyline in the treatment of patients with idiopathic fecal incontinence. Dis Colon Rectum 43:1676–1681
22. Chassagne P, Jego A, Gloc P et al (2000) Does treatment of constipation improve faecal incontinence in institutionalized elderly patients? Age Ageing 29:159–164
23. Prather CM, Camilleri M, Zinsmeister AR et al (2000) Tegaserod accelerates orocecal transit in patients with constipation-predominant irritable bowel syndrome. Gastroenterology 118:463–468
24. Tougas G, Snape WJ Jr, Otten MH et al (2002) Long-term safety of tegaserod in patients with constipation-predominant irritable bowel syndrome. Aliment Pharmacol Ther 16:1701–1708

Rehabilitation and Biofeedback

15

Filippo Pucciani

Introduction

Fecal continence depends on the interaction of many factors. Anal sphincters, pelvic floor muscles, anal sensation, rectal sensory-motor activity, and neural integrity all have determinant roles, which together provide a coordinated mechanism of gas and stool continence. The pathophysiology of fecal incontinence is, therefore, often multifactorial, and each patient has his or her own specific pathogenetic profile as a result of a mix of etiological factors. It is clear that any treatment for fecal incontinence must allow for this fundamental aspect, and each patient thus requires a clinical approach that has been modulated on his or her specific incontinence etiology. This basic fact must be considered when planning therapy for a patient with fecal incontinence.

Rehabilitative treatment using biofeedback and pelvic floor exercises is considered the first-line option in treating fecal incontinence in patients who have not responded to simple dietary advice or medication [1]. Understanding when and how to perform rehabilitative treatment is not simple because there are no international agreements on the use of the various rehabilitative techniques. The main problems are related to an absence of standards and guidelines, and the published scientific literature reflects this reality. A systematic review [1] by Norton and Kamm and a consensus conference report [2] by Whitehead et al. mention several negative factors that can be detected in many studies:

- Confusion between biofeedback and pelvic floor exercises
- A wide variety of methods within equipment and training programs
- A wide variety of outcome measures
- No predictors of outcome
- Few long-term follow-ups

Significant rehabilitative treatment results may be obtained when the patient experiences (1) perception of sensory signals associated with rectal distension and following stool loss and (2) short external anal sphincter contractions when perceiving rectal distension [3]. Moreover, the patient prerequisites of rehabilitative treatment success include motivation, intact cognition, and absence of depression [4]. Last but not least, the nurse–patient interaction is the most important variable that may influence rehabilitation success rate [3]. The treatment goes on for months, and patients need to have a person as a point of reference who is able to combine technical capacities, patience, and availability.

On these grounds, it is very hard to discuss the topic of rehabilitative fecal incontinence treatment because it will always result in being one sided and incomplete. Thus, the aim of the present study was only to provide an overview of the various approaches to fecal incontinence rehabilitative treatment. A short description of the various available rehabilitative techniques is followed by a description of multimodal rehabilitation.

Rehabilitative Techniques

The rehabilitative techniques that may be used for treating fecal incontinence are:

- Biofeedback
- Pelviperineal kinesitherapy
- Sensory retraining
- Electrostimulation

Biofeedback

Biofeedback therapy is an operant conditioning [5] that consists of pelvic floor strengthening exercises together with visual/verbal feedback training [6]. It is voluntary, employs a trial-and-error process by which learning takes place, and the subject must be aware of the desired response (signals). Two types of biofeedback training, manometric or electromyographic (EMG), can be used in fecal incontinence, but both techniques work according to the same theoretical principles of operant conditioning. Manometric biofeedback is usually performed by monitoring anal canal pressures coupled to visual/verbal signals proportional to the pressure waves. In EMG biofeedback, the EMG sensors are positioned in the anal canal or adjacent to the anus and provide measurements of the averaged EMG activity of the pelvic floor coupled to visual/verbal signals. During their first training session, patients receive instructions on how to contract the external anal sphincter and puborectalis muscle in response to or in absence of rectal distention sensation and how to improve muscle strength using modified Kegel exercises. The number of sessions is customized for each patient and may be done either in the outpatient unit using a rehabilitative work station or at home using portable devices. The sessions last 1 month, and the use of periodic reinforcement, at least during the first year of therapy, may help maintain the beneficial effects over a long period [7].

How biofeedback works is debatable, even if it is generally considered a cortical reconditioning method for the defecation reflex [8]. It can influence both the strength of the striated pelvic floor muscles and the threshold of the sphincter contraction [9]. Interestingly, some papers suggested that a marked and significant levator ani strengthening is associated with clinical improvement in response to biofeedback therapy [10], whereas the external sphincter fails to improve [11]. This could explain why the objective changes in anorectal function seem be related more to improved sensory discrimination than to resting and squeezing anal pressures [4]. Whatever the mechanism of action, about 70% of patients show a decrease in fecal incontinence episodes [12, 13].

Pelviperineal Kinesitherapy

Developed to treat genital prolapse and female urinary incontinence [14], pelviperineal kinesitherapy may also be employed in the coloproctology field for rehabilitating fecal disorders [15]. This is a type of muscular training that selectively aims at the levator ani muscles. It is applied in patients with fecal incontinence with the general aim of improving the pelvic viscera bearing and endurance and coordination of pelvic floor muscles and specific targets in order to strengthen the stress abdominal-perineal reflex and reinforce the puborectalis muscle resting tone (with positive effects on the anorectal angle) [16]. Pelviperineal kinesitherapy is useful when descending perineum syndrome [17] or pelvic floor support defects [18] are present in patients with fecal incontinence.

A cycle of pelviperineal kinesitherapy following a standard sequence is performed twice weekly in some outpatient sessions [19]. Briefly, a sequence carries the patient from a preliminary lesson on relaxed breathing and corporeal consciousness on through intermediate steps (i.e., anteversion and retroversion pelvic movements, puborectalis muscle stretch reflexes) to the final lessons, which include abdominopelvic synergy and anal contraction exercises (i.e., bending down, coughing, and Valsalva's maneuver in supine, upright, and sitting positions).

Sensory Retraining

The aim of sensory retraining is to increase the incontinent patient's ability to perceive the rectal distension induced by feces or flatus (rectal sensation) [20]. Impaired rectal sensation may be a cause of fecal incontinence. Reduced rectal sensation, with a higher than normal rectal distension conscious threshold, allows the stool to enter the anal canal and, due either to the absence or lateness of the external anal sphincter reflex contraction, incontinence may occur [4]. Conversely, an exaggerated rectal sensation, with a lower conscious threshold, may elicit fecal incontinence because it is associated with reduced rectal compliance, repetitive rectal contractions during rectal distention, and longer simultaneous sphincter relaxation [21].

In these cases, two types of sensory retraining can be used. The first type partly uses biofeedback training, as sensory retraining is coupled to sphincter strength training. In response to repeated rectal distensions induced by inflation of the catheter-mounted balloon with volumes above or below the sensory threshold, the patient contracts the anal sphincter as strongly as possible, with feedback on contraction strength [2]. The second type involves twice-daily administration of a tepid water enema (volumetric rehabilitation) [19] . The initial volume is equal to the maximally tolerated manometric volume. The patient holds the liquid using the strongest possible anal contraction for the longest period of time possible. In the days following, the enema volume is gradually either increased or decreased by 30 ml until the patient achieves a normal value of rectal sensation; the volume is increased if the patient has a resting low-conscious threshold and decreased if the resting conscious threshold is high.

Both techniques act on the above-mentioned points, suggested by Tries [3] as decisive factors in rehabilitation success. Moreover, the program can be managed successfully by advanced-practice nurses in nonhospital settings [22]. If used as an isolated rehabilitative technique, sensory retraining has the same success rate as biofeedback.

Electrostimulation

Electrical stimulation can induce muscle contraction by direct stimulation or indirectly via peripheral nerve stimulation. Anal electrical stimulation can be used to treat fecal incontinence, and the rehabilitative cycle is performed daily for some months by the patient in the home environment [19]. Patients are instructed to self-administer electrical stimulation with an anal plug probe. The device delivers a square wave of current alternating between a work period of a few seconds and a double rest period, according to a standard sequence. The daily routine is modulated on a program based on (1) current pulse (width in milliseconds and frequency in hertz) and (2) duration (minutes/day) and frequency (number/day) of sessions.

The therapeutic effects are unpredictable because they depend on current type and intensity, application time, and tissue impedance. Moreover, some scientific papers underline that electrostimulation is not a clinically effective treatment of anal incontinence and that passive electrostimulation therapy of the anal sphincter is inferior to active biofeedback training [23, 24]. A Cochrane review [25] and a recent randomized trial [26] did not alleviate these doubts. Some patients feel better after electrical stimulation, and incontinence may improve, but there is no objective effect on anal sphincter pressures. Positive effects on the anal sphincter may be due to intrinsic muscular factors that are commonly found when the electrostimulation is used in other somatic districts. Anal electrostimulation, however, could decrease the sphincteric tendency toward fatigue [23], and the compound muscle action potential of the external anal sphincter could be significantly increased by electrical stimulation [27]. After all, as the main possible mechanism of benefit, the improvement of incontinence could be conducive to better anal sensory awareness [26, 28].

Multimodal Rehabilitation

Multimodal rehabilitation is the latest news in rehabilitative treatment of fecal incontinence [19]. The algorithm for this rehabilitation management is based on the manometric reports. Biofeedback and pelviperineal kinesitherapy are indicated by low anal resting pressures or weak maximal voluntary contraction. Volumetric rehabilitation is indicated for disordered rectal sensation or impaired rectal compliance. Electrostimulation is only a preliminary step when patients need to improve sensation of the anoperineal plane. The usual procedure sequence is (1) volumetric rehabilitation, (2) electrostimulation, (3) biofeedback, and (4) pelviperineal kinesitherapy. Their combination is suggested by manometric data.

Anorectal manometry is the best diagnostic technique to identify impaired mechanisms of continence and is also a good guide to explain the pathophysiology of fecal incontinence. As stated above, each rehabilitative technique can modify specific aspects of fecal incontinence; therefore, anorectal manometry may suggest when the procedures are indicated. It is a rehabilitative treatment modulated on the incontinence pathophysiology of each patient.

The clinical outcome of multimodal rehabilitation is encouraging. Eighty-nine percent of patients show a significant improvement in incontinence score and 38% become symptom free. The worst results are obtained in patients affected by rectal prolapse and those with sphincter-saving operations. Long-term evaluation as well as prospective studies could confirm the promising results of the multimodal rehabilitation model.

Conclusion

In conclusion, the rehabilitative treatment of fecal incontinence is a good therapeutic option. Many patients may be cured and their quality of life much improved. In addition, rehabilitation techniques can be used to screen out the incontinent nonresponders, whose treatment should more appropriately include more expensive and extensive procedures (e.g., sphincteroplasty, sacral neuromodulation, artificial sphincter, dynamic graciloplasty).

References

1. Norton C, Kamm MA (2001) Anal sphincter biofeedback and pelvic floor exercises for faecal incontinence in adults. Aliment Pharmacol Ther 15:1147–1154
2. Whitehead W, Wald A, Norton J (2001) Treatment options for fecal incontinence. Dis Colon Rectum 44:131–144
3. Tries J (2004) Protocol- and therapist-related variables affecting outcomes of behavioral interventions for urinary and fecal incontinence. Gastroenterology 126 (1 Suppl 1):S152–S158
4. Bharucha AE (2003) Fecal incontinence. Gastroenterology 124:1672–1685
5. Engel BT, Nikoomanesh P, Schuster MM (1974) Operant conditioning of rectosphincteric response in the treatment of fecal incontinence. N Engl J Med 290: 646–649
6. Rao SSC, Happel J, Welcher K (1996) Can biofeedback therapy improve anorectal function in fecal incontinence? Am J Gastroenterol 91:2360–2366

7. Ozturk R, Niazi S, Stessman M, Rao SSC (2004) Long-term outcome and objective changes of anorectal function after biofeedback therapy for faecal incontinence. Aliment Pharmacol Ther 20:667–674
8. Papachrhrysostomou M, Smith AN (1994) Effects of biofeedback on obstructive defecation. Reconditioning of the defecation reflex? Gut 35:252–256
9. Chiarioni G, Bassotti G, Stanganini S et al (2002) Sensory retraining is key to biofeedback therapy for formed stool fecal incontinence. Am J Gastroenterol 97:109–117
10. Fernandex-Fraga X, Azpiroz F, Malagelada J-R (2002) Significance of pelvic floor muscles in anal incontinence. Gastroenterology 123:1441–1450
11. Miner PB, Donnelly TC, Read NW (1990) Investigation of mode of action of biofeedback in treatment of fecal incontinence. Dig Dis Sci 35:1291–1298
12. Enck P (1993) Biofeedback training in disordered defecation: a critical review. Dig Dis Sci 38:1953–1960
13. Heymen S, Jones KR, Ringel Y et al (2001) Biofeedback treatment of fecal incontinence: a critical review. Dis Colon Rectum 44:728–736
14. Kegel AH (1952) Stress incontinence and genital relaxation; a nonsurgical method of increasing the tone of sphincters and their supporting structures. Clin Symp 4:35–51
15. Pucciani F, Rottoli ML, Bologna A et al (1998) Pelvic floor dyssynergia and bimodal rehabilitation: results of combined pelviperineal kinesitherapy and biofeedback training. Int J Colorect Dis 13:124–130
16. Di Benedetto P (2004) Chinesiterapia pelvi-perineale: generalità. In: Di Benedetto P (ed) Riabilitazione uroginecologica. Edizioni Minerva Medica (II Edizione), Torino, pp 177–179
17. Harewood GC, Coulie B, Camilleri M et al (1999) Descending perineum syndrome: audit of clinical and laboratory features and outcome of pelvic floor retraining. Am J Gastroenterol 94:126–130
18. Sander P, Bjarnesen J, Mouritsen L, Fuglsang-Frederiksen A (1999) Anal incontinence after obstetric third-/fourth- degree laceration. One-year follow-up after pelvic floor exercises. Int Urogynecol J Pelvic Floor Dysfunction 10:177–181
19. Pucciani F, Iozzi L, Masi A et al (2003) Multimodal rehabilitation for faecal incontinence: experience of an Italian centre devoted to faecal disorder rehabilitation. Tech Coloproctol 7:139–147
20. Buser WD, Miner PB Jr (1986) Delayed rectal sensation with fecal incontinence. Successful treatment using anorectal manometry. Gastroenterology 91: 1186–1191
21. Sun WM, Read NW, Miner PB (1990) Relation between rectal sensation and anal function in normal subjects and patients with fecal incontinence. Gut 31:807–813
22. Bentsen D, Braun JW (1996) Controlling fecal incontinence with sensory retraining managed by advanced practice nurses. Clin Nurse Spec 10:171–175
23. Leroi AM, Karoui S, Touchais JY et al (1999) Electrostimulation is not a clinically effective treatment of anal incontinence. Eur J Gastroenterol Hepatol11:1045–1047
24. Surh S, Kienle P, Stern J, Herfarth C (1998) Passive electrostimulation therapy of the anal sphincter is inferior to active biofeedback training. Langensbeck Arch Chir Suppl Kongrssbd 115:976–978
25. Hosker G, Norton C, Brazzelli M (2000) Electrical stimulation for faecal incontinence in adults. Cochrane Database Syst Rev (2):CD0001310
26. Norton C, Gibbs A, Kamm MA (2006) Randomized, controlled trial of anal electrical stimulation for fecal incontinence. Dis Colon Rectum 49:190–196
27. Jost WF (1998) Electrostimulation in fecal incontinence. Relevance of the sphincteric compound muscle action potential. Dis Colon Rectum 41:590–592
28. Österberg A, Graf W, Eeg-Olofsson K et al (1999) Is electrostimulation of the pelvic floor an effective treatment for neurogenic faecal incontinence? Scand J Gastroenterol 34:319–324

Sphincteroplasty

16

James W. Ogilvie Jr., Robert D. Madoff

History

Fecal incontinence, as a result of trauma to the muscular sphincter complex, has long been surgically treated by approximation of healthy muscular edges on either side of the defect. In his 1923 textbook, Lockhart-Mummery described the operative procedure of mobilizing muscle lateral to the defect and sewing the "ends firmly in contact" [1]. Operative success was "usually most satisfactory," yet contingent on "proper antiseptic precautions" and "carefully performed" technique. In 1940, however, Blaisdell reported general dissatisfaction among American proctologists with this classic "plastic repair" due to infectious complications, technical challenges, and poor outcomes [2]. Blaisdell went on to describe two techniques that involved overlapping muscle edges while leaving the scarred portion of the sphincter intact. The "reefing operation" brought together muscle opposite the site of damage to narrow the circumference of the anal outlet and thus avoid manipulation of the damaged portion of the sphincter [2]. The "inversion operation" also reefed sphincter muscle together, but in this instance, damaged scar tissue was inverted into the anal canal, and healthy muscle on each side of the sphincter defect was approximated [3].

In 1971, Parks and McPartlin at St. Mark's Hospital in London published the first report of sphincteroplasty as it is known today, with deliberate overlapping of muscle edges to recreate a functional sphincter. All patients underwent complete scar excision followed by mobilization of the flanking, undamaged muscle. The freed ends of the sphincter were then secured onto each other with chromic and wire sutures. Eighteen of 20 patients experienced "excellent results," which the authors contribute to the use of preoperative diverting colostomy [4]. Popularization of this technique among American surgeons increased after Slade, Goldberg, et al. published their experience in 1977 with 37 patients over a 23-year period [5]. Of the 30 patients available for follow-up 16 had excellent results, 13 had good results, and one had fair results based on patient-reported control of solid feces, liquid feces, and flatus.

Indications

Obstetrical trauma is the most common cause of sphincter disruption. Third- and fourth-degree obstetrical tears occur in the anterior midline, and repair should be performed immediately after delivery either by simple approximation of muscle edges or via an overlapping technique [6]. If proper expertise is not available at the time of delivery, sphincter repair may be delayed for up to 24 h without significant consequences. Traditionally, most repairs are managed in the delivery suite unless there is severe contamination and/or significant tissue loss. However, given the poor results after repair of third- or fourth-degree injuries–almost 50% of women report some degree of incontinence [7]–some centers have advocated optimizing repair in the operating room with improved lighting, exposure, anesthesia, and assistance [8]. Most postpartum sphincter repairs will prove satisfactory and not require any further intervention. A small percentage of women will develop debilitating fecal incontinence and require further evaluation and treatment. Surgical repair of injuries that fail to heal, heal poorly, or are not repaired immediately should be delayed for 3–6 months after delivery until perineal inflammation and edema have completely subsided.

Complications arising from other anorectal procedures, including fistulotomy, sphincterotomy, hemorrhoidectomy, or localized external trauma, may also result in sphincter damage amenable to treatment by sphincteroplasty.

Preoperative Evaluation

In order to select patients suitable for sphincteroplasty, an appropriate preoperative evaluation is required. Clinical history should begin with documentation of the nature and duration of the incontinence, as well as its impact on the patient's daily activities. A thorough surgical, medical, and obstetrical history should be elicited in conjunction with a review of systems focused on illnesses that may contribute to urgency or increased number of bowel movements. Inflammatory bowel disease, rectal neoplasms, prolapse, dietary changes, or other causes of chronic diarrhea may all contribute to some degree of incontinence. Patients with active diarrhea or colitis should optimally be medically managed before considering any operative approaches.

Visual inspection of the perianal region will often reveal seepage and skin breakdown. The presence of scar tissue from previous sphincter repairs or trauma should also be documented. Deformity or absence of the anterior perineal body is a common finding in severe obstetrical trauma and may require perineal reconstruction in addition to sphincteroplasty. Digital rectal exam will often demonstrate laxity in the sphincter at the injury site.

Anorectal physiology tests are indicated in the majority of patients undergoing operative treatment for incontinence. Endoanal ultrasound is a highly accurate tool for defining location and extent of anatomical sphincter defects. Some centers have found alternative means, such as magnetic resonance imaging (MRI), to be useful in evaluating the entire pelvic floor. Anal manometry provides preoperative assessment of both internal and external sphincters by way of measuring resting pressure, voluntary squeeze pressure, and rectal sensation. Patients should also undergo flexible sigmoidoscopy to exclude any neoplastic or inflammatory condition. Pudendal nerve terminal motor latency (PNTML) may be performed to evaluate for pudendal neuropathy in some patients after complicated vaginal deliveries. Some [9–12] but not all [13–15] studies suggest that patients with prolonged PNTML may experience suboptimal outcomes after sphincteroplasty. For patients with incontinence of uncertain etiologies, electromyelogram (EMG), dynamic MRI, or defecography may prove useful but are not routinely required.

Operation

Although initial reports suggested that the success of sphincteroplasty was contingent on a prior colostomy, multiple series have shown equivalent results of efficacy and safety without fecal diversion [5, 16]. In the setting of multiple failed previous repairs, however, diverting ostomy may still be valuable. There are no trials that specifically define the benefit of bowel preparation and perioperative antibiotics. It is nevertheless generally accepted that patients should undergo full mechanical bowel preparation as well as perioperative broad-spectrum parenteral antibiotics.

Once in the operating room, either general or regional anesthesia may be employed. A urinary catheter is placed. We prefer to place patients in the prone jack-knife position, although others favor the lithotomy position. Prone exposure is facilitated with a large, padded roll under the pelvis and with the buttocks taped apart. After standard skin preparation, a local anesthetic is injected to provide a regional nerve block and assist with hemostasis. Our preference is 0.25% bupivacaine with epinephrine. Anterior sphincter defects are best approached with an elliptical incision around the anterior portion of the anus over the perineal body. We prefer to use a needle-tip electrocautery for dissection and a circular, self-retaining retractor for exposure. For non-obstetric-related sphincter defects, the initial incision is made directly over the defect, with enough length to facilitate exposure of healthy muscle.

The operation begins by raising an endoanal flap in the submucosal plane. Next, the posterior vaginal wall is freed from the sphincter complex anteriorly. Dissection should continue cephalad in the rectovaginal septum until the fibers of the puborectalis muscle are identified running toward the pubis. Dissection is then focused on mobilizing healthy sphincter muscle lateral to the defect. Beginning away from the scar, working laterally to medially is the easiest method to identify and mobilize the sphincter complex. Lateral dissection should continue until enough muscle is mobilized to perform the sphincteroplasty without tension. Extensive lateral dissection beyond the midcoronal line should be avoided to circumvent any damage to the inferior rectal nerves that innervate the sphincter and enter from the pudendal canal, traveling posterolaterally across the ischiorectal fossa.

Once the sphincter complex is freed from its surrounding structures, the scar is sharply divided. We adhere to the conventional wisdom that scar tissue should not be excised in order to prevent suture pull through, although no evidence exists to support or refute this practice. The taped buttocks are then released to ease tension on the subsequent repair. To recreate the muscular canal, healthy edges of muscle are wrapped onto each other and secured together with mattress sutures (Fig. 1). Our preference is to use a long-lasting, absorbable, monofilament suture, such as polydioxanone (PDS). The amount of muscle that should be overlapped has not been standardized, but the general rule is that there should be a snug sphincter mechanism without undue tension on the

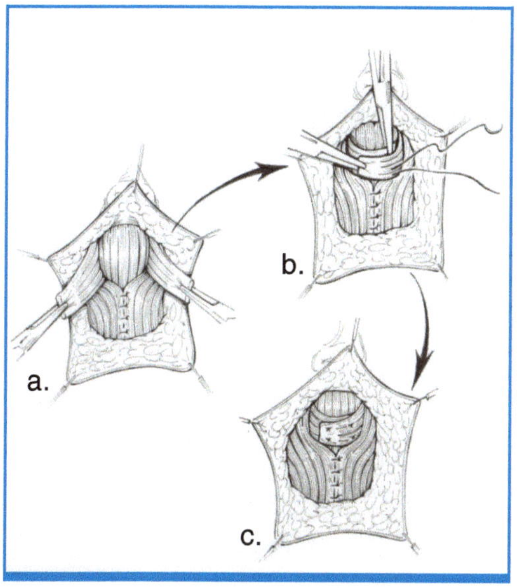

Fig. 1a–c. Sphincteroplasty. **a** Dissection begins with lateral mobilization of muscle edges, which are then **b** secured with mattress sutures through the existing scar and healthy muscle in order to **c** recreate the sphincter complex. Reprinted with permission from [17]

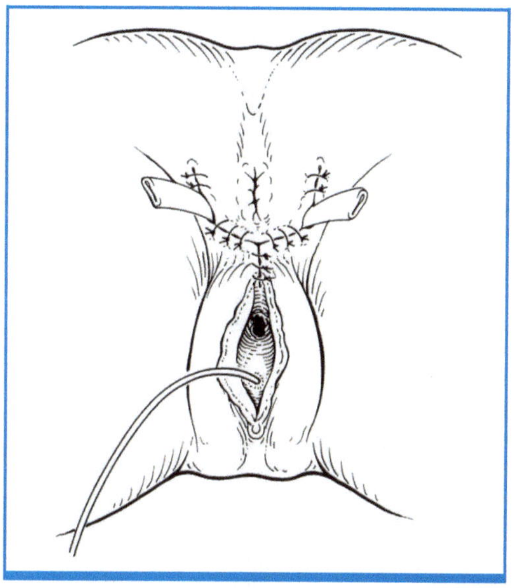

Fig. 2. Wound closure. A V-Y advancement over a Penrose drain results in a T-shaped incision and serves to lengthen the perineal body. Reprinted with permission from [18]

repair or compromise of the anal canal. Most surgeons prefer a bulk repair of both the internal and external anal sphincters, whereas others advocate separate repair of each of these muscles. There is little evidence, however, that this is beneficial.

There is disagreement on whether or not to perform an associated levatorplasty by tightening the two limbs of the puborectalis muscle cephalad to the sphincter mechanism. Advocates stress its ability to lengthen the anal canal, whereas opponents suggest it is a potential cause of dyspareunia.

In uncomplicated cases, the wound may be closed primarily with interrupted sutures in a T-shaped fashion, reapproximating the midanterior skin edges in the sagittal plane to lengthen the perineal body. Occasionally, skin flaps are raised to primarily close the wound without additional tension. Rarely, in complex cases with extensive damage to the perineal body, some form of advancement flap may be used for reconstruction and skin closure. Rotational flaps, Z-plasty closures, or V-Y advancements can all be used to close the perianal wound. Because of the large dead space that is typically present, we prefer to close the wound loosely over a Penrose drain (Fig. 2). Others prefer complete primary closure with or without suction drainage.

Postoperative Care

To ensure adequate healing and patient comfort, postoperative care should focus on pain management and avoidance of constipation. Opioid analgesics in the early postoperative period are usually required and are typically administered via epidural catheter or patient-controlled analgesia (PCA). When the patient begins oral analgesics, we routinely supplement with acetaminophen and nonsteroidal anti-inflammatory drugs to minimize opioid requirements. High-fiber diets, supplement bulking agents, and large quantities of liquids should be standard for all patients. In addition, daily use of a mild laxative or tap water enema serves to counteract the constipating effects of narcotic use and alleviate pain with defecation. In an era where diverting ostomies are not routinely performed in conjunction with sphincteroplasty, it is crucial that patients are instructed on how to take the appropriate measures to avoid damage to the sphincter repair that may result from excessive straining and passing hardened stools. Some authors have advocated the contrary, that a clear liquid diet and a bowel confinement regimen be employed postoperatively, but there been little evidence to suggest any benefits [19].

Table 1. Results after sphincteroplasty. Studies were excluded if follow-up was not designated or less than 12 months, or a more recent publication reported on the same cohort of patients

Group	Year	Number of patients	Mean age or range	Median follow-up (months)	Percent good, excellent results	Percent obstetric related
Browning [23]	1983	83	38	39	78	16
Fang [24]	1984	76	17-68	35	89	54
Christiansen [25]	1987	12	34	26	75	17
Pezim [26]	1987	40	40	67	62	58
Stern [27]	1987	11	47	7–40	73	55
Ctercteko [28]	1988	44	36	50	54	41
Abcarian [29]	1989	53	32	42	100	88
Yoshioka [30]	1989	27	34	48	26	33
Fleshman [31]	1991	55	34	12	72	87
Gibbs [32]	1993	33	47	43	73	58
Engel [33]	1994	55	42	15	76	100
Londono-Schimmer [34]	1994	94	43	59	50	64
Richard[a] [16]	1994	45/37	–	42/23	82/87	60/62
Sangalli [35]	1994	36	37	34	78	100
Simmang [11]	1994	14	66	12	71	79
Felt-Bersma [36]	1996	18	47	14	72	55
Nikiteas [14]	1996	42	–	38	67	76
Sitzler [37]	1996	31	42	12–36	74	71
Gilliland [9]	1998	77	47	24	55	69
Young [15]	1998	54	42	18	86	88
Karoui [38]	2000	74	56	40	51	83
Malouf [20]	2000	46	43	77	59	100
Osterberg [39]	2000	20	47	12	50	100
Morren[b] [40]	2001	55	39	40	56	84
Halverson [19]	2002	49	39	63	49	63
Pinta [41]	2003	39	53	22	59	100
Bravo Gutierrez [22]	2004	130	37	124	23	91
Barisic [42]	2006	65	36	80	48	72

[a]The study was divided into two groups: with and without diverting colostomy
[b]Thirteen percent were done via an end-to-end repair

Results

Successful outcomes after sphincteroplasty range between 23% and 100% (Table 1). Unfortunately, the heterogeneity of patients in individual studies has resulted in disagreement about which patient variables predict a successful outcome. Most authors would agree that patients who have severe preoperative incontinence, failed previous repairs, or who demonstrate a persistent defect on follow-up endoanal ultrasound are the least likely to have a successful outcome following sphincteroplasty. There is disagreement on other factors, such as age at time of repair or parameters of anal physiologic testing. Some authors have demonstrated correlation between successful sphincteroplasty and certain manometric parameters, such as squeeze pressure, resting pressure, and anal canal length, but data are conflicting, and many patients present clinically without a measurable defect in sphincter pressure.

Regrettably, more recent data reveal the long-term durability of overlapping sphincteroplasty to be disappointing. Initial series reported successful outcomes in between 70% and 80% of patients; however, as groups followed their patients for more than 5 years, success rates decreased to 50–60% [20, 21]. The study with the longest follow-up to date demonstrated that although 36% of their cohort was incontinent to solid stools 3 years after sphincteroplasty, 58% had become incontinent after 10 years [22]. It is unclear why such a dramatic deterioration in function occurs over time. Aging, scarring, and worsening pudendal nerve function have all been postulated as a potential mechanism.

References

1. Lockhart-Mummery JP (1923) Diseases of the rectum & colon and their surgical treatment. Macmillan, Toronto
2. Blaisdell PC (1942) Repair of the incontinent sphincter ani. Surg Gynec Obst 70:692–697

3. Blaisdell PC (1950) Plastic repair of the incontinent sphincter ani. Am J Surg 79:174–183
4. Parks AG,McPartlin JF (1971) Late repair of injuries of the anal sphincter. Proc R Soc Med 64:1187–1189
5. Slade MS, Goldberg SM, Schottler JL et al (1977) Sphincteroplasty for acquired anal incontinence. Dis Colon Rectum 20:33–35
6. Fernando R, Sultan AH, Kettle C et al (2006) Methods of repair for obstetric anal sphincter injury. Cochrane Database Syst Rev 3:CD002866
7. Sultan AH, Kamm MA, Hudson CN et al (1994) Third degree obstetric anal sphincter tears: risk factors and outcome of primary repair. BMJ 308:887–891
8. Cook TA,Mortensen NJ (1998) Management of faecal incontinence following obstetric injury. Br J Surg 85:293–299
9. Gilliland R, Altomare DF, Moreira H Jr et al (1998) Pudendal neuropathy is predictive of failure following anterior overlapping sphincteroplasty. Dis Colon Rectum 41:1516–1522
10. Oliveira L, Pfeifer J, Wexner SD (1996) Physiological and clinical outcome of anterior sphincteroplasty. Br J Surg 83:502–505
11. Simmang C, Birnbaum EH, Kodner IJ et al (1994) Anal sphincter reconstruction in the elderly: does advancing age affect outcome? Dis Colon Rectum 37:1065–1069
12. Sangwan YP, Coller JA, Barrett RC et al (1996) Unilateral pudendal neuropathy. Impact on outcome of anal sphincter repair. Dis Colon Rectum 39:686–689
13. Chen AS, Luchtefeld MA, Senagore AJ et al (1998) Pudendal nerve latency. Does it predict outcome of anal sphincter repair? Dis Colon Rectum 41:1005–1009
14. Nikiteas N, Korsgen S, Kumar D et al (1996) Audit of sphincter repair. Factors associated with poor outcome. Dis Colon Rectum 39:1164–1170
15. Young CJ, Mathur MN, Eyers AA et al (1998) Successful overlapping anal sphincter repair: relationship to patient age, neuropathy, and colostomy formation. Dis Colon Rectum 41:344–349
16. Richard C, Bernard D, Morgan S et al (1994) [Results of anal sphincteroplasty for post-traumatic incontinence: with or without colostomy]. Ann Chir 48:703–707
17. Fazio VW, Church JM, Delaney CP (eds) (2005) Current therapy in colon and rectal surgery, 2nd edn. Elsevier Mosby, Philadelphia, pp 108–109
18. Nicholls RJ, Dozois RR (eds) (1997) Surgery of the colon & rectum. Churchill Livingstone, New York, p 75
19. Nessim A, Wexner SD, Agachan F et al (1999) Is bowel confinement necessary after anorectal reconstructive surgery? A prospective, randomized, surgeon-blinded trial. Dis Colon Rectum 42:16–23
20. Malouf AJ, Norton CS, Engel AF et al (2000) Long-term results of overlapping anterior anal-sphincter repair for obstetric trauma. Lancet 355:260–265
21. Halverson AL, Hull TL (2002) Long-term outcome of overlapping anal sphincter repair. Dis Colon Rectum 45:345–348
22. Bravo Gutierrez A, Madoff RD, Lowry AC et al (2004) Long-term results of anterior sphincteroplasty. Dis Colon Rectum 47:727–31; discussion 731–732
23. Browning GG, Motson RW (1983) Results of Parks operation for faecal incontinence after anal sphincter injury. Br Med J (Clin Res Ed) 286:1873–1875
24. Fang DT, Nivatvongs S, Vermeulen FD et al (1984) Overlapping sphincteroplasty for acquired anal incontinence. Dis Colon Rectum 27:720–722
25. Christiansen J,Pedersen IK (1987) Traumatic anal incontinence. Results of surgical repair. Dis Colon Rectum 30:189–191
26. Pezim ME, Spencer RJ, Stanhope CR et al (1987) Sphincter repair for fecal incontinence after obstetrical or iatrogenic injury. Dis Colon Rectum 30:521–525
27. Stern H, Gallinger S, Rabau M et al (1987) Surgical treatment of anal incontinence. Can J Surg 30:348–350
28. Ctercteko GC, Fazio VW, Jagelman DG et al (1988) Anal sphincter repair: a report of 60 cases and review of the literature. Aust N Z J Surg 58:703–710
29. Abcarian H, Orsay CP, Pearl RK et al (1989) Traumatic cloaca. Dis Colon Rectum 32:783–787
30. Yoshioka K,Keighley MR (1989) Sphincter repair for fecal incontinence. Dis Colon Rectum 32:39–42
31. Fleshman JW, Peters WR, Shemesh EI et al (1991) Anal sphincter reconstruction: anterior overlapping muscle repair. Dis Colon Rectum 34:739–743
32. Gibbs DH,Hooks VH, 3rd (1993) Overlapping sphincteroplasty for acquired anal incontinence. South Med J 86:1376–1380
33. Engel AF, Kamm MA, Sultan AH et al (1994) Anterior anal sphincter repair in patients with obstetric trauma. Br J Surg 81:1231–1234
34. Londono-Schimmer EE, Garcia-Duperly R, Nicholls RJ et al (1994) Overlapping anal sphincter repair for faecal incontinence due to sphincter trauma: five year follow-up functional results. Int J Colorectal Dis 9:110–113
35. Sangalli MR,Marti MC (1994) Results of sphincter repair in postobstetric fecal incontinence. J Am Coll Surg 179:583–586
36. Felt-Bersma RJ, Cuesta MA,Koorevaar M (1996) Anal sphincter repair improves anorectal function and endosonographic image. A prospective clinical study. Dis Colon Rectum 39:878–885
37. Sitzler PJ,Thomson JP (1996) Overlap repair of damaged anal sphincter. A single surgeon's series. Dis Colon Rectum 39:1356–1360
38. Karoui S, Leroi AM, Koning E et al (2000) Results of sphincteroplasty in 86 patients with anal incontinence. Dis Colon Rectum 43:813–820
39. Osterberg A, Edebol Eeg-Olofsson K,Graf W (2000) Results of surgical treatment for faecal incontinence. Br J Surg 87:1546–1552
40. Morren GL, Hallbook O, Nystrom PO et al (2001) Audit of anal-sphincter repair. Colorectal Dis 3:17–22
41. Pinta T, Kylanpaa-Back ML, Salmi T et al (2003) Delayed sphincter repair for obstetric ruptures: analysis of failure. Colorectal Dis 5:73–78
42. Barisic GI, Krivokapic ZV, Markovic VA et al (2006) Outcome of overlapping anal sphincter repair after 3 months and after a mean of 80 months. Int J Colorectal Dis 21:52–56

Invited Commentary

Donato F. Altomare

Sphincteroplasty is the most immediate and intuitive approach to treating fecal incontinence following obstetric, iatrogenic, or accidental trauma to the anal sphincters and should still be considered the first step in an ideal algorithm to treat these patients. James Ogilvie and Robert Madoff must be commended for the excellent and comprehensive chapter on sphincteroplasty presented in this book, which is the result of his broad experience in the field and his natural ability to describe complex things in a simple and direct way.

I would like to briefly comment on some of the controversial points discussed by Ogilvie and Madoff. First is the variability of the success rate and its natural decline over time. We know that continence is not only the result of a well-functioning anal sphincter but is a very complex combination of a normal autonomic and somatic innervation of the anorectal region (normal sensation, compliance, and rectal motility), normal anorectum, solid luminal content, and, of course, normally functioning anal sphincters. Therefore, the reason for unreliable results after sphincteroplasty is the possible coexistence of other undetected functional anorectal abnormalities. But what worries the surgeon about the future of these patients is the common feeling that the success rate is destined to decline with time [1, 2]. Why this happens is still uncertain. Deterioration of muscle innervation and natural ageing of the tissues are the factors most commonly blamed, but the real cause is still unknown.

One of the few tests available for evaluating neural integrity of that anatomical region is pudendal nerve terminal motor latency (PNTML) developed at St. Mark's Hospital in the UK. However, the reliability of this test has recently been questioned and, despite a huge number of studies utilizing PNTML for assessing patients with fecal incontinence, there is a tendency to consider the test obsolete. Although impaired pudendal nerve function is commonly believed to be a negative prognostic factor for sphincteroplasty [3, 4], several other experiences have reported good outcomes independently of it [5, 6]. As a consequence, a reliable neurological test for evaluating innervation for the anal sphincters is not available, and a sphincteroplasty is usually carried out even in the presence of prolonged PNTML. On the other hand, a sphincter electromyography (EMG) could provide useful information, but there are no studies clearly assessing the predictive value of sphincter EMG or documenting any progressive muscle deterioration over time after sphincteroplasty.

Another controversial point is what to do after early or late failure of sphincteroplasty. This question is still really open, particularly since the introduction of the sacral nerve modulation technique, which for the first time enables the surgeon to address not only the sphincter muscles but also the other components of the physiology of continence, such as rectal sensitivity and motility. A recent paper [7] described a successful outcome of sacral nerve modulation (SNM) in patients with fecal incontinence after sphincter lesions, and a randomized controlled trial on this topic is running among centers of the Italian Group for Sacral Nerve Modulation (GINS). These data indicate that in selected cases of patients with sphincter lesions, continence can be improved by correcting the pelvic nerve function only. Furthermore, another study documented that a failed sphincteroplasty can be redone with a reasonable probability of success [8, 9].

Only in cases of resphincteroplasty or SNM failure should major surgery such as dynamic graciloplasty or artificial bowel sphincters be considered, but such procedures should be confined to severe end-stage fecal incontinence and be carried out by well-trained colorectal surgical teams in order to minimize the failure rate.

References

1. Londono-Schimmer EE, Garcia-Duperly R, Nicholls RJ et al (1994) Overlapping anal sphincter repair for faecal incontinence due to sphincter trauma: five year follow-up functional results. Int J Colorectal Dis 9:110–113

2. Barisic GI, Krivokapic ZV, Markovic VA, Popovic MA (2006) Outcome of overlapping anal sphincter repair after 3 months and after a mean of 80 months. Int J Colorectal Dis 21:52–56
3. Gilliland R, Altomare DF, Moreira H Jr et al (1998) Pudendal neuropathy is predictive of failure following anterior overlapping sphincteroplasty. Dis Colon Rectum 41:1516–1522
4. Sangwan YP, CollerJA, Barrett RC et al (1996) Unilateral pudendal neuropathy. Impact on outcome of anal sphincter repair. Dis Colon Rectum 39:686–689
5. Chen AS, Luchtefeld MA, Senagore AJ et al (1998) Pudendal nerve latency. Does it predict outcome of anal sphincter repair? Dis Colon Rectum 41:1005–1009
6. Buie WD, Lowry AC, Rothenberger DA, Madoff RD (2001) Clinical rather than laboratory assessment predicts continence after anterior sphincteroplasty. Dis Colon Rectum 44:1255–1260
7. Conaghan P, Farouk R (2005) Sacral nerve stimulation can be successful in patients with ultrasound evidence of external anal sphincter disruption. Dis Colon Rectum 48:1610–1614
8. Giordano P, Renzi A, Efron J et al (2002) Previous sphincter repair does not affect the outcome of repeat repair. Dis Colon Rectum 45:635–640
9. Vaizey CJ, Norton C, Thornton MJ et al (2004) Long-term results of repeat anterior anal sphincter repair. Dis Colon Rectum 47:858–863

Postanal Pelvic Floor Repair

17

Saleh M. Abbas, Ian P. Bissett

Historical Background

Postanal repair was developed by Sir Allan Parks in the 1970s [1] and popularised in the early 1980s for patients with neuromyopathic faecal incontinence. The original objective of this operation was to restore the anorectal angle, which was thought to be an important factor in continence. In 1975, Parks suggested the flap-valve theory that stressed the importance of the acute anorectal angle. According to this theory, a rise in intra-abdominal pressure caused the upper end of the anal canal to be occluded by anterior rectal mucosa, preventing rectal contents from entering the anal canal. Neuromyopathic faecal incontinence was associated with perineal descent and an obtuse anorectal angle, which rendered the flap-valve-like mechanism ineffective. Further investigations, however, failed to show changes of the anorectal angle, and currently, it is thought that an improvement of muscular contractility is responsible for any improvement in continence [2].

Postanal repair involves coaptation of the levator ani, puborectalis and external anal sphincter posterior to the anal canal and the anorectal junction by approximating these muscles with nonabsorbable sutures. The anatomical result of this procedure is lengthening of the anal canal and possible reduction of the anorectal angle.

Anatomic Consideration

The anal canal is 3–5 cm long, passing from the distal rectum to the anal verge. The puborectalis muscle passes posterior to the anorectal junction, forming a sling that draws the anorectal junction forwards (Fig. 1). The length of the anal canal and the sling action of the puborectalis are thought to be important parts of the continence mechanism. Patients with neuromyopathic incontinence have a shorter anal canal and a straightening of the anorectal angle. The anorectal angle is the angle between the longitudinal axis of the rectum and the anal canal. It can be assessed either by defecating proctography or magnetic resonance imaging (MRI). Normal values range from 90° to 110° at rest, increasing to about 135° during defecation. In patients with idiopathic incontinence, the angle at rest is straightened to greater than 110°.

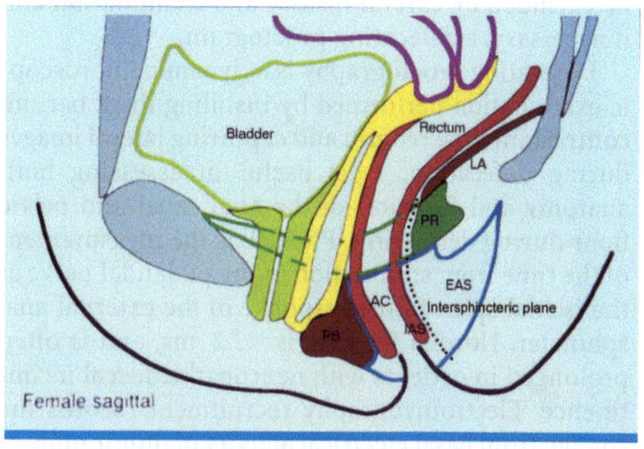

Fig. 1. Sagittal view of the pelvis on magnetic resonance imaging (MRI). Note the *dotted line* indicating the intersphincteric plane dissected in postanal repair. *AC* anal canal, *LA* levator ani, *EAS* external anal sphincter, *PR* puborectalis, *IAS* internal anal sphincter, *PB* pubic bone. (Picture by Professor Stuart Heap, University of Auckland, Department of Anatomy and Radiology)

Indications

Postanal repair is currently performed on patients with idiopathic faecal incontinence with no evidence of sphincter defect on endoanal ultrasound. It should only be offered when conservative treatment with dietary manipulation, drug therapy and physiotherapy has been implemented without success. The patients expected to benefit most from postanal repair are women with a history of multiple vaginal deliveries [2–4].

Preoperative Assessment

Operative intervention is undertaken in patients in whom appropriate assessment has been performed. This includes a careful history, clinical examination, endoanal ultrasound and anal manometry. Further tests that may be useful are a defecating proctogram, pudendal nerve terminal motor latency (PNTML) and needle electromyelogram (EMG). If these investigations identify a defect in the external sphincter, then the patient should undergo a sphincter repair rather than a postanal repair. Rectal prolapse should be excluded by careful history and examination and if necessary, a defecating proctogram.

Defecating proctography is a dynamic fluoroscopic examination performed by instilling thick barium contrast into the rectum and capturing lateral images during defecation. It is useful in assessing both anatomy and function of the anal canal and pelvic floor during defecation. PNTML is the measurement of the time from stimulation of the pudendal nerve at the ischial spine to the response of the external anal sphincter. Normal PNTML is <2.2 ms, and is often prolonged in patients with neuropathic faecal incontinence. Electromyography recruitment records the change from basal electrical activity of motor units of the external anal sphincter and levator muscles during muscle activity. This may a useful adjunct in the investigation of neuropathic incontinence.

Operative Technique

The patient is admitted on the day of surgery and prior to the operation is given an enema to empty the rectum. With induction of the anaesthetic, prophylactic antibiotics are given in the form of 1 g Cefoxitin and 500 mg metronidazole intravenously. The patient is placed in a prone jack-knife position, with the buttocks spread apart using adhesive tape. A curvilinear incision is made 6 cm posterior to the anus (Fig. 2), and dissection is directed to the intersphincteric plane, which is relatively bloodless. Fibres of the external sphincter are red in colour and contract with diathermy stimulation, while those of the internal sphincter are white and do not contract to diathermy current. Dissection is then deepened in the intersphincteric plane to the upper part of the external sphincter and puborectalis muscle, finally exposing the levator ani fascia and the mesorectal fat. This dissection is extended anteriorly to include half of the circumference of the anal canal. A deep 90° angled retractor is used to push the rectum anteriorly in order to see the highest and the most lateral part of levator ani (Fig. 3).

The levator ani is then approximated using 2/0 nonabsorbable sutures (Prolene or Ethibond). Using a small curved needle to include a large bundle of muscle fibres, three sutures are inserted at this uppermost level. The sutures are then tied loosely to

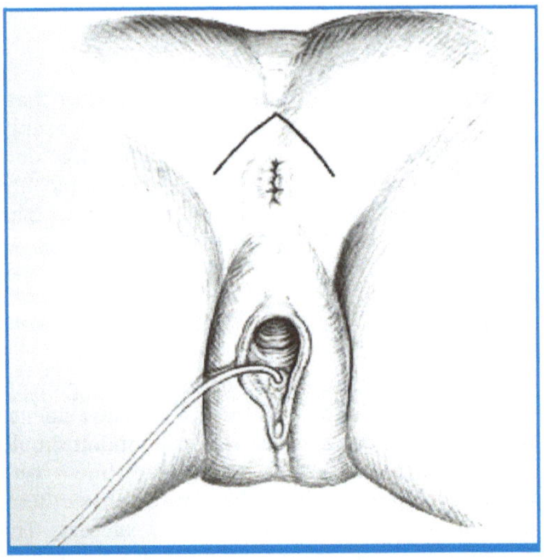

Fig. 2. Incision is curvilinear posterior to the anal canal. Reprinted with permission from Elsevier [5]

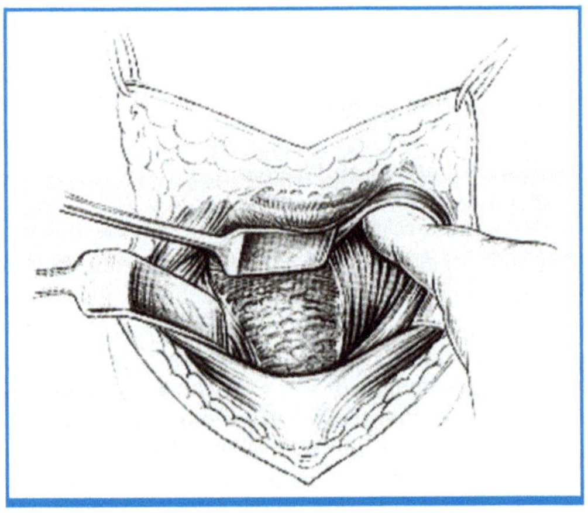

Fig. 3. Dissection in the intersphincteric plane to reveal puborectalis and levator ani. Reprinted with permission from Elsevier [5]

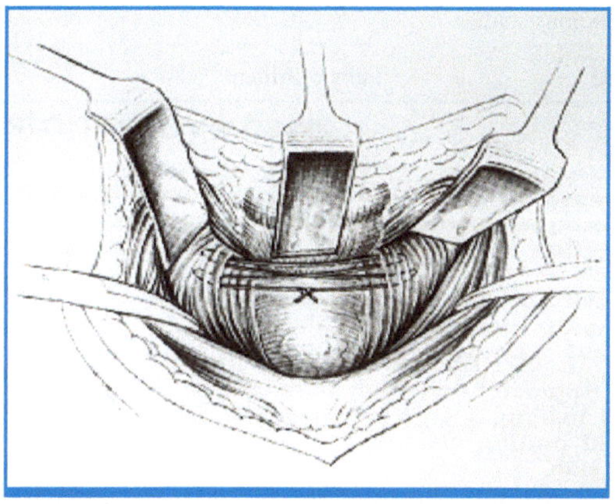

Fig. 4. Sutures in the upper levator ani are loosely tied to create a lattice behind the rectum. Reprinted with permission from Elsevier [5]

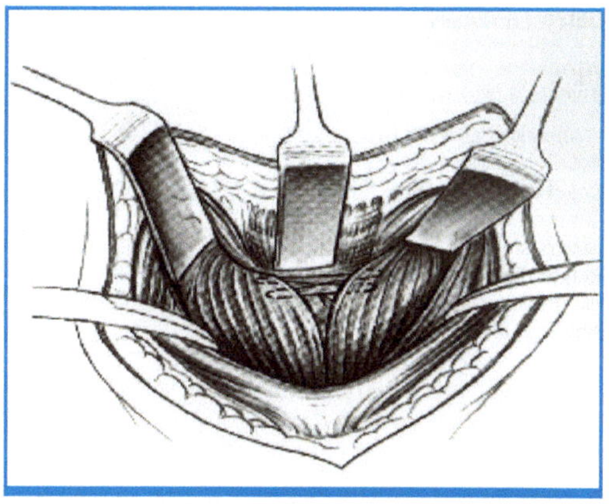

Fig. 5. Approximation of pubococcygeus by nonabsorbable sutures. Reprinted with permission from Elsevier [5]

create a lattice across the pelvis (Fig. 4). The pubococcygeus muscle is approached next and additional 2/0 nonabsorbable sutures are placed in a similar fashion by approximation of the lower fibres (Fig. 5). Sutures in the puborectalis are the most important in the repair, as this muscle is the strongest of the pelvic floor. The sutures are placed as anteriorly as possible, lifting the anorectal junction forwards. The sutures are then tied loosely approximating the two

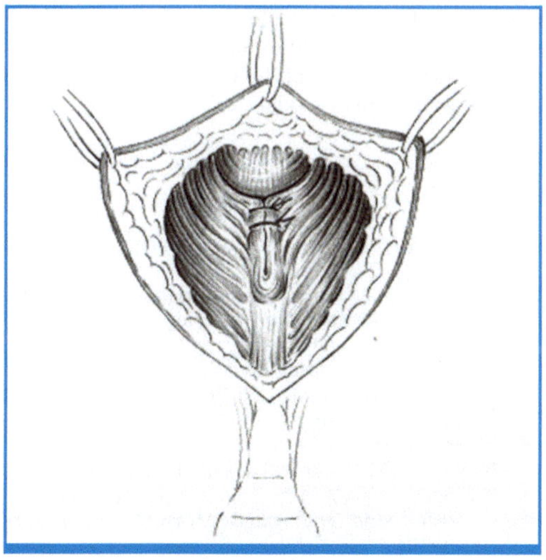

Fig. 6. Approximation of external sphincter and puborectalis. Reprinted with permission from Elsevier [5]

arms of the puborectalis. Usually, three sutures are utilised to approximate the muscles of the external sphincter. The approximation should not be tight (Fig. 6). The skin is then closed using absorbable sutures.

Postoperative Care

A urinary catheter is generally used to avoid retention and removed the following morning. Pain relief is given according to the patient's needs. Bowel softeners are used in the immediate postoperative period to avoid faecal impaction and achieve semiliquid stools; patients are instructed to avoid straining, as this may disrupt the repair. The patient is usually discharged home 24–48 h after the operation and remains on laxatives for several weeks. Long-term use of laxatives may be required.

Discussion

Parks first described postanal repair in 1975 [1], and reported very good continence results in 80% of patients. The procedure is usually performed on patients with neuropathic faecal incontinence who have an intact anal sphincter with poor sphincter contractility. Typically, the patients are older women with multiple vaginal deliveries and a weak pelvic floor.

Since its description by Parks, postanal repair has been applied in various parts of the world and re-

Table 1. Long-term results of continence for postanal repair in various studies

Study	Improvement (%)	Fully continent (%)
Womack et al. 1988 [6]	88	38
Yoshioka et al. 1989 [7]	81	34
Engel et al. 1994 [8]	50	21
Jameson et al. 1994 [9]	53	28
Athanasiadis et al. 1995 [2]	52	6
Reiger et al. 1997 [10]	58	31
Matsuoka et al. 2000 [11]	35	Not reported
Abbas et al. 2005 [12]	68	8.5

ported to accomplish modest success [9, 11]. Studies have shown improvement of 35 and 88% in faecal incontinence following postanal repair [2, 6–12] (Table 1), with only small numbers of patients achieving full continence. Factors that have been suggested to affect the outcome of postanal repair include preoperative physiological parameters such as resting anal tone, maximum squeeze pressure, PNTML, concentric needle electromyography, undetected external sphincter defects and pelvic floor descent and anorectal angle, as seen preoperatively on defecating proctography. None of these factors, however, has predicted long-term outcome, with the possible exception of maximal squeeze pressure before surgery [9–11, 13–15]. The exact mechanism of the effect of postanal repair is not fully understood, although changes in the length of the anal canal, rectal angle, change in resting anal pressure, maximum squeeze pressure and pelvic floor descent or anorectal angle following postanal repair have been proposed as possible mechanisms. These have not been proved on long-term follow-up to correlate with the outcome [2]. A randomised controlled trial by Deen et al. [14] in women with neuropathic faecal incontinence compared total pelvic floor repair with anterior levatorplasty and sphincter plication alone and postanal repair alone. Review at 6 and 24 months indicated that results were significantly better for total pelvic floor repair than either of the other procedures.

The majority of patients with faecal incontinence are found to have weak but intact external anal sphincters. This is attributed to a variety of reasons, such as diabetes and pudendal neuropathy [16]. Risk factors for idiopathic incontinence are female gender, advancing age, ill health and physical disability [17]. A recent systematic review showed a prevalence of faecal incontinence between 11% and 15% [17–19], but the proportion of those who have neuropathic incontinence is not known. A number of other treatment options are available for this type of faecal incontinence. These include conservative measures aimed at achieving symptomatic control (such as dietary manipulation, pharmacotherapy including constipating agents, and phosphate enemas) and pelvic floor retraining, also called biofeedback [20]. Newer modalities, such as sacral nerve neuromodulation, have shown promise.

Conclusion

The patients most likely to benefit from postanal repair are women with a history of multiple vaginal deliveries and a weak but intact external anal sphincter on endoanal ultrasound. Although the initial results of this procedure were promising, more recent results have been variable. The current place of postanal repair in the management of faecal incontinence patients is unclear, as there are few data comparing it with other available procedures. It is of benefit to patients with mild to moderate idiopathic faecal incontinence and can be offered in conjunction with other treatment modalities.

References

1. Parks AG (1975) Anorectal incontinence. P Roy Soc Med 68:681–690
2. Athanasiadis S, Sanchez M, Kuprian A (1995) Long-term follow-up of Parks posterior repair. An electromyographic, manometric and radiologic study of 31 patients. Langenbeck Arch Chir 380:22–30
3. Vaizey CJ, Kamm MA, Nicholls RJ (1998) Recent advances in the surgical treatment of faecal incontinence. Br J Surg 85:596–603
4. Browning GG, Parks AG (1983) Postanal repair for neuropathic faecal incontinence: correlation of clinical result and anal canal pressures. Br J Surg 70:101–104
5. Fielding LP, Goldberg SM (1993) Rob & Smith's operative surgery. Surgery of the colon, rectum and anus, 5th edn. Butterworth-Heinemann, London

6. Womack NR, Morrison JF, Williams NS (1988) Prospective study of the effects of postanal repair in neurogenic faecal incontinence. Br J Surg 75(1):48-52
7. Yoshioka K, Keighley MR (1989) Critical assessment of the quality of continence after postanal repair for faecal incontinence. Br J Surg 76:1054–1057
8. Engel AF, van Baal SJ, Brummelkamp WH (1994) Late results of postanal repair for idiopathic faecal incontinence. Eur J Surg 160:637–640
9. Jameson JS, Speakman CT, Darzi A et al (1994) Audit of postanal repair in the treatment of fecal incontinence. Dis Colon Rectum 37:369–372
10. Rieger NA, Sarre RG, Saccone GT et al (1997) Postanal repair for faecal incontinence: long-term follow-up. Aust NZ J Surg 67:566–570
11. Matsuoka H, Mavrantonis C, Wexner SD et al (2000) Postanal repair for fecal incontinence-is it worthwhile? Dis Colon Rectum 43:1561–1567
12. Abbas SM, Bissett IP, Neill ME, Parry BR (2005) Long-term outcome of postanal repair in the treatment of faecal incontinence. ANZ J Surg 75(9):783-786
13. Setti CP, Kamm MA, Nicholls RJ (1994) Long-term results of postanal repair for neurogenic faecal incontinence. Br J Surg 81:140–144
14. Deen KI, Oya M, Ortiz J, Keighley MR (1993) Randomized trial comparing three forms of pelvic floor repair for neuropathic faecal incontinence. Br J Surg 80:794–798
15. Kamm MA (1998) Fortnightly review: faecal incontinence. BMJ 316:528–532
16. Scott AD, Henry MM, Phillips RK (1990) Clinical assessment and anorectal manometry before postanal repair: failure to predict outcome. Br J Surg 77:628–629
17. Nelson R, Norton N, Cautley E, Furner S (1995) Community-based prevalence of anal incontinence. JAMA 274:559–561
18. Johanson JF, Lafferty J (1996) Epidemiology of fecal incontinence: the silent affliction. Am J Gastroenterol 91:33–36
19. Macmillan AK, Merrie AE, Marshall RJ, Parry BR (2004) The prevalence of fecal incontinence in community-dwelling adults: a systematic review of the literature. Dis Colon Rectum 47:1341–1349
20. Liavag I, Aanestad O (1985) Fecal incontinence. Diagnosis treatment. Ann Gastroent Hepato 21:247–250

Dynamic Graciloplasty

18

Cornelius G.M.I. Baeten, Jarno Melenhorst

Introduction

Fecal incontinence is a terrible burden for patients. In severe forms of incontinence, patients feel excluded from any social interaction. They prefer to stay at home close to the toilet and try to avoid shopping, attending parties, or visiting friends. If they do go into public places, they know the location of every public toilet. Even in their own homes, most of them have rules with partner and children that the moment the patient feels any urge, the toilet must be free immediately. People who are not familiar with this phenomenon can hardly understand how terrible this can be for patients. Fecal continence is so normal and taken for granted that those who have never experienced it cannot imagine how life would be if the moment arrived when he or she became incontinent. The world shrinks to a size no bigger than the patient's home. These patients have the choice of either accepting such a life or accepting a colostomy.

Fecal continence is the ability to retain feces and expel it in the appropriate place and at the appropriate time. Continence is the result of delicate cooperation of several factors: feces consistency, rectum and sigmoid peristalsis, rectum capacity and compliance, pelvic floor function, anorectal sensitivity, and anal sphincter function. When one of these factors becomes deficient, the quality of the other factors determines whether or not the patient becomes incontinent. For instance, when a patient has diarrhea, he or she stays continent as long as the sphincters are sufficient, but when sphincter and pelvic floor function diminishes, the patient is unable to hold liquid stool. For a long time, the anal sphincters were considered to be the only factor determining continence. Although this is no longer the case, integrity of the anal sphincters is still recognized as an important factor in fecal incontinence. Several operating techniques have been developed to restore dysfunctional sphincters.

Overlapping anal repair is by far the most frequently used technique to restore anal sphincters [1]. Indications are restoration of the sphincters after rupture due to obstetric causes, impalement trauma of the perineum, or complications of perineal operations. The advantage in these situations is that the ends of the sphincter are present around the anus, and the operation can be performed through one incision. The sphincters are rebuilt for sphincter function and react to the patient's own sensory input. Results are initially very good but tend to deteriorate over time [1–3]. When patients stay incontinent after anatomical restoration of the sphincter and the incontinence is not due to other factors, there are other options. A Thiersch wire or a Silastic band [4] can be brought around the anus, but these often cause problems due to erosion, so these methods are considered obsolete.

Two muscles have been used to augment the original sphincters: the gluteus muscle [5] and the gracilis muscle [6, 7]. The gluteus muscle has the advantage of being a static muscle and can contract for a longer time. However, its anatomical form and position make it less attractive for sphincter function: two gluteus muscles are needed to encircle the anus; transposition hampers the original function of the muscle, and patients are no longer able to walk stairs.

The gracilis muscle is the most ideal muscle to encircle the anus. Its form and the position of the main artery and nerve make it possible to free almost the entire length of the muscle in the medial aspect of the upper thigh. The proximal attachment of the muscle to the pubic bone, as well as the nerve and artery, remain intact. The distal part can be brought around the anus subcutaneously. This transposition causes no functional problems to the leg, and the patient is able to walk, jump, and to play sport [8]. The intrinsic characteristics of the gracilis, however, are not suitable for sphincter function. The gracilis muscle is mainly composed of type II fibers, reflecting its original function as an auxiliary muscle for adduction, flexion, and exorotation in the hip and the knee. These movements are always performed with short-term contractions of the gracilis. The gracilis consists mainly of these type II fibers, which are fast twitch and forceful but quickly fatigued. One can say that the gracilis muscle is anatomically the best muscle to encircle the anus but that its intrinsic characteristics make it one of the worst muscles to perform sphincter function. In the past, graciloplasties were performed for patients with an absent anal sphincter [9]. These patients were able to contract the anus for a short time and only when they consciously concentrated on the contraction of the gracilis. They could do this only for a short period–too short a time for the patient to find a toilet. For this reason, this transposition never became popular because the patient remained incontinent.

Studies have shown that the afferent nerve determines muscle fiber typing. When the nerve is cut and reanastomosed to another nerve, the muscle will change its composition to the demands of the "new" nerve [10, 11]. The most ideal way to proceed would be to connect the gracilis nerve to the nerve of the original external anal sphincter, which has been done [12]. The problem is that the pudendal nerve has more tasks than to "govern" the anus: it functions as nerve for the pelvic floor, the bladder, and perineal region sensibility. Cutting the pudendal nerve for innervation of the gracilis would cause many side effects. When the pudendal nerve is cut after the division of the branch to the anus, the nerve is too small for reanastomosis. In many cases of fecal incontinence, the pudendal nerve is not intact, or it is damaged and not suitable for reanastomosing to the gracilis nerve.

Another option, however, is to "trick" the gracilis nerve with low-frequency electrical stimulation. Physiologists discovered that a normal skeletal muscle fiber pattern could be changed by electrical stimulation [13]. In this way, the fiber composition of the gracilis changes, and a majority of type I fibers will appear. A predominant type I fiber muscle is less fatigable than a type II fiber muscle and can sustain long-term contraction. This makes it possible to change the transposed gracilis muscle into a muscle that has the properties of a sphincter muscle. When stimulated by an implantable stimulator, the muscle is forced to keep its contraction without the patient concentrating on this contraction. Dynamization creates a real sphincter from the transposed gracilis muscle, and the patient goes to the toilet when he or she has the urge to defecate. The stimulator can then be switched off so that no stimuli reach the muscle, and the muscle will relax, making stool passage possible. After defecation, the stimulator can be switched on again, causing the gracilis to contract. Switching the stimulator on and off can be done with an external remote control, a hand-held mini programmer carried by the patient. With this technique, continence can be restored [14].

Indication

Dynamic graciloplasty (DGP) is a major procedure and must be reserved for the most severe forms of fecal incontinence. It is indicated for patients who have a proven sphincter defect and no other reasons for incontinence. There are other therapeutic options for patients with sphincter defects, and it is necessary to investigate all factors contributing to incontinence before a decision is made.

The original sphincter can be examined with endoanal sonography to determine the extent of the defect or possible absence of the external sphincter. In cases of a major defect of the sphincter of half or more of its circumference, anal repair is not longer indicated, and DGP may be an option. The force that can be developed by the native sphincter can be seen with anal manometry. Squeeze pressure, especially, is an indicator of intactness of the external sphincter function. Absence of squeeze pressure can be an indicator for DGP. Innervation assessment can be obtained with a pudendal nerve terminal motor latency (PNTML) test, and an electromyogram (EMG) of the anal sphincter can show reinnervation as a sign of pudendopathy. It is unclear whether pudendopathy is a contraindication for anal repair [15], but it is not contraindicated for DGP because a new, well-innervated muscle is introduced. Defecography can help exclude other reasons for fecal incontinence and other diagnoses that contraindicate a DGP, for instance, intussusception, rectocele, enterocele, or rectal prolapse.

In patients who have a combination of incontinence and constipation, it is better not to perform a DGP, as it can aggravate the constipation component. When patients are incontinent for diarrhea, it is important to treat the diarrhea first. Probably, the incontinence will be solved, and if this fails, better results are seen after DGP. Anal region sensibility can be tested for touch, pain, or temperature or with electrical stimuli in the anus. Rectal sensibility can be tested with an inflatable balloon. This allows the possibility of determining whether the patient must be instructed to empty the bowel at regular times of the day. Lack of sensation can lead to stasis in the rectum after DGP and cause scybala that cannot be removed. The best indication for DGP is the patient with severe trauma that cannot be treated with other methods [14].

There is overlap with DGP and the indication for implantation with an artificial bowel sphincter (ABS) [16]. However, DGP can be used in patients with large tissue defects, such as after a severe rupture and cloaca-like gaps between anus and vagina. This is technically more demanding, and the risk of infection and erosion is much higher if such large defects are treated with an ABS. Also, patients with recurrent rectovaginal fistulas and incontinence can be helped with DGP. The gracilis muscle provides new, vital muscle tissue at the site of the defects and can serve as a replacement of the original sphincter.

Technique

DGP begins with good positioning of the patient on the operating table. With the patient in the lithotomy position, the legs are placed in movable stirrups. The patient is draped so that there is free access to the donor side in the medial aspect of the thigh and to the perineal region and lower abdomen on the same side as the leg from which the gracilis will be taken. The operation is performed under antibiotic prophylaxis. It is not necessary to clean the bowel before the operation (solid feces will stay in the bowel, and this creates less risk of infection than does watery effluent from the bowel after bowel preparation). A protective colostomy has no advantage in the prevention of infections.

The operation begins with an incision in the medial aspect of the thigh. Electrical cutting has the advantage that bleeding from varicose veins hardly occurs. The first muscle encountered is the gracilis, which is best freed half way up the upper leg by encircling the muscle with the finger. By pulling the gracilis toward the operator, the peripheral arteries and veins become visible and are cut after coagulation. The gracilis is then freed in the distal direction toward the tendon. The sartorius muscle covers this tendon. The tendon is freed in the direction of its insertion in the tuberositas tibiae. It is not necessary to go up all the way to the insertion, but the tendon can be cut 5 cm from the transition of muscle into tendon. The free gracilis tendon is grasped with a clamp and pulled toward the operator. Now it is easy to free the proximal part of the gracilis from its adhesions.

The important point is the insertion of the main neurovascular bundle. This is found approximately 8 cm from the origination of the gracilis at the pubic bone. This neurovascular bundle must stay intact. Damaging it means death of the muscle. The subcutaneous adhesions are cut toward the strong fascial layer that separates the leg from the perineum. There is one perforating artery from the muscle toward the skin that must be coagulated. The free gracilis can now be stored subcutaneously for the next phase of the operation.

Lateral to the anus, two incisions are made through which a tunnel is created dorsally of the anus with both index fingers. The lead point is the tip of the coccygeal bone. This dorsal tunnel is widened to the passage of two fingers. Then the frontal tunnel is created. This is more difficult because the layer between the rectum and vagina is very thin, and the risk of perforating the rectum always exists. In order not to perforate the rectum, it is wise to make an auxiliary incision in the backside of the vagina. Because many patients have had previous operations in this area, a good deal of scar tissue may be present. The opening in the back wall of the vagina will heal without difficulty. The frontal tunnel must be widened until three fingers can pass. This is necessary to prevent the gracilis from entrapment in the tunnel. Then, a tunnel is created from the perineum toward the wound in the thigh. The strong fascia lata must be passed, and sharp dissection is necessary. Here, also, the passage must be wide enough to prevent entrapment of the gracilis.

The freed gracilis can now be brought subcutaneously from the thigh to the perineum. There are several ways in which the gracilis can be led through the tunnels to its anchoring point: In case of a long muscular part, a gamma or epsilon loop is created; in case of a short muscular part, an alpha loop is preferred [17]. When creating an alpha loop, it is important to anchor the tendon behind the muscular part of the gracilis to prevent entrapment again. When the optimal position of the muscle is determined, the muscle is pulled back again in the thigh for two reasons. First, it is easier to place a suture through the periosteum of the pubic bone when the view is not obstructed by the gracilis. Second, it is easier to place the electrodes in the stretched muscle than in the bent muscle after the transposition.

Positioning the electrodes begins with the introduction of the anode. Where it is placed is not important, as long as it is distal to the nerve entrance. The cathode is positioned with the help of an auxiliary electrode connected to the needle. Stimulation is given, and the needle can be used to find the optimal place for the electrode. By decreasing the amplitude of the stimulation, one can find the spot where the muscle contracts at the lowest voltage. Normally, this will be very close to the nerve. Low voltage is important for longevity of the stimulator. When the optimal position is found for the cathode, the electrode is brought through the muscle and anchored to the epimysium. Both electrodes are now in position and can be stored for the next phase of the operation. The dynamized muscle is now pulled through the tunnels according to the chosen configuration. The tendon is anchored to the suture already placed through the periosteum of the pubic bone.

The two electrodes are tunneled from the thigh to a pocket created in the lower abdomen on the ipsilateral side. The pocket is created underneath the fascia of the rectus muscle. It is important to coagu-

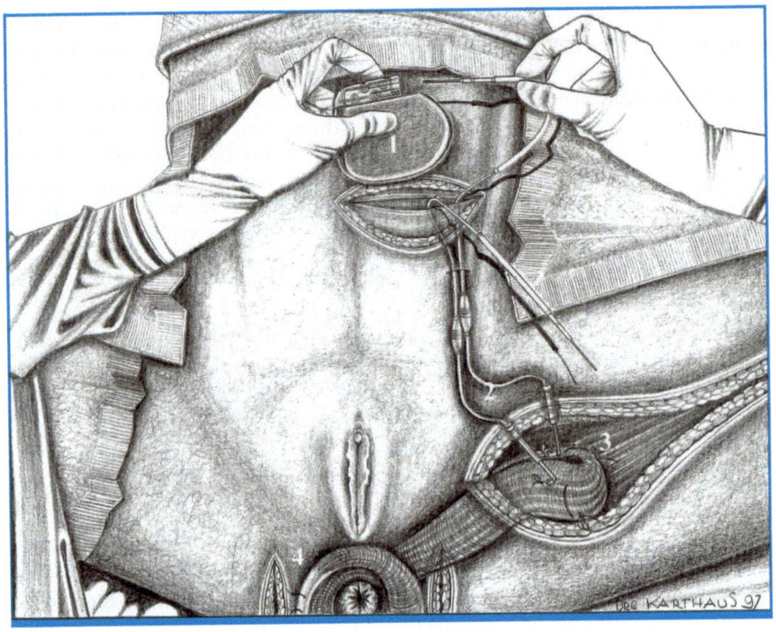

Fig. 1. Overview of the end result of dynamic graciloplasty: (*1*) implantable neurostimulator; (*2*) anode and cathode; (*3*) position of the neurovascular bundle of the gracilis muscle; (*4*) attachment of the tendon of the gracilis muscle (Image courtesy of Dr. D. Karthaus)

late possible perforating arteries and veins. The electrodes are then connected to the stimulator, and the stimulator is placed in the pocket. The fascia is closed over local antibiotics. Wounds of the thigh, lower abdomen, and lateral of the anus are all closed over local antibiotics. To prevent seromas, the leg is bandaged. An overview of the end result is shown in Figure 1.

Stimulation

After the operation, the stimulator is programmed to "off" to allow the gracilis to recover. After 1 month, training of the muscle can begin by programming the stimulator to a low frequency of 2.1 Hz. This is continued for 2 weeks and then increased to 5.2 Hz. This frequency is maintained for 2 weeks and then increased to 10 Hz. After 2 weeks, the stimulator is programmed to 15 Hz. This setting creates nonundulating muscle stimulation. The training period is now complete, and the gracilis can be stimulated "forever". The stimulator can be switched off for defecation, and the patient is advised to do the same during the night, as it will save battery life. Stimulator longevity was shown to be 8 years in a large series [14]. When the battery life ends, the stimulator must be replaced. This is a simple procedure that can be performed under local anesthesia.

Results

In the literature, several series have been published that indicate success rates from 45% to 80% [14, 18–21]. Not everyone does well after this operation, however, and many complications have been reported [17]. The most common problems are infections, constipation, and insufficient contraction of the gracilis. Infections can be minor, such as skin infections or infections around the anus, which can be treated with antibiotics. The more severe infections involve the implanted material and make explantation necessary. Constipation is seldom due to a too-tight wrap around the anus, but this is seen in about 16% of cases. The solution is often a laxative or retrograde cleaning of the bowel. Insufficient contraction of the gracilis can be caused by electrical or muscular problems. Distinction between the two is simple: Because the muscle still has its own innervation, the patient can be asked to voluntarily contract the gracilis. When there is no contraction, the problem is muscular. When there is a much weaker stimulated contraction than the voluntary one, it is a stimulation problem. The problem may be a flat battery, which then needs to be replaced. Another possibility is electrode displacement or breakage; measuring electrode impedance can identify this problem.

Conclusion

DGP is a good solution for patients with severe fecal incontinence due to sphincter malfunction when all other options are not possible. This therapy is at the end of the treatment tree before giving the patient a colostomy.

Acknowledgements

We thank Dr. D. Karthaus for providing the figure.

References

1. Sultan AH, Monga AK, Kumar D, Stanton SL (1999) Primary repair of obstetric anal sphincter rupture using the overlap technique. Br J Obstet Gynaecol 106:318–323
2. Baig MK, Wexner SD (2000) Factors predictive of outcome after surgery for faecal incontinence Br J Surg 87:1316–1330
3. Baxter NN, Bravo Guittierez A, Lowry AC et al (2003) Long-term results of sphincteroplasty for acquired faecal incontinence. Dis Colon Rectum 46:A21–A22
4. Turell R (1954) The Thiersch operation for rectal prolapse and anal incontinence. NY State J Med 54:791–795
5. Devesa JM, Vicente E, Enriquez JM et al (1992) Total fecal incontinence-a new method of gluteus maximus transposition: preliminary results and report of previous experience with similar procedures Dis Colon Rectum 35:339–349
6. Williams NS, Patel J, George BD et al (1991) Development of an electrically stimulated neoanal sphincter. Lancet 338:1166–1169
7. Baeten CG, Konsten J, Spaans F et al (1991) Dynamic graciloplasty for treatment of fecal incontinence Lancet 338:1163–1165
8. Konsten J, Baeten CG, Havenih MG, Soeters PB (1993) Morphology of dynamic graciloplasty compared with the anal sphincter. Dis Colon Rectum 36:559–563
9. Pickrell KL, Broadbent TR, Masters FW, Metzger JT (1952) Construction of a rectal sphincter and restoration of anal incontinence by transplanting the gracilis muscle: report of four cases in children. Ann Surg 135:853–862
10. Sato T, Konishi F, Kanazawa K (1996) Functional perineal colostomy with pudendal nerve anastomosis following anorectal resection: an experimental study. Surgery 119:641–651
11. Sato T, Konishi F, Noriyuki E et al (2005) Long-term outcomes of a neoanus with pudendal nerve anastomosis contemporaneously reconstructed with an abdominoperineal excision of the rectum. Surgery 137:8–15
12. Pirro N, Sielezneff I, Malouf A et al (2005) Anal sphincter reconstruction using transposed gracilis muscle with a pudendal nerve anastomosis: a preliminary anatomical study. Dis Colon Rectum 48:2085–2089
13. Pette D, Vrbova G (1992) Adaptation of mammalian skeletal muscle fibres to chronic electrical stimulation. Rev Biochem Pharmacol 120:115–202
14. Rongen MJ, Uludag Ö, El Naggar K et al (2003) Long-term follow-up of dynamic graciloplasty for faecal incontinence. Dis Colon Rectum 46:716–721
15. Chen AS, Luchtefeld MA, Senagore AJ (1998) Pudendal nerve latency. Does it predict outcome of anal sphincter repair? Dis Colon Rectum 41:1005–1009
16. Christiansen J, Lorentzen M (1987) Implantation of artificial sphincter for anal incontinence. Lancet 2:244–245
17. Geerdes BP, Heineman E, Konsten J et al (1996) Dynamic graciloplasty. Complications and management. Dis Colon Rectum 39:912–917
18. Baeten CG, Bailey HR, Bakka A et al (2000) Safety and efficacy of dynamic graciloplasty for fecal incontinence: report of a prospective, multicenter trial Dynamic Graciloplasty Therapy Study Group. Dis Colon Rectum 43:743–751
19. Penninckx F, Belgian Section of Colorectal Surgery (2004) Belgian experience with dynamic graciloplasty for fecal incontinence. Br J Surg 91:872–878
20. Wexner SD, Gonzalez-Padron A, Rius J et al (1996) Stimulated gracilis neosphincter operation. Initial experience, pitfalls, and complications. Dis Colon Rectum 39(9):957–964
21. Mander BJ, Wexner SD, Williams NS et al (1999) Preliminary results of a multicentre trial of the electrically stimulated gracilis neoanal sphincter. Br J Surg 86:1543–1548

Invited Commentary

Harald R. Rosen

Introduction

By the end of the 1980s, the introduction of electrically stimulated muscle fiber conversion [1] led to the reintroduction of an almost forgotten surgical procedure for sphincter restoration that had been published in 1952: graciloplasty. The capability to convert a skeletal muscle by controlled electrical stimulation to a muscle that was able to contract tetanically raised hope that the anal sphincter could be replaced following resection or damage leading to severe incontinence or the need for a permanent colostomy.

Due to his broad experience, Cor Baeten has described indications, technique, and results of this method in this excellent chapter. Additional comments based on our series [2], which began in 1991, follow:

Indications

Dynamic graciloplasty [as well as the artificial bowel sphincter (ABS)] should be regarded as sphincter replacement procedures to be applied only in patients in whom the defect or loss of muscle is to big to be treated by "conventional" sphincter repair methods. After the introduction of this method in the early 1990s, almost every patient with severe incontinence who failed other treatment options was regarded as a candidate for the "neosphincter" [3]. However, the introduction of sacral nerve stimulation (SNS) led to a marked decrease in the number of patients deemed eligible for this operation. Today, only patients with sphincter defects that are too large to be reconstructed (following trauma or surgery) or those who do not respond to SNS and who might have a chance for improvement by a tighter "mechanical" anal canal closure will undergo this operation. Furthermore, reversal of a colostomy following abdominoperineal rectal excision (APR) due to low rectal or recurrent anal cancer, the so-called total anorectal reconstruction (TAR)–as described by the groups of Norman Williams [4] and Enrico Cavina and Massimo Secchia [5]–emerged as another attractive indication for the application of dynamic graciloplasty. After excision of the perineal scar and pull through of the remaining colon ("neorectum", perineal colostomy), one or both gracilis muscles can be wrapped around in order to serve as a neosphincter.

Surgical Technique and Muscle-Fiber Conversion

Contrary to Baeten's technique, we and others have applied incisions anterior and posterior to the anus, which allows the possibility of doing the sometimes technically demanding dissection behind the vagina under direct sight; the blunt dissection of the lateral ischiorectal fat is rarely difficult [2, 6].

A sometimes limiting factor in this operations is the length of the gracilis muscle, and emphasis must be put on an almost complete muscular (i.e., 360°) coverage of the anus, as contact with the tendon might lead to injury and erosion of the anal canal. Adduction of the leg during the wrapping of the muscle will give additional length in this situation; however, the common sitting position during defecation with abducted legs will lead to a higher tension of the muscle and possibly anal stenosis. A possible (although not always successful) solutions is fixing the tendon to the perianal skin with a nonabsorbable suture for approximately 4 weeks, which is technically easy and allows for more flexibility for muscle fixation [5, 6]. Once the suture and the overlying part of the tendon are removed, the muscle is usually firmly anchored, and after a few weeks, a tiny scar in the skin shows the spot were the tendon can be found if revision becomes necessary in the future.

To achieve an almost guaranteed 360° muscle coverage, we introduced a modification of the muscle wrap by bringing the tendon through the muscle belly itself–the so-called split-sling technique–which is helpful in shortening the way around the anal canal [6].

Following animal and clinical studies and based on the primary original physiological publications, we were able to reduce the muscle fiber conversion period to 4 weeks. During this time, the muscle is stimulated with a frequency of 5 Hz in a continuous mode. After 4 weeks, the frequency is raised either to 16 or 21 Hz, and tetanic contraction can be achieved in almost all patients [7]. Only in those in whom intermittent muscle relaxation despite continuous stimulation is observed (due to a probably insufficient fiber conversion) must the "training period" be prolonged.

Results

As already mentioned in the chapter by Baeten and Melenhorst, continence is a function that is achieved by multiple factors. The success or failure of a sphincter replacement procedure will always depend of the presence or absence of other factors beside the mere mechanical (muscular) closure of the anal canal, e.g., reservoir and sensory function. Therefore, the success rates of dynamic graciloplasty must be analyzed, with special emphasis on the preoperatively present defects: patients with incontinence based on a muscular insufficiency will benefit most, and even complete continence can be achieved, especially if the sensory function of the rectal ampulla and the pelvic floor are not impaired.

Contrary to this, patients following total anorectal reconstruction, patients treated for incontinence following anal atresia, or patients with neurogenic defects will have much greater problems, even with a strong muscle wrap. Especially in patients following APR, satisfying results can only be achieved by regular irrigation of the perineal neoanus, thus leading to so-called pseudo continence. Therefore, some authors have more recently advocated the application of a sphincter replacement procedure (graciloplasty or ABS) only in patients with a perineal colostomy who fail to achieve a satisfying continence with irrigation alone [8].

Anal stenosis and injury are the most common problems following dynamic graciloplasty and are caused either by a technical mistake (if the wrap is fixed too tight) or due to anatomical problems (if the muscle is too short, as mentioned above). In our experience, infection of the implanted material (electrodes and pulse generator) occurred in one patient only and was successfully prevented by application of local antibiotics, as also mentioned by the authors in this chapter.

On the whole, restoration of the anal sphincter by homologous (i.e., gracilis muscle) material is the greatest advantage of this method compared with ABS (which shows comparable functional results in the literature). Especially in complicated soft-tissue situations (trauma, osteomyelitis, radiation), dynamic graciloplasty is superior to the ABS.

Conclusion

In conclusion, dynamic graciloplasty is still a well-established tool in the treatment plan for fecal incontinence due to gross and otherwise irreparable defects of the anal sphincter. However, it must be accepted that this is a technically demanding and costly procedure that requires a learning process. Due to the introduction of alternative, less invasive (and very effective) methods such as SNS for some of the former indications for dynamic graciloplasty, the number of potential candidates will be further decreased in the future, which could lead to a reduction of centers experienced in this method

References

1. Pette D, Vrbova G (1992) Adaption of mammalian skeletal muscle fibres to chronic electrical stimulation. Rev Biochem Pharmacol 120:115–202
2. Rosen HR, Urbarz C, Novi G et al (2002) Long-term results of modified graciloplasty for sphincter replacement after rectal excision. Colorectal Dis 4(4):266–269
3. Madoff RD, Rosen HR, Baeten CG et al (1999) Safety and efficacy of dynamic muscle plasty for anal incontinence: lessons from a prospective, multicenter trial. Gastroenterology 116(3):549–556
4. Mander BJ, Williams NS (1997) The electrically stimulated gracilis neo-anal sphincter. Eur J Gastroenterol Hepatol 9(5):435–441
5. Cavina E (1999) Total anorectal reconstruction after abdominoperineal resection. Int J Surg Investig 1(3):262–263
6. Rosen HR, Novi G, Zöch G et al (1998) Restoration of anal sphincter function by single-stage dynamic graciloplasty with a modified (split sling) technique. Am J Surg 175(3):187–193
7. Rosen HR, Dorner G, Feil W et al (1997) Muscle transformation of the sartorius muscle in a canine model: clinical impact for electrodynamic graciloplasty as a "neosphincter". Dis Colon Rectum 40(11):1321–1327
8. Lirici MM, Ishida M, Di Paola M et al (2004) Dynamic graciloplasty versus implant of artificial sphincter for continent perineal colostomy after Miles' procedure: Technique and early results. Minim Invasive Ther Allied Technol 13(5):347–361

19

The Artificial Bowel Sphincter in the Treatment of Severe Fecal Incontinence in Adults

Paul-Antoine Lehur, Guillaume Meurette

Introduction

Fecal incontinence is a severe disability that deeply affects the quality of life of the afflicted patient. The estimated prevalence in the general population ranges from 1% to 17%. In France, it is estimated that 350,000 persons over the age of 45 years have a severe form of fecal incontinence. In the event of ineffective medical treatment and the inability or failure of conventional surgery, the only choice for these patients until recently was to accept their condition or opt for end colostomy. However, technological progress has opened up the prospect of effective therapy for severe fecal incontinence both in terms of performance and long-term reliability. Replacement of sphincter function by an artificial bowel sphincter is one available option that has shown promising results.

This work aims to provide an overview of managing fecal incontinence by using an artificial sphincter, describe the device and how it functions, explore state-of-the-art implantation techniques and recommended patient follow-up, present the most recently published results, and discuss indications and contraindications of this treatment.

Description of the Acticon Neosphincter Artificial Bowel Sphincter

The Acticon Neosphincter artificial bowel sphincter [American Medical Systems (AMS), Minnetonka, MN, USA] is a totally implantable device made of solid silicone rubber. It comprises three parts: a perianal occlusive cuff, a control pump with a septum, and a pressure-regulating balloon. These three components are linked together by subcutaneous kink-resistant tubing. The occlusive cuff is implanted in the upper part of the anal canal, and the closing system incorporated into the cuff uses the initial part of the tubing. The cuff comes in different models with respect to length (8–14 cm) and height (2.0 cm or 2.9 cm). The choice of the cuff, an important intraoperative consideration, is determined by measurements made during the implantation procedure.

The pressure-regulating balloon, which is implanted in a pocket created in the subperitoneal space, controls the level of pressure applied on the anal canal by cuff closure. Available pressures range from 80 cm to 120 cm H_2O in 10-cm gradations. Thus, the occlusive effect of the cuff depends on its size (length and height)–that determines whether it fits more or less tightly around the anal canal–and the pressure level chosen for the balloon.

The control pump is implanted in subcutaneous tissues of the scrotum in men and of the labia majora in women. The hard upper part of the pump contains a resistance regulating the rate of fluid circulation throughout the system and a deactivation button allowing fluid cycling to be stopped by external action. The soft lower part of the pump is squeezed repeatedly to transfer fluid within the device. A septum placed at the bottom of this soft part is intended for postoperative use in case a small amount of liquid needs to be injected. The principle of this septum is similar to that of an implantable portacath (Fig. 1).

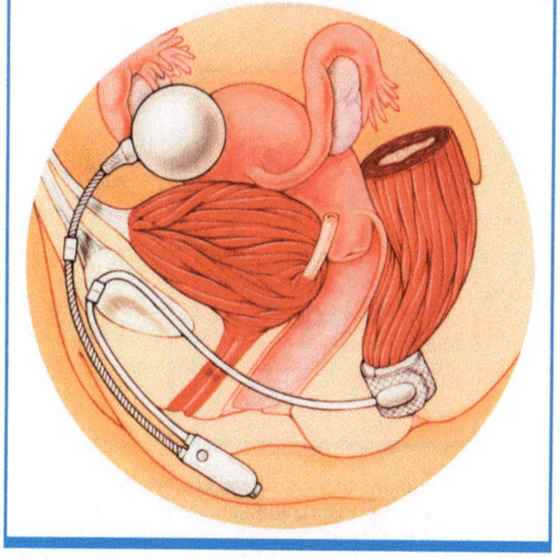

Fig. 1. Overview of the artificial bowel sphincter (ABS) used to treat severe fecal incontinence

ABS Functioning

The ABS functions semiautomatically:

1. The cuff ensures anal closure automatically and continuously at low pressures, close to physiological values of resting anal pressure. The regulating balloon transmits pressure to the occlusive cuff through the tubing, and the pressure is applied uniformly and nearly circularly to the upper part of the anal canal, restoring a barrier and isolating the rectum from outside.
2. Defecation is initiated by the patient. Anal opening is achieved by transferring the pressurized fluid from the cuff toward the balloon by means of the control pump. The fluid is transferred by 5–15 squeezes on the pump, each evacuating around 0.5 cc from the cuff, thereby lowering anal pressure and opening the anal canal to expel feces. Suitable compliance allows the volume of the pressure-regulating balloon to increase transiently to receive the several cubic centimeters of fluid contained in the cuff.
3. Anal closure occurs again automatically in 5–8 min by passive fluid transfer and a progressive return to baseline pressure in the cuff. The balloon recovers its initial volume during this period, thereby restoring equal pressure throughout the system (Fig. 2).

The system can be deactivated temporarily to allow the cuff to be empty and the anal canal to be open continuously. This arrangement can be used during the postoperative period to avoid manipulation of the cuff and pump during the healing period. Two months of deactivation are desirable after implantation to ensure tissue integration of the device. The system can then be activated simply by firmly squeezing the pump, a procedure not requiring anesthesia and that can be performed during an office visit. Deactivation of the cuff in the open position is also necessary for transanal endoscopic procedures in order to avoid any tear or damage to the cuff during the passage of the endoscope. Deactivation is a recent feature, and its absence in earlier models was responsible for some initial failures.

Implantation Technique Perioperative Care

Preoperative care includes careful cutaneous and bowel preparation over a 48-h period. Two douches of the operative field are performed daily with an iodinated solution, and complete colonic preparation is done, including X-prep and enemas, until fluid becomes clear. There is no need for a colostomy, except in the case of diarrheic patients in whom contamination of the perineal wound may occur from too rapid a resumption of bowel movements. Antibiotic prophylaxis based on a third-generation cephalosporin and an aminoglycoside is administered in a single dose at the induction of anesthesia.

The operative position of the patient should allow a combined perineal and abdominal approach. The first phase of the operation involves placement of the perianal occlusive cuff. A single preanal incision can be used, allowing rectovaginal or rectourethral separation (5–6 cm) from which a perianal tunnel can be created around the anal canal by blunt finger dissection. Alternatively, the incision can be made laterally

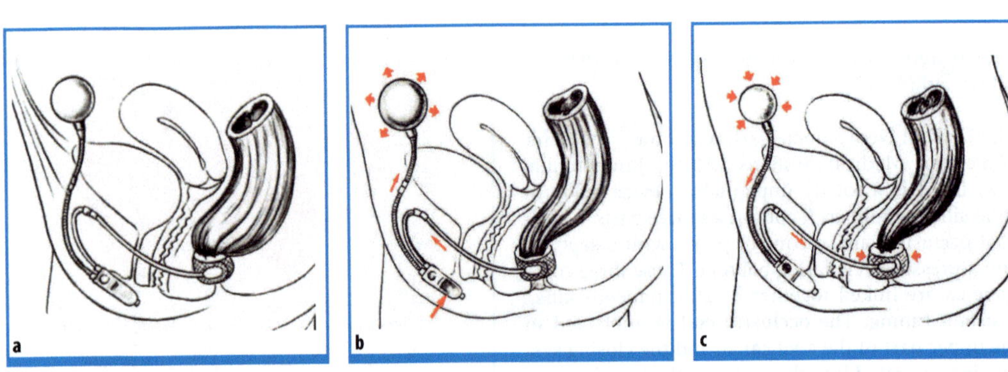

Fig. 2a–c. Functioning of the artificial bowel sphincter (ABS). **a** Anal occlusion: pressure is equilibrated throughout the system, ensuring cuff pressurization and thus automatic closure of the anal canal at a predetermined pressure level approximately equal to that of the pressure-regulating balloon selected for implantation. **b** Anal opening, controlled by the patient: pressure equilibrium in the system is interrupted by the active transfer (manipulation of the control pump) of the fluid from the cuff to the pressure-regulating balloon. **c** Progressive anal closure (*arrows* indicate the direction of fluid transfers within the system after defecation)

on both sides of the anus, following the example of graciloplasty procedure. A transvaginal approach has also been proposed recently (Patrick Lee, MD. Portland, OR, USA; personal communication). The length of the occlusive cuff is then determined using a specially designed sizer. The cuff should not narrow the anal canal, which would hinder defecation. Rectal examination is the best means of determining the caliber obtained. In the event of perforation of the vagina or rectum at this point in the dissection, implantation of the ABS should be deferred or possibly abandoned.

Once the perianal tunnel has been made, preparation of the ABS device can begin on a sterile table intended for this purpose. Tissue, blood, and any potentially aggressive surgical material are excluded from this area in order to avoid possible alteration of the device. All three components of the system are carefully bled of any air bubbles, which might prevent cycling of the pressurization fluid. This rather delicate preparation should be entrusted to a nurse trained in the technique. The pressurization fluid is an isotonic solution, as the artificial sphincter walls are semipermeable membranes and radiopaque (except in the case of iodine allergy), to allow postoperative control of fluid movements in the system. The fluid is prepared extemporaneously and composed of Telebrix 12 sodium (53%) and sterile water (47%) in our practice. Other possible solutions are described by AMS.

The perianal cuff is the first component put into place. Tubing from the cuff is then tunneled subcutaneously to the abdominal incision with a special atraumatic, long needle. The rectus abdominis is split to provide access to the subperitoneal space lateral to the bladder. A pocket is created in this space to lodge the pressure-regulating balloon. The cuff is first pressurized by connection with the balloon, which is filled with 55 cc of radiopaque fluid. The amount of fluid kept in the cuff after pressurization is carefully measured when emptying the balloon; it is usually between 4 cc and 8 cc. The balloon is implanted empty and then filled with 40 cc of radiopaque fluid, a volume at which the pressure delivered to the cuff corresponds to values determined by the manufacturer (usually between 80 cm and 100 cm of water). The aponeurosis is carefully closed during this step. The control pump is then positioned. As this is the only component that the patient will feel and manipulate, it needs to be perfectly accessible. The occlusive cuff and the pressure-regulating balloon are connected to the pump. The kink-resistant tubes are identified by a color code (black from the balloon and clear from the cuff). Connections are made with special "quick connectors", preventing any air bubbles from entering the system. After assessing that cycling is correct, the incisions are closed without drainage. The device is deactivated at the end of the procedure by pressing firmly on the deactivation button. In our experience, the entire procedure lasts around 90–120 min.

Immediately after the operation, a fluid diet only is allowed for 3 days to avoid too early a resumption of bowel movements. The anal wound is cleaned regularly. The mean length of hospital stay is 7–10 days if there are no complications. The patient is discharged once defecation has become normal and the incisions are healed. The patient is readmitted 8 weeks later for 1 day, during which the artificial sphincter is activated. A firm pressure on the control pump unblocks the deactivation button, allowing the cuff to fill and play its occlusive role. The patient is given the necessary instructions for opening the sphincter, allowing regular defecation, possibly initiated with small enemas in case of difficulty.

Recommendations for Follow-up of Patients with ABS Implants

Is it necessary to follow-up patients who have received implants? This is a debatable point, as the device is easy to operate and its use rapidly becomes natural for the patient. The patient could be instructed to return in the event of incontinence recurrence, which would be a good arrangement for persons living far from the implantation center. However, we require regular follow-up for our patients, not only for research purposes, but also to check on the proper use of the device, its efficacy in restoring satisfactory anorectal function, and the possible occurrence of complications. Postoperative evaluation is based on simple annual examinations (clinical, plain X-rays, and anorectal manometry).

Clinical evaluation relative to fecal continence and rectal evacuation is performed best by questionnaires. Efficacy of the device in restoring satisfactory quality of life can also be assessed by specific questionnaires. Such evaluations currently in progress appear to justify the financial investment involved in the use of artificial sphincters. The clinical examination checks the proper positioning of the control pump and its accessibility, the efficacy of anal closure by digital rectal exam, and the quality of anal opening after manipulation of the pump by the patient. Local tolerance of the artificial sphincter is also checked. It is important during the first postoperative months to detect any migration of the cuff. If it is too close to the anal margin, there is risk of skin damage and erosion, leading to contamination of the material and explantation. If detected early enough, this complication can be corrected by reoperation and repositioning the cuff higher in the pelvic floor. This can be achieved by redoing the perineal incision and simply unbuttoning the deactivated cuff.

Pressurization of the ABS with a radiopaque fluid allows very simple radiological monitoring. In the immediate postoperative period, device deactivation can easily be checked by plain pelvic X-rays. During activation, a series of X-rays can be used to analyze fluid transfer through the device and thus visualize the ABS function. These images can also be used for reference purposes in the event of subsequent device dysfunction. Endoanal ultrasonography can also be performed during the monitoring procedure. This examination, though not carried out routinely, is considered a valid means of assessing the thickness of tissues encircled by the cuff and detecting any possible atrophy, which would be suggestive of ulceration of the device in the anal canal.

Anal manometry, an important aspect of postimplantation monitoring, precisely and objectively estimates the efficiency of the ABS (Fig. 3). We consider it is important to determine three manometric parameters systematically:

1. Basal pressure with the ABS closed indicates the capacity of the device to create a high-pressure zone in the anal canal. A significant increase compared with preoperative values contributes to restoring fecal continence.
2. Basal pressure with the ABS opened by the patient represents residual anal pressure. When low, it is indicative of a wide anal opening and easy defecation, whereas high residual pressure could account for postoperative dyschezia.
3. The time required for the ABS to close again after being opened is also indicative of rectal evacuation quality. A sufficient period is needed to obtain complete emptying. Some patients experience a rapid closure quicker than that specified for the ABS (approximately 7 min normally), which may also be responsible for dyschezia.

Anal manometry can also be used to check whether the patient is manipulating the device correctly. Pumping quality, which needs to be slow to be efficient, and that of the resulting anal opening can be evaluated on a screen image for the patient's benefit, as during biofeedback sessions.

Recently Published Results with the ABS and Personal Series

The initial results obtained with the urinary-type device have been previously reported and discussed [1, 2]. In this review, we have concentrated on the most recent and significant published data. Several centers in Europe, the United States, and Australia have adopted the ABS to treat severe fecal incontinence not amenable to local repair. Reports with larger numbers of cases and longer follow-up have recently appeared, providing a better assessment of this innovative technique and its present place in the treatment strategy of incontinent patients.

We analyzed the most recently published experiences with the ABS, and in 2002, we reviewed our own series of 32 patients (37 implants) at our institution regarding the main outcome endpoints, including infection rate, revision surgery, and explant rate (unpublished) (Table 1). The overall incidence of permanent explantation of the ABS in the published series varied between 17% and 31% with follow-up periods of between 10 and 58 months. Revision surgery with replacement of part of or the entire device occurred in between 7% and 25% of patients. Complications leading to explantation included perioper-

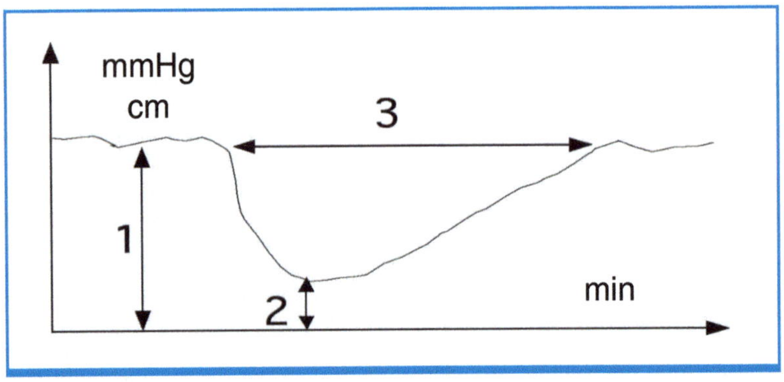

Fig. 3. Anal manometry: normal function of an artificial bowel sphincter (ABS). Measurements performed during the examination: *(1)* resting anal pressure with the cuff closed (pressurized), *(2)* resting anal pressure with the cuff open (empty), *(3)* time of anal closure

Table 1. Results with the artificial bowel sphincter (ABS)

	Number	Infection rate (%)	Revision surgery (%)	Explant rate (%)	Mean follow-up (months)
Wong et al. [3]	112	25	46	37	18
Ortiz et al. [4]	22	9	50	32	26
Altomare et al. [5]	28	18	32	25	19
Parker et al. [6]	37	34	37	40	39
Michot et al. [7]	25	7	28	20	34
Our series (unpublished)	32	0	53	31	26

ative infection, failure of wound healing, erosion of part of the device through the skin or the anal canal, late infection, and mechanical malfunction of the device due to cuff or balloon rupture. As far as function is concerned, successful results were obtained in Spain; Italy; Minneapolis, MN, USA; Rouen, France; and for us, in 15 out of 24 (62.5%), 21 out of 28 (75%), 17 out of 35 (49%), 22 out of 30 (73%), and 23 out of 32 (72%) cases espectively.

As did others, we found improvement in quality of life after ABS implantation. In a series of 16 patients consecutively receiving implants and a follow-up of 25 months, there was significant improvement in the four separate quality-of-life domains explored in the Fecal Incontinence Quality of Life (FIQL) [8]. Scores were recorded, with a linear correlation between improvement over time in the quality-of-life index and evaluation of continence measured by a clinical score.

Results from the multicenter cohort study conducted under US Food and Drug Administration (FDA) supervision showed an 85% functional success rate in patients who retained their ABS. Of 112 patients included in the trial, 51 (46%) required revision operation primarily because of infection, and 41 (37%) required complete explantation. Accordingly, the final overall intention-to-treat success rate was 53%, but this includes for a majority of the centers their initial experience with the device. Parker and coworkers [6] reported data from the University of Minnesota, one of the leader groups in the use of the ABS. They identified two patient groups: those who received implants between 1989 and 1992 (n=10; mean follow-up, 91 months) and those who received implants between 1995 and 2001 (n=37; mean follow-up, 39 months). The overall success rate in the former group was 60% (4/10 explants). The latter group had an overall success rate of 49%, with a revision and infection rate of 37% and 34%, respectively. Those patients who had successful implant procedures enjoyed a 100% functional success rate at 2 years.

The ABS has also recently been evaluated in a randomized control trial. O'Brien et al. [9] from Australia compared a group of 14 patients randomly assigned to an ABS to a similar group entering a program of best supportive care for fecal incontinence. Explant occurred once in the operative group (14%). Improvement at 6 months was significant in the ABS group in terms of continence but not in the control group. The Cleveland Clinic Score (CCS) was significantly altered in the ABS group (preoperative value, 19; postoperative value, 5–75% overall improvement) compared with the control group (preoperative value, 17; postoperative value, 14). Similar changes were observed in quality of life evaluated by different means [Short Form-36 (SF-36), FIQL, Beck Depression Inventory).

As mentioned, anal manometry is an important part of postoperative evaluation of the implanted device. The experience of Savoye et al. [10] from Rouen, France, gave very similar results to our findings (Table 2).

Table 2. Manometric assessment after artifical bowel sphincter (ABS) implantation [10]

	Mean	Range
Closed cuff		
Anal resting pressure (cm H_2O)	108	22
Maximum amplitude of voluntary contractions (cm H_2O)	26	31
Duration of voluntary contractions (s)	18	20
Open cuff		
Total duration of opening phase (s)	113[a]	8
Amplitude of decrease (% of basal pressure)	60	22
Residual pressure (cm H_2O)	40[b]	13
Time to open the cuff (s)	14	3

[a]Total duration of the opening phase in patients with obstructed defecation symptoms was significantly shorter (47 s; range, 0-65s) than in patients without obstructed defecation symptoms (178 s; range, 100-320 s) (P=0.002)
[b]Correlated with the resting pressure recorded before implantation of the ABS

ABS Reimplantation after Failure

In many series, patients have undergone successful reimplantation after failure of a previous implantation related to infection, ulceration, or mechanical breakdown. In our series of 32 patients receiving implants (unpublished), ten were explanted, but five of them underwent reimplantation with success. Part of or the entire device can be replaced when revision surgery is needed. In the series of Parker et al. [6], risk of infection following revision was 19%, lower than after primary implantation (34%). Their success rate in this setting was 65% (13/21 cases).

Patients choosing ABS therapy must be aware of the risk of revision surgery. They usually accept redo surgery in case of complications, as they greatly appreciate the benefit obtained with the device.

New Applications for the ABS

Indications for use of the ABS are broadening and have reached the complex field of anorectal reconstruction following abdominoperineal excision. Romano et al. from Italy [11] reported using the ABS in this setting. In a series of eight patients, implantation of the ABS was done at the same time as rectal excision (one case), 2 months later (five cases), and many years later (two cases). No explantation has been given to date. Among the five patients with an activated device, four are reported to have good neoanal function. Our personal experience [12] is based on three female patients aged 45, 59, and 68 years, respectively, in whom an ABS was implanted around a perineal colostomy built after curative rectal excision for T1–2 node-negative (NO) cancer. Two of them have had preoperative radiotherapy. Due to occasional leaks, the need for a strict diet, and fear of incontinence, an ABS was implanted consecutively at a mean of 4.5 years after abdominoperineal resection (APR).

Device implantation was feasible and uneventful. In one case, a superficial hematoma was drained and healed by second intention. Devices were activated 3 months after implantation. At a mean of 2.5 years' follow-up, the three patients had an activated and functional artificial sphincter. Leaks and urgency significantly decreased, but colonic retrograde enemas were maintained. Dietary restriction was loosened. Quality of life improved, and all three considered the device a useful adjunct.

In this limited experience, implantation of an artificial sphincter around a perineal colostomy following APR for cancer appeared feasible and safe, even following previous radiotherapy. Tolerance at midterm was satisfactory. Continence and quality of life significantly improved.

Indications and Contraindications for the ABS

Many factors, both anal and extra-anal, contribute to fecal continence. It is apparent that the achievement of the ABS is restoring a high-pressure zone in the anal canal in a static manner, with no ability to increase pressure in the event of a threat to continence. The ABS corrects the loss of resting anal pressure. It would thus be fallacious to assume that normal continence can be restored by this means, even though the functional results obtained are highly satisfactory.

The best indications for the ABS are lesions of the anal sphincters inaccessible to local repair and not responsive to sacral nerve stimulation (SNS) test or not indicated for such a test (Table 3). The good results in this context are the result of other extra-anal sphincter mechanisms being preserved. Thus, the ABS may be recommended, particularly in young subjects, when the chances for successful local repair are poor.

In cases of incontinence resulting from sequelae of anal agenesis, there is a lower chance of success. The lack of anal sensitivity and a rectal reservoir, and the existence of associated colonic motor disorders make all techniques of sphincteric substitution more uncertain. There are no available data predictive of ABS success in this indication, and some patients seem to have obtained better functional results with techniques of anterograde colonic enemas.

In cases of neurogenic or neurologic fecal incontinence, it is essential to take into account possible associated dyschezia and excessive perineal descent. The ABS creates an obstacle to rectal evacuation, which can sometimes cause considerable evacuation difficulties. Continence restoration should not be achieved to the detriment of evacuation capacities. However, an objective assessment of the state of preoperative transit is not always easy. Patients have often modified their diet to avoid difficulties or have had recourse to antidiarrheic treatments. Rectal prolapse or a history of surgical cure for prolapse should be carefully considered before implantation of an ABS insofar as these conditions are indicative of disturbances in the defecation process.

Contraindications to implantation of an ABS are more apparent (Table 3). Although the role of the ABS in anoperineal reconstructions after rectum amputation has not yet been fully defined, radiation therapy will probably be a limiting factor. Implantation of an ABS is possible after failure of graciloplasty and has already been reported. Likewise, reim-

Table 3. Indications and contraindications for artificial bowel sphincter (ABS)

Type of indication	Clinical settings
Good indications	Traumatic sphincter disruption; neurologic incontinence; neurogenic (idiopathic) incontinence; failure or contrindications to sacral nerve stimulation (SNS)
Relative indications	Anal imperforation; severely scarred perineum; thin rectovaginal wall; advanced age? diabetes? handling difficulties
Contraindications	Excessive perineal descent; severe constipation; irradiated perineum; perineal sepsis; Crohn's disease; anal coitus

plantation of the device can take place immediately after explantation when all or part of the device has to be replaced because of a mechanical failure, or later in the event of an infection after all inflammatory processes have disappeared.

The ABS is suitable for well-motivated, selected patients with fecal incontinence of more than a year's duration and whose condition is regarded as an important personal, familial, and/or social handicap. The technique should be proposed to the patient as an alternative to definitive colostomy. A capability to manipulate the control pump is required, as is sufficient intellectual capacity to understand the functioning of the device and ensure regular rectal evacuation. The success of this innovative technique depends on serious consideration of these selection criteria.

Place of the ABS at the Time of the Sacral Nerve Stimulation (SNS)

Recently in a systematic review from Australia [13], the role and place of the ABS have been challenged. On the basis of a full review of the literature, the authors concluded that "there was insufficient evidence on the safety and effectiveness of ABS implantation ... and for most patients, the procedure was of uncertain benefit". Such a statement is clearly not reflective of our practice, even if we agree on the exigence of ABS therapy for patients and surgical teams.

In the mean time, others have considered that the techniques relying on tightening the anal sphincter mechanism have not withstood the test of time in the era of SNS [14]. Clearly, SNS has strong and unique advantages as a minimally invasive procedure, and in terms of testing phase, allows a screening process that provides a unique patient selection and efficiency [15]. Therefore, we adopted SNS in our practice in 2001, and numerous incontinent patients are now successfully treated by this procedure (Fig. 4). But SNS does not provide a solution to all situations, and there is still a place for a sphincteric replacement technique in case of nonresponse or contraindication to SNS. In the series from Denmark [16], 32 out of 45 tested patients had an SNS functioning system, leaving 13 in whom a potential indication for the ABS exists. As we see it, a referral center in surgical treatment of fecal incontinence is incomplete if not offering a complete range of services, including ABS implantation.

Our experience with both ABS and SNS offered a unique opportunity to compare their respective

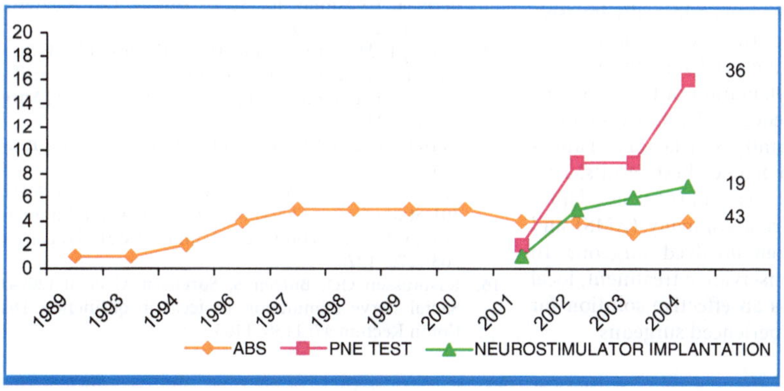

Fig. 4. Artificial bowel sphincter (ABS) and sacral nerve stimulation (SNS) procedures at our institution. *PNE* peripheral nerve evaluation

Table 4. Comparison of artificial bowel sphincter (ABS) and sacral nerve stimulation (SNS)

Score	SNS (mean ± SD)	ABS (mean ± SD)	*P* value
CCS	9.4 ± 3.3	5.6 ± 3.9	<0.01
KESS	6.3 ± 6.3	12.8 ± 5.7	<0.01
SF-36 (physical)	46.2 ± 10	47.2 ± 9.9	NS
SF-36 (emotional)	49.3 ± 8	43.3 ± 14	NS

SNS sacral nerve stimulation, *SD* standard deviation, *ABS* artificial bowel sphincter, *CCS* Cleveland Clinic Score, *KESS* Knowles-Eccersely-Scott Symptom score, *SF-36* Short Form-36

results. Among 27 patients tested in our institution between December 2001 and April 2004, 15 were successfully treated with permanent SNS (mean follow-up 15±9 months). We compared these patients in a case-control study to 15 patients treated with an ABS. Both groups were similar regarding age, gender, incontinence severity, and conservative treatment failure. Preoperative manometric studies were similar in both groups. A standardized questionnaire including incontinence (CCS) and constipation [Knowles-Eccersley-Scott-Symptom (KESS)] scoring systems and the SF-36 quality of life scale was answered by each patient. Results of the study showed that quality of life evaluation was similar in both groups, whereas incontinence and constipation scores were significantly different (Table 4). As expected, greater improvement in continence is obtained after ABS implantation but with a significant price in term of obstructed defecation burden, but quality of life after SNS is as satisfactory as after ABS implantation.

Conclusion

To conclude, the role of the ABS must be put in perspective regarding the other new, minimally invasive approaches to anal incontinence, namely, SNS. Although morbidity and the need for revision surgery is high following implantation of the ABS, outcome in terms of continence and improvement in quality of life is significantly satisfactory. Patient selection is mandatory to achieve best results. Late mechanical failure is a concern and requires adaptation from the manufacturing company (AMS) and continuous evaluation from involved surgeons. In case of nonresponse to conservative treatment, local repair, or SNS, the ABS is an effective solution for motivated patients and experienced surgeons

References

1. Christiansen J, Lorentzen M (1987) Implantation of artificial sphincter for anal incontinence. Lancet 1:244–245
2. Lehur PA, Michot F, Denis P et al (1996) Results of artificial sphincter in severe anal incontinence. Report of 14 consecutive implantations. Dis Colon Rectum 39:1352–1355
3. Wong WD, Congilosi S, Spencer M et al (2002) The safety and efficacy of the artificial bowel sphincter for faecal incontinence: results from a multicenter cohort study. Dis Colon Rectum 45:1139–1153
4. Ortiz H, Armendariz P, DeMiguel M et al (2002) Complications and functional outcome following artificial anal sphincter implantation. Br J Surg 89:877–881
5. Altomare DF, Dodi G, La Torre F et al (2001) Multicentre retrospective analysis of the outcome of artificial anal sphincter implantation for severe faecal incontinence. Br J Surg 88:1481–1486
6. Parker SC, Spencer MP, Madoff RD (2003) Artificial bowel sphincter: long-term experience at a single institution. Dis Colon Rectum 46:722–729
7. Michot F, Costaglioli B, Leroi AM, Denis P (2003) Artificial anal sphincter in severe fecal incontinence: outcome of prospective experience with 37 patients in one institution. Ann Surg 237:52–56
8. Lehur PA, Zerbib F, Glemain P et al (2002) Comparison of quality of life and anorectal function after artificial sphincter implantation. Dis Colon Rectum 45:508–513
9. O'Brien PE, Dixon JB, Skinner S et al (2004) A prospective randomised controlled clinical trial of placement of the artificial bowel sphincter (Acticon Neosphincter) for the control of fecal incontinence. Dis Colon Rectum 47(11):1852–1860
10. Savoye G, Leroi AM, Denis P, Michot F (2000) Manometric assessment of an artificial bowel sphincter. Br J Surg 87:586–589
11. Romano G, La Torre F, Cutini G et al (2003) Total anorectal reconstruction with the artificial bowel sphincter: report of eight cases. Dis Colon Rectum 46:730–734
12. Marchal F, Doucet C, Lechaux D et al (2005) Secondary implantation of an artificial sphincter after abdominoperineal resection and pseudocontinent perineal colostomy for rectal cancer. Gastroenterol Clin Biol 29:425–428
13. Mundy L, Merlin TL, Maddern GJ, Hiller JE (2004) Systematic review of safety and effectiveness of an artificial bowel sphincter for faecal incontinence. Br J Surg 91:665–672
14. Vaizey CJ (2004) Letter to the editor. Dis Colon Rectum 47:1162
15. Matzel KE, Kamm MA, Stösser M et al and the MDT 301 Study Group (2004) Sacral Spinal Nerve Stimulation for Faecal Incontinence Multicentre Study. Lancet 363:1270–1276
16. Rasmussen OO, Butzen S, Sørensen M et al (2004) Sacral nerve stimulation in fecal incontinence. Dis Colon Rectum 47: 1158–1163

Invited Commentary

Filippo La Torre

The treatment of the fecal incontinence (FI) has satisfactory indications if the incontinence is not severe. There are several traditional medical, conservative, rehabilitative, and surgical therapies available following correct diagnosis of mild to moderate FI [1]. Nevertheless, treatment success rates decrease in medium- and long-term follow-up [2]. This problem–in all the international literature [3]–is higher in cases of severe FI. All authors, in justifying the unsatisfactory long-term results, refer to the complexity of anatomical and physiological structure of the anorectal canal and pelvic floor [4, 5].

It is therefore important to show results following traditional conservative treatment of moderate FI. We suggest, for example, diet, and bulking and pharmacological supports, as described in all the gastroenterological schools. After a variable period of subjectively satisfactory results, we experienced in a large number of cases requests for more effective controls, and thus we change products and increase doses in many instances [4]. This is possible because conservative treatment allows us to change and repeat treatment and to at least suggest the option of invasive surgical treatment [4]. Because positive long-term results of conservative or rehabilitative treatment are no higher than 50%, we can offer many other treatment options. On the other hand, in the 50% of patients who experience unsatisfactory results following invasive treatment, we are left with few options [4].

Recent literature describes results following conservative treatments randomized to rehabilitative procedures in an attempt to validate them in all degrees of FI: minimally invasive procedures are proposed as better options than more invasive procedures [6].

The history of the artificial sphincter has its beginning in the treatment of urinary incontinence (UI), in which satisfactory results are reported in medium-term follow-up and many thousands of applications over 20 years [7]. The same concept applied to FI began 15 years ago, with a similar prosthesis that was changed as experience in the field grew [7]. Many individual and multicentric studies have been published describing a large number of complications following this procedure [8–15]. In the literature on UI, complication and removal rates are about 20% in more than 20,000 applications; in FI, reported complication and removal rates are greater than 50% in just a few hundred applications [16]. There was a similar experience with electrostimulated graciloplasty [17]. Surgeons obtained satisfying results in short- and medium-term follow-up (about 70%) but less than 50% in a longer follow-up [17].

The implant procedure for an artificial bowel sphincter (ABS) is very easy and quick (60–90 min), and it is very important to understand safe timing to avoid all the complications that relate to infection and skin erosion (learning curve). A multicentric Italian study (27 cases in four university hospitals) reported good results in 75% of cases in a medium-term, 24-month follow-up. However, in a review 3 years later, that rate had fallen to less than 50% [15, 18]. All complications were related to skin erosion (Fig. 1a, b), infection, and consequent fistulization (Fig. 2a, b). If infection is an early complication, the others are late complications, as are problems related to the long-term use of the prosthesis. It has also been reported that a large number of patients do not use the ABS appropriately but only when full or empty. In our experience [19] with 12 implants in nine patients in a medium-term follow-up of 48 months, we remain with only three cases with an ABS, and the complications were always those previously cited.

As reported in Prof. Lehur's chapter, the learning curve is of great importance, as is attention to a very correct procedure in order to avoid the types of complications discussed. We totally agree with his observation; nevertheless, we are observing a decreased interest from many surgeons in the ABS implant. An observation period may be appropriate during which to evaluate the future of surgical treatment of FI; this is the same consideration made about all procedures previously examined. A different perspective is the indication for and application of an ABS as a conti-

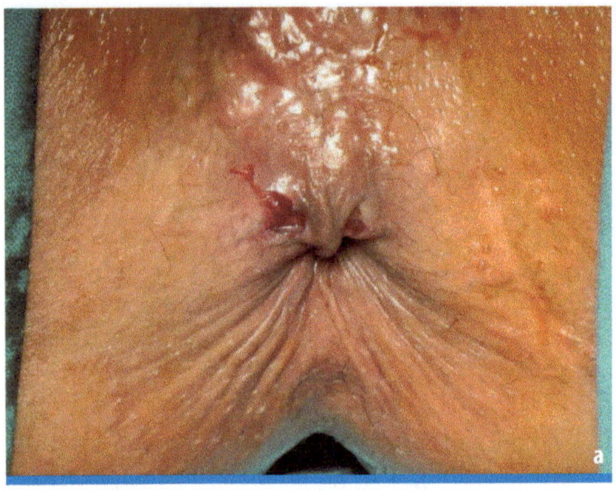

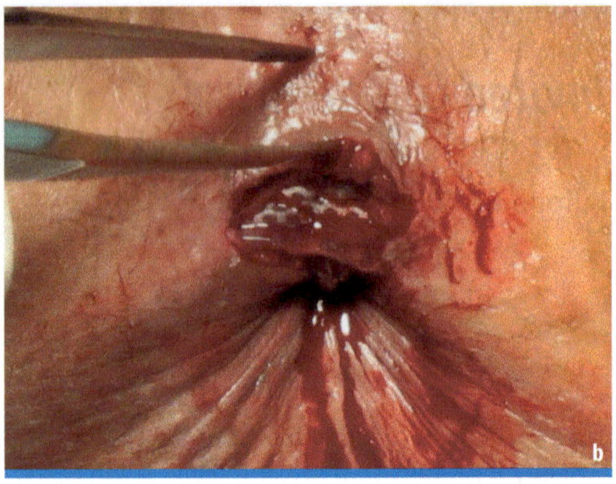

Fig. 1a, b. Skin erosion

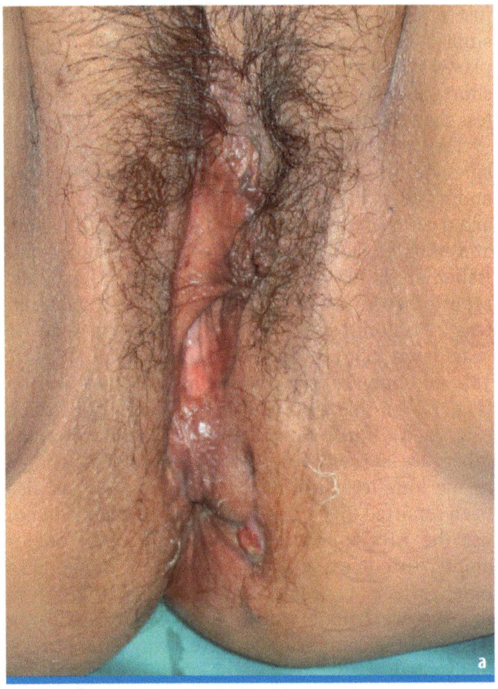

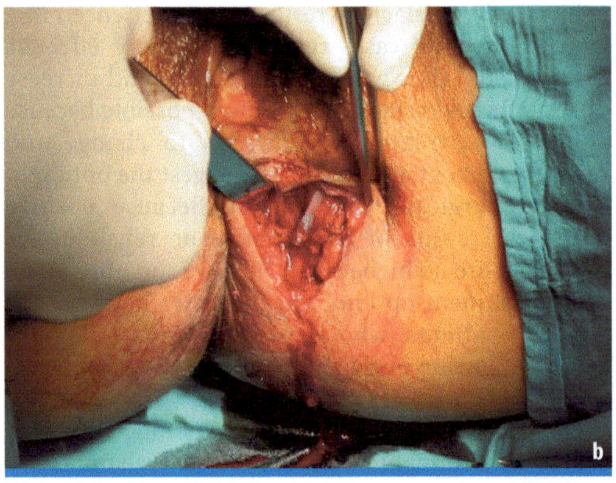

Fig. 2a, b. Fistulization

nence appliance in perineal colostomy [12]. A study reported at the American Society of Colon and Rectal Surgeons (ASCRS) described very satisfactory results in a group of patients converted from an abdominal stoma to a perineal stoma and ABS using a three-step procedure. The results in terms of quality of life were very satisfying. However, the number of applications for this technique are not increasing because the three-step procedure is costly as well as difficult for the patient: in fact, it is very difficult to find both the appropriate selection of disease-free patients or a well-motivated group.

A final opinion regarding the entire field of application of invasive surgery for FI requires a lengthy evaluation period and long-term follow-up to avoid enthusiastic reports and then disappointment. Prof. Lehur's chapter is written from the broad experience of a very dedicated and specialized surgeon. Prof. Lehur has experience in many procedures in the field of FI, and he has contributed very honest and lucid reports to the international literature, as well as his experience with the ABS implant, being one of the first in the experimental protocol. His chapter on the ABS implant is perfect for its descriptions and recommendations for all surgeons interested in the colorectal specialty and also generously describes particulars of the procedure and the function of the prostheses. All this provides very important information regarding technological research in the treatment of FI.

References

1. Ehrenpreis ED, Chang D, Eichenwald E (2007) Pharmacotherapy for fecal incontinence: a review. Dis Colon Rectum [Epub ahead of print]
2. Schiller LR (2003) Treatment of fecal incontinence. Curr Treat Options Gastroenterol 6(4):319–327
3. Coggrave M, Wiesel PH, Norton C (2006) Management of faecal incontinence and constipation in adults with central neurological diseases. Cochrane Database Syst Rev2):CD002115. Update of: Cochrane Database Syst Rev (2001) (4):CD002115
4. Bachoo P, Brazzelli M, Grant A (2000) Surgery for faecal incontinence in adults. Cochrane Database Syst Rev (2):CD001757
5. Bharucha AE (2004) Outcome measures for fecal incontinence: anorectal structure and function. Gastroenterology 126(1 Suppl 1):S90–S98
6. Norton C, Cody JD, Hosker G (2006) Biofeedback and/or sphincter exercises for the treatment of faecal incontinence in adults. Cochrane Database Syst Rev CD002111. Update of: Cochrane Database Syst Rev. (2000) (2):CD002111
7. Christiansen J, Lorentzen M (1987) Implantation of artificial sphincter for anal incontinence. Lancet 1:244–245
8. Lehur PA, Michot F, Denis P et al (1996) Results of artificial sphincter in severe anal incontinence. Report of 14 consecutive implantations. Dis Colon Rectum 39:1352–1355
9. Lehur PA, Zerbib F, Glemain P et al (2002) Comparison of quality of life and anorectal function after artificial sphincter implantation. Dis Colon Rectum 45:508–513
10. Parker SC, Spencer MP, Madoff RD (2003) Artificial bowel sphincter: long-term experience at a single institution. Dis Colon Rectum 46:722–729
11. O'Brien PE, Dixon JB, Skinner S et al (2004) A prospective randomized controlled clinical trial of placement of the artificial bowel sphincter (Acticon Neosphincter) for the control of fecal incontinence. Dis Colon Rectum 47(11):1852–1860
12. Romano G, La Torre F, Cutini G et al (2003) Total anorectal reconstruction with the artificial bowel sphincter: report of eight cases. Dis Colon Rectum 46:730–734
13. Wong WD, Congilosi S, Spencer M et al (2002) The safety and efficacy of the artificial bowel sphincter for faecal incontinence: results from a multicenter cohort study. Dis Colon Rectum 45:1139–1153
14. Ortiz H, Armendariz P, DeMiguel M et al (2002) Complications and functional outcome following artificial anal sphincter implantation. Br J Surg 89:877–881
15. Altomare DF, Dodi G, La Torre F et al (2001) Multicentre retrospective analysis of the outcome of artificial anal sphincter implantation for severe faecal incontinence. Br J Surg 88:1481–1486
16. Klutke JJ (2000) Current status of urethral occlusive devices in management of urinary incontinence. Curr Opin Obstet Gynecol 12(5):415–419
17. Madoff RD (2004) Surgical treatment options for fecal incontinence. Gastroenterology 126(1 Suppl 1):S48–S54
18. Altomare DF, Binda GA, Dodi G et al (2004) Disappointing long-term results of the artificial anal sphincter for faecal incontinence. Br J Surg 91:1352–1353
19. La Torre F, Masoni L, Montori J et al (2004) The surgical treatment of faecal incontinence with artificial anal sphincter implant. Hepatogastroenterology 51:1358–1361

20 Gluteoplasty for the Treatment of Fecal Incontinence

Lindsee E. McPhail, C. Scott Hultman

Introduction

Fecal incontinence is a devastating condition in which patients have extremely poor quality of life, with limitations in social interaction, physical activity, and employability. Defined as incomplete control of the fecal stream, fecal incontinence may be due to a number of factors, such as increased stool production, decreased rectal vault capacitance, diminished rectal distension sensibility, and anal sphincter disruption. Despite such medical therapies as motility inhibitors, stool-bulking agents, biofeedback, and Kegel exercises, these interventions may only provide limited relief from this disabling condition [1].

Disruption of the anal sphincter may be due to trauma, obstetrical injury, or iatrogenic rectal surgery, and therefore, the sphincter may be amenable to primary repair or secondary surgical reconstruction. Patients with partial sphincter function and mild to moderate symptoms may benefit from anterior overlapping sphincteroplasty, especially young women with perineal lacerations or stretch injury from childbirth [2]. If considerable damage has occurred to the pelvic floor or sphincter mechanism, functional transfer of the gracilis or gluteus muscles should be considered [3].

Introduced by Chetwood in 1902 [4], rediscovered by Bruining in 1981 [5], and further described by Guelinckx in 1996 [6], functional myoplasty with the gluteus maximus may provide adequate control of the fecal stream, improving the quality of life in carefully screened patients. Successful outcomes can be achieved, especially in patients with severe fecal incontinence (greater than one episode per day) who have good voluntary control of the reconstructed sphincter. With some training, the transferred muscle is taught to contract when the patient senses distension or filling of the rectal vault. Because the gluteus is a skeletal muscle with the potential for fatigue, patients must locate a bathroom expeditiously, as continence duration is limited.

Gracilis versus Gluteus

No randomized, controlled trials exist to compare the efficacy of the gluteus maximus muscle to the gracilis muscle in creating a neosphincter. Certain factors, such as anatomy and function, as well as the primary reason for fecal incontinence, dictate decision making. At our institution, the gluteus muscle is preferred in patients who require considerable muscle bulk, who need moderate resting tones with high squeeze pressures, who would benefit from a complete rectum wrap, and who have minimal rectovaginal scarring. Alternately, the gracilis muscle is chosen in patients who have a deficient perineal body, who have extensive scarring of the rectovaginal septum (requiring an anterior approach), who have some native sphincter function with moderate incontinence, and who have minimal needs for high squeeze pressures [7–22].

Anatomy and Function

The gluteus maximus muscle arises from the outer surface of the os ileum, sacrum, coccyx, and sacrotuberous ligament and inserts into the iliotibial tract and gluteal tuberosity of the femur. Motor innervation is derived from the inferior gluteal nerve, which is composed of nerve roots L5, S1, and S2; therefore, fecal incontinence secondary to spina bifida or myelomeningocele are absolute contraindications to gluteoplasty [23]. The superior and inferior gluteal arteries supply blood to the muscle at its proximal origin, making gluteoplasty contraindicated in those with Leriche syndrome [6]. Because the neurovascular bundle is proximal, distal muscle transposition has little or no adverse effect [23].

Running, climbing stairs, and standing up from a sitting position are all actions facilitated by the gluteus maximus. Thus, the gluteus as opposed to the gracilis, which plays a supportive role in thigh adduction and hip flexion, is more amenable to reeducation [6]. A natural synergy exists between the gluteus and the external anal sphincter; contracting the gluteus is a reflexive action in response to rectal distention, and hip adduction is not [6]. Furthermore, gluteus muscle bulk generates significantly higher squeeze pressures than the gracilis muscle and provides a generous amount of tissue in which to implant electrodes and seal rectal microperforations [6].

Despite the reported success of gluteoplasty for fecal incontinence, graciloplasty is more frequently performed, for reasons that include ease of harvest, anterior approach, and patient positioning [7–22]. Minimal donor-site morbidity can be achieved via endoscopic harvest or through minimal-access incisions [22]. Disadvantages of the gracilis flap include early muscle fatigue, difficulty training them to contract (which is accomplished via thigh adduction), incomplete rectum wrap, inability to generate a high squeeze pressure, and frequent constipation due to distortion of the anorectal angle. The gracilis may, in fact, serve as a static sling with some contractile properties, whereas the gluteus can generate significant sustained squeeze pressures and add considerable bulk to the perirectal space.

History

In 1902, Chetwood first described the use of the gluteus maximus muscle as an anal neosphincter. Transposing the gluteus muscles by crossing them underneath the ligamentous connection between the anus and the coccyx, Chetwood successfully treated a patient who developed fecal incontinence secondary to trauma [4]. Today, some argue that his reported results are a product of fibrosis as opposed to functionality [5]. In 1944, Bistrom also utilized the gluteus muscle in treating fecal incontinence. He created a hole in the detached origin of the muscle, through which he brought the rectal stump [24].

Over the next half century, attention turned from the gluteus maximus muscle as a potential neosphincter and focused on the gracilis muscle. In 1981, Bruining reintroduced the gluteus, describing a technique in which this muscle is detached from the femur and elevated to the level of the proximal neurovascular pedicle. Both muscles are then wrapped around the rectum, after splitting the distal ends, to form a "scissors-like" neosphincter [5]. An alternate method was described by Hentz in 1982 in which the gluteus is detached at its sacral origin, split, and wrapped around the rectum [25]. Also in 1982, Prochiantz and Gross published a series of 15 patients with fecal incontinence who underwent gluteoplasty with a proximally based muscle flap that functioned as a contractile sling [26].

In 1985, Orgel and Kucan introduced the technique utilized at our institution–the right inferior double-split gluteus maximus muscle procedure. For this operation, the inferior half of one gluteus muscle (typically the right, which is technically easier to harvest for right-handed surgeons) is mobilized at its insertion at the iliotibial band and posterior gluteal tubercle of the femur, divided longitudinally in the direction of its fibers, tunneled around the sphincter, and attached to the contralateral ischial tuberosity. This method, which involves mobilizing only one muscle, has the advantage of decreasing the potential for hip instability [27].

Since 1985, several more studies were conducted investigating the use of gluteoplasty. The vast majority–Yuli in 1987 [28], Pearl in 1991 [23], Devasa in 1992 [29], Christiansen in 1995 [30], Meehan in 1997 [31], and Yoskioka in 1999 [32]–employed the technique first introduced by Hentz: bilateral distally based muscle flap fashioned in a contractile sling about the rectum. Only Guelinckx in 1996 deviated from this majority [6]. His unilateral, proximally based muscle flap, which is tunneled around the rectum and attached to the contralateral ischial tuberosity, resulted in an 82% continence rate, and this procedure is employed at our institution today [6].

A comprehensive review of published cases reveals a limited number of studies with large sample size and objective assessment of long-term outcomes [3–6, 23, 25–35]. Combined data from 17 reports identified 149 patients who underwent functional gluteoplasty for fecal incontinence. This procedure was successful or partially successful in 73% of patients, with a combined major and minor complication rate of 38%. These results are comparable with those of our institution, where we demonstrated a success rate or partial success rate of 88%. Our complication rate, though, was notably higher than that of the combined series, at 64% [36]. However, these studies represent a diverse group of patients in terms of operative technique, with three series using unilateral flaps and 14 using bilateral flaps. Six reports described proximally based flaps, while nine described distally based flaps. Regarding flap fixation, 12 series noted the creation of a sling without boney anchoring, and four reported the use of the ischial tuberosity to secure the gluteal slips.

Surgical Approach and Operative Technique

At our institution, preoperative evaluation includes assessment by a multidisciplinary team that comprises members from general surgery, plastic surgery, urogynecology, and gastroenterology. Workup involves a combination of sigmoidoscopy, endorectal ultrasound, rectal manometry, and pudendal nerve studies. The information provided by these studies helps identify patients with fecal incontinence who are suitable operative candidates, specifically those individuals with good rectal vault capacitance, intact sensibility with rectal distension, and favorable anatomy for transposition of the gluteus muscle. Selected patients may benefit from preoperative biofeedback and training of the gluteus.

After obtaining informed consent and providing discussion of the potential benefits and risks, patients receive a mechanical bowel preparation and are kept on clear liquids for several days prior to their procedure. Temporary diverting colostomy should be strongly considered in high-risk patients with rectovaginal or perirectal fistulas, inflammatory bowel disease, or severe perirectal scarring with perineal deficiency. Topographic landmarks, including the sacrum, infragluteal crease, and borders of the gluteus, are marked in the preoperative holding area (Fig. 1a).

Following intubation and induction of general anesthesia, the patient is transferred to the prone, jack-knife position (Fig. 1b). Perirectal incisions are made laterally at the junction of the skin and anoderm, exposing the contralateral ischial tuberosity (usually the left), which is marked with a braided, permanent suture that is anchored in periosteum and later attached to the tendon of the transferred muscle Anterior and posterior rectal tunnels are developed with blunt and sharp dissection, avoiding rectal perforation. The lower third of the gluteus maximus muscle is then harvested through a sigmoid incision placed near the infragluteal crease. Effort is made to preserve the posterior cutaneous nerve of the thigh. The gluteus is detached from its insertion on the posterior gluteal tubercle of the femur, saving a strip of tendon and periosteum for later fixation to the ischial tuberosity (Fig. 1c)

After identifying and preserving the inferior gluteal nerve and vascular pedicle (Fig. 1d), the infe-

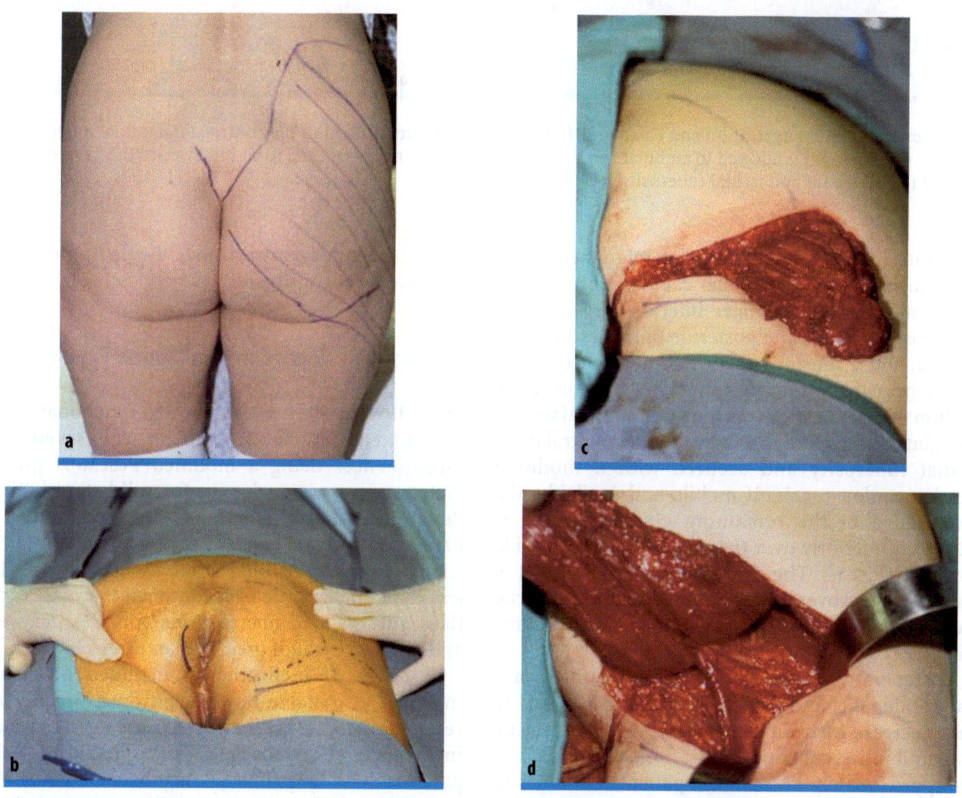

Fig. 1a–g. A 48-year-old woman with severe fecal incontinence (greater than one episode/day) from an obstetrical stretch injury who had a previously failed anterior overlapping sphincteroplasty. She underwent reconstruction of the anal sphincter with a proximally based, unilateral, split gluteus muscle as a functional transfer. She is now able to maintain continence long enough to get to a bathroom, by contracting the gluteus neosphincter when she senses rectal vault distension. **a** Marks in the preoperative holding area. **b** Jack-knife position. **c** The gluteus is detached. **d** Identifying and preserving the inferior gluteal nerve and vascular pedicle (*continued*)

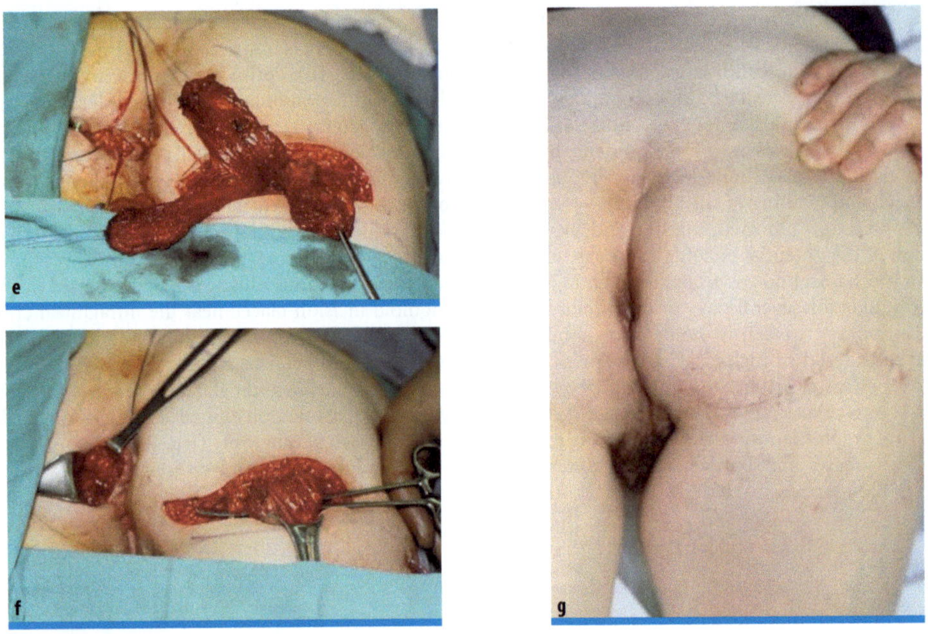

Fig. 1. *(continued)* **e** Transposition and balancing. **f** The gluteal slips are brought to the contralateral ischial tuberosity and secured. **g** The patient is allowed to ambulate on the second day but is not permitted to sit for 2 weeks; thus avoiding pressure on the perineum and ischial tuberosity

rior gluteal flap is elevated from lateral to medial and subsequently split with bipolar cautery. This maneuver creates a slightly longer inferior slip, which is transposed through the posterior tunnel around the rectum, and a shorter superior slip, which is transposed through the anterior tunnel in the rectovaginal septum (Fig. 1e). After transposition and balancing, the gluteal slips are brought to the contralateral ischial tuberosity and secured with a modified Kessler tendon repair. If mobile and available, the lower edge of the remaining gluteus muscle is advanced inferiorly over the sciatic nerve to provide coverage (Fig. 1f). The gluteal donor site is closed in multiple layers over a fluted drain, and the perirectal incision is similarly closed, with vaginal packing placed.

Postoperatively, the patient is maintained on a low-residue diet and given narcotics for analgesia to help decrease gastrointestinal motility. Prophylactic oral antibiotics, covering enteric flora, are prescribed for approximately 1 week. The patient is allowed to ambulate on the second day after the procedure but is not permitted to sit for 2 weeks, thus avoiding pressure on the perineum and ischial tuberosity (Fig. 1g). Within 4 weeks, most patients can perform voluntary contraction of the gluteus, although biofeedback has been necessary in a minority of our patients to guide contraction of the neosphincter and improve fecal continence.

University of North Carolina Clinical Experience

From 1996 to 2004, we performed functional unilateral gluteoplasty in 25 patients with severe fecal incontinence. Using a modified Pescatori grading system to assess continence for solid stool [37], we determined that gluteoplasty was successful in 18 patients (72%) and partially successful in four (16%). Gluteoplasty was defined as successful if patients had less than one episode of incontinence per week, partially successful if one to three episodes per week, and not successful if greater than three per week.

Etiology of incontinence included obstetrical injury (13), irritable bowel syndrome (3), previous rectal surgery (3), Crohn's disease (3), traumatic impalement (1), rectocele (1), and idiopathic (1). Five patients with a primary diagnosis of obstetrical injury also had a secondary diagnosis of irritable bowel syndrome. Gender distrtibution was 22 women and three men, with a mean age of 42 years and a range of 23–65 years. Mean length of follow-up was 20.6 months, with a range of 3–68 months.

Although gluteoplasty was efficacious in improving continence in 22/25 patients (88%), significant morbidity was observed. Two patients required permanent colostomy for refractory incontinence. In terms of donor-site complications, 16/25 patients (64%) developed a combination of posterior thigh numbness (7), dysesthesias (5), cellulitis (5), irregular contour (3), abscess (2), severe chronic pain (2), and hematoma (1), but there was no altered gait or hip dysfunction. Regarding perirectal complications, 14/25 patients (56%) had sinus tract formation (3), flap dehiscence requiring reoperation (2), perirectal abscess requiring temporary fecal diversion (2), chronic pelvic pain (2), vaginal perforation with delayed healing (1), recurrent fistula (1), and rectal prolapse (1). Six patients required readmission for wound care, intravenous antibiotics, or operative intervention.

Despite this high incidence of donor-site and perirectal complications, we concluded that the risk–benefit profile for functional gluteoplasty remains favorable. Although a continence rate of 88% was observed in our series, patients must be adequately counseled and prepared for significant potential morbidity. We believe that careful patient selection, preoperative education, biofeedback, and surgical technique refinement are important determinants of successful outcome.

Future surgical approaches to the management of fecal incontinence include the development of mechanical artificial sphincters [38, 39] and the exploration of alternative muscle flaps, such as the sartorius and rectus femoris, with the goal of improving efficacy and reducing morbidity [40–42]. Furthermore, dynamic stimulation of the muscle flap via implantable electrodes (to help decrease muscle fatigue and by recruiting slow-twitch fibers), shows considerable promise in clinical trials [6, 13–21]. Finally, randomized clinical trials comparing the results of graciloplasty and gluteoplasty would be of considerable value in terms of guiding patient selection and elucidating the efficacy of these two procedures in anal sphincter reconstruction for fecal incontinence.

References

1. Whitehead W, Wald A, Norton N (2001) Treatment options for fecal incontinence. Dis Colon Rectum 44:131–144
2. Oliveira L, Pfeifer J, Wexner SD (1996) Physiological and clinical outcome of anterior sphincteroplasty. Br J Surg 83:502–505
3. Madoff RD, Rosen HR, Baeten CG et al (1999) Safety and efficacy of dynamic muscle plasty for anal incontinence: lessons from a prospective, multicenter trial. Gastroenterology 116:549–556
4. Chetwood CH (1902) Plastic operation for restoration of the sphincter ani with report of a case. Med Rec 61:529
5. Bruining HA, Bos KE, Colthoff EG et al (1981) Creation of an anal sphincter mechanism by bilateral proximally based gluteal muscle transposition. Plast Reconstr Surg 67:70–72
6. Guelinckx PJ, Sinsel NK, Gruwez JA (1996) Anal sphincter reconstruction with the gluteus maximus muscle: anatomic and physiologic considerations concerning conventional and dynamic gluteoplasty. Plast Reconstr Surg 98:293–302
7. Pickrell KL, Broadbent TR, Masters FW et al (1952) Construction of a rectal sphincter and restoration of anal continence by transplanting the gracilis muscle. Ann Surg 135:853–862
8. Niriella DA, Deen KI (2000) Neosphincters in the management of faecal incontinence. Br J Surg 87:1617–1628
9. Akoz T, Civelek B, Gorgu M et al (1998) Anal sphincter reconstruction with bilateral gracilis muscle flap. Plast Reconstr Surg 102:1777–1778
10. Kumar D, Hutchinson R, Grant E (1995) Bilateral gracilis neosphincter construction for treatment of faecal incontinence. Br J Surg 82:1645–1647
11. Williams NS, Patel J, George BD et al (1991) Development of an electrically stimulated neoanal sphincter. Lancet 338:1166–1169
12. Baeten CGMI, Geerdes BP, Adang EMM et al (1995) Anal dynamic graciloplasty in the treatment of intractable fecal incontinence. N Engl J Med 332:1600–1605
13. Wexner SD, Gonzalez-Padron A, Rius J et al (1996) Stimulated gracilis neosphincter operation: initial experience, pitfalls, and complications. Dis Colon Rectum 39:957–964
14. Christiansen J, Rasmussen OO, Lindorff-Larsen K (1998) Dynamic graciloplasty for severe anal incontinence. Br J Surg 85:88–91
15. Mander BJ, Wexner SD, Williams NS et al (1999) Preliminary results of a multicentre trial of the electrically stimulated gracilis neoanal sphincter. Br J Surg 86:1543–1548
16. Matzel KE, Madoff RD, LaFontaine LJ et al (2001) Complications of dynamic graciloplasty: incidence, management, and impact on outcome. Dis Colon Rectum 44:1427–1435
17. Baeten CGMI, Uludag O, Rongen MJ (2001) Dynamic graciloplasty for fecal incontinence. Microsurgery 21:230–234
18. Ruckauer KD (2001) Dynamic graciloplasty in children with fecal incontinence: a preliminary report. J Pediatr Surg 36:1036–1039
19. Williams NS, Ogunbiyi OA, Scott SM et al (2001) Rectal augmentation and stimulated gracilis anal neosphincter. Dis Colon Rectum 44:192–198
20. Zonnevijlle EDH, Somia NN, Abadia GP et al (2000) Sequential segmental neuromuscular stimulation reduces fatigue and improves perfusion in dynamic graciloplasty. Ann Plast Surg 45:292–297
21. Bouamrirene D, Micallef JP, Rouanet P et al (2000) Electrical stimulation-induced changes in double-wrapped muscles for dynamic graciloplasty. Arch Surg 135:1161–1167

22. Ramakrishnan V, Southern S, Hart NB et al (1998) Endoscopically assisted gracilis harvest for use as a free and pedicled flap. Br J Plast Surg 51:580–583
23. Pearl RK, Prasad ML, Nelson RL et al (1991) Bilateral gluteus maximus transposition for anal incontinence. Dis Colon Rectum 34:478–481
24. Bistrom O (1944) Plastischer ersatz des m sphincter ani. Acta Chir Scand 90:431
25. Hentz VR (1982) Construction of a rectal sphincter using the origin of the gluteus maximus muscle. Plast Reconstr Surg 70:82–85
26. Prochiantz A, Gross P (1982) Gluteal myoplasty for sphincter replacement: principles, results and prospects. J Pediatr Surg 17:25–30
27. Orgel MG, Kucan JO (1985) A double-split gluteus maximus muscle flap for reconstruction of the rectal sphincter. Plast Reconstr Surg 75:62–67
28. Yuli C, Xueheng Z (1987) Reconstruction of rectal sphincter by transposition of gluteus muscle for fecal incontinence. J Pediatr Surg 22:62–64
29. Devesa JM, Vicente E, Enriquez JM et al (1992) Total fecal incontinence: a new method of gluteus maximus transposition: preliminary results and report of previous experience with similar procedures. Dis Colon Rectum 35:339–349
30. Christiansen J, Ronholt Hansen C, Rasmussen O (1995) Bilateral gluteus maximus transposition for anal incontinence. Br J Surg 82:903–905
31. Meehan JJ, Hardin WD, Georgeson KE (1997) Gluteus maximus augmentation for the treatment of fecal incontinence. J Pediatr Surg 32:1045–1048
32. Yoshioka K, Ogunbiyi OA, Keighley MRB (1999) A pilot study of total pelvic floor repair or gluteus maximus transposition for postobstetric neuropathic fecal incontinence. Dis Colon Rectum 42:252–257
33. Abou-Zeid AA, Marzouk DM (2000) Gluteus maximus neosphincter is a viable option for patients with end-stage fecal incontinence. Dis Colon Rectum 43:1635
34. Devesa JM, Madrid JM, Gallego BR et al (1997) Bilateral gluteoplasty for fecal incontinence. Dis Colon Rectum 40:883–888
35. Skef Z, Radhakrishnan J, Reyes HM (1983) Anorectal continence following sphincter reconstruction utilizing the gluteus maximus muscle: a case report. J Pediatr Surg 18:779–781
36. Hultman CS, Zenn MR, Agarwal T et al (2006) Restoration of fecal continence after functional gluteoplasty: Long-term results, technical refinements, and donor-site morbidity. Ann Plast Surg 56:65–71
37. Pescatori M, Anastasio G, Bottini C et al (1992) New method of grading anal incontinence: evaluation of 335 patients. Dis Colon Rectum 35:482–487
38. Christiansen J, Sparso B (1992) Treatment of anal incontinence by an implantable prosthetic anal sphincter. Ann Surg 215:383–386
39. Lehur PA, Michot F, Denis P et al (1996) Results of artificial sphincter in severe anal incontinence. Dis Colon Rectum 39:1352–1355
40. Hallan RI, Williams NS, Hutton MRE et al (1990) Electrically stimulated sartorius neosphincter: canine model of activation and skeletal muscle transformation. Br J Surg 77:208–213
41. Konsten J, Baeten CGMI, Havenith MG et al (1994) Canine model for treatment of faecal incontinence using transposed and electrically stimulated sartorius muscle. Br J Surg 81:466–469
42. Girsch W, Rab M, Mader N et al (1998) Considerations on stimulated anal neosphincter formation: an anatomic investigation in search of alternatives to the gracilis muscle. Plast Reconstr Surg 101:889–898

Sacral Nerve Stimulation

21

Klaus E. Matzel

Introduction

Fecal incontinence is a socially disabling problem that is underestimated but widespread. Approximately 2% of the general population suffer from the inability to control bowel emptying [1], and this rate rises with age: up to 11% of men and 26% of women over age 50 [2]. Its impact on society is substantial. Only a small portion of this population has to be treated surgically.

With better diagnostic methods, understanding the physiology and pathophysiology of the continence organ components has improved in recent years. Maintenance of fecal continence is an integrated result of the reservoir system of the rectum and the distal colon, outlet resistance of the sphincteric complex, and the sensory lining of the anal canal. Their functional interaction is attained by a convergence of somatomotor, somatosensory, and autonomic innervation mediated by fibers traveling with the sacral spinal nerves. Sacral nerve stimulation (SNS) potentially affects all of these functions.

The concept of recruiting residual function of an inadequate anorectal continence organ by electrostimulation of its peripheral nerve supply, i.e., the sacral spinal nerves, was adapted from the field of urology in the early 1990s. The rationale for applying SNS to fecal incontinence was based on both clinical observations and anatomic considerations (from the former, the beneficial effect on bowel habits and anorectal continence function and increased anorectal angulation and anal canal closure pressure seen in urologic patients; from the latter, the demonstration by dissection of a dual peripheral nerve supply of the striated pelvic floor muscles that govern these functions) [3]. It was thought that because the sacral spinal nerve site is the most distal common location of this dual nerve supply, stimulation there could both enhance physiologic function [3] and improve the symptoms of fecal incontinence. Subsequently, in 1994, SNS was first applied for the treatment of fecal incontinence [4] in patients with functional deficits of the anal sphincter but no morphologic defect. Patients were selected because conservative treatment had failed, traditional surgical options such as sphincter repair were conceptually questionable, or the benefit of sphincter-replacement procedures, such as artificial bowel sphincter and dynamic graciloplasty, with their high morbidity, would not outweigh the risk in this population [5, 6].

Since then, the technique has undergone continuous development, the patient selection process has been modified, and the spectrum of indications has expanded. Today, the treatment can be considered part of the armamentarium for treating fecal incontinence; however, our knowledge and understanding of its underlying mechanism of action is only slowly improving.

Patient Selection and Indications

Today, fecal incontinence from a variety of causes can be treated with SNS. The current spectrum of applications reflects the evolution and expansion of the initial indication. Initially, SNS was confined to patients with deficient function of the striated anal sphincter and levator ani but with no morphologic defect [4], as residual function of the continence organ would be recruited by electrical stimulation. Thus, initial patient selection for the SNS protocol was based on clinical and physiologic finding of reduced or absent voluntary sphincteric function but existing reflex activity, indicating an intact nerve–muscle connection (confirmed by intact anocutaneous reflex activity or by muscular response to pudendal stimulation with the St. Mark's electrode) [7]. In this group of patients, the causes varied and covered a spectrum from postoperative sphincteric weakness consequent to anal and rectal procedures to total lack of voluntary sphincteric control as a sequela of cauda syndrome secondary to lumbar spine fracture. The latter suggested the potential use of SNS in neurogenic incontinence (Table 1) [6]. The common denominator of the heterogeneous etiologies addressed was reduced function and intact morphology.

Table 1. Sacral nerve stimulation for fecal incontinence: clinical results

Report	Patients	Prestimulation	Stimulation			Follow-up
			Temporary	Permanent[a]	(months)	
Frequency of incontinence episodes to solid or liquid stool over a 7-day period						
Initial concept						
Matzel [7]	6	9 (2–19)	1.5 (1–5)	0 (0–1)	59 (5–70)	
Leroi [8]	6	2 (1–7)	0 (0–4)	0.5 (0–2)	6 (3–6)	
Ganio [9]	5	3(2–14)	0	0	14 (5–37)	
Ganio [10]	16	5.5 (1–19)	–	0. (0–1)	10.5 (3–45)	
Matzel [11]	34	8.3 (1.7–78.7)	–	0.75 (0–25)	23.9 (1–36)	
Modified Concept						
Vaizey [12]	9	8 (2–58)	0 (0–10)	–	–	
Malouf [13]	5	(see Cleveland Clinic Incontinence Score)				
Current Concept						
Rosen [14]	16	2 (1–5)	–	0.7 (0–5)	15 (3–26)	
Kenefick [15]	15	11 (2–30)	0 (0–7)	0 (0–4)	24 (3–80)	
Ripetti [16]	4	12[b]	–	2[b,c]	24	
Uludag [17]	50	7.5 (1–18)	0.67(0–4)	0.8(0–5)[c]	12.0[b]	
Altomare [18]		14	14 (11–14)[d]	–	0.5 (0–2)[d]	14 (6–48)
Jarrett [19]	46	7.5 (1–78)	–	1 (0–39)	12 (1–72)	
		Cleveland Clinic Incontinence Continence Score[e]				
Malouf [13]	5	16 (13–20)	–	2 (0–13)	16	
Matzel [20]	16	16 (12–19)	–	2 (0–7)	32.5(3–99)	
Rasmussen [21]	10	19.5 (14–20)	–	5.5 (0–20)	4.5 (1–12)	
Altomare [18]		14	15 (12.5–17.5)	–	5.7 (2–6)[d]	14 (6–48)

Data presented as median value unless otherwise indicated, – Not available, [a]Data at last follow-up, [b]Median value, standard deviation (SD) and range not available, [c]Follow-up value: median of values at published follow-up intervals, [d]Median values during a 2-week period, [e]Cleveland Clinic Incontinence Score [30]: 0 continent, 20 incontinent

This initial spectrum of indications and the positive clinical outcome were confirmed by single-center reports [6, 8, 10, 22] and recently in a prospective multicenter study (Table 2) [11]. Clinical symptoms, measured as number of episodes with involuntary loss of stool, were significantly improved during permanent stimulation. Approximately 90% of patients experienced a substantial (>50%) improvement, and 50% of patients gained full continence. In a recently published prospective multicenter trial, not only was the number of incontinent episodes or days with incontinence improved during the period of observation, but the ability to postpone defecation intentionally was significantly increased [7, 11, 23].

Recording anorectal activity during temporary

Table 2. Permanent sacral nerve stimulation for fecal incontinence, clinical results; quality of life

Report	Patients	Short Form (SF)-36	Fecal Incontinence Quality of Life			
		Categories improved	Lifestyle coping/behavior		Depression/self-perception embarrassment	
Malouf [13]	5	SF, RE, MH, RF	–	–	–	–
Rosen [14]	16	–	Increased[a]	Increased[a]	Increased[a]	Increased[a]
Kenefick [15]	15	All[a] except HT	–	–	–	–
Ripetti [16]	4	SF[a], RE[a], PF[a]	–	–	–	–
Matzel [20]	16	–	Increased[a]	Increased[a]	Increased[a]	Increased[a]
Altomare [18]	14	–	Increased[a]	Increased[a]	Increased[a]	Increased[a]
Matzel [11]	34	SF[a], MH, RE, RP, BP	Increased[a]	Increased[a]	Increased[a]	Increased[a]

SF 36: *RE* role-emotional, *GH* general health, *MH* mental health, *BP* bodily pain, *RP* role-physical, *SF* social function, *V* vitality, *HAT* health transition, *PF* physical functioning, – Not available, [a]Significant, (adapted from [7])

Table 3. Permanent sacral spinal nerve stimulation for fecal incontinence: anorectal physiologic findings

Report	Patients	Resting Pressure	Squeeze Pressure	Threshold Volume	Urge Volume	Maximal Tolerable Volume
Malouf [13]	5	No effect	No consistent change	No effect	No effect	Increased
Matzel [7]	6	No effect	Increased[a]	No effect	No effect	No effect
Ganio [9]	16	Increased	Increased	Decreased	Decreased	–
Leroi [8]	6	No effect	No consistent change	–	–	Decreased
Rosen [14]	16	Increased[a]	Increased[a]	Decreased	Decreased	No effect
Uludag [17]	50	No effect	No effect	–	–	–
Kenefick [15]	15	No effect	Increased[a]	Decreased[a]	No effect	Decreased
Ripetti [16]	4	Increased	Increased	Decreased	No effect	–
Matzel [20]	16	No effect	Increased[a]	Decreased	No effect	Increased
Altomare [18]	14	No effect	No effect	No effect	Decreased	No effect
Ganio [10]	16	Increased[a]	Increased[a]	Decreased	Decreased[a]	–

– Not available, [a]Significant, (adapted from [7])

testing suggested that the effect of SNS was not limited to the striated sphincter muscle [12]. Subsequently, indications for permanent SNS were expanded to patients suffering from fecal incontinence owing to a deficiency of the smooth muscle internal anal sphincter, to limited structural defects, and to functional deficits of the external and internal sphincters. As with the initial group of patients, the causes varied widely and included scleroderma, degeneration or disruption of the internal anal sphincter with or without concomitant external anal sphincter dysfunction, and idiopathic causes of sphincteric weakness. The symptomatic improvement in these patients was comparable with the outcome in the initial group (Table 1) [13, 15].

During the initial work, it became apparent that the two-step selection of patients with two phases of diagnostic stimulation–acute and temporary–was highly predictive of the therapeutic effect of permanent SNS [7, 23]. Consequently, patient selection was no longer based on a conceptual consideration of the potential mechanism of action but on a more pragmatic, trial-and-error approach. Test stimulation was indicated not by an underlying physiologic condition but by the existence of an anal sphincter and residual sphincteric or reflex function. Contraindications included pathologic conditions of the sacrum preventing adequate electrode placement (such as spina bifida), skin disease at the area of implantation, anal sphincter damage amenable to direct repair or requiring a sphincter substitute (e.g., artificial bowel sphincter, dynamic graciloplasty), trauma sequelae with micturition disorders or low bladder capacity, pregnancy, bleeding complications, psychological instability, low mental capacity, and the presence of a cardiac pacemaker or implantable defibrillator.

This pragmatic, trial-and-error selection process resulted in numerous publications [7, 23]. Most studies have represented patients with very heterogeneous pathophysiologic conditions, thus outlining the range of patients who might benefit from SNS. In only one study is a more defined patient population described: 75% of participants suffered from fecal incontinence of neurologic origin [14].

Most commonly, clinical outcome is reported as an improvement in incontinent episodes or days with incontinence during the observation period and in quality of life. The studies vary with regard to design and number of patients, but there is general agreement regarding the two-step stimulation for permanent implant selection. The short- and long-term effects of SNS have been demonstrated in multiple single- and multicenter trials (Table 3). The favorable clinical outcome data (Table 3) confirm this pragmatic selection process.

Technique

Because no other predictors of SNS outcome exist at present, patients are uniformly selected for operative implantation of a permanent neurostimulation device on the basis of clinical improvement during test stimulation, which is documented with standardized questionnaires and diaries. The testing procedure is most commonly considered therapeutically effective if the frequency of fecal incontinence episodes documented by a bowel-habit diary is alleviated by at least 50% and if the improvement is reversible after discontinuation.

The method of choice for permanent stimulation is unilateral implantation of a foramen electrode on the spinal nerve site demonstrated to be therapeutically effective during the test stimulation phase. Bilateral foramen electrodes can be considered if unilateral stimulation is insufficient and bilateral test stimulation reveals acceptable results [24].

Technical Evolution

The technique has been described extensively [25]. In short, after successful acute stimulation with needle electrodes placed at the target nerve(s) through the sacral foramen, electrodes are placed temporarily to test the clinical benefit of low frequency. Two technical options are used for subchronic percutaneous nerve evaluation (PNE): a temporary, percutaneously placed, test stimulation lead (or multiple leads) (Medtronic model 041830, temporary screening lead; Medtronic, MN, USA) that will be removed at the end of this phase or operative placement of a quadripolar lead, the so-called foramen electrode (Medtronic model 3886). Recently, a less invasive technique that uses a foramen electrode with a modified anchoring device, the so-called tined lead, placed through a trocar (Medtronic model 3550-18), has been increasingly used [26]. Both types of leads are connected to an external pulse generator for screening (Medtronic Screener 3625), the latter with a percutaneous extension cable.

Percutaneous placement of temporary test stimulation leads can be done on just one sacral spinal nerve or on multiple spinal nerves to offer the option of testing the effect of stimulating different sides and levels or of synchronous stimulation of multiple nerves in an awake patient [27]. Placement of the foramen electrode or tined lead is usually limited to one site.

At the end of the screening phase, the percutaneously placed temporary test stimulation lead is removed. If placement was successful, a permanent system consisting of an electrode, connecting cable, and pulse generator is implanted. The operatively placed foramen electrode is either removed if unsuccessful or connected to an implanted pulse generator (so-called two-stage implant [28]) if successful, offering the advantage of identical positioning of the electrode during screening and therapeutic stimulation. Bilateral placement of foramen electrodes, if performed, is based either on improved outcome of bilateral stimulation during the screening phase [24] or on conceptual considerations [29].

Stimulation parameters applied are those from the use of SNS in urology, sometimes with slight modifications. The combination most effective with regard to required voltage and the patient's perception of perineum and anal sphincter muscle contraction is commonly chosen for permanent stimulation: pulse width, 210 μs; frequency, 15 Hz; on/off, 5–1 s; or continuous stimulation. Stimulation level is usually adapted to be above the individual patient's perception of muscular contraction or perianal sensation and adjusted if necessary.

Results

As noted above, in most studies, quantitative measures are used to describe the clinical benefit, such as days with incontinent episodes/period of observation, absolute numbers of incontinent episodes/period of observation, ability to postpone defecation (in minutes), and percentage of improvement. Even though published reports differ with regard to patient population, a general pattern of outcome can be observed (Table 1). Results of the screening phase are reproduced with the permanent implant. When compared with baseline status, the clinical outcome is highly significant.

The complication rate is relatively low [7, 23]. These have comprised pain at the site of the electrode or pulse generator, electrode dislodgement or breakage, infection, loss of effect, or deterioration in bowel symptoms. In only approximately 5% has discontinuation of treatment with device removal been necessary because of loss of effect, deterioration of symptoms, pain, lead dislocation, or infection. When infection has necessitated removal, reimplantation at a later date has been successful [13].

As with indications, outcome assessment has also evolved. Initially, the usual measures were the number of incontinent episodes or days with incontinence during a set observation period (based on bowel-habit diary). Subsequently, aspects of quality of life were added to the evaluation: Cleveland Clinic Incontinence Score (CCIS) [30], Short Form-36 (SF-36) [31], and the Fecal Incontinence Quality of Life (FIQL) index [32]. The therapeutic impact of SNS is most evident when disease-specific quality-of-life instruments are applied. The disease-specific FIQL showed highly significant improvement in all four categories–lifestyle, coping/behavior, depression/self-perception, embarrassment-in both single- and multicenter studies (Table 2) [7, 23].

Anorectal Physiology

Numerous efforts have been made to correlate the clinical outcome of SNS with results of anorectal physiology studies, but the effect of chronic stimulation varies greatly among published reports (Table 3) [7, 23]. Data are in part contradictory, inconclusive, and sometimes not reproducible. The most common finding was an increase in striated muscle function, expressed as improved squeeze pressure. In one study, the duration of voluntary contraction was shown to be increased [33]. The effect on resting pressure and rectal perception is inconsistent, although a trend toward decreased sensory and urge thresholds is apparent. Rectal hyposensitivity improved during chronic stimulation [34].

Rectal manometry (24 h) has indicated that the effect of SNS is not limited to sphincteric function and rectal perception. Reduction of spontaneous rectal motility complexes [12, 17] and spontaneous anal sphincter relaxation [33] are qualitative changes in anal and rectal motility. Changes in blood flow recorded by rectal Doppler flowmetry during stimulation give further indication that SNS affects distal bowel autonomic function [35]. Improvement in anal sensory function and sensibility of the perianal and perineal skin during SNS has been reported in one study [14]. Recently, it has been demonstrated that the physiologic changes induced by SNS can be observed not only on the target organ but also in the central nervous system [36, 37].

Thus, the clinical effect of SNS is likely multifactorial based on multiple physiologic functions. Understanding of the relative importance of each of these functions and their dependence on pathophysiologic preconditions is unclear. It may simply be that SNS works differently in different patients. The number of studies with a homogenous patient population is limited, and most studies represent a heterogeneous aggregation of patients with a wide variety of underlying pathophysiologic conditions selected by pragmatic means; thus, any firm conclusion regarding the underlying mechanism of action is unreasonable. A potential placebo effect is unlikely, and long-term benefit has been shown to be sustainable. Patients who experienced clinical deterioration had their therapeutic benefit restored after technical problems with the neurostimulator, of which they were not aware, were corrected; and lastly, the clinical effect has been confirmed in double-blind trials [11, 38].

Future Directions

The future direction of SNS in the context of anorectal dysfunction is in part already outlined by current research. Various interrelated clinical and technical issues are addressed by ongoing research efforts aimed at increasing our knowledge of the appropriate use of SNS and its mechanism of action.

A broad spectrum of patients is today successfully selected by the current pragmatic approach. Recently, some small case series and individual case reports have investigated the effect of SNS in groups of patients presenting with distinct conditions or well-defined anorectal physiologic findings, e.g., muscular dystrophy [39], a history of rectal resection and neoadjuvant chemoradiation [40], a sphincteric gap requiring surgical repair [41], neurologic dysfunction [42], rectal prolapse repair [43], and rectal resection for cancer [44]. Initial results are promising but need to be confirmed in large prospective trials. This approach hopes to pinpoint clinical predictors of responders, potentially obviating test stimulation; also, by focusing on a distinct pathophysiologic condition, it may be helpful to our understanding of how SNS works.

By applying SNS to patients with sphincteric disruption [42] in whom surgical repair is planned, and thus potentially avoiding repair, the current treatment algorithm for fecal incontinence is challenged. This is of special interest, as we have learned in recent years that the short-term benefit of sphincteric repair deteriorates over time; indeed, after 5 years, it has been shown to be less favorable [45, 46]. However, data of the long-term efficacy and durability of SNS are themselves limited.

Not only are surgical treatment options challenged by SNS, the role of SNS in the treatment algorithm needs to be reconsidered. It is currently viewed as an option if conservative therapy has failed. However, because test stimulation is a highly predictive diagnostic procedure with very limited morbidity, it is used much more liberally to explore potential future patient groups. It will be worthwhile to compare the very early use of SNS in the treatment algorithm with results of conservative treatment.

Electrostimulation of the sacral nerve depends on appropriate placement of the electrode to the target nerve, and anatomic pathophysiology may prevent this. This problem could be overcome with stimulation at the pudendal nerve level with a minimally invasive microstimulator [47]. Although further research is required to prove the efficacy and reliability of pudendal stimulation for anorectal dysfunction, recent work indicates that an even more peripheral stimulation, i.e., tibial, may be beneficial [48].

To increase its efficacy, SNS has been applied bilaterally in only a few patients. It remains to be determined whether bilateral stimulation per se leads to an improved and more durable clinical response. The observed increased effectiveness of bilateral SNS or unilateral stimulation of more than one nerve may depend on the patient's individual innervation pattern [49]. The validity, accuracy, and reproducibility of electrophysiologic testing, whether during treatment to monitor functional changes or during the initial operation to optimize electrode placement, must continue to be investigated to further improve outcome and longevity of the pulse generator.

It is noteworthy that the stimulation parameters, especially subsensory threshold stimulation, are also under investigation. Not only may variations therein increase efficacy by prolonging the battery life of the stimulator; they may provide insight into the clinical effect of SNS, which may in some patients not be dependent on the perception of stimulation [50]. However, a placebo effect is not likely [38].

Outcome has been measured quantitatively by focusing separately on frequency of fecal incontinence episodes and quality-of-life parameters. The indication for a permanent implant has only been based on the clinical effect on incontinence during test stimulation, not on the impact of SNS on quality of life. It is hoped that integrating the effect of SNS on incontinence and quality of life into the decision-making process in a defined manner will be a valid option.

The indications for SNS have been expanded beyond the field of fecal incontinence to slow-transit constipation and outlet obstruction. Preliminary data indicate that it may be beneficial [51] and that this benefit is unlikely to be a placebo effect [52]. Based on these findings, a prospective multicenter trial is ongoing. Not only is the effect of SNS on functional disorders of the colorectum and anus of interest, in the future, its interaction with the anterior and middle compartment of the pelvis and pelvic floor will be important to identify further conditions in which SNS can be of clinical value.

The use of SNS has constantly evolved since its first application for the treatment of fecal incontinence. From selection based on conceptual physiologic considerations, it became a technique applied by a pragmatic approach. Based on the positive outcome, the technique established its place in the current treatment algorithm and is-by exploring new indications with the help of the minimally invasive test stimulation, which can be considered a diagnostic investigation-not only expanding it, but also challenging some paradigms of traditional surgical thinking. However, despite its very positive clinical outcome, increased use, and broadened acceptance, further distribution is hampered by economic considerations. Proof of cost effectiveness is varied [53].

Our knowledge of its mechanism of action remains limited. Further research should be performed on patient selection (based on defined morphologic and physiologic conditions), new indications (with the staged diagnostic approach) and new techniques, long-term outcome, increased efficacy (either by technical modifications or an individualized approach based on physiologic findings), and further determination of the role of SNS in the treatment algorithm. This is a dynamic process with a relatively new treatment concept, and we must constantly reconsider our understanding of anorectal physiology and neurostimulation in the treatment of anorectal functional disorders.

References

1. Nelson R, Norton N, Cautley E, Furner S (1995) Community based prevalence of anal incontinence. JAMA 274:559–561
2. Roberts RO, Jacobsen SJ, Reilly WT (1999) Prevalence of combined fecal and urinary incontinence: a community-based study. J Am Geriatr Soc 47:837–841
3. Matzel KE, Schmidt RA, Tanagho EA (1990) Neuroanatomy of the striated muscular anal continence mechanism: Implications for the use of neurostimulation. Dis Colon Rectum 33:666–673
4. Matzel KE, Stadelmaier U, Hohenfellner M, Gall FP (1995) Electrical stimulation for the treatment of faecal incontinence. Lancet 346:1124–1127
5. Baeten C, Bailey RA, Bakka A et al (2000) Safety and efficacy of dynamic graciloplasty for fecal incontinence: Report of a prospective multicenter trial. Dis Colon Rectum 43:743–751
6. Wong WD, Congliosi SM, Spencer MP et al (2002) The safety and efficacy of the artificial bowel sphincter for fecal incontinence: results from a multicenter cohort study. Dis Colon Rectum 45:1139–1153
7. Matzel KE, Stadelmaier U, Hohenberger W (2004) Innovations in fecal incontinence: Sacral nerve stimulation. Dis Colon Rectum 47:1720–1728
8. Leroi AM, Michot F, Grise P, Denis P (2001) Effect of sacral nerve stimulation in patients with fecal and urinary incontinence. Dis Colon Rectum 44:779–789
9. Ganio E, Luc AR, Clerico G, Trompetto M (2001) Sacral nerve stimulation for treatment of fecal incontinence Dis Colon Rectum 44:619–623
10. Ganio E, Ratto C, Masin A et al (2001) Neuromodulation for fecal incontinence: outcome in 16 patients with definitive implant. The initial Italian Sacral Neurostimulation Group (GINS) experience. Dis Colon Rectum 44:965–970
11. Matzel KE, Kamm MA, Stösser M et al MDT 301 Study Group (2004) Sacral nerve stimulation for fecal incontinence: a multicenter study. Lancet 363:1270–1276
12. Vaizey CJ, Kamm MA, Turner IC et al (1999) Effects of short term sacral nerve stimulation on anal and rectal function in patients with anal incontinence. Gut 44:407–412
13. Malouf AJ, Vaizey CJ, Nicholls RJ, Kamm M (2000) Permanent sacral nerve stimulation for fecal incontinence. Ann Surg 232:143–148
14. Rosen HR, Urbarz C, Holzer B et al (2001) Sacral nerve stimulation as a treatment for fecal incontinence. Gastroenterology 121:536–541
15. Kenefick NJ, Vaizey CJ, Cohen CG et al (2002) Medium-term results of permanent sacral nerve stimulation for faecal incontinence. Br J Surg 89:896–901
16. Ripetti V, Caputo D, Ausania F et al (2002) Sacral nerve neuromodulation improves physical, psychological and social quality of life in patients with fecal

incontinence. Tech Coloproctol 6:147–52
17. Uludag Ö, Koch S, van Gemert WG et al (2004) Sacral neuromodulation in patients with fecal incontinence: A single-center study. Dis Col Rectum 47:1350–1357
18. Altomare DF, Rinaldi M, Petrolino M et al (2004) Permanent sacral nerve modulation for fecal incontinence and associated urinary disturbances. Int J Colorectal Dis 19: 203–209
19. Jarrett MED, Varma JS, Duthie GS (2004) Sacral nerve stimulation for faecal incontinence in the UK. Br J Surg 91:755–761
20. Matzel KE, Bittorf B, Stadelmaier U et al (2003) Sakralnervstimulation in der Behandlung der Stuhlinkontinenz. Chirurg 74:26–32
21. Rasmussen O, Christiansen J (2002) Sakralnervestimulation ved analinkontinens. Ugeskr Laeger 164:3866–3868
22. Matzel KE (2001) Sacral spinal nerve stimulation in treatment of fecal incontinence. Semin Colon Rectal Surg 12:121–130
23. Tjandra JJ, Lim JF, Matzel KE (2004) Sacral nerve stimulation - an emerging treatment for faecal incontinence. ANZ J Surg 74:1098–1106
24. Matzel KE, Stadelmaier U, Bittorf B et al (2002) Bilateral sacral spinal nerve stimulation for fecal incontinence after low anterior resection. Int J Colorectal Disease 17:430–434
25. Hohenfellner M, Matzel KE, Schultz-Lampel D et al (1997) Sacral neuromodulation for treatment of micturition disorders and fecal incontinence. In: Hohenfellner R, Fichtner J, Novick A (eds) Innovations in urologic surgery, ISIS Medical Media, Oxford, p 129
26. Spinelli M, Giardiello G, Arduini A, van den Hombergh U (2002) New percutaneous technique of sacral nerve stimulation has high initial success rate: preliminary results. Eur Urol 208:1–5
27. Stadelmaier U, Dahms S, Bittorf B et al (2001) Efferent innervation patterns during sacral nerve stimulation. Dis Colon Rectum 44(4):A2
28. Janknegt RA, Weil EHJ, Eerdmans PHA (1996) Improving neuromodulation technique for refractory voiding dysfunctions: two-stage implant. Urology 49:358–362
29. Ratto C, Grillo E, Parello A et al (2005) Sacral neuromodulation in treatment of fecal incontinence following anterior resection and chemoradiation for rectal cancer. Dis Colon Rectum 48:1027–1036
30. Jorge JMN, Wexner SD (1993) Etiology and management of fecal incontinence. Dis Colon Rectum 36:77–79
31. Ware JE (1993) SF-36 Health Survey, Manual and Interpretation, The Health Institute, New England Medical Center, Boston
32. Rockwood TH, Church JM, Fleshman JW et al (2000) Fecal incontinence quality of life scale: quality of life instrument for patients with fecal incontinence. Dis Colon Rectum 43:9–16
33. Leroi AM, Michot F, Grise P, Denis P (2001) Effect of sacral nerve stimulation in patients with fecal and urinary incontinence. Dis Colon Rectum 44:779–789
34. Rosen H (2004) SNS-How does it work. European Association of Coloproctology, Geneva
35. Kenefick NJ, Emmanuel A, Nicholls RJ, Kamm MA (2003) Effect of sacral nerve stimulation on autonomic nerve function. Br J Surg 90:1256–1260
36. Braun PM, Baezner H, Seif C et al (2002) Alterations of cortical electrical activity in patients with sacral neuromodulator. Eur Urol 41:562–566
37. Malaguti S, Spinelli M, Giardiello G et al (2003) Neurophysiological evidence may predict the outcome of sacral neuromodulation. J Urol 170:2323–2326
38. Leroi AM, PArc Y, Lehur PA et al (2005) Efficacy of sacral nerve stimulation for fecal incontinence. Ann Surg 242:662–669
39. Buntzen S, Rasmussen OO, Ryhammer AM et al (2004) Sacral nerve stimulation for treatment of fecal incontinence in a patient with muscular dystrophy: report of a case. Dis Colon Rectum 47:1409–1411
40. Ratto C, Grillo E, Parello A et al (2005) Sacral neuromodulation in treatment of fecal incontinence following anterior resection and chemoradiation for rectal cancer. Dis Colon Rectum 48:1027–1036
41. Conaghan P, Farouk R (2005) Sacral nerve stimulation can be successful in patients with ultrasound evidence of external anal sphincter disruption. Dis Colon Rectum 48:1610–1614
42. Jarrett ME, Matzel KE, Christiansem J et al (2005) Sacral nerve stimulation for faecal incontinence in patients with previous partial spinal injury including disc prolapse. Br J Surg 92:734–739
43. Jarrett ME, Matzel KE, Stosser M et al (2005) Sacral nerve stimulation for fecal incontinence following surgery for rectal prolapse repair: a multicenter study. Dis Colon Rectum 48:1243–1248
44. Jarrett ME, Matzel KE, Stosser M et al (2005) Sacral nerve stimulation for faecal incontinence following a rectosigmoid resection for colorectal cancer. Int J Colorectal Dis 20:446–451
45. Malouf AF, Norton CS, Engel AF et al (2000) Long-term results of overlapping anterior anal sphincter repair for obstetric trauma. Lancet 366:260–265
46. Halverson AL, Hull TL (2002) Long-term outcome of overlapping anal sphincter repair. Dis Colon Rectum 45:345–348
47. Matzel KE, Stadelmaier U, Besendörfer M, Hohenberger W (2005) Pudendal stimulation for anorectal dysfunction-the first application of a fully implantable microstimulator. Colorectal Dis 7
48. Queralto M, Portier G, Cabarrot PH et al (2006) Preliminary results of peripheral transcutaneous neuromodulation in the treatment of idiopathic fecal incontinence. Int J Colorectal Dis 21:670–672
49. Matzel, KE, Stadelmaier U, Hohenfellner M et al (1999) Asymmetry of pudendal motor function assessed during intraoperative monitoring. Gastroenterology 116:G4508
50 Koch SM, van Gemert WG, Baeten CG (2005) Determination of therapeutic threshold in sacral nerve modulation for faecal incontinence. Br J Surg 92:83–87
51. Jarrett MED, Mowatt G, Glazener CMA et al (2004) Systematic review of sacral nerve stimulation for faecal incontinence and constipation. Br J Surg 91:1559–1569
52. Kenefick NJ, Vaizey CJ, Cohen CR (2002) Double-blind placebo-controlled crossover study of sacral nerve stimulation for idiopathic constipation. Br J Surg 89:1570–1571
53. Hetzer FH, Bieler A, Hahnloser D et al (2006) Outcome and cost analysis of sacral nerve stimulation for fecal incontinence. Br J Surg 93:1411–1417

Invited Commentary

Franc H. Hetzer

Sacral nerve stimulation (SNS) was developed and initially used in patients with urinary bladder dysfunction by Prof. Tanagho et al. during the 1980s [1, 2]. However, in 1990, to Prof. K. Matzel's great credit, the technique was adapted for use in patients with severe anal incontinence [3]. After anatomical considerations and clinical observations, he applied SNS successfully in patients with functional sphincter deficit [4].

Initially, SNS was a treatment for a highly select group of patients with no morphological defect of the sphincter, a deficit also known as idiopathic fecal incontinence [5]. However, in recent years, indications for its use have dramatically increased. This evolution was possible due to the development of the minimally invasive and highly predictive test stimulation. I agree with Prof. Matzel that patient selection is no longer based on morphological and physiological findings or conceptual considerations; it is a trial and error approach.

Due to the minimally invasive technique and the predictive test stimulation, SNS has become a very early option in the algorithm of surgical treatment of fecal incontinence. Complicated neosphincter procedures, such as dynamic graciloplasty or artifical bowel sphincter, have nearly vanished because of SNS. Even the classic sphincter repair, with its moderate long-term results, is being replaced by SNS. Additionally, an ongoing study evaluates SNS use for moderate fecal incontinence and compares it with the best conservative treatment (diet, medication, biofeedback, and pads) (personal communication by Prof. J.J. Tjandra, 2005).

In my opinion, there are a few things that need to be considered: First, I agree with Prof. Matzel that most new indications (e.g., muscular dystrophy, fecal incontinence after low anterior rectum resection and radiotherapy, and multiple sclerosis) are either based on case reports or single-center studies and have to be confirmed in larger series. Second, SNS is still a young technique without long-term follow-up. This lack of knowledge about long-term results makes a comparison with, for example, overlapping sphincter repair difficult. However, to my knowledge, there is also no randomized study available comparing SNS to classic sphincter repair or to a neosphincter procedure. Third, new medical treatments or technical approaches for fecal incontinence must not only prove their efficiency and safety but show cost-effectiveness. All studies label SNS as a highly safe treatment. The published complication rate is about 20% [6], and most of these complications are minor (e.g., test electrode dislodgement or a break of an extension during test stimulation). On the other hand, SNS is a costly treatment due to the expensive neurostimulator (6,200 euros) and electrode (1,800 euros). Additionally, complications such as an infection at the stimulator pocket can dramatically increase costs. This infection is normally not life threatening, but the infected stimulator and the electrode have to be removed immediately. Fortunately, a couple of weeks after successfully treating the infection, a new devise can be implanted.

As part of the expanded indications, the technique of SNS has changed, as described by Prof. Matzel. Recently, a new, smaller-sized neurostimulator (InterStim II model 3058, Medtronic) has become available, which simplifies implantation and increases patient acceptance. The slightly modified permanent electrode (white marker tip on an all-tinned lead, which provides for correct connection with the neurostimulator) can now be directly connected to the new stimulator. A special extension is no longer needed. Also, to vary the implantation position of the stimulator (e.g., gluteally or abdominally), different lengths of the permanent electrode (28-, 33-, or 41-cm leads, models 3093 and 3889, Medtronic) are available. Furthermore, there is a new patient programmer available (InterStim iCon Patient Programmer, Medtronic) that comes with an easy to read liquid crystal display (LCD) and allows to store four preset programs of stimulation. The patient is able to change those programs if necessary. However, in my experience, the more complicated the electronic tool, the more confusion there is for these, most often, elderly patients. Also, it needs to be considered that whereas it may be reasonable and useful in patients with urinary bladder dysfunction, the benefit of switching between different stimulation patterns is questionable in patients with fecal incontinence.

In addition, a great improvement was accomplished through the development of a new introducing kit by Spinelli et al. [7]. Therefore, I would like to highlight the minimally invasive technique and the advantage of this two-stage procedure. Despite the fact that the tinned lead electrode (model 3889, Medtronic; 1,800 euros) is more expensive than the conventional screening electrode (model 30576SC, Medtronic; 130 euros), published data shows that the success rate of the screening phase is significantly improved, between 30% and 90%, when using the tinned lead [7–9] compared with 26% and 71% when using the conventional test electrode [10, 11]. Two aspects of the electrode may explain these findings: First, the tinned lead electrode is designed for both screening and permanent stimulation; therefore, a change of electrode is no longer necessary at the time of neurostimulator implantation. The electrode position is precisely the same as where it achieved positive screening results, thus, failures after permanent implantation are avoided. Second, the quadripole tinned lead allows for changing the location (pole) of the stimulation during the screening test to correct slight dislocations that may occur in the first days after introducing the electrode. This ability prevents false negative screening tests and increases the success rate of the first stage.

Due to the minimally invasive technique, the implantation of the permanent electrode can be easily performed under local anesthesia. General anesthesia may simplify the procedure for the surgeon but it increases costs. Additionally, we were able to demonstrate that the test electrode placement is more precise in awake patients, as they can report sensitive responses during the procedure. In addition to the visualization of the pelvic floor contraction, patients under local anesthesia were able to tell us intraoperatively if the response was symmetric and whether or not disturbing sensations in the lower extremities were present [8]. The conversion to general anesthesia was rare in our series (3 out of 41 electrode implantations). Limiting factors for the use of local anesthesia are small sacral foramina, which makes the introduction of the foramen needle (model 141828, Medtronic) or the electrode (model 3889, Medtronic) painful. The danger of sacral-root blockade does not allow the injection of local anesthesia in the foramen itself. Both the use of local anesthesia and a tinned lead electrode for the screening process allowed the SNS procedure to be performed in an outpatient setting.

SNS is now a confirmed therapy option in fecal incontinence. Its use in other bowel dysfunctions, such as outlet obstruction and slow-transit constipation, are under evaluation. Complex pelvic floor deficits arise as new targets of chronic stimulation. Urinary and fecal incontinence are often combined symptoms in patients older than 50 years (women ~9% and men ~6%) [12]. Other authors found a double incontinence in up to 25% of patients [13, 14]. For those patients, SNS is a promising therapy option because no other surgical treatment is similarly effective for both forms of incontinence. In the future, the challenge will be to assess pelvic floor disorders and select patients who may benefit from SNS. To do this, an interdisciplinary approach, as that found in pelvic-floor centers, is warranted. Additionally, by concentrating the treatment of SNS in such centers, the success and cost-effectiveness of the procedure will be guaranteed.

References

1. Tanagho EA, Schmidt RA (1982) Bladder pacemaker: scientific basis and clinical future. Urology 20:614–619
2. Tanagho EA, Schmidt RA, Orvis BR (1989) Neural stimulation for control of voiding dysfunction: a preliminary report in 22 patients with serious neuropathic voiding disorders. J Urol 142:340–345
3. Matzel KE, Schmidt RA, Tanagho EA (1990) Neuroanatomy of the striated muscular anal continence mechanism. Implications for the use of neurostimulation. Dis Colon Rectum 33:666–673
4. Matzel KE, Stadelmaier U, Hohenfellner M, Gall FP (1995) Electrical stimulation of sacral spinal nerves for treatment of faecal incontinence. Lancet 346:1124–1127
5. Kenefick NJ, Christiansen J (2004) A review of sacral nerve stimulation for the treatment of faecal incontinence. Colorectal Dis 6:75–80
6. Hetzer FH, Hahnloser D, Clavien P-A, Demartines N (2007) Quality of life and morbidity after permanent sacral nerve stimulation for fecal incontinence. Arch Surg 142:8–13
7. Spinelli M, Giardiello G, Arduini A, van den Hombergh U (2003) New percutaneous technique of sacral nerve stimulation has high initial success rate: preliminary results. Eur Urol 43:70–74
8. Hetzer FH, Hahnloser D, Knoblauch Y et al (2005) New screening technique for Sacrale Nerve Stimulation in local anaesthesia. Tech Coloproctol 9:25–28
9. Scheepens WA, Van Koeveringe GA, De Bie RA et al (2002) Long-term efficacy and safety results of the two-stage implantation technique in sacral neuromodulation. BJU Int 90:840–845
10. Ganio E, Luc AR, Clerico G, Trompetto M (2001) Sacral nerve stimulation for treatment of fecal incontinence: a novel approach for intractable fecal incontinence. Dis Colon Rectum 44:619–629
11. Uludag O, Darby M, Dejong CH et al (2002) Sacral neuromodulation is effective in the treatment of fecal

incontinence with intact sphincter muscles; a prospective study. Ned Tijdschr Geneeskd 146:989–993
12. Roberts RO, Jacobsen SJ, Reilly WT et al (1999) Prevalence of combined fecal and urinary incontinence: a community-based study. J Am Geriatr Soc 47:837–841
13. Soligo M, Salvatore S, Milani R et al (2003) Double incontinence in urogynecologic practice: a new insight. Am J Obstet Gynecol 189:438–443
14. Meschia M, Buonaguidi A, Pifarotti P et al (2002) Prevalence of anal incontinence in women with symptoms of urinary incontinence and genital prolapse. Obstet Gynecol 100:719–723

Injectable Bulking Agents

22

Carolynne J. Vaizey, Yasuko Maeda

Introduction

Faecal incontinence is a common but complex problem that can be difficult to treat successfully. Whereas some patients are helped by antidiarrhoeal drugs such as loperamide or codeine phosphate, this is a holding measure rather than a cure. Surgical treatments are limited, and some are complex with a high morbidity rate. The search for minimally invasive therapies continues. Sacral nerve stimulation is becoming the preferred option in many cases of internal and external anal sphincter dysfunction, but it is expensive and involves a two-stage procedure.

In 1938, an obstetric registrar called Murless reported on the use of paraurethral injections of sodium morrhuate to stimulate the formation of fibrous tissue. Twenty cases of stress urinary incontinence were said to have achieved a "fair degree of success" [1]. Sclerosants have not been used to treat faecal incontinence, but radiofrequency energy has been applied to cause scarring of the anal canal. This treatment, known as the Secca procedure, creates thermal lesions deep to the mucosa at multiple sites and levels in the anal canal. More popular in the United States than in Europe, it has been reported to improve passive incontinence, but long-term follow up is lacking.

Since 1964, urologists have also used injectable bulking agents to close down the bladder neck. The first report of this therapy for passive faecal leakage was nearly 30 years later, in 1993 [2]. Polytetrafluoroethylene (Teflon or Polytef) injected into the anal submucosa in 11 patients resulted in short-term improvement in all. Two years later, the same author used autologous fat harvested from the abdominal wall to bulk up the anal canal. Again, the small number of patients was said to have had good short-term results following submucosal injection [3]. Three years later, there was a case report on the use of injected fat to treat a woman with obstetric-related incontinence. In this case, there had been a failed overlapping sphincter repair, and repeated injections were said to have improved her symptoms [4].

Following the trend in urology, the next agent to be trialled was glutaraldehyde cross-linked collagen injection, or Contigen. This was followed shortly after by trials on Bioplastique, a silicone-based product known as Macroplastique in urinary incontinence. There are currently more reports using this material than any other for treating faecal incontinence, although experience is still limited and injection techniques still evolving. The largest series comes from Australia: 82 patients were randomised to receive silicone injections with or without ultrasound guidance [5]. Pilot studies in faecal incontinence have also been conducted using carbon-coated zirconium oxide beads known as Durasphere and injectable self-detaching cross-linked silicone microballoons.

For a technique described more than a decade ago, relatively little has been published in the literature on the use of injectable bulking agents for faecal incontinence. Even more notable is the lack of randomised trials and long-term follow-up. Many new agents are still undergoing investigation in urology and coloproctology to determine both their clinical efficacy and long-term safety.

The Injectable Bulking Agents

In broad terms, an agent should be biocompatible, nonmigratory, nonallergic, nonimmunogenic, noncarcinogenic, easy to inject and able to produce durable results. Such an agent probably does not yet exist. Scientific studies have looked at particle size in relation to their potential for local and distant migration. It would appear that particles should be at least 80 mm in diameter to avoid phagocytosis and transport throughout the body.

As with sacral nerve stimulation, there is no consistent evidence that this form of treatment results in a significant increase in either resting or squeeze pressures. Objective assessment of outcomes therefore relies entirely on incontinence diaries, scoring systems and quality-of-life questionnaires. Patients are known to be very haphazard in filling out diary cards. The use of quality-of-life instruments in the setting of faecal incontinence may also be questionable, as it appears that any offer of help to these desperate patients, whether successful or not, may be reflected in an increase in scores.

Polytef [polytetrafluoroethylene paste (Teflon PTFE)]: Dupont, Shiner, TX, USA

The main problem with this substance is the small particle size, which leads to distant migration. The particles range in size from 4 μm to 100 μm, with 90% being in the 4- to 40-μm range. Animal studies have shown that particles can be found in the lymph nodes, lungs, kidneys, spleen and brain. Migration leads to poor local durability and, more seriously, to the possibility of chronic granuloma formation at the migration site. Orthopaedic, laryngologic and urological reports have confirmed migration in humans, but no carcinogenic potential has yet been established.

Autologous Fat

Whilst this bulking agent may be readily available, nonallergenic, nonimmunogenic and may have a certain aesthetic appeal for the larger patient, there has been a reported mortality following injection of autologous fat in a urological patient [6]. Pulmonary adipose tissue and lipid droplet embolism was found at post mortem following periurethral injection. There have also been reports of strokes, including fatalities, following autologous fat injection into the face [7, 8]. A further urological case had multiple pulmonary emboli diagnosed on ventilation perfusion scanning. The patient survived after being resuscitated and ventilated for several hours [9].

Results in urology suggest that 6-month outcomes are considerably less positive than those of collagen and no better than saline injections at 6 months. It is unlikely to be trialled again in faecal incontinence using present techniques given the poor outcomes in urology and relatively poor safety record. However, the use of autologous fat continues to be reported in the fields of otorhinolaryngology and plastic surgery.

GAX [(glutaraldehyde cross-linked) collagen; Contigen]: Bard, Covington, GA, USA

Glutaraldehyde cross-linked (GAX) collagen is purified from bovine dermis, enzymatically treated to eliminate telopeptides to decrease antigenicity, and chemically cross-linked with glutaraldehyde to help resist breakdown by collagenases. It is easy to inject through a 21-gauge needle and does not appear to cause problems with granuloma formation. However, in vivo degradation appears to limit its long-term efficacy, and there was also a report of a urethrovaginal fistula following periurethral injection for stress urinary incontinence [10]. A further problem is its antigenicity; therefore, skin testing must be performed prior to definitive treatment injections.

In urinary incontinence, the long-term results of periurethral collagen injections have been described as disappointing and particularly poor in women with intrinsic sphincter deficiency. Even medium-term results were described as only being acceptable. A Cochrane Review found no studies that compared collagen injection with conservative treatment in urinary incontinence [11]. A recent randomised clinical trial comparing collagen injections with surgery for stress urinary incontinence showed injection success rate was 19% lower than surgery 1 year after the intervention [12].

Comparative studies have shown equivalent results with collagen and with silicone particles and carbon spheres at 1-year follow up [13]. Compared with calcium hydroxylapatite, twice as much collagen appears to be required for equivalent results.

PTQ Implants: Uroplasty BV, Geleen, The Netherlands

This agent consists of solid, textured polydimethylsiloxane particles suspended in a bioexcretable hydrogel carrier of polyvinylpyrrolidone [povidone (PVP)]. When its use in faecal incontinence was first reported, it was known as Bioplastique. Since then, the name has been changed to PTP implants and then to PTQ implants. It is the same substance as that used in urology, known as Macroplastique. This is the only injectable bulking agent licensed for use in faecal incontinence in the UK.

The particle size generally falls within the 100- to 450-μm range, but there are smaller particles within the gel. Potential for migration of smaller particles has been suggested, and this could potentially lead to the possibility of granuloma formation. However, animal studies have shown minimal local reaction and a lack of distal migration. There have also been concerns about a possible link between silicone and autoimmune disease, but again, recent data appear to refute this. One disadvantage of this product is its high viscosity, which makes it difficult to inject, with difficulty increasing with needle length. A specially designed gun is supplied for injection into the anal canal, and the agent's smooth deployment may improve with experience.

In 2003, a systematic review of Macroplastique's efficacy in stress urinary incontinence found only two randomised controlled trials. There were 11 pre-experimental and observational studies; no firm conclusions could be made because of poor-quality methodology [14].

This product was licensed for use in faecal incontinence on the evidence of small pilot studies, but more recently, larger studies are beginning to emerge. A recent report noted significant improvement in incontinence score and maximum anal resting pressure following injection under endoanal ultrasound guidance [5]. However, the incontinence score did not incorporate the use of concurrent constipating medication, which is effective in many patients with internal anal sphincter dysfunction. The practicality and efficacy of using endoanal ultrasound outside a trial setting also warrants further debate.

Microballoons: American Medical Systems, Minnetonka, MN, USA

These injectable, self-detaching, cross-linked silicone microballoons with a biocompatible filler material have previously proved successful for treating stress urinary incontinence. Only one study was done in faecal incontinence [15]. Six patients had microballoons implanted into the anal canal submucosa, and all showed good improvement in Wexner's score. The balloons have now been withdrawn from the market because of difficulties with sterilisation.

Durasphere: Carbon Medical Technologies, St. Paul, MN, USA

This product is composed of pyrolytic carbon-coated zirconium oxide beads ranging in size from 212 μm to 500 μm suspended in a water-based carrier gel containing beta-glucan. Pyrolytic carbon is a nonreactive product that has been used in medical devices, including heart valves, for the past 30 years. Injection requires an 18-gauge needle, and the product is radio-opaque. The beads are not biodegradable, but a urological study has shown evidence of significant migration to the local and distant lymph nodes as well as into the urethral mucosa [16]. There was also a recent report of four patients with periurethral mass formation 12–18 months following a Durasphere injection. The patients exhibited symptoms of irritation, pelvic pain or difficulty voiding [17]. Pilot studies conducted using Durasphere in faecal incontinence have recorded mixed results [18].

Calcium Hydroxylapatite/Coaptite: Bioform, Franksville, WI, USA

Calcium hydroxylapatite is a normal constituent of bones and teeth. In its synthetic form, it has been used in dental and orthopaedic reconstruction and in replacement heart valves. Hydroxylapatite ceramic microspheres (CaHA) 75- to 125-μm in diameter are suspended in a carrier gel of sodium carboxylmethylcellulose, glycerine and water. It is nonantigenic and noninflammatory. After injection, the particles become enmeshed within a nonencapsulated, stable, soft collagen matrix, which is said to result in volume maintenance even after the solid particles have been slowly degraded and resorbed.

This product is easy to inject through a 21-gauge needle and is also radio-opaque. However, there is a report of massive urethral mucosa prolapse due to granulomatous reaction 3 months after the transurethral injection [19].

Known as Radiance FN in plastic surgery, this product is best known as a facial soft-tissue filler. A small pilot study in urology showed a substantial improvement in seven of ten women at 1-year follow-up [20].

Deflux [dextranomer/hyaluronic acid (Dx/HA) copolymer; Zuidex]: Q-Med, Uppsala, Sweden

Dextranomer consists of cross-linked molecules of dextran, a glucose-based polysaccharide used as a plasma expander. Dextranomer (Dx) microspheres are 120-μm in diameter suspended in nonanimal stabilised hyaluronic acid (NASHA). It is nonallergenic, nonimmunogenic and nonmigratory. Following degradation, it is said to retain its bulking effects through endogenous soft-tissue fibrosis formation with ingrowth of fibroblasts, inflammatory cells, blood vessels and then collagen.

Dextranomer has been used successfully in treating vesicoureteral reflux in children as young as neonates. One study in adults reported on the long-term results of treatment of stress incontinence. Seventeen of 20 patients had objective improvement or cure at the 6-month follow-up, and over half of the patients available for further follow-up demonstrated sustained improvement after six and a half years [21]. No studies have yet been published on the use of Deflux in faecal incontinence.

Permacol: Tissue Sciences Laboratories (TSL), Covington, GA, USA

Cross-linked porcine dermal collagen is now being introduced as an alternative biocompatible, nonallergenic collagen product with improved durability through revascularisation and cell ingrowth. It is relatively easy to inject.

It has been used in pilot studies for facial contour augmentation and has also been compared with Macroplastique in treating urinary incontinence. At 6 weeks, 64% of patients receiving Permacol were improved on quantified pad losses compared with 54% of those patients injected with Macroplastique. At a 6-month follow-up, results were sustained for the Permacol patients but not for the Macroplastique patients [22].

A prospective study of 32 patients with stress urinary incontinence showed good results in nearly two thirds of patients after 6 months, with an average of 1.1 treatments, and the improvement was sustained at 1 year [23]. There is no literature on its use in faecal incontinence.

Bulkamid: Contura, Soeborg, Denmark

This is a new bulking agent, which is a polyacrylamide hydrogel composed of water bound to cross-linked polyacrylamide. It is easy to inject and nonresorbable. It has an infinite molecular size, which means it is migration resistant. As a homogeneous hydrogel with no particles, it is said to retain elasticity and does not cause hard-tissue fibrosis. It is also nonallergenic.

It is known as Aquamid in the plastic surgical literature. There is one report of its use in urinary incontinence. Of 21 patients injected for stress urinary incontinence, 12 had subjective and objective improvement [24].

Uryx and Enteryx: Boston Scientific, Natick, MA, USA

Uryx and Enteryx are ethylene vinyl alcohol copolymers. Uryx was approved by the US Food and Drug Administration (FDA) as a urethral bulking agent in December 2004, and a report from a multicentre randomised controlled trial showed one third less injected volume than collagen, with both subjective and objective improvement at 1 year after the treatment [25].

An identical ethylene vinyl alcohol copolymer has been used to treat gastrointestinal reflux disease; in this setting, it was known as Enteryx. The technical difficulty of performing this procedure resulted in 11 oesophageal perforations. In one case, death occurred in an elderly patient due to puncture of the aorta. Enteryx was then recalled from distribution in September 2005 [26].

Stem Cells

Muscle-derived stem cells (MDSC) have been injected into the external urethral sphincter. Initial trials in animals showed an increase in leak-point pressure, and there is now a report on the use of MDSC in 42 patients with urinary stress incontinence [27]. Fibroblasts mixed with a small amount of collagen as a carrier were injected into the urethral submucosa, and myoblasts were directly injected into the sphincter. All patients were said to have been either completely cured or improved, with no complications.

A pluripotent population of processed lipoaspirate (PLA) cells has also been investigated in a pilot study [28].

Techniques for Bulking Agent Injection

There is no general agreement as to the ideal method of injection around the anal canal. Two major questions need to be answered. The first is the sites at which the bulking agents should be placed. There are two different groups into which these patients fall. One is the group with a defect in the internal anal sphincter, and the other is the group with a weak but intact internal anal sphincter. With the first group, it is not known whether the agent should just be placed into the defective area or whether the bulk should be distributed more circumferentially. The second group obviously needs circumferential injections, but how many injections should be used? Should the operator try to recreate the haemorrhoidal cushions using injections at the 3, 7 and 11 o'clock positions, or perhaps use four quadrant injections?

The ideal track of the injection needle is also unresolved. There are two main options. The first is to use a method similar to that for injecting oily phenol into piles, where the product is injected via a proctoscope into the submucosa above the dentate line. The second method is trans-sphincterically through a long tract to avoid product back leakage. Under local or general anaesthesia, a longer needle is used to pass through the skin and both sphincter muscles, the tip of the needle being directed to the submucosa above the dentate line.

A further debate may surround the use of either the index finger or endoanal ultrasound to guide the position of the needle tip and accurately place the agent. Should ultrasound guidance really prove to be the optimal method of injection, it will limit the use of these agents to colorectal centres who have this equipment and even further to those who have spare equipment available for use in theatres.

Table 1. Comparison of the different injection methods for treating faecal incontinence

Durasphere study [18]	PTQ implants [29]	PTQ implants [5]
Outpatient department	Outpatient department	Day case
No local anaesthetic	Local anaesthetic	Sedation and local anaesthetic
No antibiotic cover	Antibiotics given	Antibiotics given
Not specified	Laxatives given	Enema
Left lateral position	Left lateral position	Left lateral position
Direct injection	Trans-sphincteric or intersphincteric injection	Trans-sphincteric injection
Submucosal	Submucosal	Intersphincteric space
Site of defect	Above dentate line	Above dentate line
Performed through a proctoscope	Guided by the index finger	Endoanal ultrasound guided or by index finger
Haemorrhoidal injection needle	1-or 2½-in. needle and gun	2½-in. needle and gun
1–4 sites	At a single site for localised defect or multiple circumferential injections for weakness	2, 4, 8 and 10 o'clock positions for weak internal anal sphincter, or 3×2.5 ml into defect plus one injection contralateral to a defect
Maximum 2 ml at each site	Total between 5 and 11.5 ml	Maximum 10 ml
Method of needle withdrawal not specified	Slow withdrawal of needle	Method of needle withdrawal not specified

Table 1 is a comparison of the three methods described for Durasphere and PTQ implant injection. Slow, twisting removal of the needle and hydrodissection, opening up the submucosal plane using a local anaesthetic, have been described as technical advances in urology. The technique we currently use is shown in Figure 1 and Figure 2.

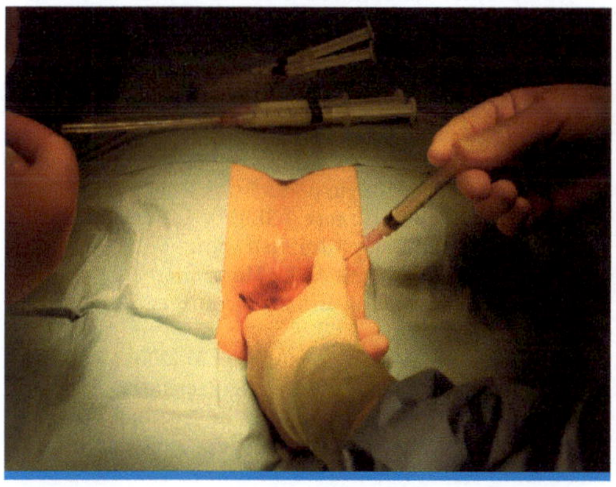

Fig. 1. Markings at 3, 7 and 11 o'clock positions. The needle is inserted trans-sphincterically under digital guidance

Conclusion

Many colorectal surgeons are experimenting with injectable bulking agents for the treatment of passive faecal leakage. This is being done in the absence of good scientific supporting evidence. Fortunately, using nonautologous agents appears to be a relatively safe practice and does not compromise further therapy should it be needed. Until irrefutable evidence is available, all cases injected should be audited, including details on efficacy and safety.

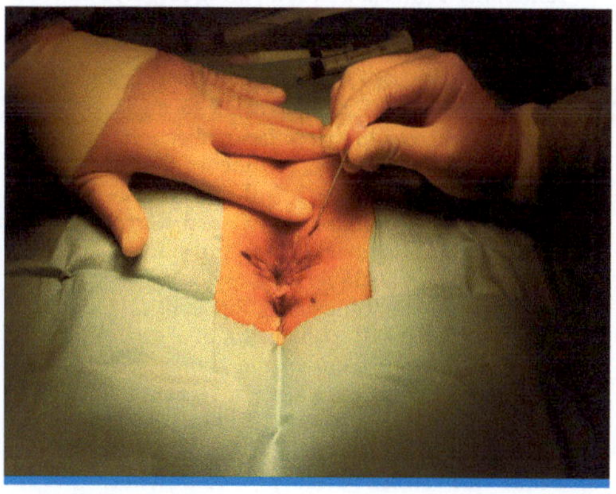

Fig. 2. Needle withdrawal. The needle is pulled out slowly with a rotating movement

References

1. Murless BC (1938) The injection treatment of stress incontinence. J Obstet Gynaecol Br Emp 45:67–73

2. Shafik A (1993). Polytetrafluoroethylene injection for the treatment of partial fecal incontinence. Int Surg 78(2):159–161
3. Shafik A (1995) Perianal injection of autologous fat for treatment of sphincteric incontinence. Dis Colon Rectum 38(6):583–587
4. Bernardi C, Favetta U, Pescatori M (1998) Autologous fat injection for treatment of fecal incontinence: manometric and echographic assessment. Plast Reconstr Surg 102(5):1626–1628
5. Tjandra JJ, Lim JF, Hiscock R, Rajendra P (2004) Injectable silicone biomaterial for fecal incontinence caused by internal anal sphincter dysfunction is effective. Dis Colon Rectum 47(12):2138–2146
6. Currie I, Drutz HP, Deck J, Oxorn D (1997) Adipose tissue and lipid droplet embolism following periurethral injection of autologous fat: case report and review of the literature. Int Urogynecol J Pelvic Floor Dysfunct 8(6):377–380
7. Yoon SS, Chang DI, Chung KC (2003) Acute fatal stroke immediately following autologous fat injection into the face. Neurology 61(8):1151–1152
8. Thaunat O, Thaler F, Loirat P (2004) Cerebral fat embolism induced by facial fat injection. Plast Reconstr Surg 113(7):2235–2236
9. Sweat SD, Lightner DJ (1999) Complications of sterile abscess formation and pulmonary embolism following periurethral bulking agents. J Urol 161(1):93–96
10. Carlin BI, Klutke CG (2000) Development of urethrovaginal fistula following periurethral collagen injection. J Urol 164:124
11. Pickard R, Reaper J, Wyness L (2003) Periurethral injection therapy for urinary incontinence in women. Cochrane Database Syst Rev 2:CD003881
12. Corcos J, Collet JP, Shapiro S et al (2005) Multicenter randomized clinical trial comparing surgery and collagen injections for treatment of female stress urinary incontinence. Urology 65(5):898–904
13. Chrouser KL, Fick F, Goel A et al (2004) Carbon coated zirconium beads in beta-glucan gel and bovine glutaraldehyde cross-linked collagen injections for intrinsic sphincter deficiency: continence and satisfaction after extended followup. J Urol 171(3):1152–1155
14. ter Meulen PH, Berghmans LC, van Kerrebroeck PE (2003) Systematic review: efficacy of silicone microimplants (Macroplastique) therapy for stress urinary incontinence in adult women. Eur Urol 44(5):573–582
15. Feretis C, Benakis P, Dailianas A et al (2001) Implantation of microballoons in the management of fecal incontinence. Dis Colon Rectum 44(11):1605–1609
16. Pannek J, Brands FH, Senge T (2001) Particle migration after transurethral injection of carbon coated beads for stress urinary incontinence. J Urol 166(4):1350–1353
17. Madjar S, Sharma AK, Waltzer WC et al (2006) Periurethral mass formations following bulking agent injection for the treatment of urinary incontinence. J Urol 175(4):1408–1410
18. Davis K, Kumar D, Poloniecki J (2003) Preliminary evaluation of an injectable anal sphincter bulking agent (Durasphere) in the management of faecal incontinence. Aliment Pharmacol Ther 18(2): 237–243
19. Palma PC, Riccetto CL, Martins MH et al (2006) Massive prolapse of the urethral mucosa following periurethral injection of calcium hydroxylapatite for stress urinary incontinence. Int Urogynecol J Pelvic Floor Dysfunct 17(6):670–671
20. Mayer R, Lightfoot M, Jung I (2001) Preliminary evaluation of calcium hydroxylapatite as a transurethral bulking agent for stress urinary incontinence. Urology 57(3):434–438
21. Stenberg AM, Larsson G, Johnson P (2003) Urethral injection for stress urinary incontinence: long-term results with dextranomer/hyaluronic acid copolymer. Int Urogynecol J Pelvic Floor Dysfunct 14(5):335–338; discussion 338
22. Bano F, Barrington JW, Dyer R (2005) Comparison between porcine dermal implant (Permacol) and silicone injection (Macroplastique) for urodynamic stress incontinence. Int Urogynecol J Pelvic Floor Dysfunct 16(2):147–150; discussion 150
23. Teo R, Mayne C, Barrington J, Freeman R (2004) An open clinical evaluation of Permacol injection as new urethral bulking agent: an updated 12 month follow-up. In: International Continence Society (ICS) 34th annual meeting. Paris
24. Lose G (2004) A new bulking agent (Aquamid) in treating female stress urinary incontinence. In: International Continence Society (ICS) 34th Annual Meeting. Paris
25. Dmochowski R, Herschorn S, Karram M et al (2004) Multicenter randomized controlled trial to evaluate Uryx urethral bulking agent in treating female stress urinary incontinence: comparison of initial and expansion phases of trial. In: International Continence Society (ICS) 34th Annual Meeting. Paris
26. Schultz DG (2005) FDA Preliminary Public Health Notification*: Recall of Boston Scientific procedure kits and injector single packs for treatment of gastroesophageal reflux disease (GERD). In: Health CfDaR (ed) Food and Drug Administration
27. Strasser H, Marksteiner R, Margreiter E et al (2004 Stem cell therapy for urinary incontinence. Urologe A 43(10):1237–1241
28. Jack GS, Almeida FG, Zhang R et al (2001) Processed lipoaspirate cells for tissue engineering of the lower urinary tract: implications for the treatment of stress urinary incontinence and bladder reconstruction. J Urol 174(5):2041–2045
29. Malouf AJ, Vaizey CJ, Norton CS, Kamm MA (2001) Internal anal sphincter augmentation for fecal incontinence using injectable silicone biomaterial. Dis Colon Rectum 44(4):595–600

Invited Commentary

Joe J. Tjandra

At the community level, passive fecal incontinence is the most common cause of fecal incontinence [1]. Dietary management, bulking agents, and pelvic floor exercises have only limited efficacy and at best are holding measures rather than a cure. Injectable therapy has the attraction of being simple and safe, and it appears to be effective.

Of the agents that have undergone trial for fecal incontinence, injectable PTQ implant (Uroplasty BV, Geleen, The Netherlands) is the best studied. The treatment by injectable PTQ implant is most effective if administered under guidance of endoanal ultrasound rather than by digital palpation [2]. In the largest reported series [2], the injection is directed into the intersphincteric space in the four quadrants. If there is a defect of the internal anal sphincter, three injections are directed into the defect, with the fourth injection into the contralateral site to provide symmetry. Overall, 68% of patients have >50% improvement in Wexner incontinence score at 12 months after injection. The improvement becomes clinically apparent around 6–8 weeks after injection to allow ingrowth of collagen tissues. Clinical improvement continues up to 12 months after injection. There is, however, deterioration in function with time in that by 3 years after injection, the median Wexner incontinence score deteriorated from 4.5 to 8.5 [3]. Reinjection can be performed safely, with further improved function [4].

A randomized trial comparing injectable PTQ implant with Durasphere (Carbon Medical Technologies, St. Paul, MN, USA) has recently been completed and reported in the 2007 Annual Meeting of the American Society of Colon and Rectal Surgeons [5]. At 12 months after injection, injectable PTQ implant was significantly more effective than Durasphere. In addition, Durasphere was associated with significantly more toxicity, including type III hypersensitivity reaction in a patient [5]. Permacol (TSL, Covington, GA, USA) and Bulkamid (Contura, Soeborg, Denmark) have only been evaluated in small pilot studies and do not appear to have significant efficacy based on these small studies (personal communication).

Injectable therapy is simple and effective. Its role, however, is largely limited to patients with passive fecal incontinence or fecal seepage due to internal sphincter dysfunction. This is not the therapy for severe fecal incontinence, which is better treated with more vigorous therapy such as sacral nerve stimulation [1]. Injectable PTQ implant appears to be the most effective injectable agent available thus far. Logically, other, newer injectable agents ought to be compared against the injectable PTQ implant. A major concern with all injectable bulking agents is the cost of the agent, which might deter a wider adoption of it use.

References

1. Tjandra JJ, Tan JJY (2007) Evolving therapy for fecal incontinence. Dis Colon Rectum (in press)
2. Tjandra JJ, Lim JF, Hiscock R, Rajendra P (2004) Injectable silicone biomaterial for fecal incontinence due to internal anal sphincter dysfunction is effective. Dis Colon Rectum 47:2138–2146
3. Tjandra JJ, Tan J, Lim JF, Murray-Green C (2006) Long-term results of injectable silicone biomaterial for passive fecal incontinence – a randomized trial. Dis Colon Rectum 49:730–731
4. Tan JJ, Tjandra J (2006) Reinjection of injectable silicone biomaterial (PTQ™) is not as effective as the initial injection. Dis Colon Rectum 49:761
5. Tjandra JJ, Yeh H, Chan M (2007) Injectable silicone biomaterial is more effective than Durasphere® in treating passive fecal incontinence – a randomized trial. Dis Colon Rectum (*in press*)

Radiofrequency

23

Jenny Speranza, Steven D. Wexner

Radiofrequency

Radiofrequency energy delivery (Secca® procedure; Curon Medical) is a newer modality for treating fecal incontinence originally used for treating gastroesophageal reflux disease [1], benign prostatic hyperplasia [2], and joint-capsule laxity [3]. After being found a safe and effective means of strengthening tissues, its beneficial effects were first used within the anal canal in Mexico in 1999. Since then, demonstrated improvements have prompted further investigation, with promising results, for use within the anal canal. The radiofrequency generator produces heat by a high-frequency, alternating current that flows from two electrodes–active and dispersive–causing frictional movement of ions and tissue heating [4]. This procedure is not an option for obvious sphincter defects but can be used with a weak or thinned anal sphincter complex. Patients with a history of inflammatory bowel disease (IBD), extensive perianal disease, or chronic diarrhea should not be offered this treatment.

The exact mechanism of action is unknown, although the current hypothesis is that the temperature-controlled energy heats the tissue causing collagen contraction and initiates focal wound healing in the sphincter muscle, actually tightening the tissue [5]. Preliminary animal studies demonstrated small areas of fibrosis within the anal sphincter [6]. In a prospective follow-up study of ten women, Takahashi et al. [7] showed that symptomatic improvement persists for 2 years after delivery of radiofrequency energy to the anal canal. The patients answered questionnaires including the Cleveland Clinic Florida Fecal Incontinence (CCF-FI) scale, Fecal Incontinence Quality of Life (FIQOL) score, and the Short Form-36 (SF-36) at baseline and at 1, 2, 3, 6, 12, and 24 months after the procedure. At 24 months, the CCF-FI score improved from 13.8 to 7.3. The FIQOL score also improved significantly. There was no decrease in effect shown from 12 to 24 months postprocedure. Of note, manometric studies show a significant reduction in initial and maximal rectal volumes, although resting and squeeze pressures have not been demonstrated to change after treatment [7].

Patients who may be candidates for this treatment should have no definite sphincter defect, as overlapping sphincteroplasty is still the optimal treatment. Radiofrequency can still be used as an adjunct post sphincter repair. Patients who have IBD, chronic diarrhea, anal fissure, or abscesses should not undergo this treatment.

The procedure itself is simple to perform, requires minimal sedation, and can be performed in an ambulatory setting requiring no hospital admission. The patient is placed in the prone jackknife position with the buttocks taped apart. The handheld disposable anoscope (Fig. 1) is inserted into the anal canal 1 cm distal to the anal verge. The needle electrodes are deployed, and the radiofrequency energy is delivered deep within the muscle, while the mucosa and submucosa are cooled by constant external irrigation. The needle electrodes contain sensors to prevent overheating and tissue desiccation. The energy is

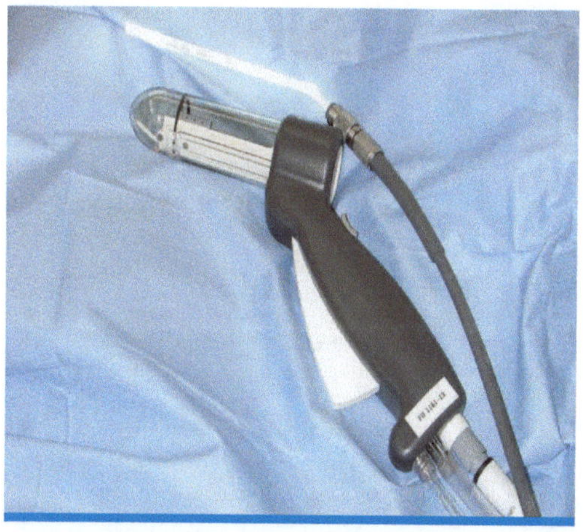

Fig. 1. Handheld disposable anoscope is inserted into the anal canal 1 cm distal to the anal verge

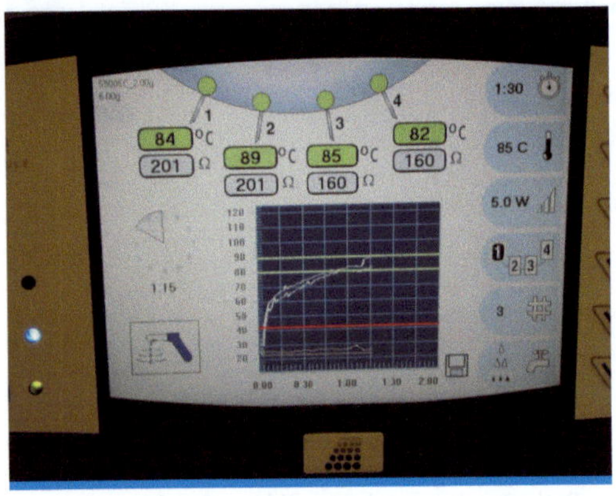

Fig. 2. The main control unit displays the time elapsed and tissue and mucosal surface temperature

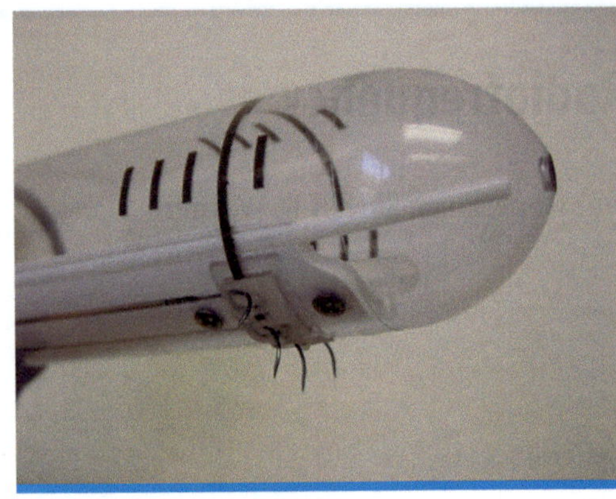

Fig. 3. The main control unit also displays the resistance of each electrode

deployed for 90 s to achieve a temperature of 85 °C. If the resistance or the mucosal tissue becomes too high, the energy being delivered to the tissue will be automatically discontinued. The main control unit (Fig. 2) displays the time elapsed, tissue and mucosal surface temperature, and the resistance of each electrode (Fig. 3). This procedure is carried out in 0.5-cm increments proximally along the distance of the internal sphincter and then repeated in each quadrant of the anal canal. By the end of the procedure, approximately 16–20 thermal lesions are created along the internal anal sphincter (Fig. 4).

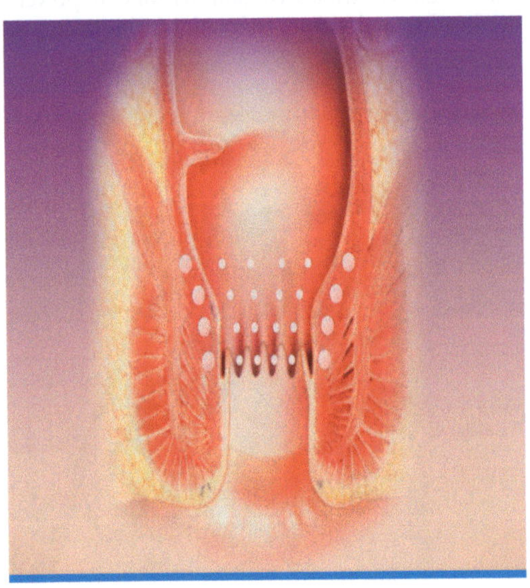

Fig. 4. By the end of the procedure, 16–20 thermal lesions have been created along the internal anal sphincter

Radiofrequency energy has proven to be an effective modality in treating fecal incontinence. In a multicenter study, Efron et al. [8] demonstrated a significant improvement in both CCF-FI and FIQOL scores. Fifty patients at five centers were enrolled. Initially and 6 months postprocedure, patients completed the CCF-FI score, the FIQOL score, the SF-36, and visual analog scale (VAS). At 6 months, the CCF-FI score improved from 14.5 to 11.1 ($p<0.0001$). FIQOL scores all improved significantly, although anal manometry and anal ultrasound showed no changes. Complications were minimal and included mucosal ulceration and delayed bleeding in one patient.

Radiofrequency energy delivery is minimally invasive requiring only sedation and can be performed on an outpatient basis. It is ideal as a preliminary step in a patient with multiple comorbidities who may not be able to tolerate a lengthier procedure. Radiofrequency energy delivery has been shown to be a relatively safe treatment with minimal morbidity, including mucosal ulceration and bleeding [8]. It is a simple procedure that can be used alone or in conjunction with other modalities in the challenging, often difficult realm of treating fecal incontinence. The Secca procedure is approved by the US Federal Drug Administration for use in the United States. However, the Curon Company filed bankruptcy on November 15, 2006, and therefore this technology is not available at the time of publication of this chapter.

References

1. Triadafilopoulos G, DiBaise JK, Nostrant TT et al (2002) The Stretta procedure for the treatment of

GERD: 6 and 12 month follow-up of the U.S. open label trial. Gastrointest Endosc 55:149–156

2. Issa MM, Oesterling JE (1996) Transurethral needle ablation (TUNA): an overview of radiofrequency thermal therapy for the treatment of benign prostatic hyperplasia. Curr Opin Urol 6:20–27
3. Hecht P, Hayashi K, Cooley AJ et al (1998) The thermal effect of monopolar radiofrequency energy on the porperties of joint capsule. An in vivo histologic study using a sheep model. Am J Sports Med 26:808–814
4. Person B, Wexner S (2005) Advances in the surgical treatment of fecal incontinence. Surg Innovation 12:7–21
5. Gustavson KH (1964) On the chemistry of collagen. Fed Proc 23:613–617
6. Takahashi T, Garcia-Osogobio S, Valdovinos M et al (2002) Radio-frequency energy delivery to the anal canal for the treatment of fecal incontinence. Dis Colon Rectum 45:915–922
7. Takahashi T, Garcia-Osogobio S, Valdovinos M et al (2003) Extended two-year results of radio-frequency energy delivery for the treatment of fecal incontinence(the Secca Procedure). Dis Colon Rectum 46:711–715
8. Efron, JE, Corman ML, Fleshman J et al (2003) Safety and effectiveness of temperature-controlled radio-frequency energy delivery to the anal canal (Secca® procedure) for the treatment of fecal incontinence. Dis Colon Rectum 46:1606–1616

Physiological Parameters Predicting the Outcome of Surgical and Nonsurgical Treatment of Fecal Incontinence

24

Donato F. Altomare, Marcella Rinaldi

Introduction

Fecal incontinence is a multifactorial disease. Anorectal physiology studies play an outstanding role in the evaluation of its etiology and severity, the two main factors that constitute the basis for the correct choice of treatment. However, the prognostic role of clinical factors and anorectal physiological tests in predicting the outcome to either conservative or surgical treatment is questionable.

Conservative Treatment

Biofeedback training, in association with kinesitherapy and electrostimulation, is an effective first-line treatment for anal incontinence in patients with no important sphincteric defect, leading to improvement rates ranging between 50% and 92% in different studies [1] (65–75% in reviews). Several clinical conditions; physiological anorectal tests, especially anal manometry, pundendal nerve terminal motor latency (PNTML), anal sphincter electromyogram (EMG), and transanal ultrasound (US) and different treatment methods have been investigated for their possible prognostic value. However, their significance is still uncertain due to the wide range of variability in the definition of fecal incontinence, in treatment protocols, and in the definition of a successful outcome; the short duration of the follow-up or the lack of follow-up data are other aspects contributing to the confusion. Patient age, and duration and severity of the fecal incontinence were not found to be predictive of the response; on the contrary, patient motivation and etiology of the fecal incontinence (postsurgical or traumatic) were found to be associated with outcome [2, 3].

Manometric Parameters

Manometric parameters are the most extensively studied factors. In a group of 28 incontinent patients treated with biofeedback, Sangwan et al. [4] found that, except for increased cross-sectional asymmetry in the high-pressure zone, which may be a forerunner of an adverse outcome, manometric parameters (resting and squeezing anal canal pressure, pressure volume, sphincter length, sphincter fatigue rate) before biofeedback failed to reveal any statistically significant differences between responders and nonresponders. Improvement in continence may be independent of resting and squeezing pressures achieved after biofeedback therapy.

In a retrospective analysis of 145 consecutive patients, Fernandez-Fraga et al. [5] found that response to biofeedback training, performed by means of a manometric technique, was not influenced by basal anal pressures, anal canal length, or squeeze pressures. The rectoanal inhibitory reflex was normal in all patients. In a prospective study of 30 patients treated with electromyographic-based biofeedback training, Rieger et al. [6] found that pretreatment resting or squeezing pressures were unable to predict therapy results. Chiarioni et al. [7] studied 24 patients with frequent solid-stool incontinence; sensory discrimination training and sphincter strengthening training were both provided. Baseline measures that predicted a positive treatment response were lower (closer to normal) sensory threshold (for first sensation and urge to defecate), and lower thresholds for the rectoanal inhibitory reflex and for automatic external anal sphincter contractions during sensory testing, which were significant predictors of biofeedback response. Neither anal squeeze pressure nor incontinence severity was predictive of treatment outcome. Improved rectal sensation, expressed by a decreased threshold to rectal distension volume inducing sphincter contraction during biofeedback training, was found to be consistently associated with a good outcome in two other studies [2, 8].

Pudendal Nerve Terminal Motor Latencies and Anal Ultrasound

PNTML and anal US are included in the standard pretreatment evaluation of fecal incontinence patients, but there is conflicting evidence about their predictive value of the outcome after biofeedback therapy. In a study by Rieger et al. [6] of 30 patients who demonstrated anal sphincter disruption, a positive result to biofeedback training was achieved in six patients with sphincter injury, indicating that a sphincter defect does not preclude symptom improvement. Similarly, evidence of pudendal neuropathy using PNTML (7/14) did not preclude symptom improvement (3/7) after biofeedback therapy.

In agreement with Rieger et al. [6], Leroi et al. [9] found that improvement may be expected despite an external anal sphincter defect demonstrated at endoanal US. Incontinence severity and the occurrence of pudendal neuropathy, shown by an abnormal PNTML, should be considered poor prognostic factors after biofeedback therapy. This negative impact of pudendal neuropathy on the outcome of biofeedback therapy is confirmed by other authors [2, 3], who found that patients with traumatic or iatrogenic sphincter injury have better results after biofeedback therapy than do patients with neurogenic fecal incontinence in which both the afferent and efferent pathways are impaired. In the authors' conclusions, PNTML has an important prognostic role prior to biofeedback therapy, and the latter is not the therapy of choice for fecal incontinence related to pudendal neuropathy.

Surgical Treatment

It is very difficult to identify parameters predicting the outcome of surgical therapy for fecal incontinence because of the variety of currently available surgical options, which can be subdivided into procedures that repair or strengthen the sphincter mechanism, and neosphincter construction procedures using autologous tissue or artificial devices. Finally, a technique of sacral root neuromodulation may be performed.

Postanal Repair

Posterior levatorplasty is intended to improve continence by sharpening the anorectal angle while lengthening the anal canal. Early success rates range between 32% and 87%, but in a long-term analysis, it dropped to 33% [10]. The authors found that pudendal neuropathy was the only predictor of a negative outcome after postanal repair. However, this was not confirmed in a subsequent study by Mavrantonis et al. of the Cleveland Clinic (Florida) [11], in which neither clinical nor physiological variables were predictive of success.

Sphincteroplasty

Overlapping sphincteroplasty is the operation of choice in patients with an anterior external anal sphincter defect, especially in postobstetric trauma. Overlapping without excision of the scar tissue, as suggested by Slade et al. [12], significantly improves functional results compared with initial reports. This is the most extensively investigated procedure for treatment of fecal incontinence, and many studies have analyzed the prognostic value of anal physiology tests. Whereas the absence of a correlation between preoperative manometric, ultrasonographic, and electromyographic parameters and outcome is commonly accepted, many authors have considered the role of pudendal neuropathy, and despite conflicting results, some suggest that it may be predictive of a poor outcome.

Laurberg et al. [13] were the first to demonstrate the correlation between the absence of pudendal neuropathy and the success of sphincteroplasty in a group of 19 patients, achieving 80% positive results in those without pudendal neuropathy versus 11% in patients with neuropathy. Similar results were subsequently published by other authors [14–21]. In particular, Sangwan et al. [19] described good results after sphincteroplasty only in patients in whom both pudendal nerves were normal. The relationship between pudendal nerve condition and repair success is not universally accepted [22, 23]. In a group of 42 patients, Nikiteas et al. found no correlation between failure and pudendal neuropathy, nor did a manometric preoperative evaluation have a predictive value [24]; Rasmussen et al. [25] Young et al. [26], and Chen et al. confirmed the absence of a relationship between pudendal nerve status and surgical procedure success [27]. In their conclusions, Buie et al. [28] found clinical factors rather than the laboratory assessment to be predictive of outcome in a group of 191 patients who underwent anterior sphincteroplasty. There was no significant difference in postoperative continence among patients with normal, unilaterally abnormal, or bilaterally abnormal pudendal latency. In the authors' opinion, this result was due to more than one cause: the first was that PNTML is able to measure the conduction time of the fastest remaining nerve fibers but does not quantify the amount of nerve damage; the second was that the two pudendal nerves may not provide symmetric sphincter innervation, and this anatomical factor may explain the greater deficit caused by unilateral damage. Furthermore, the clinical rele-

Table 1. Success rate after sphincteroplasty according to the presence or not of pudendal neuropathy

Author	Year	No. patients	Success rate (%)		
			No neuropathy	Neuropathy	*P* value
Laurberg [13]	1988	19	80	11	<0.05
Wexner [14]	1991	16	92	50	n.s.
Engel [22]	1994	55	–	–	n.s.
Simmang [18]	1994	10	70	20	n.s.
Londono-Schimmer [17]	1994	94	55	30	<0.001
Sitzler [21]	1996	31	67	63	n.s.
Felt-Bersma [23]	1996	18	–	–	n.s.
Sangwan [19]	1996	15	100	14	<0.005
Gilliland [16]	1998	77	63	10	<0.01
Buie [28]	2001	89	61	71	n.s.

n.s. not significant

vance of unilateral or bilateral neuropathy is questionable due to the lack of homogeneity in literature definitions of normal ranges of PNTML. In conclusion, it is possible that above a certain value, PNTML may be predictive of a negative surgical outcome (Table 1).

Total Pelvic Floor Repair

This procedure is a combination of anterior sphincter plication with levatorplasty and postanal repair. There are currently few reports on this procedure, which describe only small groups of patients, with no physiological investigations.

Dynamic Graciloplasty

Transposition of the gracilis muscle to replace the anal sphincter was first proposed by Pickrell in 1952 [29]. This procedure was subsequently modified by the introduction of muscle electrostimulation in order to transform an easily fatigued muscle into one fatigue resistant, which led to dynamic graciloplasty.

This is the treatment of choice in patients with end-stage fecal incontinence secondary to trauma, neurological abnormalities, or anorectal malformations for whom conventional surgical procedures have failed or are not expected to be useful. Long-term success rates vary widely–from 50% to 70%–according to the surgical center's experience and the definition of success. Obstructed defecation, in fact, is a significant problem after dynamic graciloplasty, and for this reason, some authors suggest the association of an antegrade colonic enema procedure. Identification of prognostic factors for obstructed defecation would be helpful, but on this topic, the literature is completely silent.

All studies of dynamic graciloplasty report a high incidence of complications, especially due to infection or technical problems; furthermore, this procedure is very expensive and technically demanding. For these reasons, better knowledge of factors predictive of outcome is urgently required to help select the most appropriate candidates.

Korsgen and Keighley noted that poor rectal sensation is predictive of a negative outcome due to incomplete evacuation and the need for repeated enema washouts; they suggested that normal rectal sensitivity and compliance have an important role in predicting success after dynamic graciloplasty [30]. Baeten et al. also reported poor results in patients with impaired rectal sensation [31]. In a recent study in patients with an anorectal malformation, Koch et al. suggested that results are worse in such patients than in patients affected by incontinence of different etiologies. In their series, the best results were achieved in patients with a minor anorectal malformation compared with patients with a severe malformation, confirming the predictive value of the rectal sensitivity threshold [32].

Rectal sensitivity and type of malformation are indicated as prognostic factors for outcome. All the above authors believe that no other data obtained from physiological investigations are predictive of the outcome.

Sacral Nerve Modulation

This procedure was first described in 1960 for urinary difficulties and was then applied in 1995 by Matzel et al. [33] in patients with functional deficits of the anal sphincter but with no morphological defect. Subsequently, this procedure spread rapidly, and continuous technical improvements were made and indications extended. Recently, good results have been reported in patients with fecal incontinence caused by scleroderma, partial spinal cord injury, idiopathic sphincter degeneration, and low anterior resection of the rectum [34, 35]. Current data show that sacral nerve modulation (SNM) is a successful treatment for fecal incontinence, featuring a 70–80% success rate and an overall complication (minor) rate of 5–10% in a recent review by Kenefick and Christiansen [36] and Jarrett et al. [37].

Although real mechanisms of action are still partly unknown, pelvic and central nervous system neural pathway integrity is generally believed to be a necessary condition for a positive response. Effectiveness of the SNM procedure is preliminarily tested by means of a peripheral nerve evaluation (PNE), a simple procedure with minimal morbidity performed under local anesthesia that has a high predictive value. The permanent implant is performed only in cases of a positive PNE. To determine the predictive value of the electrophysiological anal tests–usually performed as part of the diagnostic workup–in predicting the clinical outcome of the PNE, we retrospectively studied 82 incontinent patients who underwent PNE after complete assessment of their anorectal physiology [38]. Data analysis showed that the functional level of the external anal sphincter, expressed by the EMG, can predict PNE outcome with an acceptable positive predictive value and sensitivity. The neurophysiological basis underlying this positive correlation is difficult to interpret because the effects of SNM on the external anal sphincter are not well understood, and some studies [39, 40] do not confirm the effects of SNM on squeezing and anal resting pressures demonstrated by early reports [33]. Furthermore, another recent study in experimental animals demonstrated that external anal sphincter activation is mediated by a cerebral response rather than being a direct effect of electrostimulation [41]. This central nervous system involvement would require an intact afferent and efferent neural pathway, but PNTML provides information only on the integrity of the efferent (motor) endings of the pudendal nerves. If these are abnormal, the EMG is pathological. The low number of patients who have undergone motor-evoked sacral potentials (MEPs) precludes the possibility of an in-depth analysis of this aspect.

On the basis of our results, we concluded that only simple anal sphincter EMG can predict PNE outcome with a good positive predictive value and specificity in patients with fecal incontinence. Other, more expensive, tests such as PNTML and MEPs do not add further prognostic information.

Conclusion

In conclusion, to date the literature does not provide sufficiently consistent data indicating which preoperative variables may predict a positive or negative outcome of conservative or surgical treatment of fecal incontinence.

References

1. Enck P (1993) Biofeedback training in disordered defecation: a critical review. Dig Dis Sci 38:1953–1560
2. Cerulli MA, Nikoomanesh P, Schuster MM (1979) Progress in biofeedback conditioning for fecal incontinence. Gastroenterology 76:742–746
3. Wald A (1981) Biofeedback therapy for fecal incontinence. Ann Intern Med 95:146–149
4. Sangwan YP, Coller JA, Barrett RC et al (1995) Can manometric parameters predict response to biofeedback therapy in fecal incontinence? Dis Colon Rectum 38:1021–1025
5. Fernandez-Fraga X, Azpiroz F, Aparici A et al (2003) Predictors of response to biofeedback treatment in anal incontinence. Dis Colon Rectum 46:1218–1225
6. Rieger NA, Wattchow DA, Sarre RG et al (1997) Prospective trial of pelvic floor retraining in patients with fecal incontinence. Dis Colon Rectum 40:821–826
7. Chiarioni G, Bassotti G, Stegagnini S et al (2002) Sensory retraining is key to biofeedback therapy for formed stool fecal incontinence. Am J Gastroenterol 97:109–117
8. Rao SS, Welcher KD, Happel J (1996) Can biofeedback therapy improve anorectal function in fecal incontinence? Am J Gastroenterol 91:2360–2366
9. Leroi AM, Dorival MP, Lecouturier MF et al (1999) Pudendal neuropathy and severity of incontinence but not presence of an anal sphincter defect may determine the response to biofeedback therapy in fecal incontinence. Dis Colon Rectum 42:762–769
10. Setti-Carraro P, Kamm MA, Nicholls RJ (1994) Long-term results of postanal repair for neurogenic faecal incontinence. Br J Surg 81:140–144
11. Mavrantonis C, Matsuoka H, Wexner SD et al (2000) Postanal repair for fecal incontinence: is it worthwhile? Dis Colon Rectum 43:1561–1567.
12. Slade MS, Goldberg SM, Schottler JL et al (1977) Sphincteroplasty for acquired anal incontinence. Dis Colon Rectum 20:33–35
13. Laurberg S, Swash M, Snooks SJ, Henry MM (1988) Neurologic cause of idiopathic incontinence. Arch Neurol 45:1250–1253
14. Wexner SD, Marchetti F, Jagelman DG (1991) The role of sphincteroplasty for fecal incontinence re-evaluated: a prospective physiologic and functional review. Dis Colon Rectum 34:22–30
15. Oliveira L, Pfeifer J, Wexner SD (1996) Physiological and clinical outcome of anterior sphincteroplasty. Br J Surg 83:502–505
16. Gilliland R, Altomare DF, Moreira H Jr et al (1998) Pudendal neuropathy is predictive of failure following anterior overlapping sphincteroplasty. Dis Colon Rectum 41:1516–1522

17. Londono-Schimmer EE, Garcia-Duperly R, Nicholls RJ et al (1994) Overlapping anal sphincter repair for faecal incontinence due to sphincter trauma: five year follow-up functional results. Int J Colorectal Dis 9:110–113
18. Simmang C, Birnbaum EH, Kodner IJ et al (1994) Anal sphincter construction in the elderly: does advancing age affect outcome? Dis Colon Rectum 37:1065–1069
19. Sangwan YP, CollerJA, Barrett RC et al (1996) Unilateral pudendal neuropathy. Impact on outcome of anal sphincter repair. Dis Colon Rectum 39:686–689
20. Jacobs PP, Scheuer M, Juijpers JH, Vingerhoets MH (1990) Obstetric fecal incontinence: role of pelvic floor denervation and results of delayed sphincter repair. Dis Colon Rectum 33:494–497
21. Sitzler PJ, Thomson JPS (1996) Overlap repair of damaged anal sphincter. A single surgeon's series. Dis Colon Rectum 39:1356–1360
22. Engel AF, Kamm MA, Sultan AH, (1994) Anterior anal sphincter repair in patients with obstetric trauma. Br J Surg 81:1231–1234
23. Felt-Bersma RJF, Ciesta MA, Koorevaar M (1996) Anal sphincter repair improves anorectal function and endosonographic image. A prospective clinical study. Dis Colon Rectum 39:878–885
24. Nikiteas N, Korsgen S, Kumar D, Keighley MRB (1996) Audit of sphincter repair. Factors associated with poor outcome. Dis Colon Rectum 39:1164–1170
25. Rasmussen OO, Colstrup H, Lose G, Christiansen J (1990) A technique for the dynamic assessment of anal sphincter function. Int J Colorectal Dis 5:135–141
26. Young CJ, Mathur MN, Eyers AA, Solomon MJ (1998) Successful overlapping anal sphincter repair: relationship to patient age, neuropathy and colostomy formation. Dis Colon Rectum 41:344–349
27. Chen AS, Luchtefeld MA, Senagore AJ et al (1998) Pudendal nerve latency. Does it predict outcome of anal sphincter repair? Dis Colon Rectum 41:1005–1009
28. Buie WD, Lowry AC, Rothenberger DA, Madoff RD (2001) Clinical rather than laboratory assessment predicts continence after anterior sphincteroplasty. Dis Colon Rectum 44:1255–1260
29. Pickrell KL, Broadbent TR, Masters FW, Metzger JT et al (1952) Construction of a rectal sphincter and restoration of anal continence by transplanting the gracilis muscle. Ann Surg 135:853–862
30. Korsgen S, Keighley MRB (1995) Stimulated gracilis neosphincter-not as good as previously thought. Report of four cases. Dis Colon Rectum 38:1331–1333
31. Baeten CG, Geerdes BP, Adang EM Et al (1995) Anal dynamic graciloplasty in the treatment of intractable fecal incontinence. N Engl J Med 332:1600–1605
32. Koch SM, Uludag O, Rongen MJ et al (2004) Dynamic graciloplasty in patients born with an anorectal malformation. Dis Colon Rectum 47:1711–1719
33. Matzel KE, Stadelmaier U, Hohenfellner M, Gall FP (1994). Electrical stimulation of sacral spinal nerves for treatment of faecal incontinence. Lancet 346:1124–1127
34. Matzel KE, Stadelmaier U, Bittorf B et al (2002) Bilateral sacral spinal nerve stimulation for fecal incontinence after low anterior rectum resection. Int J Colorectal Dis 17:430–434
35. Ratto C, Grillo E, Parello A et al (2005) Sacral neuromodulation in treatment of fecal incontinence following anterior resection and chemoradiation for rectal cancer. Dis Colon Rectum 48:1027–1036
36. Kenefick NJ, Christiansen J (2004) A review of sacral nerve stimulation for the treatment of faecal incontinence. Colorectal Dis 6:75–80
37. Jarrett MED, Mowatt G, Glazener CMA et al (2004) Systematic review of sacral nerve stimulation for faecal incontinence and constipation. Br J Surg 91:1559–1569
38. Altomare DF, Rinaldi M, Petrolino M et al (2004) Reliability of electrophysiologic anal tests in predicting the outcome of sacral nerve modulation for fecal incontinence. Dis Colon Rectum 47:853–857
39. Malouf AJ, Vaizey CJ, Nicholls RJ, Kamm MA (2000) Permanent sacral nerve stimulation for fecal incontinence. Ann Surg 232:143–148
40. Leroi AM, Michot F, Grise P, Denis P (2001) Effect of sacral nerve stimulation in patients with fecal and urinary incontinence. Dis Colon Rectum 44:779–789
41. Fowler CJ, Swinn MJ, Goodwin RJ et al (2000) Studies of the latency of pelvic floor contraction during peripheral nerve evaluation show that the muscle response is reflexly mediated. J Urol 163:881–883

SECTION IV

Selected Clinical Conditions

Rectal Resection

25

Giovanni B. Doglietto, Carlo Ratto, Angelo Parello, Lorenza Donisi, Francesco Litta

Introduction

The frequency of fecal incontinence (FI) in patients submitted to rectal resection (RR) for cancer ranges between 2% and 40% [1–6]. In fact, despite the significant improvements registered over the last few decades in the treatment of rectal cancer, not only in the control of the neoplasm itself and sparing of the anal sphincters but also in the preservation of urinary and sexual function [6–19], FI can occur, with severe detrimental effects on patients' quality of life. In these patients, FI is a disabling clinical condition, the etiology of which is complex and not yet fully elucidated. It is regarded as a component of "anterior resection syndrome," including an increased number of daily bowel movements, clustering, FI, and soiling after this operation [20–22]. In some cases, urinary incontinence also contributes to worsening of the clinical condition. Even if these patients are comforted by the fact that they have won their fight against the cancer, their personal and social life suffers considerably. Unfortunately, the minimalist attitude of some physicians prevents these patients from exploring the possibilities of treatment other than an appropriate diet or stimulating systems to empty the bowel completely.

Hypothesis of Pathophysiology

Various causes (including reduction of the rectal ampulla, iatrogenic internal sphincter lesions, autonomic nerve lesions, influence of chemoradiation) could play a role in determining this dysfunction.

A sphincter-saving RR significantly reduces the rectal ampulla; frequently, excision of the entire rectum is necessary, and coloanal anastomosis is performed [5, 23–27]. Even if a colonic pouch is constructed, FI may still occur [5, 23, 28]. However, the role of methods of reconstruction appears essential. At present, the J-pouch remains the gold standard for routine clinical practice, thanks to good results at long-term follow-up, but the transverse coloplasty and side to end anastomosis assure a superposable intestinal function in many trials [29–34].

The transanal introduction of a stapler or anal dilatation may be a cause of iatrogenic lesion of the internal anal sphincter in a high percentage of patients (18% at endoanal ultrasound evaluation) [2, 35, 36], but the external sphincter does not appear lesioned by the procedure. Internal anal sphincter fragmentation can cause a decrease of resting anal pressure. On the other hand, transabdominal anastomosis minimized the risk of sphincter damage and showed a good degree of continence [36–38].

Despite the warning that great care should be taken regarding nerve sparing, sympathetic and parasympathetic fibers can be interrupted, with significant deregulation of the nervous inputs and outputs to and from the pelvis, particularly the remaining rectum, anus, and perirectal structures [11]. On the other hand, the preservation of autonomic nerve structures during total mesorectal excision (TME) can decrease the risk of FI and urogenital disturbances. The pelvic organs are innervated by sympathetic and parasympathetic nerve fibers. The sympathetic supply arises from L1 to L3, which contribute to the superior hypogastric plexus that extends to the sacral promontory. This plexus gives origin to the right and left hypogastric nerves. The parasympathetic nerve fibers arise from S2 to S4. They emerge through the sacral foramina (nerves erigentes) and join the sympathetic hypogastric nerves to constitute the right and left inferior pelvic plexuses sited at the pelvic sidewall anteriorly and laterally to the lower third of the rectum. From each pelvic plexus, nerve fibers (both sympathetic and parasympathetic) reach the pelvic viscera.

Identification of the nerve fibers is more difficult for the parasympathetic nerves that extend deep into the pelvis, whereas visualization of the sympathetic system is easier. However, damage could occur along the entire nerve fiber branchings: periaortic/pericaval, superior hypogastric plexus, hypogastric nerves, S2–S4 parasympathetic nerves, inferior pelvic plexuses, and distal nerve fibers. Other factors can also influence nerve sparing: male gender, tumor size, intraoperative blood loss, and surgeon expertise. When urinary incontinence and/or disturbances of sexual function occur as secondary effects of nerve damage, they contribute to worsening of the patient's clinical condition [39].

Pelvic radiotherapy can play an important role in the pathogenesis of functional disturbances of continence [40–42]. In patients treated with pelvic radiotherapy for prostate, gynecological, bladder, anal, or rectal cancer, the incidence of FI is 3–53% [43]. This is despite progress in irradiation procedure. The patient's age and presence of "anal symptoms" are described as risk factors. In their review article, Putta and Andreyev [43] assessed that rectal cancer seems to present the highest incontinence rate, probably due to the additive effects of surgery to those of radiotherapy. In this work, only 8–56% of incontinent patients were found affected in their quality of life. The authors interpreted this finding because patients "do not feel or seem ill, will not report symptoms, as they believe they are inevitable consequences of radiotherapy treatment, of being old, or that there is nothing that can be done". With the aim of investigating bowel dysfunctions, Peeters et al. [44] sent a questionnaire to 597 patients enrolled in the prospective randomized TME trial (5×5 Gy before TME surgery vs. TME surgery alone), with a median follow-up of 5.1 years after the treatment. Irradiated patients compared with nonirradiated patients reported increased rates of FI (62% vs. 38%, respectively; $p<0.001$), pad wearing as a result of incontinence (56% vs. 33%, respectively; $p<0.001$), anal blood loss (11% vs. 3%, respectively; $p=0.004$), and mucus loss (27% vs. 15%, respectively; $p=0.005$). Satisfaction with bowel function was significantly lower and the impact of bowel dysfunction on daily activities was greater in irradiated patients compared with patients who underwent TME alone. Pollack et al. [45] recently reported results of a randomized trial within the Stockholm Radiotherapy Trials on 64 patients submitted to low anterior resection with or without preoperative radiotherapy (21 and 43 patients, respectively) followed up with quality-of-life questionnaires, clinical examination, anorectal manometry, and endoanal ultrasound. An impaired anorectal function was common after low anterior resection for rectal cancer, and the risk was increased after radiotherapy. Irradiated patients had significantly more symptoms of FI (57% vs. 26%, $p=0.01$), soiling (38% vs. 16%; $p=0.04$), and bowel movements per week (20 vs. 10; $p=0.02$). Significantly lower resting (35 mmHg vs. 62 mmHg; $p<0.001$) and squeeze pressures (104 mmHg vs. 143 mmHg; $p=0.05$) and more scarring of the anal sphincters (33% vs. 13%; $p=0.03$) were documented in irradiated patients. A worse quality of life affected incontinent patients.

Multiple factors are supposed to produce the effects of radiotherapy on the pelvic structures involved in the continence mechanisms, including radiotherapy dose as well as physical, patient-related, treatment, and genetic factors [43]. Effects could be found on both anal canal structures and the rectum. In most studies, anal maximum resting pressure decreased following pelvic irradiation [46–54], hypothetically due to damage of endovascular cushions, internal anal sphincter thinning or atrophy, or both. However, disagreement exists on manometric assessment of resting pressure, as it was unchanged in other reports [50, 55–57]. Even if pressure increment due to squeezing is decreased in most studies [47, 48, 50, 51–54, 57, 58] and thickness of the external anal sphincter has been reported after radiotherapy for prostate cancer [54], the influence of pudendal neuropathy in a change of muscle morphology is unclear. A significant prolonged pudendal nerve terminal motor latency (PNTML) has been observed in patients treated with neoadjuvant chemoradiation (irrespective to the inclusion or not of the anal canal to the irradiation field) and is associated to the FI severity score [57]. Moreover, being that the pudendal nerve is also responsible for anal sensitivity, damage to it can be a significant cause of fecal seepage.

A lumbosacral plexopathy may be a concomitant cause of incontinence and can cause perianal anesthesia and alterations to the pudendal nerve [59]. Myenteric plexus degeneration within the bowel wall has been thought to influence continence [46]. The rectal sensation to distension is primarily transmitted along the S2, S3, and S4 parasympathetic nerves, which traverse the pelvic splanchnic nerves. Damage to these nerves induced by radiotherapy could alter rectal compliance. Regarding rectal physiology, most studies report a significant decrease in threshold volume and maximum tolerated volume in incontinent patients following pelvic irradiation [46–52, 54, 56, 58]. Moreover, radiotherapy induces an inflammatory response within the pelvic vessels and an increased secretion of growth factors, with consequent damage to the microcircle of the rectum.

Diagnostic Assessment

In patients submitted to RR for cancer, clinicians must dedicate attention in investigating defecation disorders. In fact, a variety of dysfunctions can occur considering the multifactorial etiology of FI in these patients, particularly when integrated therapies have been associated to surgery. Increased bowel frequency only or associated with fecal soiling or seepage should be of concern. Tenesmus is not infrequent, and incontinence to gas could coexist. In more severe cases, incontinence to liquid and/or solid feces is reported, up to many episodes per day, altering significantly daily activities and quality of life. FI severity index could be very high in these patients. Calculation of a specific score is usually useful not only to measure baseline FI severity but also to compare this to the condition reached after a given treatment. In each case, special efforts must be made to assess alteration of rectoanal sensitivity, and patients must be asked about their ability to distinguish gas from liquid and solid stools, defer defecation, and feel the bowel completely empty.

The aim of clinical examination is to investigate perianal/perineal scars, patulous anus, perineal soiling, anal ectropion, sphincter deficit, loss of perineal body, and perineal descent. During digital examination, resting and squeeze tones must be evaluated, whereas the puborectalis muscle needs to be assessed at rest, squeezing, and straining. Proctoscopy or, if necessary, colonoscopy is needed to ascertain absence of tumor recurrence or other bowel neoplasms. Physiology evaluation is of utmost importance. Anorectal manometry can offer information about alterations in resting and squeeze pressures, sphincter asymmetry by vector manometry, anomalies of rectoanal inhibitory reflex (sometimes absent, sometimes normal, sometimes not identifiable when resting pressure is very low), and rectal compliance. Assessment of rectal sensation (measuring threshold, urge, and maximum tolerated volumes) could be of help in interpreting pathophysiology in these patients. Endoanal ultrasound (or magnetic resonance, as an alternative) is mandatory to detect sphincter lesions. Electrophysiology study can investigate anal and rectal sensory and PNTML.

Treatment

Due to the multifactorial pathogenesis of FI following RR with or without (chemo)radiotherapy, primary aims of any treatment should be intervention on the underlying causes to restore or, at least, significantly improve continence. Although various therapies (medical and surgical) are available as effective treatment of FI, a gold standard has not yet been established.

Medical Therapy

A number of therapeutic agents and options have been proposed (bulking agents and high-fiber diet, valproate sodium, diazepam, topical phenylephrine, biofeedback [60–65]). Theoretically, loperamide should have the best mechanism of action when compared with other antidiarrheal drugs, because it potentially can improve internal anal sphincter pressure [66]. Biofeedback and pelvic floor training could have the best possibilities of success if dysfunctional external anal sphincter or puborectalis is one of the main reasons of FI following RR, although only few reports have been published in this specific clinical condition [65].

Surgery

When intractable FI occurs, surgical treatment must be considered. Traditionally, two assumptions have guided treatment choice. First, stoma formation represents the "radical" approach, but the impact on patient's quality of life, as yet undetermined, should be questioned. Second, a few alternatives for surgical sphincter repair (sphincteroplasty) or substitution (gracilis/gluteus transposition, artificial sphincter) could be considered, but this approach is often thought hazardous because of the high risk of nonhealing, infection, chronic pain, and fistula formation [43, 67]. Finally, a palliative approach, i.e., anal plugs and rectal irrigation, will only minimize the effects of FI. A new, promising treatment could be sacral nerve stimulation.

Dynamic Graciloplasty

In 1990, Baeten and Spaans and Williams et al. [68, 69] introduced a new technique for the treatment of FI in the presence of large sphincter defects: the dynamic graciloplasty. Cavina applied this therapy after abdominoperineal resection of the rectum [70]. This "sphincterial" substitution can be achieved as a synchronous procedure or after several years and can involve one or both gracilis muscles [71–73]. The primary reconstruction is more frequently applied because more technical difficulties can be encountered during such a sphincter restoration in a previously "mutilated" pelvic floor. At the long-term follow-up, about two thirds of the patients with dynamic graciloplasty after abdominoperineal resection of the rectum achieved satisfactory continence. However, no reports are available on the application of dynamic graciloplasty following sphincter-saving RR for cancer.

Artificial Sphincter

Indications for application of an artificial sphincter are very similar to those for dynamic graciloplasty. Even if reports on this approach have documented positive impact on restoration of continence in the majority of patients [74–77], postoperative and short-term morbidity as well as long-term results reduce the overall efficacy of this treatment. Unfortunately, no series has been reported of FI patients treated with artificial sphincter following RR for rectal cancer. Only a case report is documented, in which the device needed to be explanted due to intense perineal pain [74].

Sacral Nerve Stimulation

Electrical stimulation of sacral nerves has been thought to excite these nerves and thus "modulate" specific functions due to this complex nerve supply. Expected results of such stimulation should be to stimulate additional impulses not only to an inadequate pelvic floor musculature and pelvic organs but also to the sensitive pelvic fibers. This therapeutic approach is called sacral nerve stimulation (SNS). It presents peculiar characteristics if compared with other surgical options for FI treatment. The first step, the percutaneous nerve evaluation (PNE), is both a diagnostic procedure and a test of therapeutic efficacy. It permits implantation of an electrode adjacent to the sacral nerves (through the sacral foramina, the S3 foramen being generally preferred (Fig. 1) to both evaluate the nerves' response to stimulation during the implantation procedure and during the following period and to assess the clinical efficacy on defecation disturbances. Indeed, the PNE test, when affecting significant improvement, allows a 100% positive predictive value of response to permanent chronic stimulation. Actually, there is a tendency to use the new-model self-fixing definitive quadripolar electrode for the PNE test. The electrode can be implanted by a percutaneous technique (Fig. 2) under local anesthesia and connected to the external stimulator during the test period. The second step is permanent implant of the sacral neuromodulation (SNM) system. Only if the PNE test produced good results in improving FI can a permanent implant be considered. When the quadripolar electrode has already been implanted, only the definitive electrostimulator has to be placed into a subcutaneous pocket located in the gluteal area (Fig. 3) and connected to the electrode. This procedure is usually performed under local anesthesia. One or two electrodes can be placed, which are connected to a single electrostimulator.

Primarily, inclusion criteria for SNS were poor FI (at least one episode of either solid or liquid stool leakage per week) and failure of conservative treatment. Thereafter, functional defects of the striated pelvic musculature (without sphincter lesion) were the main criteria used in the early studies [20]. Enrolled patients had decreased manometric squeeze pressure but normal PNTML. More recently, other, more precise, indications have been investigated suc-

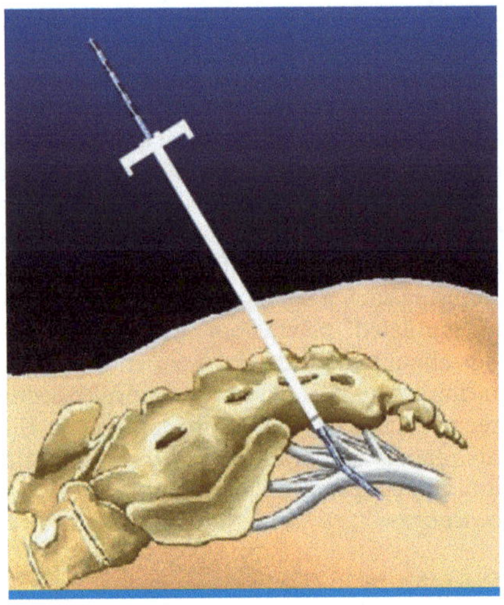

Fig. 1. Schema of percutaneous implantation of self-fixing definitive quadripolar electrode for sacral nerve stimulation (SNS). Courtesy of Medtronic S.p.A, Italy

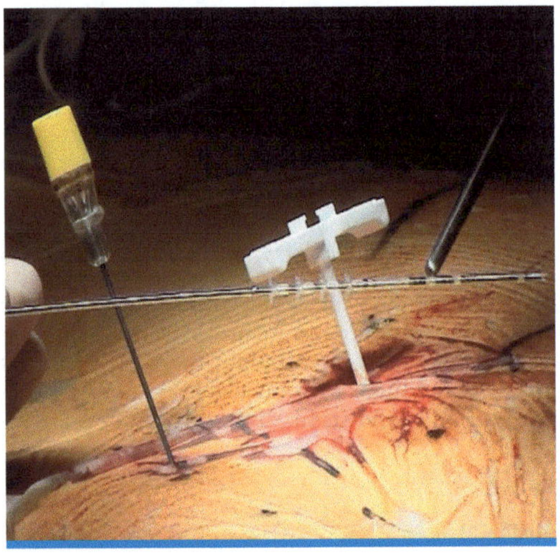

Fig. 2. Percutaneous implantation of self-fixing definitive quadripolar electrodes for sacral nerve stimulation (SNS), under local anesthesia, in a patient with fecal incontinence (FI) following chemoradiotherapy and rectal resection (RR) for rectal cancer. Reprinted with permission from [80]

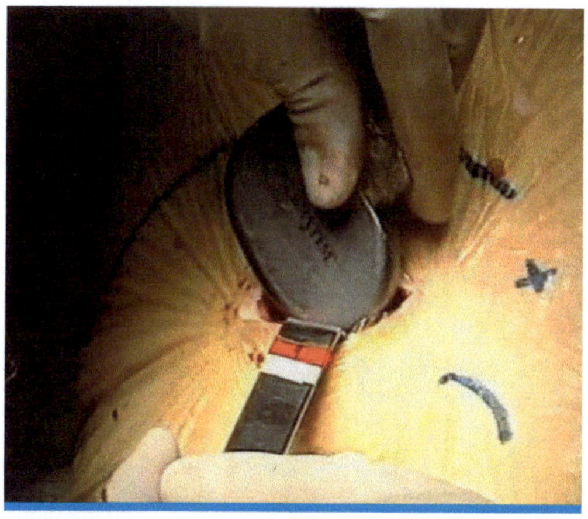

Fig. 3. Electrostimulator implant for sacral nerve stimulation (SNS) in a patient with fecal incontinence (FI) following chemoradiotherapy and rectal resection (RR) for rectal cancer. Reprinted with permission from [80]

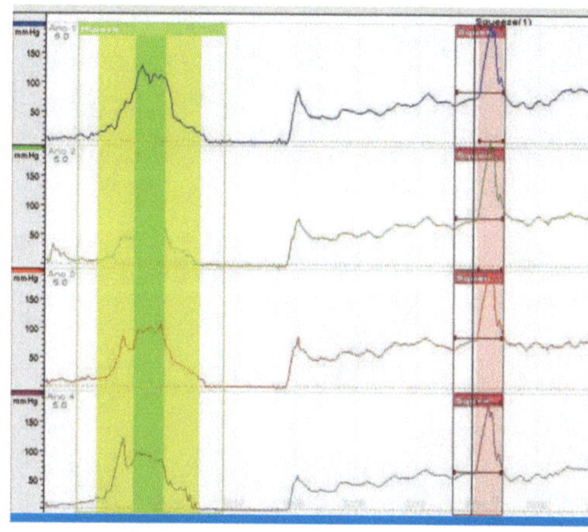

Fig. 4. Anorectal manometry: normal resting and squeeze pressure profiles in a patient with fecal incontinence (FI) following chemoradiotherapy and rectal resection (RR) for rectal cancer

cessively, including FI due to idiopathic sphincter degeneration, iatrogenic internal sphincter damage, partial spinal cord injury, scleroderma, limited lesions of internal or external anal sphincters, rectal prolapse repair, and low anterior resection of the rectum.

In the 2002, Matzel et al. [78] described a single case report of SNS for FI after low anterior rectum resection. Two sacral electrodes were used. Complete resolution of FI was reported 18 months after the implant, with significant improvement not only in the continence score but also in the quality-of-life score. Moreover, squeeze pressure improved, and resting pressure and neorectal sensation parameters appeared not to be affected. Our preliminary experience concerning definitive SNS implant in four patients has been published [79]. After device implantation, the mean FI scores decreased, and the mean number of incontinence episodes dropped from 12.0 to 2.5 per week ($p<0.05$). Permanent implant resulted in a significant improvement in fecal continence in three patients, and incontinence was slightly reduced in the fourth. Manometric parameters agreed with clinical results: maximum and mean resting tone and the squeeze pressure were normal in three patients and reduced in one. In these same three patients, neorectal sensation parameters increased when the preoperative value was normal or below normal and decreased when the preoperative value was higher than normal, whereas in one patient in whom extremely low values were recorded, all parameters decreased significantly.

At present, in our series, a PNE test was performed in eight patients after chemoradiation and RR for rectal cancer. Patients were evaluated with anorectal manometry (Fig. 4), endoanal ultrasound (Fig. 5), and electrophysiology study. In one of these patients, functional results were poor and the PNE test was interrupted; in another, they were not very good, and the test was also stopped. The other six patients had an excellent functional recovery of FI, so the definitive implant was completed. At long-term follow-up, the results are very good and have been stable over time (unpublished data).

Conclusion

Patients presenting with FI following RR with or without neoadjuvant therapy must be carefully evaluated. Skepticism by patients and clinicians negatively affects the possibility to rightly assess the clinical condition and to plan therapy. In this view, an accurate clinical and physiological evaluation is mandatory. Even if traditional therapeutic procedures are not always successful, they can be attempted in selected patients. If suspected "neurogenic" FI is confirmed by the physiological tests, SNS may be proposed and tested. Positive results of the PNE test suggest that a permanent SNM device must be implanted. Long-term results of SNS are encouraging. Failure of this approach does not prevent the use of other, more aggressive, forms of treatment.

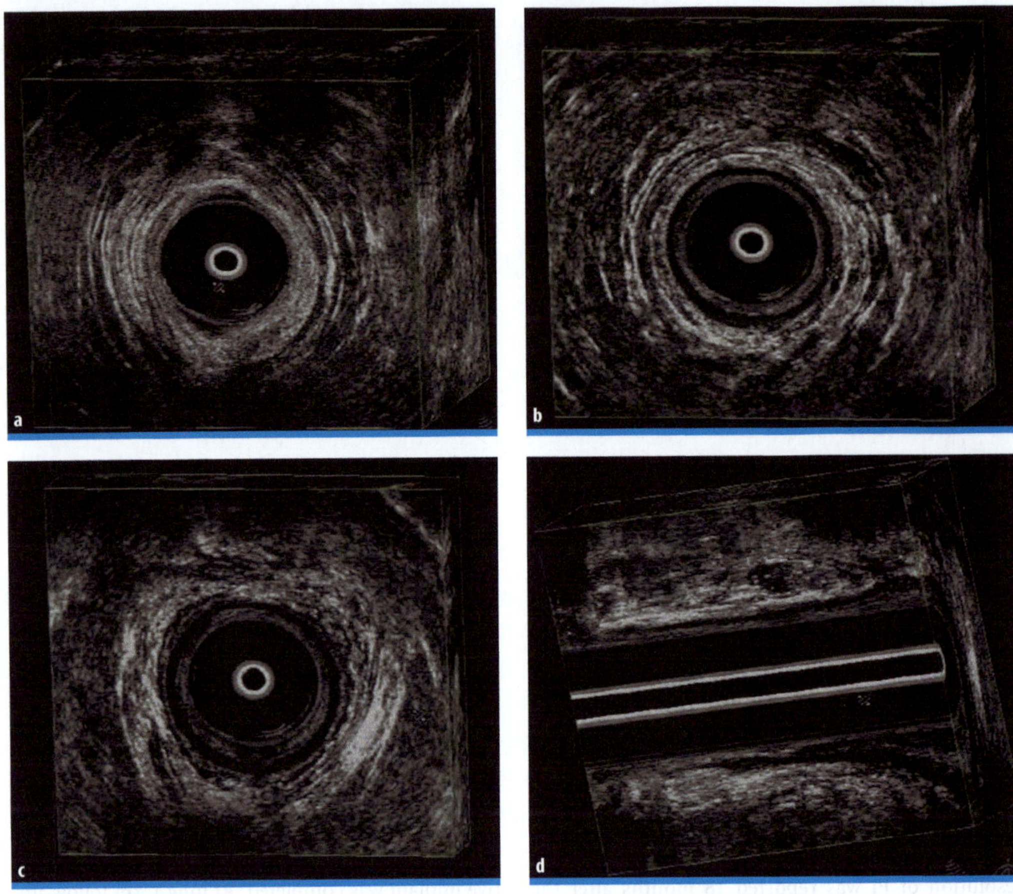

Fig. 5a-d Endoanal ultrasound in a patient with fecal incontinence (FI) following chemoradiotherapy and rectal resection (RR) for rectal cancer: absence of internal and external sphincter lesions. **a** Lower anal canal (coronal view), **b** middle anal canal (coronal view), **c** upper anal canal (coronal view), **d** midline anal canal (sagittal view)

References

1. Hautefeuille P, Valleur P, Perniceni T et al (1988) Functional and oncologic results after coloanal anastomosis for low rectal carcinoma. Ann Surg 207:61–64
2. Horgan PG, OConnell PR, Shinkwin CA et al (1989) Effect of anterior resection on anal sphincter function. Br J Surg 76:783–786
3. Paty PB, Enker WE, Cohen AM et al (1994) Long-term functional results of coloanal anastomosis for rectal cancer. Am J Surg 167:90–84
4. Vassilakis JS, Pechlivanides G, Zoras OJ et al (1995) Anorectal function after low anterior resection of the rectum Int J Colorectal Dis 10:101–106
5. Fichera A, Michelassi F (2001) Long-term prospective assessment of functional results after proctectomy with coloanal anastomosis. J Gastrointest Surg 5:153–157
6. Duijvendijk P, Slors F, Taat CW et al (2003) A prospective evaluation of anorectal function after total mesorectal excision in patients with a rectal carcinoma. Surgery 133:56–65
7. Kapiteijn E, Marijnen CA, Nagtegaal ID et al (2001) Dutch Colorectal Cancer Group: preoperative radiotherapy combined with total mesorectal excision for resectable rectal cancer. N Engl J Med 345:638–646
8. Kapiteijn E, Putter H, van de Velde CJ (2002) Cooperative investigators of the Dutch Colorectal Cancer Group: impact of the introduction and training of total mesorectal excision on recurrence and survival in rectal cancer in The Netherlands. Br J Surg 89:1142–1149
9. Wibe A, Moller B, Norstein J et al (2002) Norwegian Rectal Cancer Group. A national strategic change in

treatment policy for rectal cancer-implementation of total mesorectal excision as routine treatment in Norway. A national audit. Dis Colon Rectum 45:857–866
10. Richard CS, Phang PT, McLeod RS (2003) Canadian Association of General Surgeons Evidence Based Reviews in Surgery. 5. Need for preoperative radiation in rectal cancer-preoperative radiotherapy combined with total mesorectal excision for resectable rectal cancer. Can J Surg 46:54–56
11. Havenga K, Enker WE (2002) Autonomic nerve preserving total mesorectal excision. Surg Clin North Am 82:1009–1018
12. Hanna NN, Guillem J, Dosoretz A et al (2002) Intraoperative parasympathetic nerve stimulation with tumescence monitoring during total mesorectal excision for rectal cancer. J Am Coll Surg 195:506–512
13. Kim NK, Aahn TW, Park JK et al (2002) Assessment of sexual and voiding function after total mesorectal excision with pelvic autonomic nerve preservation in males with rectal cancer. Dis Colon Rectum 45:1178–1185
14. Junginger T, Kneist W, Heintz A (2003) Influence of identification and preservation of pelvic autonomic nerves in rectal cancer surgery on bladder dysfunction after total mesorectal excision. Dis Colon Rectum 46:621–628
15. Theodoropoulos G, Wise WE, Padmanabhan A et al (2002) T-level downstaging and complete pathologic response after preoperative chemoradiation for advanced rectal cancer result in decreased recurrence and improved disease-free survival. Dis Colon Rectum 45:895–903
16. Valentini V, Coco C, Picciocchi A et al (2002) Does downstaging predict improved outcome after preoperative chemoradiation for extraperitoneal locally advanced rectal cancer? A long-term analysis of 165 patients. Int J Radiat Oncol Biol Phys 53:664–674
17. Garcia-Aguilar J, Hernandez de Anda E, Sirivongs P et al (2003) A pathologic complete response to preoperative chemoradiation is associated with lower local recurrence and improved survival in rectal cancer patients treated by mesorectal excision. Dis Colon Rectum 46:298–304
18. Ratto C, Valentini V, Morganti AG et al (2003) Combined-modality therapy in locally advanced primary rectal cancer. Dis Colon Rectum 46:59–67
19. Crane CH, Skibber JM, Feig BW et al (2003) Response to preoperative chemoradiation increases the use of sphincter-preserving surgery in patients with locally advanced low rectal carcinoma. Cancer 97:517–524
20. Williamson ME, Lewis WG, Holdsworth et al (1994) Decrease in the anorectal pressure gradient after low anterior resection of the rectum. A study using continuous ambulatory manometry. Dis Colon Rectum 37:1228–1231
21. Kakodkar R Gupta S, Nundy S (2006) Low anterior resection with total mesorectal excision for rectal cancer: functional assessment and factors affecting outcome. Colorectal Dis 8:650–656
22. Desnoo L Faithfull S (2006) A qualitative study of anterior resection syndrome: the experiences of cancer survivors who have undergone resection surgery. Eur J Cancer Care 15:244–251
23. Benoist S, Panis Y, Boleslawski E et al (1997) Functional outcome after coloanal versus low colorectal anastomosis for rectal carcinoma. J Am Coll Surg 185:114–119
24. Matzel KE, Stadelmaier U, Muehldorfer S et al (1997) Continence after colorectal reconstruction following resection: impact of level of anastomosis. Int J Colorectal Dis 12:82–87
25. Lee SJ, Park YS (1998) Serial evaluation of anorectal function following low anterior resection of the rectum. Int J Colorectal Dis 13:241–246
26. Gamagami R, Istvan G, Cabarrot P et al (2000) Fecal continence following partial resection of the anal canal in distal rectal cancer: long-term results after coloanal anastomoses. Surgery 127:291–295
27. Temple LK Bacik J, Savatta SG et al (2005) The development of a validated instrument to evaluate bowel function after sphincter-preserving surgery for rectal cancer. Dis Colon Rectum 48:1353–1365
28. Dehni N, McNamara DA, Schlegel RD et al (2002) Clinical effects of preoperative radiation therapy on anorectal function after proctectomy and colonic J-pouch-anal anastomosis. Dis Colon Rectum 45: 1635–1640
29. Lazorthes F Chiotasso P, Gamagami RA et al (1997) Late clinical outcome in a randomized prospective comparison of colonic J pouch and straight coloanal anastomosis. Br J Surg 84:1449–1451
30. Machado M, Nygren J, Goldman S et al (2003) Similar outcome after colonic pouch and side-to-end anastomosis in low anterior resection for rectal cancer: a prospective randomized trial. Ann Surg 238:214–220
31. Pimentel JM, Duarte A, Gregorio C et al (2003) Transverse coloplasty pouch and colonic J-pouch for rectal cancer-a comparative study. Colorectal Dis 5:465–470
32. Furst A, Suttner S, Agha A et al (2003) Colonic J-pouch vs. coloplasty following resection of distal rectal cancer: early results of a prospective, randomized, pilot study. Dis Colon Rectum 46:1161–1166
33. Hida J, Yoshifuji T, Tokoro T et al (2004) Comparison of long-term functional results of colonic J-pouch and straight anastomosis after low anterior resection for rectal cancer: a five-year follow-up. Dis Colon Rectum 47:1578–1585
34. Hida J, Yoshifuji T, Okuno K et al (2006) Long-term functional outcome of colonic J-pouch reconstruction after low anterior resection for rectal cancer. Surg Today 36:441–449
35. Farouk R, Drew PJ, Duthie GS et al (1996) Disruption of the internal anal sphincter can occur after transanal stapling. Br J Surg 83:1400
36. Farouk R, Duthie GS, Lee PW et al (1998) Endosonographic evidence of injury to the internal anal sphincter after low anterior resection: long-term follow-up. Dis Colon Rectum 41:888–891
37. Ho YH Tsang C, Tang CL et al (2000) Anal sphincter injuries from stapling instruments introduced transanally: randomized, controlled study with endoanal ultrasound and anorectal manometry. Dis Colon Rectum 43:169–173
38. Jiang JK, Yang SH, Lin JK (2005) Transabdominal anastomosis after low anterior resection: A prospective, randomized, controlled trial comparing long-

term results between side-to-end anastomosis and colonic J-pouch. Dis Colon Rectum 48:2100–2108
39. Kim NK, Aahn TW, Park JK et al (2002) Assessment of sexual and voiding function after total mesorectal excision with pelvic autonomic nerve preservation in males with rectal cancer. Dis Colon Rectum 45:1178–1185
40. Dahlberg M, Glimelius B, Graf W et al (1998) Preoperative irradiation affects functional results after surgery for rectal cancer: results from a randomized study. Dis Colon Rectum 41:543–551
41. Gervaz PA, Wexner SD, Pemberton JH (2002) Pelvic radiation and anorectal function: introducing the concept of sphincter-preserving radiation therapy. J Am Coll Surg 195:387–394
42. Ammann K, Kirchmayr W, Klaus A et al (2003) Impact of neoadjuvant chemoradiation on anal sphincter function in patients with carcinoma of the mid rectum and low rectum. Arch Surg 138:257–261
43. Putta S, Andreyev HJ (2005) Faecal incontinence: A late side-effect of pelvic radiotherapy. Clin Oncol (R Coll Radiol) 17:469–477
44. Peeters KC, van de Velde CJ, Leer JW et al (2005) Late side effects of short-course preoperative radiotherapy combined with total mesorectal excision for rectal cancer: increased bowel dysfunction in irradiated patients-a Dutch colorectal cancer group study. J Clin Oncol 23:6199–6206
45. Pollack J, Holm T, Cedermark B et al (2006) Long-term effect of preoperative radiation therapy on anorectal function. Dis Colon Rectum 49:345–352
46. Varma J, Smith A, Busuttil A (1985) Correlation of clinical and manometric abnormalities of rectal function following chronic radiation injury. Br J Surg 72: 875–878
47. Yeoh E, Horowitz M, Russo A et al (1993) Effect of pelvic irradiation on gastrointestinal function. Am J Med 95:397–406
48. Yeoh E, Sun W, Russo A (1996) A retrospective study of the effects of pelvic irradiation for gynaecological cancer on anorectal function. Int J Radiat Oncol Biol Phys 35:1003–1010
49. Iwamoto T, Nakahara S, Mibu R et al (1997) Effect of radiotherapy on anorectal function in patients with cervical cancer. Dis Colon Rectum 40:693–697
50. Kim G, Lim JJ, Park W et al (1998) Sensory and motor dysfunction assessed by anorectal manometry in uterine cervical carcinoma patients with radiation-induced late rectal complications. Int J Radiat Oncol Biol Phys 4:835–841
51. Ho Y, Lee K, Eu K et al (2000) Effects of adjuvant radiotherapy on bowel function and anorectal physiology after low anterior resection for rectal cancer. Tech Coloproctol 4:13–16
52. Berndtsson I, Lennernas B, Hulten L (2002) Anorectal function after modern conformal radiation therapy for prostate cancer: a pilot study. Tech Coloproctol 6:101–114
53. Kushwaha R, Hayne D, Vaizey C et al (2003) Physiologic changes of the anorectum after pelvic radiotherapy for the treatment of prostate and bladder cancer. Dis Colon Rectum 46:1182–1188
54. Yeoh E, Holloway R, Fraser R et al (2004) Anorectal dysfunction increases with time following radiation therapy for carcinoma of the prostate. Am J Gastroenterol 99:361–369
55. Birnbaum E, Dresnik Z, Fry R et al (1994) Chronic effects of pelvic radiation therapy on ano-rectal function. Dis Colon Rectum 37:909–915
56. Yeoh E, Botten R, Russo A et al (2000) Chronic effects of therapeutic irradiation for localised prostatic carcinoma on anorectal function. Int J Radiat Oncol Biol Phys 47:915–924
57. Lim JF, Tjandra JJ, Hiscock R et al (2006) Preoperative chemoradiation for rectal cancer causes prolonged pudendal nerve terminal motor latency. Dis Colon Rectum 49:12–19
58. Broens P, Van Limbergen E, Penninckx F et al (1998) Clinical and manometric effects of combined external beam irradiation and brachytherapy for anal cancer. Int J Colorectal Dis 13:68–72
59. Iglicki F, Coffin B, Ille O et al (1996) Fecal incontinence after pelvic radiotherapy: evidence for lumbosacral plexopathy: report of a case. Dis Colon Rectum 39:465–467
60. Sentovich SM, Rivela LJ, Blatchford GJ et al (1995) Pattern of male fecal incontinence. Dis Colon Rectum 38:281–285
61. Keighley MR (1993) Fecal incontinence. In: Keighley MR, Williams NS, eds. Surgery of the anus, rectum and colon. Saunders, London, pp 516–607
62. Kusunoki M, Shoji Y, Ikeuchi H et al (1990) Usefulness of valproate sodium for treatment of incontinence after ileoanal anastomosis Surgery 107:311–315
63. Maeda K, Maruta M, Sato H et al (2002) Effect of oral diazepam on anal continence after low anterior resection: a preliminary study. Techn Coloproctol 6:15–18
64. Carapeti EA, Kamm MA, Phillips RK (2000) Randomized controlled trial of topical phenylephrine in the treatment of fecal incontinence. Br J Surg 87:38–42
65. Ho YH, Chiang JM, Tan M et al (1996) Biofeedback therapy for excessive stool frequency and incontinence following anterior resection or total colectomy. Dis Colon Rectum 39:1289–1292
66. Read M, Read NW, Barber DC et al (1982) Effects of loperamide on anal sphincter function in patients complaining of chronic diarrhea with fecal incontinence and urgency. Dig Dis Sci 27:807–814
67. Marks G, Mohiudden M (1983) The surgical management of the radiation-injured intestine. Surg Clin North Am 63:81–96
68. Baeten CG, Spaans F (1990) Construction of a neorectum and neoanal sphincter. Br J Surg 77:473–474
69. Williams NS, Hallan RI, Koeze TH et al (1990) Restoration of gastrointestinal continuity and continence after abdominoperineal excision of the rectum using an electrically stimulated neoanal sphincter. Dis Colon Rectum 33:561–565
70. Cavina E (1996) Outcome of restorative perineal graciloplasty with simultaneous excision of the anus and rectum for cancer. A ten-year experience with 81 patients. Dis Colon Rectum 39:182–190
71. Geerdes BP, Zoetmulder FA, Baeten CG (1995) Double dynamic graciloplasty and coloperineal pull-through after abdominoperineal resection. Eur J Cancer 31A(7–8):1248–1252

72. Rosen HR, Urbarz C, Novi G et al (2002) Long-term results of modified graciloplasty for sphincter replacement after rectal excision. Colorectal Dis 4: 266–269
73. Violi V, Boselli AS, De Bernardinis M et al (2005) Anorectal reconstruction by electrostimulated graciloplasty as part of abdominoperineal resection. Eur J Surg Oncol 31:250–258
74. Lehur PA, Michot F, Denis P et al (1996) Results of artificial sphincter in severe anal incontinence. Report of 14 consecutive implantations. Dis Colon Rectum 39:1352–1355
75. Madoff RD, Baeten CG, Christiansen J et al (2000) Standards for anal sphincter replacement. Dis Colon Rectum 43:135–141
76. Wong WD, Congliosi SM, Spencer MP et al (2002) The safety and efficacy of the artificial bowel sphincter for fecal incontinence: results from a multicenter cohort study. Dis Colon Rectum 45:1139–1153
77. Lehur PA, Zerbib F, Neunlist M et al (2002) Comparison of quality of life and anorectal function after artificial sphincter implantation. Dis Colon Rectum 45:508–513
78. Matzel KE, Stadelmaier U, Bittorf B et al (2002) Bilateral sacral spinal nerve stimulation for fecal incontinence after low anterior rectum resection. Int J Colorectal Dis 17:430–434
79. Ratto C, Grillo E, Parello A et al (2005) Sacral neuromodulation in treatment of fecal incontinence following anterior resection and chemoradiation for rectal cancer. Dis Colon Rectum 48:1027–1036
80. Ratto C, Parello A, Donisi L (2007) Sacral neuromodulation in the treatment of defecation disorders. Acta Neurochir 97 (Suppl):341–350

Iatrogenic Sphincter Lesions

26

Oliver M. Jones, Ian Lindsey

Introduction

Iatrogenic faecal incontinence can be split into two broad categories by aetiology. The largest group comprises patients undergoing proctological surgery for haemorrhoids, fissures, sepsis, rectoceles and local excision of rectal neoplasia. A second surgical group includes patients who have received anal instrumentation for the purpose of performing an anastomosis in the pelvis, most commonly by transanal insertion of a stapling device.

Proctological Procedures

General Introduction

Studies often underestimate iatrogenic incontinence, as follow-up is often short and trials are powered to show difference in intervention efficacy, not effect on continence. Anal-canal pressures decrease with age, and the initial iatrogenic injury may be compounded by subsequent obstetric injury [1]. Therefore, incontinence resulting from the proctological procedure may not be unmasked for a number of years.

We recently published our experience of patients with incontinence after proctological procedures [2]. This study evaluated a cohort of patients referred for investigation and treatment of faecal incontinence having undergone a proctological procedure. Ninety-three patients were evaluated: 27 after manual anal dilatation, 17 after lateral sphincterotomy, 20 after fistulotomy and 29 after haemorrhoidectomy. As expected, internal sphincter defects were found in patients who had undergone sphincterotomy and many who had had fistula surgery. However, less expected was the finding of an additional, unexpected, external sphincter injury in around one third of patients. From the anatomy of this injury, the aetiology was thought to be poorly performed surgery or occult obstetric injury. Patients who had undergone haemorrhoidectomy and had symptoms of incontinence were also found to have sphincter defects. Twenty-six of 29 patients had an internal anal sphincter injury, and external anal sphincter injuries were seen in 19 patients. From the distribution of the external sphincter injury, we considered that obstetric injury was the likely cause of external sphincter damage in 12 patients, whilst in the other seven, the damage appeared to be related to haemorrhoidectomy injury.

Manual Anal Dilatation

Anal dilatation has been a mainstay of treatment of many colorectal diseases and was popularised for treating haemorrhoids by Lord [3]. Techniques have been variable. Watts et al. used four fingers in the anal canal to provide lateral distraction "with considerable force" and reported "occasionally some bleeding from the mucocutaneous junction" [4]. Others have tried to standardise the procedure, using a Parks' retractor opened to a set distance [5].

There have been many reports of incontinence after manual anal dilatation. This appears to be related to internal anal sphincter fragmentation. A study from St. Mark's Hospital in the UK of 12 men with incontinence after manual anal dilatation found that resting anal pressures were low. Eleven of the men had a disrupted internal anal sphincter, with fragmentation in ten of these cases (Figs. 1 and 2). Three patients also had external anal sphincter fragmentation [6]. A further study [7] examined 32 consecutive patients who had undergone manual dilatation and found minor anal incontinence in 12.5%. Of 20 patients who agreed to endoanal ultrasound, sphincteric defects were found in 13. In a retrospective study of 100 patients undergoing anal stretch in a single centre in Scotland [8], clinical indication was anal fissure in 46 patients, first- or second-degree haemorrhoids in 22 patients and anal stenosis in seven patients. In 25 patients, manual dilatation was performed without a diagnosis. Incontinence episodes occurred in 27 patients, of whom 21 were women. Other authors report lower incontinence

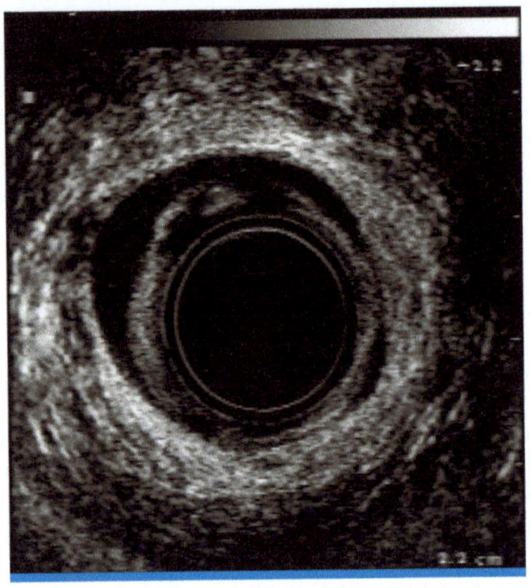

Fig. 1. Endoanal ultrasound appearances after manual anal dilatation showing internal anal sphincter fragmentation (deficient between 2 and 3 o'clock and 4 and 8 o'clock). Reprinted with permission from [2]

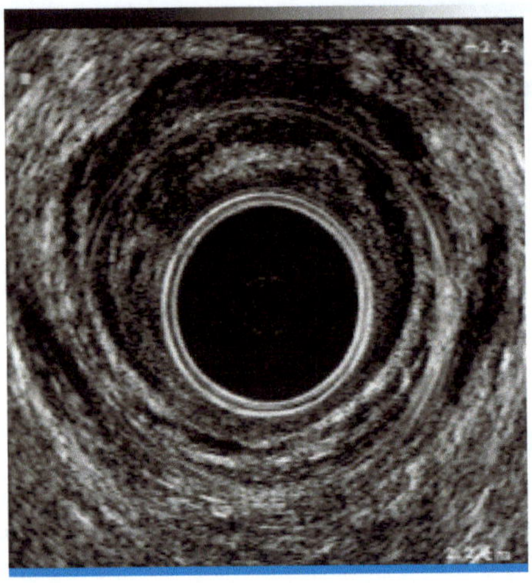

Fig. 2. Gross disruption and fragmentation of both internal and external anal sphincters following manual anal dilatation. Reprinted with permission from [2]

rates. A retrospective single-centre review analysed 241 patients who had undergone manual dilatation for anal fissure. Patients were contacted either by phone or by postal questionnaire [9]. Nine patients (3.8%) were reported to have persistently impaired continence as a result of the dilatation and eight patients had temporary symptoms of incontinence. None of these patients had either manometric or endoanal ultrasound evidence of sphincter disruption. Reports from other centres suggest very low rates of significant incontinence [10]. Despite a recent review suggesting that manual dilatation "should probably be abandoned" as a treatment for anal fissure [11], there is little doubt that it is still a widely practised procedure [12].

Lateral Sphincterotomy

Lateral sphincterotomy aims to divide the internal anal sphincter. This causes a reduction in anal resting pressure [13], and it is generally thought that it overcomes sphincter spasm and results in better anal canal perfusion to allow fissure healing.

Incontinence to flatus may be seen in around one third of patients undergoing sphincterotomy [14, 15]. Other studies have suggested lower rates of incontinence: Vafai and Mann [16] reported an incidence of 1% permanent partial incontinence to faeces after closed lateral internal sphincterotomy, and Hoffmann and Goligher [17] reported a 6% rate of flatus incontinence and 1% faecal incontinence. The true incidence of incontinence may be difficult to assess, as it has been suggested that patients underreport their symptoms to their surgeon [18].

Surgical and anaesthetic technique may play a role in the incidence of incontinence. Closed internal sphincterotomy has been suggested to be marginally safer than open sphincterotomy [15]. Combining sphincterotomy with other anorectal procedures seems to be higher risk [19]. Keighley et al. [20] recommended that sphincterotomy should be performed only under general anaesthesia.

Sphincterotomy length is closely related to symptoms of incontinence. Garcia-Aguilar et al. [21] compared 13 patients with symptoms of incontinence after sphincterotomy to 13 control patients who had undergone the same operation without symptoms. They found that whilst manometric characteristics and rectal sensory parameters were similar in both groups, sphincterotomy length was significantly greater in the incontinent group (75% vs. 57%). Furthermore, the external sphincter was also thinner at the site of sphincterotomy in patients with incontinence, raising the concern that iatrogenic damage to this structure might also contribute to symptoms.

A similar study from St. Mark's Hospital reported on ten women and five men after lateral sphincterotomy [22]. Of the women, endoanal ultrasound showed that the entire length of the internal sphincter had been divided in nine, three of whom had flatus incontinence (Fig. 3). The sphincterotomy was only partial in the men. This discrepancy was thought to be related to the shorter anal sphincter in women.

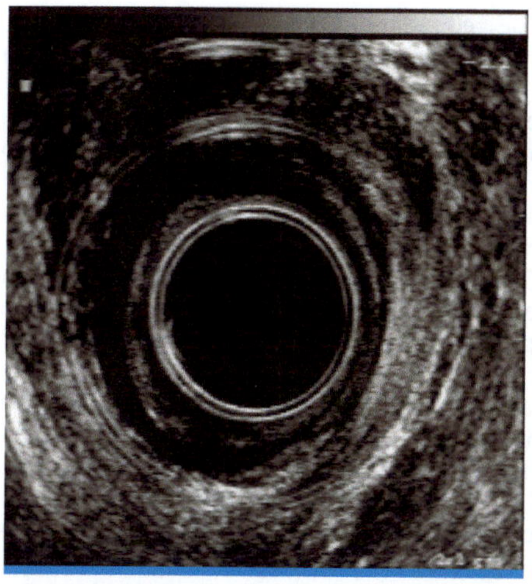

Fig. 3. A full-length deficiency of the internal sphincter between 2 and 6 o'clock up to the level of the puborectalis sling, with bunching of the sphincter fibres on the contralateral side following lateral internal sphincterotomy. Reprinted with persmission from [2]

Newer pharmacological therapies for anal fissure are displacing sphincterotomy and manual dilatation as first-line therapies for anal fissure. They do not appear to have a long-term detrimental impact on sphincter function [23].

Anal Fistula Surgery

Anal fistula surgery represents a compromise between the need to drain sepsis and lay open tracts whilst minimising sphincter muscle division. Incontinence rate estimates after fistula surgery vary widely. A study from St. Mark's Hospital [24] prospectively audited results in 98 patients, 86 of whom had fistulas of cryptoglandular origin. Eleven (11%) had superficial fistulas, 30 (31%) had intersphincteric fistulas, 52 (53%) had transsphincteric fistulas, three (3%) had suprasphincteric fistulas and two (2%) had extrasphincteric fistulas. Fistula recurrence occurred in four (4%) cases, whilst nine (9%) cases still had a seton drain in situ at the end of the audit period. However, incontinence was seen in ten (10%) patients, and interestingly, nine (9%) of these patients had undergone previous fistula surgery prior to the audit. A similar study from Wolverhampton in the UK [25] of 63 patients treated over a 4-year period suggested that clinic review might underestimate the prevalence of incontinence in patients after fistula surgery. They reported that 50% of patients had a degree of incontinence to flatus or liquid after all techniques of fistula treatment, though this was missed at routine clinic review and detected only with a detailed continence questionnaire.

A study of 110 patients who had undergone fistulotomy in a single centre suggested that faecal incontinence, as measured by the Faecal Incontinence Severity Index (FISI), was a good predictor of quality of life after fistula surgery [26]. Linear regression analysis further suggested that only the amount of external sphincter divided correlated with the FISI.

There is little doubt, however, that patients with fistula recurrence or persistence may also exhibit high dissatisfaction levels. A further retrospective study on 624 patients who had undergone surgical treatment of anal fistulas addressed this specific issue [27]. Three hundred and seventy-five patients responded to the questionnaire. The authors attempted to identify factors that affected patients' lifestyles and satisfaction levels. Interestingly, patients with fistula recurrence reported the highest level of dissatisfaction (61%), which was significantly higher than patients with incontinence (24%).

The aetiology of incontinence following fistula surgery is probably multifactorial. Sphincter division is an inevitable part of laying open many fistulas, and this is undoubtedly central to incontinence in many cases. Seton drains, fibrin glue and advancement flaps are all attempts to conserve sphincter anatomy in fistula treatment. In patients with a disease underlying their perianal sepsis, such as Crohn's disease, incontinence symptoms may be exacerbated by colitis and alterations in stool frequency and consistency. It has also been suggested that patients who experience post-fistula-surgery incontinence may have disordered rectal sensation, with an increase in maximal rectal volume threshold [28].

Inadvertent anal dilatation during fistula surgery probably also plays a role. A randomised trial comparing the Parks' and Scott anal retractors suggested that the Parks' retractor caused significant deterioration in continence and a fall in resting anal pressures [29]. Neither of these parameters changed with use of the Scott retractor. The authors concluded that internal anal sphincter damage was responsible for the incontinence.

Surgical Haemorrhoidectomy

In a retrospective multicentre study of 507 patients undergoing Milligan-Morgan haemorrhoidectomy, anal incontinence was reported by 33%, most of whom attributed this incontinence to the haemorrhoidectomy itself [30]. The incontinence mechanism is uncertain, though it has been noted that patients with incontinence symptoms tend to have

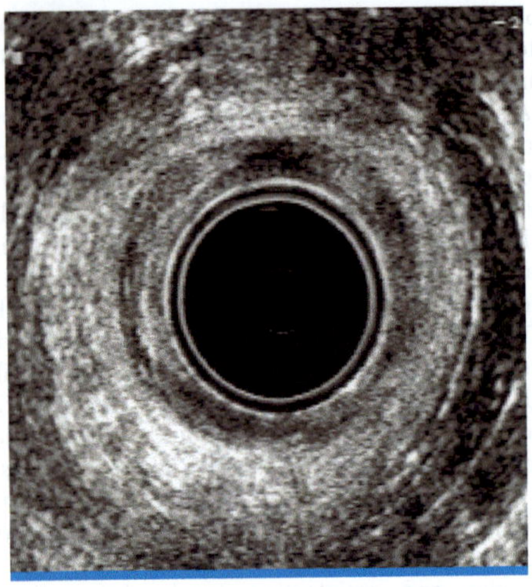

Fig. 4. Patchy internal sphincter defects at surgical haemorrhoidectomy sites. Reprinted with persmission from [2]

abnormally low sphincter pressures [31]. However, in the majority of patients undergoing haemorrhoidectomy, the fall in sphincter pressures was often from a high to a normal level. Often, sphincter pressures increased at around 3–6 months after surgery. Interestingly, the rectoanal inhibitory reflex appears to be unaltered by haemorrhoidectomy, though ultraslow waves do appear to be abolished [32].

Inadvertent sphincter dilatation by anal retractors during haemorrhoidectomy might also play a role. A randomised trial comparing haemorrhoidectomy performed "perineally" to that performed using a Parks' anal retractor suggested that resting pressure decreased by 8% in the perineal group but by 23% in the retractor group. This difference was statistically significant [33].

Direct surgical trauma to the sphincters may also be a factor. In a paper evaluating ten patients with incontinence after haemorrhoidectomy, the authors reported that endoanal ultrasound found an internal sphincter defect in five patients, a combined internal and external sphincter defect in two patients and an isolated external sphincter defect in one patient (Fig. 4) [34].

Stapled Haemorrhoidectomy

This technique employs a circular intraluminal stapling device that is introduced into the anal canal to excise redundant rectal mucosa and interrupt the superior haemorrhoidal arteries above the base of the haemorrhoids, causing a shrivelling of external haemorrhoids and skin tags. Although results of long-term follow-up are not yet available, this procedure appears to be less painful than conventional Milligan–Morgan haemorrhoidectomy and allows an earlier return to work [35, 36].

There have been concerns that stapled haemorrhoidectomy may damage the anal sphincter, perhaps through excessive anal canal dilatation to accommodate the stapling device and its associated dilator. Another concern is that the mucosal purse string might incorporate fibres of the internal anal sphincter. In a report of five patients with persistent pain and faecal urgency persisting after stapled haemorrhoidectomy, four patients had some muscle incorporated into the stapler doughnuts compared with only one of 11 patients operated on by the same surgeon with a good functional result [37]. However, other centres have reported few complications (and specifically no anal incontinence) after the procedure though inevitably as with any new procedure, many of the studies are small and with short follow-up [38].

However, reports on effects on continence following stapled haemorrhoidectomy are conflicting. In a recent study [39] of 20 patients undergoing surgery, there was no significant effect on either resting pressures or squeeze pressure after surgery and little significant effect on the rectoanal inhibitory reflex. Three-dimensional ultrasonography did not demonstrate any changes in internal anal sphincter thickness. Interestingly, the ability of the anal mucosa to discriminate hot from cold water was actually improved in five patients.

A recent trial of 100 patients randomised between open and stapled haemorrhoidectomy has shown that patients undergoing stapled haemorrhoidectomy had more difficulty maintaining continence to liquid stools in the early days after surgery. After 30 days, however, their continence score was superior to the group undergoing open haemorrhoidectomy [40]. Another randomised trial compared closed and stapled haemorrhoidectomy [41]. In the stapled group, maximum anal resting pressure and squeeze pressure were reduced at 3 months compared with preoperative values, though these values returned to baseline at 6 months. Again, the mechanism of temporary reduction in sphincter function remains unclear. Dilatation is a possibility, as is inclusion of muscle fibres within the stapling doughnut, proven histologically in this study. Interestingly, a similar number of patients had muscle fibres excised by closed haemorrhoidectomy.

Rectocele Surgery

Patients with rectocele may have associated physiological abnormalities, including chronic constipation and incontinence. Incontinence aetiology is variable but includes rectoanal intussusception, complete rectal prolapse, sphincter disruption and atrophy [42]. There are a number of surgical approaches to correcting the defect, including the transvaginal, transanal and transperineal approaches.

Most published papers on rectocele surgery comprise retrospective data. There are few randomised trials [43]. There are concerns about continence following the transanal approach to rectocele repair. A prospective study of the transanal approach has been reported. Anal dilatation was limited to a maximum of 4 cm. After 6 months, no patient complained of incontinence, though interestingly, there were significant reductions in both resting and squeeze pressures [44]. However, as already mentioned, the pathophysiology of rectocele is complex, and incontinence may be seen in patients undergoing transvaginal repair in whom there is presumably little or no anal digitation and instrumentation [45].

Transanal Endoscopic Microsurgery (TEM)

Transanal endoscopic microsurgery (TEM) is a new technique that is finding a place in the local management of benign rectal tumours and selective T1 and T2 malignancies [46, 47]. The procedure involves inserting a large-diameter (4 cm) operating sigmoidoscope into the anal canal, producing significant anal dilatation, often for prolonged periods of time.

In a recent study [48], anorectal manometry showed a significant fall in resting pressure after TEM from 104±32 cm water to 73±30 cm water, though there was no significant effect on squeeze pressure. However, this was a small study and postoperative evaluation was short (6 weeks). Interestingly, the fall in resting pressure was correlated with length of operating time. Overall, there was no significant effect on continence score, however. An isolated effect of TEM on resting pressure without effect on squeeze pressure has been reported in other studies [49]. Such findings suggest that the predominant injury after TEM is to the internal anal sphincter, and this has been borne out by anorectal ultrasound studies that have shown endosonographic evidence of internal sphincter function in 29% of patients [50].

Certainly, there is evidence from other studies that any effect on anal resting pressure may be transient. In one such study, manometric pressure falls observed 3 months after surgery were restored after 1 year, correlating with improvements in continence [51].

Anal Instrumentation for Anastomosis

General Introduction

Anterior resection and proctectomy with ileoanal pouch formation are the two main operations performed in the pelvis that involve anastomosis performed either by inserting a staple gun transanally or by hand-sewn transanal colo- or ileoanal anastomosis.

Anterior Resection

Transanal stapling devices have allowed easier performance of low anastomoses and led to a reduction in the number of abdominoperineal excisions [52]. Use of these stapling devices, however, may be associated with disturbance of continence [53]. Whilst lower anterior resections are associated with more significant incontinence symptoms [54], quality of life appears to be superior when compared with patients who have had an abdominoperineal excision [55]. In a study from Basingstoke in the UK [56], 93 elderly patients were evaluated after anterior resection: 78 denied significant bowel symptoms, 14 had some symptoms but did not consider them serious enough to warrant a stoma and one had opted for a stoma for functional reasons.

The aetiology of this impairment may be multifactorial, but dilatation either manually prior to stapler insertion or by the stapler gun itself is probably central. Anatomically, much of this injury is predominantly at the site of the internal anal sphincter. In a prospective study of 39 patients undergoing low anterior resection [57], patients were evaluated preoperatively with endoanal ultrasound and at 3, 6, 9, 12 and 24 months. There was no evidence of internal sphincter defect in any patient preoperatively, though three of the female patients had evidence of external sphincter defects consistent with past obstetric history. After surgery, seven patients had endosonographic evidence of internal sphincter defects that persisted at a mean of 2 years' follow-up. The nature of the injury was a thinned internal sphincter with minor areas of disruption, though in three patients, there was disruption of the entire length of the internal sphincter at one site. Of these patients, two did not have their covering ileostomies reversed because of anastomotic leak. Of the remaining five, all had incontinence postoperatively, though in two continence recovered.

A recent study examined the use of glyceryl trinitrate (GTN) paste to induce internal anal sphincter relaxation prior to staple-gun insertion [58]. In this study, 60 patients without previous evidence of sphincter damage were randomised in a double-blind manner to receive either GTN paste or placebo. Surgery and anaesthesia were standardised as far as possible, and low anterior resection was performed using a double-stapling technique with a 31-mm transanal stapling gun, with the use of gentle two-finger digital dilatation selectively in patients in whom this was required to insert the staple gun. Intraoperative mean resting pressures (mmHg) were significantly reduced by nitroglycerin compared with prenitroglycerin levels ($P = 0.002$) or controls ($P = 0.001$). Twenty-one of the 28 controls (75%) but only four of the 32 patients in the nitroglycerin group (12.5%) required digital dilatation to insert the stapling instrument ($P = 0.003$). Squeeze pressures were unaltered by the intervention, but mean resting pressures were higher in the nitroglycerin group postoperatively, and incontinence scores were lower in the nitroglycerin group at 3 ($P = 0.003$) and 12 ($P = 0.002$) months.

There are reports of employing transabdominal anastomosis after anterior resection for mid and low rectal cancers. The technique's enthusiasts have reported it is safe, with little long-term effect on continence or manometric parameters [59]. Transabdominal anastomosis after low anterior resection remains a technical challenge and may not be safer in terms of anastomotic integrity when compared with stapling.

Radiotherapy may further compromise continence after anterior resection [60]. A recent study evaluated patients from the Stockholm trials and compared patients who had preoperative radiotherapy with those who had not [61]. Whilst the indications for radiotherapy in these trials were a little outdated and regimens often included sphincter irradiation, this study had the advantage of a long follow-up (mean 14 years). It suggested that irradiated patients had significantly greater symptoms of faecal incontinence and soiling and more bowel movements per week. Although there was no preoperative data, patients in the irradiated group had significantly lower resting and squeeze pressures and more evidence of scarring on endoanal ultrasound. Similar detrimental effects of radiotherapy on continence and function amongst patients from the Swedish trial have also been reported [62].

The use of colonic pouches to improve bowel function and continence has been widely promoted. Some reports have suggested improved functional outcome compared with straight anastomosis [63–65]. Data in this area is contradictory, however. A recent report of a 2-year follow-up of patients randomised between a colonic pouch or a side-to-end anastomosis showed an improvement in neorectal volume in the J-pouch group. Functional outcome was assessed and found to be similar in both groups. The authors concluded that male gender, low anastomosis, pelvic sepsis and the postoperative decrease in sphincter pressures were more independent factors in more incontinence symptoms [66].

Other factors have been shown to impact continence after anterior resection. Anastomotic leakage has been shown to reduce functional outcomes and continence after anterior resection [67]. This is probably the effect of fibrosis at the anastomosis causing a reduction in neorectal reservoir function [68]. The rectoanal inhibitory reflex may be impaired by anterior resection, and this doubtless relates to disruption of the descending local reflex arc responsible for this. Reflex recovery may be mirrored by an improvement in continence [69].

Ileoanal Pouch

Prospective data on patients undergoing ileoanal pouch surgery has shown that in patients with low maximum anal resting pressures pre- and postoperatively [70], seepage and incontinence were worse, and this was associated with a poorer quality of life.

In this surgery, there are differences in technique, with some authors preferring the stapled ileal pouch–anal anastomosis and others a mucosectomy and hand-sewn ileal pouch–anal anastomosis. The hand-sewn technique appears to be associated with poorer function in terms of daytime and nighttime continence [71], pad usage and avoidance of ileostomy [72]. Manometric pressures have been shown to be better preserved in patients undergoing stapled pouch–anal anastomosis compared with those having hand-sewn anastomoses with mucosectomy [73].

The mechanism of incontinence development after stapled pouch–anal anastomosis is uncertain. In a study of 20 patients, maximum anal resting pressure was found to be significantly reduced 3 months postoperatively, though this returned to preoperative values when reassessed 7 and 12 months after surgery. The rectoanal inhibitory reflex, which had been present in all patients preoperatively, was absent at 3 months of follow-up but was observed in all but one patient at 12 months of follow-up. Anorectal sampling was also seen in 16 patients preoperatively, only one patient at 3 months of follow-up, but in 17 patients at 12 months of follow-up [74].

Loss of rectoanal inhibitory reflex was also seen in a smaller study of 17 patients undergoing ileoanal pouch surgery [75].

Conclusion

Iatrogenic faecal incontinence is a significant problem in surgery. The increasing use of stapling techniques for pelvic surgery and a move towards more sphincter-preserving rectal-cancer surgery is commendable but is achieved often at the cost of leaving a patient with imperfect continence.

Overall strategies for reducing iatrogenic incontinence include avoiding outdated, high-risk procedures such as manual dilatation of the anus. Sphincter-preserving techniques for proctological conditions such as botulinum toxin injection for anal fissure and anal flaps for high anal fistulas will further reduce incontinence.

Before being submitted to a procedure that risks iatrogenic incontinence, patients should be assessed for preexisting incontinence symptoms and evidence of previous occult obstetric injury. In selected cases, endoanal ultrasound and manometry may be helpful. This enables the surgeon to help the patient make an informed decision about surgery in the light of risks of iatrogenic faecal incontinence.

References

1. Jameson JS, Chia YW, Kamm MA et al (1994) Effect of age and parity on anorectal function. Br J Surg 81:1689–1692
2. Lindsey I, Jones OM, Smilgin-Humphreys MM et al (2004) Patterns of faecal incontinence after anal surgery. Dis Colon Rectum 47:1643–1649
3. Lord PH (1968) A new regime for the treatment of haemorrhoids. Proc R Soc Med 61:935–036
4. Watts JM, Bennett RC, Goligher JC (1964) Stretching of anal sphincters in the treatment of fissure-in-ano. Br Med J 2:342–343
5. Sohn N, Eisenberg MM, Weinstein MA et al (1992) Precise anorectal dilatation-its role in the therapy of anal fissures. Dis Colon Rectum 35:322–327
6. Speakman CT, Burnett SJ, Kamm MA et al (1991) Sphincter injury after anal dilatation demonstrated by anal endosonography. Br J Surg 78:1429–1430
7. Nielsen MB, Rasmussen OO, Pedersen JF et al (1993) Risk of sphincter damage and anal incontinence after anal dilatation for fissure-in-ano. An endosonographic study. Dis Colon Rectum 36:677–680
8. MacDonald A, Smith A, McNeill AD et al (1992) Manual dilatation of the anus. Br J Surg 79:1381–1382
9. Strugnell NA, Cooke SG, Lucarotti ME et al (1999) Controlled digital dilatation under total neuromuscular blockade for chronic anal fissure: a justifiable procedure. Br J Surg 86:651–656
10. Weaver RM, Ambrose NS, Alexander-Williams J et al (1987) Manual dilatation of the anus vs. subcutaneous sphincterotomy in the treatment of chronic fissure-in-ano. Results of a prospective, randomized, clinical trial. Dis Colon Rectum 30:420–423
11. Nelson R (2005) Operative procedures for fissure-in-ano. The Cochrane Database of Systematic Reviews, Issue 2. Art. No.:CD002199
12. Karandikar S, Brown GM, Carr ND et al (2003) Attitudes to the treatment of chronic anal fissure in ano after failed medical treatment. Colorectal Dis 5:569–572
13. Hancock BD (1977) The internal sphincter and anal fissure. Br J Surg 64:92–95
14. Khubchandani IT, Reed JF (1989) Sequelae of internal sphincterotomy for chronic fissure in ano. Br J Surg 76:431–434
15. Garcia-Aguilar J, Belmonte C, Wong WD et al (1996) Open vs. closed sphincterotomy for chronic anal fissure: long-term results. Dis Colon Rectum 39:440–443
16. Vafai M, Mann CV (1987) Closed lateral internal anal sphincterotomy as an office procedure for the treatment of anal fissures. Coloproctology I:49–52
17. Hoffmann DC, Goligher JC (1970) Lateral subcutaneous internal sphincterotomy in treatment of anal fissure. Br Med J 3:673–675
18. Casillas S, Hull TL, Zutshi M et al (2005) Incontinence after a lateral internal sphincterotomy: are we underestimating it? Dis Colon Rectum 48:1193–1199
19. Leong AF, Husain MJ, Seow-Choen F et al (1994) Performing internal sphincterotomy with other anorectal procedures. Dis Colon Rectum 37:1130–1132
20. Keighley MR, Greca F, Nevah E et al (1981) Treatment of anal fissure by lateral subcutaneous sphincterotomy should be under general anaesthesia. Br J Surg 68:400–401
21. Garcia-Aguilar J, Belmonte Montes C, Perez JJ et al (1998) Incontinence after lateral internal sphincterotomy: anatomic and functional evaluation. Dis Colon Rectum 41:423–427
22. Sultan AH, Kamm MA, Nicholls RJ et al (1994) Prospective study of the extent of sphincter division during lateral sphincterotomy. Dis Colon Rectum 37:1031–1033
23. Lindsey I, Jones OM, Cunningham C et al (2004) Chronic anal fissure. Br J Surg 91:270–279
24. Malouf AJ, Buchanan GN, Carapeti EA et al (2002) A prospective audit of fistula-in-ano at St Mark's Hospital. Colorectal Dis 4:13–19
25. Joy HA, Williams JG (2002) The outcome of surgery for complex anal fistula. Colorectal Dis 4:254–261
26. Cavanaugh M, Hyman N, Osler T (2002) Fecal incontinence severity index after fistulotomy: a predictor of quality of life. Dis Colon Rectum 45:349–353
27. Garcia-Aguilar J, Davey CS, Le CT et al (2000) Patients satisfaction after surgical treatment for fistula-in-ano. Dis Colon Rectum 43:1206–1212
28. Pescatori M, Ayabaca S, Caputo D (2004) Can anal manometry predict anal incontinence after fistulectomy in males? Colorectal Dis 6:97–102
29. Zimmerman DD, Gosselink MP, Hop WC et al (2003) Impact of two different types of anal retractor on fecal continence after fistula repair: a prospective, randomized, clinical trial. Dis Colon Rectum 46:1674–1679
30. Johannsson HO, Graf W, Pahlman L (2002) Long-term results of haemorrhoidectomy. Eur J Surg 168:485–489
31. Read MG, Read NW, Haynes WG et al (1982) A prospective study of the effect of haemorrhoidectomy

on sphincter function and faecal incontinence. Br J Surg 69:396–398
32. Roe AM, Bartolo DC, Vellacott KD et al (1987) Submucosal versus ligation excision haemorrhoidectomy: a comparison of anal sensation, anal sphincter manometry and postoperative pain and function. Br J Surg 74:948–951
33. Van Tets WF, Kuijpers JH, Tran K et al (1997) Influence of Parks' anal retractor on anal sphincter pressures. Dis Colon Rectum 40:1042–1045
34. Abbasakoor F, Nelson M, Beynon J et al (1998) Anal endosonography in patients with anorectal symptoms after haemorrhoidectomy. Br J Surg 85:1522–1524
35. Rowsell M. Bello M, Hemingway DM (2000) Circumferential mucosectomy (stapled haemorrhoidectomy) versus conventional haemorrhoidectomy: randomised controlled trial. Lancet 355:779–781
36. Mehigan BJ, Monson JR, Hartley JE (2000) Stapling procedure for haemorrhoids versus Milligan–Morgan haemorrhoidectomy: randomised controlled trial. Lancet 355:782–785
37. Cheetham MJ, Mortensen NJ, Nystrom PO et al (2000) Persistent pain and faecal urgency after stapled haemorrhoidectomy. Lancet 356:730–733
38. Singer MA, Cintron JR, Fleshman JW et al (2002) Early experience with stapled haemorrhoidectomy in the Untied States. Dis Colon Rectum 45:360–367
39. Altomare DF, Rinaldi M, Sallustio PL et al (2001) Long-term effects of stapled haemorrhoidectomy on internal anal function and sensitivity. Br J Surg 88:1487–1491
40. Ganio E, Altomare DF, Gabrielli F et al (2001) Prospective randomized multicentre trial comparing stapled with open haemorrhoidectomy. Br J Surg 88:669–674
41. Khalil KH, O'Bichere A, Sellu D (2000) Randomized clinical trial of sutures versus stapled closed haemorrhoidectomy. Br J Surg 87:1352–1355
42. Pucciani F, Rottoli ML, Bologna A et al (1996) Anterior rectocele and anorectal dysfunction. Int J Colorectal Dis 11:1–9
43. Sand PK, Koduri S, Lobel R et al (2001) Prospective randomized trial of polyglactin 910 mesh to prevent recurrence of cystoceles and rectoceles. Am J Obstet Gynecol 184:1357–1364
44. Ho YH, Ang M, Nyam D et al (1998) Transanal approach to rectocele repair may compromise anal sphincter pressures. Dis Colon Rectum 41:354–358
45. Kahn MA, Stanton SL (1997) Posterior colporrhaphy: its effects on bowel and sexual function. Br J Obstet Gynecol 104:82–86
46. Cook TA, Mortensen NJ (1998) Management of faecal incontinence following obstetric injury. Br J Surg 85:293–299
47. Saclarides TJ (1997) Transanal endoscopic microsurgery. Surg Clin North Am 77:229–239
48. Kennedy ML, Lubowski DZ, King DW (2002) Transanal endoscopic microsurgery excision: is anorectal function compromised? Dis Colon Rectum 45:601–604
49. Banerjee AK, Jehle EC, Kreis ME et al (1996) Prospective study of the proctographic and functional consequences of transanal endoscopic microsurgery. Br J Surg 83:211–213
50. Herman RM, Richter P, Walega P et al (2001) Anorectal sphincter function and rectal barostat study in patients following transanal endoscopic microsurgery. Int J Colorectal Dis 16:370–376
51. Kreis ME, Jehle EC, Huag V et al (1996) Functional results after transanal endoscopic microsurgery. Dis Colon Rectum 39:1116–1121
52. Kirwan WO, O'Riordan MG, Waldron R (1989) Declining indications for abdomino-perineal resection. Br J Surg 76:1061–1063
53. Williams NS, Price R, Johnston D (1980) The long-term effect of sphincter preserving operations for rectal carcinoma on function of the anal sphincter in man. Br J Surg 67:203–208
54. Efthimiadis C, Basdanis G, Zatagias A et al (2004) Manometric and clinical evaluation of patients after low anterior resection for rectal cancer. Tech Coloproctol 8(Suppl 1):205–207
55. Guren MG, Eriksen MT, Wiig JN et al (2005) Quality of life and functional outcome following anterior or abdominoperineal resection for rectal cancer. Eur J Surg Oncol 31:735–742
56. Phillips PS, Farquharson SM, Sexton R et al (2004) Rectal cancer in the elderly: patients' perceptions of bowel control after restorative surgery. Dis Colon Rectum 47:287–290
57. Farouk R, Duthie GS, Lee PWR et al (1998) Endosonographic evidence of injury to the internal anal sphincter after low anterior resection. Dis Colon Rectum 41:888–891
58. Winter DC, Murphy A, Kell MR et al (2004) Perioperative topical nitrate and sphincter function in patients undergoing transanal stapled anastomosis: a randomized placebo-controlled, double-blinded trial. Dis Colon Rectum 47:697–703
59. Jiang JK, Yang SH, Lin JK (2005) Transabdominal anastomosis after low anterior resection: a prospective, randomized, controlled trial comparing long-term results between side-to-end anastomosis and colonic J-pouch. Dis Colon Rectum 48:2100–2108
60. Welsh FK, McFall M, Mitchell G et al (2003) Pre-operative short-course radiotherapy is associated with faecal incontinence after anterior resection. Colorectal Dis 5:563–568
61. Pollack J, Holm T, Cedermark B et al (2006) Long-term effect of pre-operative radiation on anorectal function. Dis Colon Rectum 49:345–352
62. Dahlberg M, Glimelius B, Graf W et al (1998) Pre-operative irradiation affects functional results after surgery for rectal cancer: results from a randomized study. Dis Colon Rectum 41:543–549
63. Hida J, Yoshifuji T, Tokoro T et al (2004) Comparison of long-term functional results of colonic J-pouch and straight anastomosis after low anterior resection for rectal cancer: a five year follow-up. Dis Colon Rectum 47:1578–1585
64. Williams N, Seow-Cheon F (1998) Physiological and functional outcome following ultra-low anterior resection with colon pouch-anal anastomosis. Br J Surg 85:1029–1035
65. Halbrook O, Pahlman L, Krog M et al (1996) Randomized comparison of straight and colonic J pouch anastomosis after low anterior resection 224:58–65

66. Machado M, Nygren J, Goldman S et al (2005) Functional and physiological assessment of the colonic reservoir or side-to-end anastomosis after low anterior resection for rectal cancer: a two-year follow-up. Dis Colon Rectum 48:29–36
67. Nesbakken A, Nygaard K, Lunde OC (2001) Outcome and late functional results after anastomotic leakage following total mesorectal excision for rectal cancer Br J Surg 88:400–404
68. Hallbook O, Sjodahl R (1996) Anastomotic leakage and functional outcome after anterior resection of the rectum 83:60–62
69. O'Riordain WG, Molloy RG, Gillen P et al (1992) Rectoanal inhibitory reflex following low stapled anterior resection of the rectum. Dis Colon Rectum 35:974–978
70. Braun J, Treutner KH, Harder M et al (1991) Anal sphincter function after intersphincteric resection and stapled ileal pouch-anal anastomosis. Dis Colon Rectum 34:8–16
71. Curran FT, Hill GL (1990) Results of 50 ileoanal J pouch operations. Aust N Z J Surg 60:579–583
72. Remzi FH, Chursh JM, Bast J et al (2001) Mucosectomy vs. stapled ileal pouch-anal anastomosis in patients with familial adenomatous polyposis: functional outcome and neoplasia control. Dis Colon Rectum 44:1590–1596
73. Tuckson WB, McNamara MJ, Fazio VW et al (1991) Impact of anal manipulation and pouch design on ileal pouch function. J Natl Med Assoc 83:1089–1092
74. Sagar PM, Holdsworth PJ, Johnston D (1991) Correlation between laboratory findings and clinical outcome after restorative proctocolectomy: serial studies in 20 patients with end-to-end pouch-anal anastomosis. Br J Surg 78:67–70
75. Sun WM, Read NW, Katsinelos P et al (1994) Anorectal function after restorative proctocolectomy and low anterior resection with coloanal anastomosis. Br J Surg 81:280–284

Rectal Prolapse

27

Michael E.D. Jarrett

Introduction

The term rectal prolapse can be associated with three different clinical entities: full-thickness rectal prolapse, mucosal prolapse and internal rectal intussusception. Full-thickness rectal prolapse is the most commonly recognised type and is defined as protrusion of the full thickness of the rectal wall through the anus. In mucosal prolapse, only the rectal mucosa protrudes from the anus. Internal intussusception may be a full thickness or a partial rectal-wall disorder, but the prolapsed tissue does not pass beyond the anal canal and does not pass out of the anus. This chapter focuses on full-thickness rectal prolapse with specific regard to associated faecal incontinence.

Faecal incontinence is the most common symptom in patients with full-thickness rectal prolapse, apart from the presence of the prolapse itself. It affects 50–80% of patients [1–3]. Of those who complain of faecal incontinence, about one third will continue to be incontinent after rectopexy [4–7]. The cause of the ongoing incontinence may be a result of anal sphincter disruption from dilatation by the prolapsing bowel or from a pudendal neuropathy caused by repeated traction on the pudendal nerves during prolapse or both [8, 9].

Women with rectal prolapse outnumber men by ten to one [10, 11]. Amongst women, the incidence rises with age, with more than 50% of female patients with prolapse being over the age of 70 years [12]. This is not mirrored in men [13, 14]. The incidence of prolapse does not appear to be confined to parous women, with one third of elderly patients with prolapse being nulliparous [15, 16]. Nulliparae appear to be less likely to suffer from incontinence (22%) when compared with those who have had a vaginal delivery (85%) [17]. It is rare for men with a prolapse to suffer from incontinence.

Rarely, children can develop a rectal prolapse; usually before the age of 3 years. The evaluation and treatment of children with rectal prolapse is different from that for adults and will not be discussed.

Rectal prolapse is an intussusception of the rectum through the anal sphincters and often has other associated abnormalities especially related to a weak pelvic floor [18]. A deep pouch of Douglas, lax lateral ligaments and/or loss of attachment of the rectum to the sacrum are commonly present and lead to genital prolapse in 25% of patients [12] and urinary incontinence in 30% [17, 19, 20].

Symptoms and Signs

Typically, patients complain of prolapse, mucus discharge, bleeding and either incontinence or constipation. The diagnosis of full-thickness rectal prolapse, although suggested by the history, needs to be confirmed on examination to rule out partial-thickness rectal prolapse, prolapsing haemorrhoids and the like. Ideally, the patient should be placed on a toilet or commode and encouraged to bear down in order to demonstrate the prolapse, as embarrassment and fear of soiling often prevents demonstration of the prolapse in the consultation room. Incontinence should be specified, as mucus or minor soiling from the surface of the prolapsing rectum is often reported as faecal incontinence.

Investigations

Investigation should be targeted to the individual, with the underlying principle being one of selecting a procedure that will best correct the rectal prolapse whilst addressing both any problems associated with concurrent pelvic floor insufficiency and functional disturbances, if present.

Flexible Sigmoidoscopy

Flexible sigmoidoscopy should be carried out to exclude a solitary rectal ulcer, rectal polyp, tumour or mucosal disease. Colonoscopy may be carried out if more proximal colonic pathology is suspected, and transit studies may be useful in patients with constipation to elicit whether a resection rectopexy is indicated.

Defecating Proctography

Defecating proctography is not routinely required if a full-thickness rectal prolapse is evident clinically, although it may be used to predict return of continence. A narrow anorectal angle during pelvic floor contraction, minimal pelvic floor descent during contraction and a long anal canal at rest and during contraction all increase the chance of return of continence after prolapse fixation [21].

Anal Manometry

Anal manometry is not routinely carried out in all patients with rectal prolapse. However, in patients with associated faecal incontinence, it has some predictive value in identifying patients who are likely to remain incontinent following rectal prolapse repair [22]. Patients with rectal prolapse have a reduced resting anal canal pressure [4, 5, 23, 24]. Those with rectal prolapse and incontinence have both reduced resting and squeeze pressures, which improve significantly following operation. Patients who remain incontinent after surgery have a significantly lower preoperative resting anal pressure and maximum voluntary contraction pressure than do patients who improve or regain continence. Preoperative resting anal pressure below 10 mmHg and maximum voluntary contraction pressure below 50–60 mmHg are associated with persisting incontinence after surgery [25, 26].

Pudendal Nerve Terminal Motor Latency

Pudendal nerve terminal motor latency (PNTML) is being carried out less and less. Although it is often prolonged in patients with associated incontinence, its relevance to further management is not well understood.

Endoanal Ultrasound

Endoanal ultrasound often reveals an early thickened internal anal sphincter and submucosa [27] and, with long-standing prolapse, a torn or even fragmented internal anal sphincter and/or external sphincter [28, 29]. The feeling is that the internal sphincter thickens initially in response to the prolapse in order to try to contain it but eventually fails from traumatic disruption. In the incontinent patient, baseline endoanal ultrasound and physiological measurements are useful to ascertain the likelihood of ongoing problems of faecal incontinence following rectal prolapse fixation.

Operative Intervention

Operative treatment is usually indicated for full-thickness rectal prolapse if the primary problem is not one of excessive straining. More than 100 different procedures have been described to treat the condition [30] but can be broadly divided into those that are abdominal (open or laparoscopic) or perineal in approach. The latter are often favoured for the frail and the infirm and in young males to minimise operative trauma and the risk of nerve damage. Continence restoration rates are similar between the two

Table 1. Large studies (>50 patients) involving open abdominal repair of full-thickness rectal prolapse

Study	Patients	Procedure	Improved continence (%)	Recurrence rate (%)
Morgan [31]	150	Ivalon	52	3.2
Penfold and Hawley [2]	95	Ivalon	55	3
Mann and Hoffman [32]	51	Ivalon	38	0
McCue and Thomson [33]	53	Ivalon	38	3.8
Keighley et al. [3]	86	Marlex	64	0
Launer et al. [34]	54	Ripstein		12
Holmstrom et al. [35]	97	Ripstein	39	4.1
Tjandra et al. [36]	142	Ripstein	48	8
Watts et al. [16]	102	Resection	77	1.9
Kim et al. [37]	161	Resection	55	5

Table 2. Large studies (>50 patients) involving perineal repair of full-thickness rectal prolapse

Study	Patients	Procedure	Improved continence (%)	Recurrence rate (%)
Lechaux et al. [38]	85	Delorme's	69	13.5
Watts and Thompson [39]	113	Delorme's	40	26.5
Watkins et al. [40]	52	Delorme's	83	10
Williams et al. [41]	114	Altemeier	46	10
Ramanujam et al. [42]	72	Altemeier	67	5.5
Kim et al. [37]	183	Altemeier	53	15.8
Kimmins et al. [43]	63	Altemeier	50	6.4

groups. In the larger studies (>50 patients), 38–77% of patients achieved improved continence with an abdominal procedure, as did 40–83% of those following a perineal procedure (Tables 1 and 2). It would seem that with prolapse resolution, continence restoration follows suit independent of the procedure undertaken. Recurrence rates, however, do vary markedly, and one would anticipate that with prolapse recurrence, incontinence would also recur. Laparoscopic procedures give a wide range of improved continence, with from 31–90% of patients getting improvement. Recurrence rates seem similar to those of open abdominal surgery (Table 3).

Persistent Postoperative Incontinence

If a full-thickness rectal prolapse is treated quickly and effectively, there is a good chance that continence will be restored. The management of persistent postoperative incontinence, however, remains a difficult problem in what is often an elderly population, and treatment needs to be tailored accordingly.

Conservative Therapy

Treatment of persistent faecal incontinence is primarily conservative. Initially, dietary advice and titration of antidiarrhoeal medication such as loperamide or codeine phosphate are suggested. This aims to firm the patient's stool but not render them constipated, thus allowing the continence mechanism to have conditions such that it can work to the best of its ability. Physical and behavioural therapy [48–51] (e.g. pelvic floor muscle training and biofeedback) also aim to support the patient and optimise sphincter function. Advice on the use of absorbent pads or anal plugs may also be given. Whereas these measures are effective in many patients, a proportion remains with persistent severe incontinence that requires more intensive treatment.

Sacral Nerve Stimulation

Sacral nerve stimulation may be considered at this stage and has the advantages of having a peripheral nerve evaluation phase to evaluate whether a permanent implant is likely to be successful. It is also a minimally invasive procedure and may be carried out under local anaesthetic. Four female patients with persisting faecal incontinence following full-thickness rectal prolapse repair have shown improvement in incontinent episodes from 14 to two per week [52]. Two other papers [53, 54] studying sacral nerve stimulation in a more general population included three patients with ongoing resistant faecal incontinence

Table 3. Large studies (>50 patients) involving laparoscopic abdominal repair of full-thickness rectal prolapse

Study	Patients	Procedure	Improved continence (%)	Recurrence rate (%)
Auguste et al. [44]	54	Laparoscopic	72.4	7.4
D'Hoore et al. [45]	42	Laparoscopic	90	5
Lechaux et al. [46]	48	Laparoscopic	31	4
Kariv et al. [47]	111	Laparoscopic	48	9.3

following rectal prolapse surgery. All three were reported as showing improvement. It appears to be an effective therapy in this subgroup of patients, although numbers reported remain small.

Injectable Bulking Agents

Another minimally invasive procedure involves the injection of sphincter bulking biomaterials. Some benefit has been noted, but studies again remain small and follow-up short [55, 56].

Postanal Repair, Dynamic Graciloplasty, Artifical Bowel Sphincter, Stoma

More invasive surgery includes postanal repair, which has been tried with limited success, and most series have been small, especially with regard to faecal incontinence following prolapse repair [57]. The dynamic graciloplasty procedure and artificial bowel sphincter implants may also be attempted, but both are major operations that have a high morbidity and failure rate [58, 59]. Permanent stoma placement is another surgical option.

Discussion

The majority of patients with full-thickness rectal prolapse experience faecal incontinence [4, 5, 60]. Once the prolapse has been dealt with surgically, approximately one third of these patients continue to suffer from faecal incontinence [4–7]. Treatment is largely conservative in what is often an elderly group of patients. Minimally invasive procedures, such as sacral nerve stimulation, and other more invasive procedures, including stoma formation, should be reserved for the carefully selected minority or patients with ongoing symptoms significantly affecting their quality of life.

References

1. Kupfer CA, Goligher JC (1970) One hundred consecutive cases of complete prolapse of the rectum treated by operation. Br J Surg 57(7):482–487
2. Penfold JC, Hawley PR (1972) Experiences of Ivalon-sponge implant for complete rectal prolapse at St. Mark's Hospital, 1960-70. Br J Surg 59(11):846–848
3. Keighley MR, Fielding JW, Alexander-Williams J (1983) Results of Marlex mesh abdominal rectopexy for rectal prolapse in 100 consecutive patients. Br J Surg 70(4):229–232
4. Broden G, Dolk A, Holmstrom B (1988) Recovery of the internal anal sphincter following rectopexy: a possible explanation for continence improvement. Int J Colorectal Dis 3(1):23–28
5. Sainio AP, Voutilainen PE, Husa AI (1991) Recovery of anal sphincter function following transabdominal repair of rectal prolapse: cause of improved continence? Dis Colon Rectum 34(9):816–821
6. Keighley MR, Shouler P (1984) Clinical and manometric features of the solitary rectal ulcer syndrome. Dis Colon Rectum 27(8):507–512
7. Ramanujam PS, Venkatesh KS, Fietz MJ (1994) Perineal excision of rectal procidentia in elderly high-risk patients. A ten-year experience. Dis Colon Rectum 37(10):1027–1030
8. Neill M, Parks A, Swash M (1981) Physiology studies of the pelvic floor in idiopathic faecal incontinence and rectal prolapse. Br J Surg 68:531–536
9. Lubowski DZ, Swash M, Nicholls RJ, Henry MM (1988) Increase in pudendal nerve terminal motor latency with defaecation straining. Br J Surg 75(11):1095–1097
10. Duthie GS, Bartolo DC (1992) Abdominal rectopexy for rectal prolapse: a comparison of techniques. Br J Surg 79(2):107–113
11. Agachan F, Pfeifer J, Joo JS et al (1997) Results of perineal procedures for the treatment of rectal prolapse. Am Surg 63(1):9–12
12. Loygue J, Nordlinger B, Cunci O et al (1984) Rectopexy to the promontory for the treatment of rectal prolapse. Report of 257 cases. Dis Colon Rectum 27(6):356–359
13. Nicholls JR, Banarjee A (1997) Rectal prolapse and solitary rectal ulcer syndrome. In: Nicholls JR, Dozois RR, eds, Surgery of the colon and rectum. Churchill Livingstone, New York, pp 709–737
14. Kupfer CA, Goligher JC (1970) One hundred consecutive cases of complete prolapse of the rectum treated by operation. Br J Surg 57(7):482–487
15. Mortensen NJ, Vellacott KD, Wilson MG (1984) Lahaut's operation for rectal prolapse. Ann R Coll Surg Engl 66(1):17–18
16. Watts JD, Rothenberger DA, Buls JG et al (1985) The management of procidentia. 30 years' experience. Dis Colon Rectum 28(2):96–102
17. Keighley MR, Williams NS (2001) Surgery of the anus rectum and colon, 2nd edn. W.B. Saunders, London
18. Yoshioka K, Heyen F, Keighley MR (1989) Functional results after posterior abdominal rectopexy for rectal prolapse. Dis Colon Rectum 32(10):835–838
19. Vongsangnak V, Varma JS, Watters D, Smith AN (1985) Clinical, manometric and surgical aspects of complete prolapse of the rectum. J R Coll Surg Edinb 30(4):251–254
20. Hudson CN (1988) Female genital prolapse and pelvic floor deficiency. Int J Colorectal Dis 3(3):181–185
21. Yoshioka K, Hyland G, Keighley MR (1989) Anorectal function after abdominal rectopexy: parameters of predictive value in identifying return of continence. Br J Surg 76(1):64–68
22. Williams JG, Wong WD, Jensen L et al (1991) Incontinence and rectal prolapse: a prospective manometric study. Dis Colon Rectum 34(3):209–216
23. Matheson DM, Keighley MR (1981) Manometric evaluation of rectal prolapse and faecal incontinence. Gut 22(2):126–129

24. Williams JG, Wong WD, Jensen L et al (1991) Incontinence and rectal prolapse: a prospective manometric study. Dis Colon Rectum 34(3):209–216
25. Keighley MR, Shouler PJ (1984) Abnormalities of colonic function in patients with rectal prolapse and faecal incontinence. Br J Surg 71(11):892–895
26. Glasgow SC, Birnbaum EH, Kodner IJ et al (2006) Preoperative anal manometry predicts continence after perineal proctectomy for rectal prolapse. Dis Colon Rectum 49(7):1052–1058
27. Dvorkin LS, Chan CL, Knowles CH et al (2004) Anal sphincter morphology in patients with full-thickness rectal prolapse. Dis Colon Rectum 47(2):198–203
28. Damon H, Henry L, Roman S (2003) Influence of rectal prolapse on the asymmetry of the anal sphincter in patients with anal incontinence. BMC Gastroenterol 3:23
29. Woods R, Voyvodic F, Schloithe AC et al (2003) Anal sphincter tears in patients with rectal prolapse and faecal incontinence. Colorectal Dis 5(6):544–548
30. Wassef R, Rothenberger DA, Goldberg SM (1986) Rectal prolapse. Curr Probl Surg 23(6):397–451
31. Morgan CN, Porter NH, Klugman DJ (1972) Ivalon (polyvinyl alcohol) sponge in the repair of complete rectal prolapse. Br J Surg 59(11):841–846
32. Mann CV, Hoffman C (1988) Complete rectal prolapse: the anatomical and functional results of treatment by an extended abdominal rectopexy. Br J Surg 75(1):34–37
33. McCue JL, Thomson JP (1991) Clinical and functional results of abdominal rectopexy for complete rectal prolapse. Br J Surg 78(8):921–923
34. Launer DP, Fazio VW, Weakley FL et al (1982) The Ripstein procedure: a 16-year experience. Dis Colon Rectum 25(1):41–45
35. Holmstrom B, Broden G, Dolk A (1986) Results of the Ripstein operation in the treatment of rectal prolapse and internal rectal procidentia. Dis Colon Rectum 29(12):845–848
36. Tjandra JJ, Fazio VW, Church JM et al (1993) Ripstein procedure is an effective treatment for rectal prolapse without constipation. Dis Colon Rectum 36(5):501–507
37. Kim DS, Tsang CB, Wong WD et al (1999) Complete rectal prolapse: evolution of management and results. Dis Colon Rectum 42(4):460–466
38. Lechaux JP, Lechaux D, Perez M (1995) Results of Delorme's procedure for rectal prolapse. Advantages of a modified technique. Dis Colon Rectum 38(3):301–307
39. Watts AM, Thompson MR (2000) Evaluation of Delorme's procedure as a treatment for full-thickness rectal prolapse. Br J Surg 87(2):218–222
40. Watkins BP, Landercasper J, Belzer GE et al (2003) Long-term follow-up of the modified Delorme procedure for rectal prolapse. Arch Surg 138(5):498–502
41. Williams JG, Rothenberger DA, Madoff RD, Goldberg SM (1992) Treatment of rectal prolapse in the elderly by perineal rectosigmoidectomy. Dis Colon Rectum 35(9):830–834
42. Ramanujam PS, Venkatesh KS, Fietz MJ (1994) Perineal excision of rectal procidentia in elderly high-risk patients. A ten-year experience. Dis Colon Rectum 37(10):1027–1030
43. Kimmins MH, Evetts BK, Isler J, Billingham R (2001) The Altemeier repair: outpatient treatment of rectal prolapse. Dis Colon Rectum 44(4):565–570
44. Auguste T, Dubreuil A, Bost R et al (2006) Technical and functional results after laparoscopic rectopexy to the promontory for complete rectal prolapse. Prospective study in 54 consecutive patients. Gastroenterol Clin Biol 30(5):659–663
45. D'Hoore A, Cadoni R, Penninckx F (2004) Long-term outcome of laparoscopic ventral rectopexy for total rectal prolapse. Br J Surg 91(11):1500–1505
46. Lechaux D, Trebuchet G, Siproudhis L, Campion JP (2005) Laparoscopic rectopexy for full-thickness rectal prolapse: a single-institution retrospective study evaluating surgical outcome. Surg Endosc 19(4):514–518
47. Kariv Y, Delaney CP, Casillas S et al (2006) Long-term outcome after laparoscopic and open surgery for rectal prolapse: a case-control study. Surg Endosc 20(1):35–42
48. Norton C, Kamm MA (1999) Outcome of biofeedback for faecal incontinence. Br J Surg 86(9):1159–1163
49. Cheetham MA, Kenefick NJ, Kamm MA (2001) Non-surgical treatment of faecal incontinence. Hosp Med 62(9):538–541
50. Norton C, Kamm MA (2001) Anal sphincter biofeedback and pelvic floor exercises for faecal incontinence in adults—a systematic review. Aliment Pharmacol Ther 15(8):1147–1154
51. Rosen HR, Urbarz C, Holzer B et al (2001) Sacral nerve stimulation as a treatment for fecal incontinence. Gastroenterology 121(3):536–541
52. Jarrett ME, Matzel KE, Stosser M et al (2005) Sacral nerve stimulation for fecal incontinence following surgery for rectal prolapse repair: a multicenter study. Dis Colon Rectum 48(6):1243–1248
53. Matzel KE, Bittorf B, Stadelmaier U, Hohenberger W (2003) Sakralnervstimulation in der Behandlung der Stuhlinkontinenz. Chirurg 74:26–32
54. Kenefick NJ, Vaizey CJ, Cohen RG et al (2002) Medium-term results of sacral nerve stimulation for faecal incontinence. Br J Surg 89(7):896–901
55. Vaizey CJ, Kamm MA (2005) Injectable bulking agents for treating faecal incontinence. Br J Surg 92(5):521–527
56. Kenefick NJ, Vaizey CJ, Malouf AJ et al (2002) Injectable silicone biomaterial for faecal incontinence due to internal anal sphincter dysfunction. Gut 51:225–228
57. Setti CP, Nicholls RJ (1994) Postanal repair for faecal incontinence persisting after rectopexy. Br J Surg 81(2):305–307
58. Baeten CG, Bailey HR, Bakka A et al (2000) Safety and efficacy of dynamic graciloplasty for fecal incontinence: report of a prospective, multicenter trial. Dynamic Graciloplasty Therapy Study Group. Dis Colon Rectum 43(6):743–751
59. Lehur PA, Glemain P, Bruley D et al (1998) Outcome of patients with an implanted artificial anal sphincter for severe faecal incontinence. A single institution report. Int J Colorectal Dis 13(2):88–92
60. Williams JG, Rothenberger DA, Madoff RD, Goldberg SM (1992) Treatment of rectal prolapse in the elderly by perineal rectosigmoidectomy. Dis Colon Rectum 35(9):830–834

Sphincter Atrophy

28

Richelle J.F. Felt-Bersma

Introduction

The term "sphincter atrophy" refers mostly to external anal sphincter (EAS) atrophy, as the EAS is the most important factor for maintaining fecal continence. EAS atrophy, often due to pudendal neuropathy caused by stretch injury during childbirth [1] or chronic constipation [2, 3], is an important cause of fecal incontinence. When a woman is fecally incontinent and there is a history of a difficult childbirth with prolonged labor or chronic constipation as well as a sphincter rupture, there is always a chance that, besides the rupture, some atrophy is present in the EAS.

The importance of differentiating between the contribution of a defect or neuropathy/atrophy to the fecal incontinence lies in the fact that only patients with a significant sphincter defect are offered a sphincter repair. There is some, although not unanimous, evidence that severe atrophy interferes with a good result after sphincter repair.

It has been suggested that patients with low anal pressures and poor innervation to the pelvic floor and elderly patients have less favorable results with postanal repair [4, 5] and anal sphincter repair [6–8]. However, prospective studies are lacking. Reviewing the recent literature, Gearhart et al. [9], Pinta et al. [10], and Engel et al. [11] could not find a relationship between pudendal nerve terminal motor latency (PNTML) and anal repair. Birnbaum et al. [12] found a relationship between PNTML and the results of rectopexy. Establishing (the amount of) atrophy, at least the extreme cases, seems of clinical importance when selecting patients for sphincter repair.

Diagnosing External Anal Sphincter Atrophy

Establishing atrophy of the anal sphincter complex has been evaluated with endoanal magnetic resonance imaging (MRI) [13–17]. Studies with endoanal MRI have demonstrated that severe atrophy of the EAS corresponded with a poor clinical outcome [15] and histopathology in biopsies taken from the EAS during surgery [13]. In general, atrophy can be established by measuring EAS thickness and surface area, and the subjective evaluation of the amount of fat. Another study found no relationship between fat content and anorectal function [18]. One study described the aspect of the EAS with anal endosonography in comparison with endoanal MRI, but without three-dimensional (3D) application and without transversal or longitudinal sphincter measurements [18]. With 3D anal endosonography (3D-AE), it is possible to measure EAS length on the lateral view and subsequently perform volume measurements. The high expectations of EAS volume measurements were not met, as no discrimination was found between healthy controls and patients with fecal incontinence [19]. In a subsequent study, using volume measurement was found to be unsuccessful in predicting EAS atrophy in patients with fecal incontinence. Another issue was that in all patients, MRI mentioned atrophy but no histology was performed [20].

A recent study in 18 women with fecal incontinence compared 3D endoanal ultrasound (EUS) and MRI to evaluate EAS atrophy [21]. Atrophy of the EAS with EUS was judged upon its reflection of the outer interface (border of the EAS and subadventitial fat), reflection pattern, and length. Atrophy was scored as none (clearly visible outer interface, mixed reflection pattern), moderate (partly visible outer interface, intermediate reflection, moderate shortening), and severe (hardly visible outer interface, hyperechogenic reflection pattern, severe shortening). These criteria were derived from Williams et al. [17]. Examples of normal and atrophic anal sphincters are shown in Figures 1–5. EAS atrophy with MRI was defined as diffuse thinning of the EAS muscle or diffuse replacement of EAS muscle by fat. EAS atrophy was graded as none (no thinning of the EAS and no replacement of EAS muscle by fat), moderate ($\geqslant$50% thinning of the EAS and/or replacement of EAS muscle by fat), or severe (?50% thinning of the EAS and/or replace-

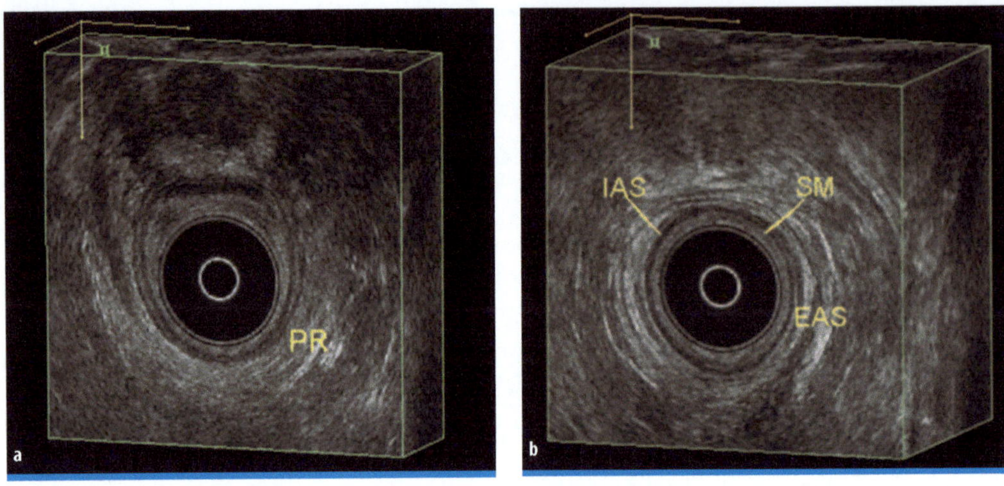

Fig. 1a, b. Endoanal ultrasonography (EAS). Normal anatomy of the anal sphincter and puborectalis muscle in three-dimensional (3D) imaging. **a** Frontal view of puborectalis muscle. **b** Frontal view of the anal sphincters. *PR* puborectalis muscle, *SM* submucosa, *IAS* internal anal sphincter, *EAS* external anal sphincter

ment of EAS muscle by fat). Three-dimensional AE and MRI did not significantly differ for the detection of EAS atrophy (p=0.25) and defects (p=0.38): 3D-AE demonstrated EAS atrophy in 16 patients; MRI detected EAS atrophy in 13 patients. Also, 3D-AE agreed with MRI in 15 of 18 patients in detecting EAS atrophy. Using the grading system, eight of the 18 patients scored the same grade. It was concluded that both endoanal techniques are comparable in detecting EAS atrophy and EAS defects, although there is a substantial difference in grading EAS atrophy. Exact thickness and length measurements do not really contribute to atrophy score. This indicates that this imaging technique can be added as a diagnostic tool for EAS atrophy in patients with fecal incontinence. Limitations of this study are the small number of patients and the absence of a gold standard. Further prospective studies should consist of more patients, healthy controls, and evaluation with surgery and histology.

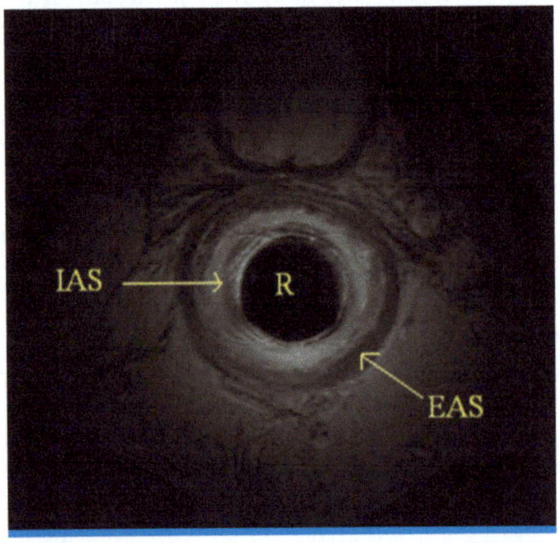

Fig. 2. Magnetic resonance imaging (MRI) (axial view). Normal anatomy of the internal and external anal sphincter. *R* rectum, *IAS* internal anal sphincter, *EAS* external anal sphincter

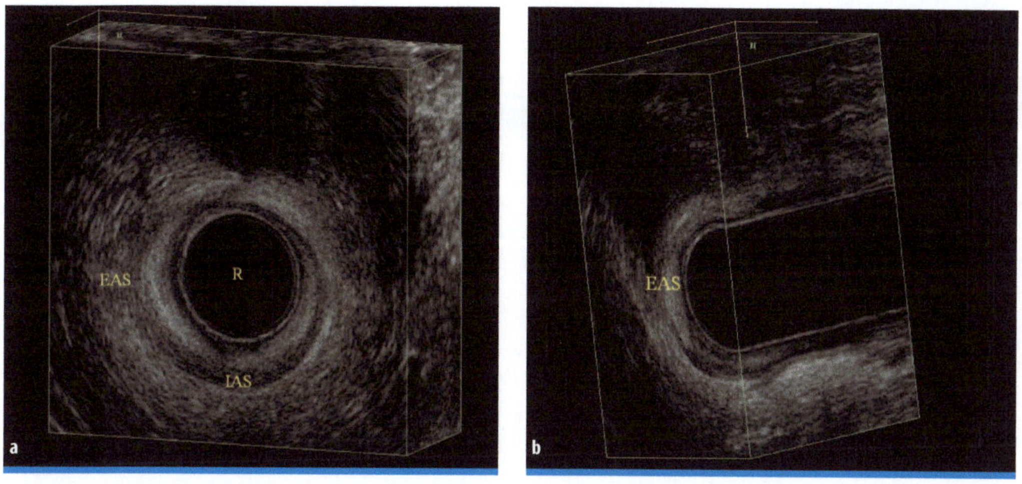

Fig. 3a, b. Endoanal ultrasound (EUS) image of external anal sphincter atrophy. **a** Frontal and **b** lateral views. *R* rectum, *IAS* internal anal sphincter, *EAS* external anal sphincter

Internal Anal Sphincter Atrophy

Internal anal sphincter (IAS) atrophy will often occur combined with EAS atrophy. Although the IAS is innervated by autonomic nerves, often the same injuries can afflict both somatic and autonomic nerves. Generally, IAS problems will lead more to soiling (leakage) of fecal fluid or mucous. Several reports have emerged about rare causes of fecal incontinence, such as primary IAS degeneration in passive fecal incontinence [22] and IAS sclerosis in mixed connective tissue disease [23] and systemic sclerosis [24]. In these patients, there is diffuse thinning (<0.2 mm) of the IAS. Clinical consequence is small, as no causative therapy is available, and general measurements such as defecation regulation and local hygiene are the only options.

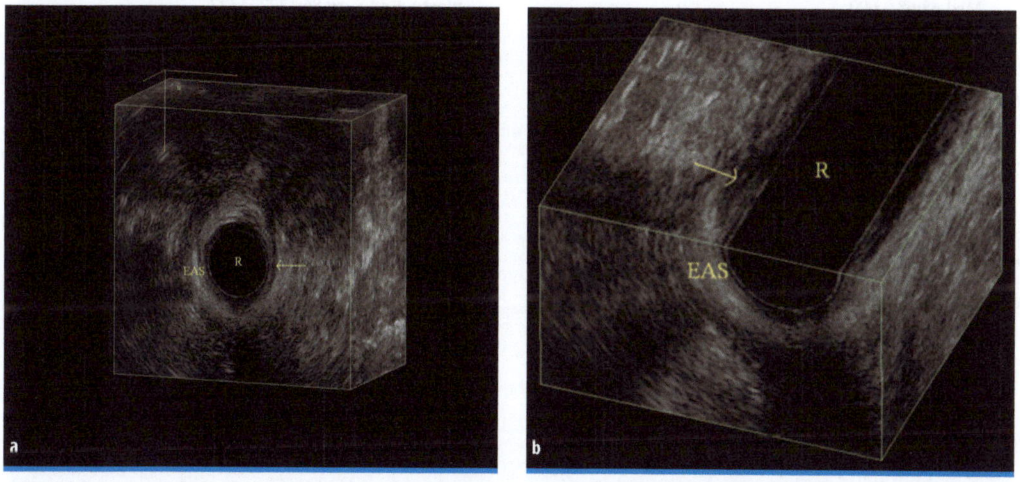

Fig. 4a, b. Endoanal ultrasound (EUS) image of external and internal anal sphincter atrophy. **a** Frontal and **b** lateral views. *R* rectum, *EAS* external anal sphincter. The IAS is hardly visible and is also atrophic (*arrow*)

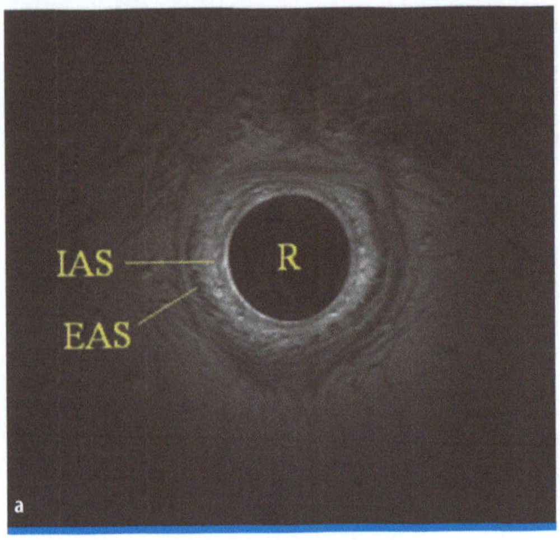

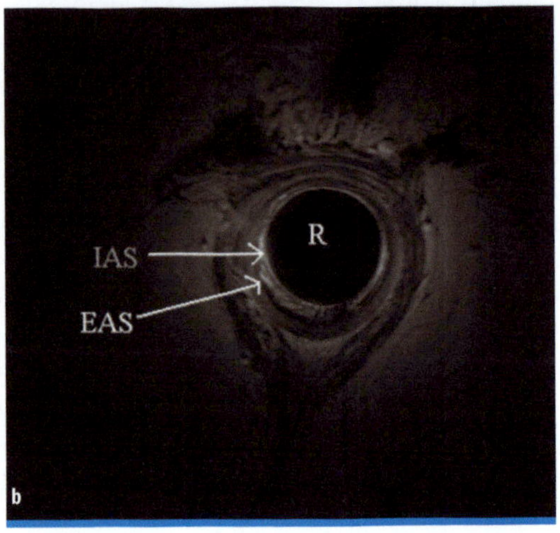

Fig. 5a, b. Magnetic resonance imaging (MRI) (axial) of external anal sphincter atrophy in two different patients. *R* rectum, *IAS* internal anal sphincter, *EAS* external anal sphincter

References

1. Snooks SJ, Swash M, Henry MM, Setchell M (1986) Risk factors in childbirth causing damage to the pelvic floor innervation. Int J Colorectal Dis 1:20–24
2. Snooks SJ, Barnes PR, Swash M, Henry MM (1985) Damage to the innervation of the pelvic floor musculature in chronic constipation. Gastroenterology 89:977–981
3. Lubowski DZ, Swash M, Nicholls RJ, Henry MM (1988) Increase in pudendal nerve terminal motor latency with defaecation straining. Br J Surg 75:1095–1097
4. Parks AG (1975) Anorectal incontinence. Proc R Soc Med 68:681–690
5. Keighley MRB, Fielding JWL (1983) Management of faecal incontinence and results of surgical treatment. Br J Surg 70:463–468
6. Fang DT, Nivatvongs S, Vermeulen FD et al (1984) Overlapping sphincteroplasty for acquired anal incontinence. Dis Col Rectum 27:720–722
7. Browning GGP, Parks AG (1983) Postanal repair for neuropathic faecal incontinence: correlation of clinical results and anal canal pressures? Br J Surg 70:101–104
8. Motson RW (1985) Sphincter injuries: indications for, and results of sphincter repair. Br J Surg 72:S19–S21
9. Gearhart S, Hull T, Floruta C et al (2000) Anal manometric parameters: predictors of outcome following anal sphincter repair? J Gastrointest Surg 9:115–120
10. Pinta T, Kylanpaa-Back ML, Salmi T et al (2003) Delayed sphincter repair for obstetric ruptures: analysis of failure. Colorectal Dis 5:73–78
11. Engel AF, Kamm MA, Sultan AH et al (1994) Anterior anal sphincter repair in patients with obstetric trauma. Br J Surg 81:1231–1234
12. Birnbaum EH, Stamm L, Rafferty JF et al (1996) Pudendal nerve terminal motor latency influences surgical outcome in treatment of rectal prolapse. Dis Colon Rectum 39:1215–1221
13. Briel JW, Zimmerman DD, Stoker J et al (2000) Relationship between sphincter morphology on endoanal MRI and histopathological aspects of the external anal sphincter. Int J Colorectal Dis 15:87–90
14. deSouza NM, Puni R, Zbar A et al (1996) MR imaging of the anal sphincter in multiparous women using an endoanal coil: correlation with in vitro anatomy and appearances in fecal incontinence. AJR Am J Roentgenol 167:1465–1471
15. Briel JW, Stoker J, Rociu E et al (1999) External anal sphincter atrophy on endoanal magnetic resonance imaging adversely affects continence after sphincteroplasty. Br J Surg 86:1322–1327
16. Rociu E, Stoker J, Eijkemans MJ, Lameris JS (2000) Normal anal sphincter anatomy and age- and sex-related variations at high-spatial-resolution endoanal MR imaging. Radiology 217:395–401
17. Williams AB, Malouf AJ, Bartram CI et al (2001) Assessment of external anal sphincter morphology in idiopathic fecal incontinence with endocoil magnetic resonance imaging. Dig Dis Sci 46:1466–1471
18. Williams AB, Bartram CI, Modhwadia D et al (2001) Endocoil magnetic resonance imaging quantification of external anal sphincter atrophy. Br J Surg 88:853–859
19. West RL, Felt-Bersma RJ, Hansen BE et al (2005) Volume measurements of the anal sphincter complex in healthy controls and fecal-incontinent patients with a three-dimensional reconstruction of endoanal ultrasonography images. Dis Colon Rectum 48:540–548
20. West RL, Dwarkasing S, Briel JW et al (2005) Can three-dimensional endoanal ultrasonography detect external anal sphincter atrophy? A comparison with endoanal magnetic resonance imaging. Int J Colorectal Dis 20:328–333

21. Cazemier M, Terra MP, Stoker J et al (2006) Atrophy and defects detection of the external anal sphincter: comparison between three-dimensional anal endosonography and endoanal magnetic resonance imaging. Dis Colon Rectum 49:20–27
22. Vaizey CJ, Kamm MA, Bartram CI (1997) Primary degeneration of the internal anal sphincter as a cause of passive faecal incontinence. Lancet 349:612–615
23. Engel AF, Kamm MA, Talbot IC (1994) Progressive systemic sclerosis of the internal anal sphincter leading to passive faecal incontinence. Gut 35:857–859
24. Daniel F, De Parades V, Cellier C (2005) Abnormal appearance of the internal anal sphincter at ultrasound: a specific feature of progressive systemic sclerosis? Gastroenterol Clin Biol 29:597–599

29

Obstetric Lesions: The Coloproctologist's Point of View

Jill C. Genua, Steven D. Wexner

Introduction

During the nineteenth century, at the current location of the famous Waldorf-Astoria Hotel in New York City, stood the first hospital in the world dedicated to the care of women with obstetric fistulas and complications [1]. By the end of that century, advances in obstetrics had dramatically decreased the severe complications of labor and delivery, and the hospital was closed. Currently, hospitals dedicated to the treatment of obstetric injury, particularly obstetric fistulas, exist in areas of the world that continue to struggle with the devastating effects of prolonged childbirth, obstructed labor, and maternal mortality [2].

The obstetric lesions encountered by a modern coloproctologist, while not as dramatic or life threatening as in the past, can be devastating for the patient and challenging for the physician. Obstetric trauma to the perineum contributes to a large number of cases of incontinence. Incontinence has been called the "unvoiced symptom" [3], the "silent affliction" [4], and "a physically and psychologically distressing handicap" [5]. The fear of social embarrassment and the personal isolation that accompany incontinence can severely limit a woman's personal potential. The additional financial burden of making lifestyle accommodations or receiving treatment for incontinence can be substantial. Mellgren et al. analyzed the costs for evaluation and treatment of 63 patients with fecal incontinence after childbirth and reported that despite an average evaluation and treatment cost of US $17,166 per patient in 1996, several patients had persistent incontinence at follow-up [6].

Many papers have been published regarding obstetric lesions as they relate to incontinence. However, it is difficult to accurately quantify the prevalence of obstetric injury and its effect on the incidence of incontinence. Differences in study populations, in the method of investigation, and in the length of follow-up make it difficult to correlate the clinical significance of the injuries. Labor and vaginal delivery have two potential effects: damage to the sphincter complex, and damage to pelvic-floor innervation. The progression of these effects to fecal incontinence is not clearly defined and is probably the result of multiple contributing factors over time.

An estimated 4–6% of women who undergo vaginal delivery will suffer from fecal incontinence [7]. The incidence of obstetric trauma to the perineum is 5% [8]. Generally, less than 3% of vaginal deliveries are complicated by sphincter tears, which are recognized and repaired at the time of delivery [9–14]. Studies that include primiparous women often report higher incidences of sphincter tears (approximately 13–14%) [12, 15]. Forty percent of women who have sphincter tears repaired at the time of delivery will develop later incontinence [11, 16, 17].

Diagnostic Tools: Endoanal Ultrasound

Since the early 1990s, anal ultrasound has become an important tool in studying the anal sphincter complex. The technique's popularity began after a publication by Law and Bartram in 1989 [18]. Ultrasound gained popularity in visualizing, defining, and describing the anatomy of the anal canal and the sphincter complex [19, 20]. The ultrasonographic findings were compared and correlated to electromyography (EMG) and manometry. Law et al. [21] studied 15 patients with fecal incontinence due to perineal trauma. There was high correlation in identifying and detailing sphincter defects, and the ultrasound was observed to be a more tolerable test for the patient, confirming its usefulness in assessing traumatic defects of the anal sphincter. Felt-Bersma et al. also reported agreement between ultrasound and EMG in mapping the external anal sphincter [22]. Tjandra and colleagues [23] demonstrated the correlation between ultrasound and EMG and described additional agreement between ultrasound and operative findings during sphincter repair.

As the use of ultrasound became more popular, it revealed an almost alarming rate of extent of damage to the sphincter following childbirth [24]. In a frequently referenced study by Sultan and colleagues in

1993 [25], ultrasound at 6 weeks postpartum revealed sphincter injuries in 35% of primiparous women and 44% of multiparous women.

However, there are several difficulties in the use of ultrasound to evaluate fecal incontinence in women following childbirth. In one study, the prevalence of sphincter defects on ultrasound was 65% in incontinent patients; however, sphincter defects were also found in 43% of continent women after childbirth [26]. Sentovich and colleagues reported that even in experienced hands and with a strict protocol of imaging and interpretation, identification of sphincter defect was falsely positive in 5–25% of cases [27]. Study of normal sphincter anatomy has revealed a natural defect anteriorly that has been suggested to complicate the interpretation of ultrasound and result in false positive anterior defects [28].

The Sultan study revealed a common incidence of occult sphincter injury, meaning sphincter injuries unrecognized at the time of delivery, some of which are asymptomatic. For example, 13% of primiparous women reported incontinence or urgency 6 weeks after vaginal delivery; however, 35% of primiparous women had sphincter defects demonstrated on ultrasound at 6 weeks postpartum. A more recent US-based study of anal sphincter morphology and function of primiparous women before and after delivery found a 20% incidence of occult sphincter injuries [12]. The fact that the clinical consequences of occult sphincter injury, particularly asymptomatic injury, are uncertain is another difficulty in the use of ultrasound. Patients with occult injuries do not always develop fecal incontinence.

Oberwalder and colleagues [29] performed a meta-analysis of five published studies to associate postpartum sphincter defects diagnosed by endoanal ultrasonography with fecal incontinence [25, 30–33]. This meta-analysis of 717 vaginal deliveries has three notable results: First, the incidence of anal sphincter defects in primiparous women was 26.9%. Second, multiparous women had an 8.5% incidence of new sphincter defects. Third, the calculated probability that postpartum fecal incontinence was due to a sphincter defect was 76.8–82.8%. A more recent study of a group of primiparous women detected sphincter defects and evaluated the consequences at 6-year follow-up [34]. The presence of an anal sphincter defect after the index vaginal delivery was significantly associated with the presence of fecal incontinence 6 years later.

Sphincter Defect Classification

The role of occult sphincter injury likely plays a role in the development of fecal incontinence, but it is unclear which women will be asymptomatic at first but subsequently develop fecal incontinence. A decrease in sphincter strength, anal canal pressure, and rectal compliance with aging has been described [35–39]. It is possible that occult sphincter defects are initially asymptomatic because the muscle can compensate for this defect; over decades, however, the aging muscle compensates less and the symptoms of incontinence develop [24]. In women with a history of vaginal delivery earlier in life who presented with late-onset fecal incontinence, 71% were found to have an anatomical sphincter defect [40]. Data therefore suggest careful follow-up of women with obstetric injuries because with aging and time, they are at a high risk of developing fecal incontinence [41].

Although there is some discrepancy in the details of classifying obstetric anal sphincter injury, a third-degree tear involves the anal sphincter and a fourth-degree tear involves the sphincter and the anal mucosa [42]. The reported incidence of third- and fourth-degree tears is 0.6–5% of all vaginal deliveries [43, 44]. These overt sphincter injuries are identified and repaired at the time of delivery; however, the success of these primary repairs has been questioned. Fitzpatrick et al. detected residual sphincter defects in 66% of women following primary sphincter repair [45]. Poen and colleagues found 88% of women had residual sphincter defects on endoanal ultrasound and 40% had symptoms of anal incontinence following primary repair [46]. Pinta and colleagues compared two groups of women following vaginal delivery: the study group consisted of 52 women with a third- or fourth-degree perineal laceration, and the control group consisted of women with no tears at delivery [47]. A persistent sphincter defect was seen on ultrasound in 75% of the study group women following primary sphincter repair; 20% of women in the control group had an ultrasonographic external sphincter defect with no recognized obstetric tear. Following primary sphincter repair, 61% of women had symptoms of anal incontinence and 20% had fecal incontinence. Oppong and Freeman studied 50 postpartum women who presented to a pelvic-floor clinic after primary repair of third- and fourth-degree perineal tears and found that 54.2% had a persistent gap on ultrasound [48].

Surgical Results: Outcomes of Primary Repair

Several factors contribute to the outcome of primary repair. Fernando and colleagues [42] found wide variation in the experience of acute anal sphincter repairs in a survey of obstetricians and gynecologists in the UK. At the time of delivery and injury, edema and blood may prevent adequate exposure to the muscle, complicating identification of the muscle layers and therefore preventing an optimal repair [49].

Different techniques are used to primarily repair the acute sphincter tear. Primary repair most commonly involves simple approximation of the muscle ends with two to three figure-of-eight sutures of chromic or Polyglactin [43]. An overlap technique and separation, with internal and external sphincter identification and separation, has been suggested as a more effective primary repair to reduce future incontinence [50]. A randomized prospective trial comparing primary vs. overlap primary repair of third-degree tears sustained in 112 primiparous women was performed. At 3-month follow-up, no significant difference in symptoms of incontinence, anal manometry, or ultrasound findings were detected [45]. The authors concluded that approximation and overlap repair outcomes were similar: both repairs resulted in residual sphincter defect, but symptomatic outcome was good. At least one other study concluded that despite the presence of a persistent defect on ultrasound following primary repair, the symptoms of this residual defect were minimal within a 3-year study period [51]. The literature is inconclusive regarding antibiotic prophylaxis and medical bowel confinement after primary repair; the practices and recommendations of surveyed UK physicians vary on these points [42]. Other variables in the technique of primary repair include the use of postrepair antibiotics and bowel confinement.

The demonstrated persistence of defects despite primary repair has implications for future continence [48]. It has therefore been suggested that a colorectal surgeon preferentially perform repairs for acute obstetric anal sphincter injuries because of their training and experience with sphincter repair in other settings. One paper describes the short-term involvement of a colorectal team in the acute management of third-degree tears [52]. In this study, four women with acute tears that extended to the anal canal or rectum underwent acute repair by a colorectal surgeon. The repair involved identification of both the internal and external sphincters, the use of a nerve stimulator to identify the external sphincter, imbrication of the internal sphincter, and overlapping repair of the external sphincter. At the 3-month and 1-year follow-ups, ultrasound showed intact repairs, and only one of the four women had flatus incontinence and occasional seepage. Based on this experience, the authors suggest that involving the colorectal surgeon may improve long-term outcome of primary repairs. However, no prospective data convincingly demonstrate who would offer "the best hope of repair" [52].

The presence of a colorectal surgeon at the time of delivery is potentially disruptive to both the staff and to the needs of the mother and newborn baby and may not be feasible within the organization of a delivery ward. However, there is widespread agreement that interdisciplinary cooperation and integrated follow-up is necessary. Counseling by a continence advisor and offering consultation with a colorectal surgeon [51], sphincter repair workshops [48], clinical evaluation by a proctologist every 6 months to determine if a repair should be repeated [47], and the use of anorectal physiology to plan future deliveries [52] have all been suggested. Follow-up of all women with sphincter tears will identify symptomatic women early enough to allow them to be treated and to advise them regarding future deliveries [53].

Risk Factors for Sphincter Injuries

Risk factors for the development of tears include parity, instrumental delivery (particularly forceps), prolonged second stage of labor, large babies, abnormal fetal presentation, and episiotomy [43, 49, 54]. Primiparity has been associated with a higher incidence of sphincter injuries [12, 25, 55]. Repeat vaginal deliveries have a cumulative effect and cause repeated damage to the sphincter, increasing the risk of incontinence with each delivery [56]. In a study of primiparous women who sustained a fourth-degree laceration at first delivery, the incidence of severe incontinence was significantly higher in women who had two or more vaginal deliveries [57]. Instrumental delivery has been associated with increased perineal trauma and development of anal incontinence [58–60]. Some studies show that these symptoms decrease over time as the perineum recovers; however, a larger fetal head size has been shown to be a risk factor for persistent incontinence [58, 61]. Multiple studies report that greater than 60% of vaginal delivery with forceps results in anal sphincter injury [25, 31, 54, 55, 62]. Vacuum deliveries have been demonstrated to be less traumatic to the anal sphincter than forceps [62–64].

In a prospective study of healthy primiparous women, deParedes and colleagues suggest that anal sphincter injury may be overestimated [65]. This study revealed that less than 13% of patients had a sphincter defect on ultrasound following forceps delivery. The prevalence of anal incontinence was 22% in this patient population; there was no significant relationship between visible ultrasound defect and anal incontinence. The study had several limitations: a large number of eligible patients were not included, the type of forceps and technique may differ from those used outside of France, and the follow-up was very short (6 weeks). In a different type of study, Bollard and colleagues identified women from a 1964 delivery database and assessed the prevalence of incontinence 34 years later [66]. They found a strong association between forceps delivery and sphincter defect on ultrasound but no significant increase in incontinence following forceps delivery.

Episiotomy was at one time believed to be protective to the perineum during childbirth and was used to prevent the occurrence of third- and fourth-degree tears [67]. There is now evidence that episiotomy not only fails to protect the perineum [68] but has been associated with increased tearing and anal sphincter injury [69–72]. Signorello and colleagues [73] studied the relationship between episiotomy and postpartum anal incontinence. They found no protective benefit but found impaired continence. The authors compared women who had episiotomies with women who had an intact perineum and women who spontaneously tore; in all comparisons, episiotomy doubled or tripled the risk of incontinence.

In addition to direct trauma to the sphincter muscle, pudendal neuropathy is another consequence of vaginal delivery, which contributes to fecal incontinence. The pudendal nerve is believed to be damaged by the fetal head, which compresses the nerve, causing ischemia or stretching its branches [74, 75]. The result is partial denervation of the external sphincter muscle and muscles of the pelvic floor. Pudendal damage is particularly a problem with a prolonged, complicated delivery of a large baby. In some women, this damage manifests early after delivery as incontinence, then reinnervation occurs and the symptoms spontaneously disappear; this suggests that early intervention is not necessary [74, 76]. In other cases, repeated pregnancies and deliveries add to the damage, the neuropathy progresses as the woman ages, and the worsening over time causes significant fecal incontinence that presents between 50 and 60 years of age [77, 78]. Different patterns of neuropathy have been demonstrated on physiologic testing, contributing to variation in symptoms and differing responses to treatment [79]. Pudendal neuropathy may be an isolated consequence of delivery, or patients may have "a double pathology", both a direct sphincter injury and pudendal nerve damage [74].

Cesarean section has been advocated as an option to protect the pelvic floor and reduce the incidence of postpartum fecal incontinence; however, this issue is controversial [80]. Cesarean section performed after cervical dilation, especially if performed late in the second stage of labor, is not entirely protective against direct sphincter trauma or pudendal neuropathy [77, 81, 82]. However, the risk of pelvic floor morbidity has become an impetus for women to choose elective cesarean section [42, 82]. Reducing pelvic floor morbidity by increasing the cesarean section rate would require a large number of cesareans be done to prevent a small number of tears. At this time, the best practice seems to be evaluation of a woman's risk factors, informed consent regarding her risk of pelvic floor trauma from vaginal delivery, proper recognition of injury at the time of delivery [53, 83, 84], and effective postpartum evaluation [80].

Treating Sphincter Injuries: The Colorectal Surgeon's Role

Women with incontinence due to childbirth present in three categories [49]. First are women who have an injury that was recognized and acutely repaired. Second are those who present with incontinence within the first year after a delivery and a primary sphincter repair. Third are those who present many years from the time of delivery, usually in middle age. The first group, the acute setting and primary repair of injuries, has been discussed. The colorectal surgeon most frequently evaluates and manages the second and third groups of women.

Evaluation

The evaluation begins as a comprehensive history. Questions to define the patients' symptoms and their onset and to exclude other causes of fecal incontinence are essential. An obstetric history includes number and mode of deliveries, birthweight, complications of the pregnancy or labor, whether an episiotomy was performed, perineal wound complications, and postpartum infections. Prior anorectal surgery is noted. Concomitant symptoms of urinary continence and/or organ prolapse are also components of a colorectal surgeon's evaluation, as there is evidence that combining sphincter repair with procedures for treating urinary incontinence and pelvic organ prolapse is cost effective, with favorable outcomes [85].

To quantify symptom severity and the impact of incontinence on the woman's life, a number of scoring systems have been developed. One popular system is the Wexner Cleveland Clinic Florida Fecal Incontinence (CCF-FI) score [37, 86]. Five areas are scored: incontinence to solid stool, incontinence to liquid stool, incontinence to gas, use of pads, and alteration of lifestyle. A total score is obtained by adding the frequency of each area (0 = never, 1 = less than once per month, 2 = less than once per week but greater than once per month, 3 = less than once per day but greater than once per week, 4 = at least once per day). A score of 0 indicates perfect continence; a score of 20 indicates complete incontinence. The fecal incontinence score is very helpful in guiding treatment decisions based on lifestyle alterations and allows assessment of treatments both individually and for research purposes [37] (Table 1).

A thorough physical examination is performed, the key portions of which are the perianal and rectal examination. The perianal area is inspected for soiling, evidence of infectious diseases, skin excoriation, or poor hygiene. Presence of a patulous anus, skin tag, episiotomy scars, spontaneous hemorrhoidal prolapse, drainage, fistulas, or fissures are noted. The patient is asked to strain so that prolapse or perineal descent can be evaluated, and anal sensation is tested. External palpation excludes fissure, masses, abscesses, or fistulas. Digital rectal examination evaluates for masses or tenderness and assesses resting sphincter tone. The patient is asked to squeeze, and the examiner feels for concentric contraction of the sphincter muscle and estimates squeeze pressure. Upon relaxation, contraction of the puborectalis muscle is assessed for paradox. Anoscopy enables visualization of the mucosa and provides further assessment of hemorrhoids. A bidigital exam assesses the thickness of the perineal body. If there is suspicion of a rectovaginal fistula, a speculum examination will facilitate inspection of the vagina; a tampon test using methylene blue may be employed at this time. An office flexible sigmoidoscopy may be used at this time to exclude proctosigmoiditis, inflammatory conditions, polyps, or tumors. However, full colonoscopic examination is performed according to presenting symptoms and standard screening guidelines. Following the history and physical, physiologic testing including anal ultrasound, pudendal nerve testing, EMG, anal manometry, and defecography are helpful.

After the surgeon has excluded other medically treatable causes of incontinence and the incontinence has been defined, the first variable determining treatment is severity. For patients who are continent to solid stool but have difficulties with control of liquid stool or flatus, aggressive medical therapy consisting of high-fiber diet, fiber supplementation, and antimotility agents may be successful. Perineal muscle strengthening exercises are another conservative option for patients with mild symptoms [37]. Biofeedback therapy is a more formal method of perineal muscle strengthening [87, 88]. A trained therapist monitors the voluntary contraction of the external anal sphincter and guides the patient in more effectively contracting. Patient motivation, commitment, and cooperation is necessary; however for the proper patient, this is a good option.

For women with more severe incontinence, the first question a colorectal surgeon asks is whether there is defect of the sphincter muscle. A sphincter defect in the setting of significant incontinence following vaginal delivery is usually repaired. The patient is preoperatively assessed for pudendal neuropathy, which has been a predictor of poor success of sphincter repair in treating incontinence [49, 89, 90]. However, all patients with fecal incontinence and an external sphincter defect can be offered sphincter repair as long as the expectations of success are realistic [89]. With concomitant pudendal neuropathy, even if the sphincter repair is successful, success may be transient. The patient should realize that either repeat sphincter repair or other surgical options may subsequently be required. They should also realize that even with "success", function may be suboptimal (Table 2).

Surgical Treatment: Sphincter Repair

There are three methods of repairing the sphincter: apposition, plication/reefing, and overlapping sphincteroplasty [37]. Apposition has classically been associated with low success rates [91]. Scar tissue

Table 1. Cleveland Clinic Florida Fecal Incontinence (CCF-FI) score[a]. From [37]

Type of incontinence	Frequency				
	Never	<1/month	<1/week ≥1/month	<1/day ≥1/week	≥1/day
Solid	0	1	2	3	4
Liquid	0	1	2	3	4
Gas	0	1	2	3	4
Wears pads	0	1	2	3	4
Lifestyle alteration	0	1	2	3	4

[a]0 = perfect continence, 20 = complete incontinence

Table 2. Influence of pudendal neuropathy on success of sphincter repair

Author	Year	Number	Success without neuropathy	Success with neuropathy	*P* value
Laurberg [92]	1988	19	42%	5%	<0.05
Londono-Schimmer [93]	1994	94	60%	14%	<0.001
Sitzler [94]	1996	29	48%	24%	–
Gilliland [89]	1998	72	51%	3%	<0.01

excision was later implicated in the failure of the apposition technique [37]. More recently, in a study of 40 patients with sphincter trauma over a 15-year period, an end-to-end apposition was performed with excellent results [95]. The technique involves minimizing dissection of the injured muscle to preserve vascularity and the preservation of scar tissue to help anchor the overlapped muscle. The authors advocate the apposition repair because of its simplicity and effectiveness. Plication or reefing can be performed anteriorly (vaginal mobilization, external sphincter division, levator ani plication followed by puborectalis and external sphincter repair, or posterior plication of the external sphincter and levators) [96]. In 1975, Parks described the "postanal repair" for incontinence associated with rectal prolapse and idiopathic incontinence [97]. The postanal repair involves posterior plication of the puborectalis muscle to restore the normal anorectal angle. The postanal repair is used when pudendal neuropathy rather than sphincter trauma is the cause of incontinence.

The most popular repair method, which has been shown to improve symptoms of continence and physiologic studies, is dividing and preserving the anterior sphincter and overlapping the muscle [94, 98–101]. In a randomized controlled trial of overlapping sphincter repair vs. direct end-to-end anterior repair, no benefit of the overlapping repair was demonstrated [101]. However, most authors maintain their practice of overlapping scarred, fibrotic muscle. Short-term results of anterior repair are quite successful, with rates between 69% and 97% [102]. At least one study demonstrated no significant change in short-term and long-term success [103]. However, most studies of long-term success of overlapping anterior repair demonstrate a decrease over time to a 35–50% success rate [104–106]. Some studies cite age as a factor predicting poorer outcome [107]. However, other studies report outcomes in elderly women are comparable with those in younger women [98, 108] (Tables 3 and 4).

Our preferred method of repairing sphincter defects is the overlapping sphincteroplasty. The patient undergoes full mechanical and antibiotic bowel preparation and receives prophylactic antibiotics. After induction of general or spinal anesthesia, a Foley catheter is placed, and the patient is positioned in the prone jackknife position. A mixture of 0.5% Xylocaine, 0.25% bupivacaine, and 1:400,000 U epinephrine is injected; this solution facilitates dissection by defining planes of scar and normal muscle and tissue. An anterolateral circumanal incision of approximately 120° is made with diathermy. Allis clamps are placed on the anoderm and vaginal

Table 3. Overlapping sphincter repair: short-term results

Author	Year	Number	Obstetric/ operative trauma (%)	Results (%)		
				Excellent/good	Fair	Poor
Fleshman [100]	1991	55	100	72	22	6
Wexner [50]	1991	16	100	76	19	5
Fleshman [99]	1991	28	100	75	21	4
Engel [109]	1994	55	100	79	–	21
Oliveira [98]	1996	55	99	71	9	20
Felt-Bersma [110]	1996	18	94	72	–	28
Nikiteas [111]	1996	42	88	60	17	24
Sitzler [94]	1996	31	87	74	–	26
Ternent [112]	1997	16	100	44	31	25
Zorcolo [102]	2005	93	100	65	9	27
Barisic [105]	2006	65	86	74	17	9

Table 4. Overlapping sphincter repair: long-term results

Author	Year	Number	Obstetric/ operative trauma (%)	Results (%)		
				Excellent/good	Fair	Poor
Engel [113]	1994	28	92	75		25
Londono-Schimmer [93]	1994	94	90	50	26	24
Vaizey [103]	2004	21	100	52	10	38
Gutierrez [106]	2004	130	91	22	19	57
Zorcolo [102]	2005	73	100	63	19	18
Barisic [105]	2006	65	86	48	13	39

aspects to separate these two areas. During dissection, a finger is periodically placed in both the anus and the vagina to avoid inadvertent injuries. Dissection of the external anal sphincter muscle commences laterally in the ischiorectal fat then proceeds medially where most of the scar will be encountered. The edges of the muscle have usually retracted laterally to the right and left; when the two ends are identified, they are grasped and further defined using cautery dissection. Once the edges of the muscle have been defined, attention is turned to the intersphincteric groove where the internal and external muscles are separated. The injured internal sphincter muscle is repaired separately and adds an extra layer of strength overall to the repair.

Next, the surgeon decides the optimal configuration of overlap of the ends of the external sphincter muscles (right over left vs. left over right). Horizontal mattress sutures are used to secure the overlap configuration. In general, four to six sutures of Polydioxanone are used. The senior author of this chapter has demonstrated Polydioxanone as the optimum suture choice; experience revealed Polypropylene had a tendency to cause persistent sinuses and Polyglactin absorbed too quickly for a solid repair. Ultimately, the overlapping repair creates a cube of tissue. An overlap of 3–4 cm of the ends of the muscle is ideal. Caudad to cephalad, a new high-pressure zone of at least 2–3 cm is created. Hemostasis is confirmed, and the skin is partially reapproximated with Polyglactin suture, leaving the central portion open for drainage. Perioperative antibiotic coverage is given; oral antibiotics are continued beyond this period only if clinically warranted. No postoperative bowel confinement is used. A regimen of fiber supplementation, Sitz baths, and analgesia is prescribed, and the wound generally heals within 4–6 weeks.

Anovaginal and Rectovaginal Fistula Repair

Anovaginal and rectovaginal fistulas are uncommon injuries resulting from vaginal delivery; however, obstetric injury is the most common cause of these fistulas [114]. Injury to the perineum during vaginal delivery and poor healing of primary repair of perineal tears are the main causes of the obstetric-induced rectovaginal fistula [115]. A small percentage will heal spontaneously; after resolution of acute edema and inflammation, if the fistula is still present, there is usually well-vascularized tissue that permits successful healing following repair [116]. A patient will classically complain of the passage of stool or flatus via the vagina; physical exam usually reveals the fistula. However, fistula symptoms may mask or confuse incontinence symptoms. Anal ultrasound and physiologic testing must be performed to evaluate for concomitant sphincter damage, which would require a sphincter repair in addition to surgical treatment of the fistula [117].

If a rectovaginal fistula is present in addition to a sphincter defect, our earlier technique of overlapping sphincteroplasty is modified slightly into a transperineal repair. The same technique is applied with emphasis on separating the rectum and vagina and careful cephalad dissection through the fistulous communication and above the scarring. The vaginal defect is cored to remove any granulation tissue, and the defect is closed by imbrication. The rectal defect is excised if distal; if quite large or cephalad, it is repaired with an endorectal advancement flap. The sphincters are repaired as described earlier, and the result is a multilayer repair that simultaneously repairs the fistulous defects, separates the anorectal and vaginal components, and repairs the muscle defect.

Conclusion

Modern advances in obstetric care have dramatically decreased maternal morbidity and mortality. However, when a significant intrapartum event occurs or when the consequences of childbirth lead to incontinence, a woman's life is severely affected. Childbirth and vaginal delivery have two consequences: injury to the anal sphincter and injury to and innervation of the pelvic floor. While severe perineal trauma resulting in overt sphincter injury is rare, occult sphincter injury following vaginal delivery is well documented by endoanal ultrasound in a significant number of cases. Not all sphincter defects translate into incontinence, and the development of incontinence is probably the result of multiple factors over time, including age and repeated deliveries. A cooperative and interdisciplinary approach is recommended to decrease the chance of incontinence following vaginal delivery. This method should involve an endoanal ultrasound following complicated vaginal deliveries to identify potentially problematic sphincter defects, inquiry about symptoms of incontinence during the postpartum period, and establishing follow-up clinics for continence assessment of women at highest risk. Obstetricians are the most experienced to deal with acute obstetric anal sphincter injury and their primary repair. There is no convincing prospective evidence of improved outcomes by involving a colorectal surgeon at the time of delivery, and this involvement is likely not feasible, appropriate, or beneficial.

Colorectal surgeons are most often asked to evaluate two categories of incontinent women following childbirth: women who develop incontinence shortly after a vaginal delivery that was, usually, complicated by a primarily repaired tear or episiotomy, and women who develop incontinence later in life, usually at middle age. A colorectal consultation includes a thorough history, which clarifies the symptoms and quantifies the degree of incontinence and its effect on the woman's life; a physical exam; physiologic studies; and counseling regarding future deliveries, surveillance, and treatment. If a sphincter defect is identified, it is repaired preferably with anterior overlapping sphincteroplasty. Concomitant pudendal nerve injury may decrease the success of sphincteroplasty in achieving full continence; however, a colorectal surgeon will continue along a treatment algorithm that involves new and promising procedures such as injectable sphincter bulking agents, sacral nerve stimulation, stimulated or nonstimulated gracilis transposition, and the artificial bowel sphincter. Rectovaginal fistulas are rarer complications of vaginal delivery but are associated with great morbidity. Incontinence and a concomitant sphincter injury should always be addressed; failure to do so will result in decreased success of treatment.

References

1. Hamlin EC, Little J (2001) The hospital by the river: a story of hope. Pan MacMillan, Sydney
2. Arrowsmith S, Hamlin EC, Wall LL (1996) Obstructed labor injury complex: obstetric fistula formation and the multifaceted morbidity of maternal birth trauma in the developing world. Obstet Gynecol Sur 51(9):568–574
3. Leigh RJ, Turnberg LA (1982) Faecal incontinence: the unvoiced symptom. Lancet 1:1349–1351
4. Johanson JF, Lafferty J (1996) Epidemiology of fecal incontinence: the silent affliction. Am J Gastroenterol 91:33–36
5. Rothbarth J, Bemelman WA, Meijerink WJHJ et al (2001) What is the impact of fecal incontinence on quality of life? Dis Colon Rectum 44:67–71
6. Mellgren A, Jensen LL, Zetterstrom JP (1999) Long-term cost of fecal incontinence secondary to obstetric injuries. Dis Colon Rectum 42:857–867
7. Keighley MR, Bick D, MacArthur C (1995) Prevalence and obstetric factors in childbirth related fecal incontinence (meeting abstract). Dis Colon Rectum 38:P14
8. Venkatesh KS, Ramanujam PS, Lason DM, Haywood MA (1989) Anorectal complications of vaginal delivery. Dis Colon Rectum 32:1039–1041
9. Haadem K, Dahlstrom JA, Ling L, Ohrlander S (1987) Anal sphincter function after delivery room rupture. Obstet Gynecol 70:53–56
10. Borgotta L, Piening SL, Cohen WR (1989) Association of episiotomy and delivery position with deep perineal laceration during spontaneous delivery in nulliparous women. Am J Obste Gynecol 160:294–297
11. Fornell EK, Berg G, Hallbook O et al (1996) Clinical consequences of anal sphincter rupture during vaginal delivery. J Am Coll Surg 183:553–558
12. Zetterstrom J, Mellgren A, Jensen L et al (1999) Effect of delivery on anal sphincter morphology and function. Dis Colon Rectum 42:1253–1260
13. BuekensP, Lagasse R, Dramaix M, Wollast E (1985) Episiotomy and third degree tears. Br J Obstet Gynaecol 92:820–823
14. Moller Bek K, Laurberg S (1992) Intervention during labor: risk factors associated with complete tear of the anal sphincter. Acta Obstet Gynecol Scand 71:520–524
15. Zetterstrom J, Lopez A, Anzen B et al (1999) Anal incontinence after vaginal delivery–a prospective study in primiparous women. Br J Obstet Gynaecol 106:324–330
16. Sultan AH, Kamm MA, Hudson CN, Bartram CI (1994) Third degree obstetric anal sphincter tears:risk factors and outcome of primary repair. BMJ 308:887–891
17. Tetzschner T, Sorensen M, Lose G, Christiansen J (1996) Pudendal nerve recovery after a non-instrumented vaginal delivery. Int Urogynecol J Pelvic Floor Dysfunct 7:102–104
18. Law PJ, Bartram CI (1989) Anal endosonography: technique in normal anatomy. Gastrointest Radiol 14:349–353
19. Gerdes B, Kohler HH, Zielke A et al (1997) The anatomical basis of anal endosonography. Surg Endosc 11:986–990
20. Eckardt VF, Jung B, Fischer B, Lierse W (1994) Anal endosonography in healthy subjects and patients with idiopathic fecal incontinence. Dis Colon Rectum 37:235–242
21. Law PJ, Kamm MA, Bartram CI (1990) A comparison

between electromyography and anal endosonography in mapping external anal sphincter defects. 33:370–373
22. Felt-Bersma RJF, Cuesta MA, Koorevaar M et al (1992) Anal endosonography: relationship with anal manometry and neurophysiological tests. Dis Colon Rectum 35:944–949
23. Tjandra JJ, Milsom JW, Schroeder T, Fazio V (1993) Endoluminal ultrasound is preferable to electromyography in mapping anal sphincter defects. Dis Colon Rectum 36:689–692
24. Hull T (2002) Invited commentary. Dis Colon Rectum 45:1450–1451
25. Sultan AH, Kamm MA, Hudson CN et al (1993) Anal-sphincter disruption during vaginal delivery. N Eng J Med 329:1905–1911
26. Karoui S, Savoye-Collet, Koning C et al (1999) Prevalence of anal sphincter defects revealed by sonography in 335 incontinent patients and 115 continent patients. AJR Am J Roentgenol 173:389–392
27. Sentovich S, Wong WD, Blatchford GJ (1998) Accuracy and reliability of transanal ultrasound for anterior anal sphincter injury. Dis Colon Rectum 41:1000–1004
28. Bollard RC, Gardiner A, Lindow S et al (2002) Dis Colon Rectum 45:171–175
29. Oberwalder M, Connor J, Wexner SD (2003) Meta-analysis to determine the incidence of obstetric anal sphincter damage. Br J Surg 90:1333–1337
30. Abramowitz L, Sobhani I, Ganansia R et al (2000) Are sphincter defects the cause of anal incontinence after delivery? Dis Colon Rectum 43:590–598
31. Varma A, Gunn J, Gardiner A et al (1999) Obstetric anal sphincter injury: prospective evaluation of incidence. Dis Colon Rectum 42:1537–1543
32. Fynes M, Donnelly V, Behan M et al (1999) Effect of second vaginal delivery on anorectal physiology and fecal continence: a prospective study. Lancet 354:983–986
33. Faltin DL, Boulvain M, Irion O et al (2000) Diagnosis of anal sphincter tears by postpartum endosonography to predict fecal incontinence. Obstet Gynecol 95:643–647
34. Damon H, Bretones S, Henry L et al (2005) Long-term consequences of first vaginal delivery-induced anal sphincter defect. Dis Colon Rectum 48:1772–1776
35. Beck DE, Wexner SD (eds) (1998) Fundamentals of anorectal surgery, 2nd edn. W.B. Saunders, London
36. Laurberg S, Swash M (1989) Effects of aging on the anorectal sphincters and their innervation. Dis Colon Rectum 32:737–742
37. Jorge JMN, Wexner SD (1993) Etiology and management of fecal incontinence. Dis Colon Retum 36:77–97
38. Bannister JJ, Abouzekry L, Read NW (1987) Effect of aging on anorectal function. Gut 28:353–357
39. McHugh SM, Diamant NE (1987) Effect of age, gender and parity on anal canal pressures. Dig Dis Sci 32:726–736
40. Oberwalder M, Dinnewitzer A, Baig K et al (2004) The association between late-onset fecal incontinence and obstetric anal sphincter defects. Arch Surg 139:429–432
41. Haadem K, Dahlstrom A, Ling L, Ohrlander AS (1987) Anal sphincter function after delivery rupture. Obstet Gynecol 70:53–57
42. Fernando RJ, Sultan AH, Radley S et al (2002) Management of obstetric anal sphincter injury: a systematic review and national practice survey. BMC Health Serv Res 2:9
43. Sultan AH, Kamm MA, Hudson CN, Bartram CI (1994) Third degree obstetric anal sphincter tears: risk factors and outcome of primary repair. BMJ 308:887–891
44. Khanduja KS, Yamashita HJ, Wise WE et al (1994) Delayed repair of obstetric injuries of the anorectum and vagina. Dis Colon Rectum 37:344–349
45. Fitzpatrick M, O'Connell PR, O'Herlihy C (2000) A randomized clinical trial comparing primary overlap with approximation repair of third-degree obstetric tears. Am J Obstet Gynecol 183:1220–1224
46. Poen AC, Felt-Bersma RF, Strijers RL et al (1998) Third degree obstetric perineal tear: long-term clinical and functional results after primary repair Br J Surg 85:1433–1438
47. Pinta TM, Kylanpaa M-L, Salmi TK et al (2004) Primary sphincter repair:are the results of the operation good enough? Dis Colon Rectum 47:18–23
48. Oppong FC, Freeman RM (2004) Prospective audit of third- and fourth-degree obstetric anal sphincter injuries. BR J Surgery 91:24
49. Cook TA, Mortensen NJ (1998) Management of fecal incontinence following obstetric injury. Br J Surg 85:293–299
50. Wexner SD, Marchetti F, Jagelman DG (1991) The role of sphincteroplasty for fecal incontinence reevaluated: A prospective physiologic and functional review. Dis Colon Rectum 34:22–30
51. Rieger N, Perera S, Stephens J et al (2004) Anal sphincter function and integrity after primary repair of third-degree tear: uncontrolled prospective analysis. ANZ J of Surg 74:122–124
52. Cook T, Keane D, Mortensen N (1999) Is there a role for the colorectal team in the management of acute severe third-degree vaginal tears? Colorectal Dis 1:263–266
53. Byrd LM, Hobbiss J, Tasker M (2005) Is it possible to predict or prevent third degree tears? Colorectal Dis 7:311–318
54. Abramowitz L, Sobhani I, Ganansia R et al (2000) Are sphincter defects the cause of anal incontinence after vaginal delivery? Results of a prospective study. Dis Colon Rectum 43:590–596
55. Belmonte-Montes C, Hagerman G, Vega-Yepez PA et al (2001) Anal sphincter injury after vaginal delivery in primiparous females. Dis Colon Rectum 44:1244–1248
56. Ryhammer AM, Bek KM, Laurberg S (1995) Multiple vaginal deliveries increase the risk of permanent incontinence of flatus and urine in normal premenopausal women. Dis Colon Rectum 38:1206–1209
57. Sze E (2005) Prevalence and severity of anal incontinence in women with and without additional vaginal deliveries after a fourth-degree perineal laceration. Dis Colon Rectum 48:66–69
58. Mazounia C, Bretelle F, Battar S et al (2005) Frequency of persistent anal symptoms after first instrumental delivery. Dis Colon Rectum 48:1432–1436
59. Hall W, McCracken K, Osterweil P, Guise JM (2003) Frequency and predictors for postpartum fecal incon-

tinence. Am J Obstet Gynecol 188:1205–1207
60. Sultan AH, Johanson RB, Carter JE (1998) Occult anal sphincter trauma following randomized forceps and vacuum delivery. Int J Gynaecol Obstet 61:113–119
61. Nazir M, Carlsen E, Nesheim BI (2002) Do occult anal sphincter injuries, vector volume manometry and delivery variables have any predictive value for bowel symptoms after first time vaginal delivery without third and fourth degree rupture? A prospective study. Acta Obstet Gynecol Scan 81:720–726
62. Sultan AH, Kamm MA, Bartram CI, Hudson CN (1993) Anal sphincter trauma during instrumental delivery. Int J Gynecol Obstet 43:263–270
63. Johanson RB, Rice C, Doyle M et al (1993) A randomized prospective study comparing the new vacuum extractor policy with forceps delivery. Br J Obstet Gynaecol 100:524–350
64. Sultan AH, Johanson RB, Carter JE (1998) Occult anal sphincter trauma following randomized forceps and vacuum delivery. Int J Gynaecol Obstet 61:113–119
65. deParedes V, Etienney I, Thabut D et al (2004) Anal sphincter injury after forceps delivery: myth or reality? A prospective ultrasound study of 93 females. Dis Colon Rectum 47:24–34
66. Bollard R, Gardiner A, Duthie GS, Lindow SW (2003) Anal sphincter injury, fecal and urinary incontinence. A 34-year follow-up after forceps delivery. Dis Colon Rectum 46:1083–1088
67. Thacker SB, Banta HD (1983) Benefits and risks of episiotomy: an interpretive review of the English language literature. Obstet Gynecol Surv 38:322–338
68. Thorp JM Jr, Bowes WA Jr (1993) Episiotomy: can its routine use be defended? Am J Obstet Gynecol 160:1027–1030
69. Thorp JM Jr, Bowes WA Jr, Brame RG, Cefalo R (1987) Selected use of midline episiotomy: effect on perineal trauma. Obstet Gynecol 70:260–262
70. Helwig JT, Thorp JM Jr, Bowes WA Jr (1993) Does midline episiotomy increase the risk of third- and fourth-degree lacerations in operative vaginal deliveries? Obstet Gynecol 82:276–279
71. Walker MPR, Farine D, Rolbin SH, Ritchie JWK (1991) Epidural anesthesia, episiotomy, and obstetric laceration. Obstet Gynecol 77:668–671
72. Klein MC, Gauthier RJ, Robbins JM et al (1994) Relationship of episiotomy to perineal trauma and morbidity, sexual dysfunction, and pelvic floor relaxation. Am J Obstet Gynecol 171:591–598
73. Signorello LB, Harlow BL, Chekos AK, Repke JT (2000) Midline episiotomy and anal incontinence: retrospective cohort study. BMJ 320:86–90
74. Jacobs PPM, Scheuer M, Kuijpers, JHC, Vingerhoets MH (1990) Obstetric fecal incontinence. Role of pelvic floor denervation and results of delayed sphincter repair. Dis Colon Rectum 33:494–497
75. Snooks SJ, Swash M, Henry MM (1986) Risk factors in childbirth causing damage to the pelvic floor innervation. Int J Colorect Dis 1:20–24
76. Snooks SJ, Swash M, Henry MM et al (1985) Injury to the innervation of the pelvic floor musculature in childbirth. Lancet 2:546–550
77. Goldberg RP, Kwon C, Gandhi S (2003) Prevalence of anal incontinence among mothers of multiples and analysis of risk factors. Am J Obstet Gynecol 189:1627–1631
78. Snooks SJ, Swash M, Henry SE (1990) Effect of vaginal delivery on the pelvic floor: a 5-year follow-up. Br J Surg 77:1358–1360
79. Fitzpatrick M, O'Brien C, O'Connell PR. O'Herlihy C (2003) Patterns of abnormal pudendal nerve function that are associated with postpartum fecal incontinence. Am J Obstet Gynecol 189: 730–735
80. O'Boyle AL, Davis GD, Calhoun BC (2002) Informed consent and birth:protecting the pelvic floor and ourselves. Am J Obstet Gynecol 187:981–983
81. Liebling RE, Swingler R, Patel RR et al (2004) Pelvic floor morbidity up to one year after difficult instrumental delivery and cesarean section in the second stage of labor: a cohort study. Am J Obstet Gynecol 191:4–10
82. Al-Mufti R, McCarthy A, Fisk NM (1996) Obstetrician's personal choice and mode of delivery. Lancet 347:544
83. McKenna DS, Ester JB, Fischer JR (2003) Elective cesarean section delivery for women with a previous anal sphincter rupture. Am J Obstet Gynecol 189:1262–1266
84. Lal M, Mann CH, Callender R et al (2003) Does cesarean delivery prevent anal incontinence? Obstet Gynecol 101:305–312
85. Halverson A, Hull T, Paraiso MF, Floruta C (2001) Outcome of sphincteroplasty combined with surgery for urinary incontinence and pelvic organ prolapse. Dis Colon Rectum 44:1421–1326
86. Person B, Wexner SD (2005) Advances in the surgical treatment of fecal incontinence. Surg Innovation 12:7–21
87. Engel BT, Nikoomanesh P, Schuster MM (1974) Operant conditioning to rectosphincteric responses in the treatment of fecal incontinence. N Eng J Med 29:646–649
88. Macleod JH (1987) Management of anal incontinence by biofeedback. Gastroenterology 93:291–294
89. Gilliland R, Altomare DF, Moreira H et al (1998) Pudendal neuropathy is predictive of failure following anterior overlapping sphincteroplasty. Dis Colon Rectum 41:1516–1522
90. Gardiner A, Kaur G, Cundall J, Duthie GS (2004) Neural network analysis of anal sphincter repair. Dis Colon Rectum 47:192–197
91. Blaisdell PC. (1940) Repair of the incontinent sphincter ani. Surg Gynecol Obstet 70:692–697
92. Laurberg S, Swash M, Henry MM (1988) Delayed external sphincter repair for obstetric tear. Br J Surg 75(8):786–788
93. Londono-Schimmer EE, Garcia-Duperly R, Nicholls RJ et al (1995) Overlapping anal sphincter repair for faecal incontinence due to sphincter trauma: five year follow-up functional results. Int J Colorectal Dis 10(2):123
94. Sitzler PJ, Thomson JPS (1996) Overlap repair of damaged anal sphincter: a single surgeon's series. Dis Colon Rectum 39:1356–1360
95. Arnaud A, Sarles JC, Sielezneff I et al (1991) Sphincter repair without overlapping for fecal incontinence. Dis Colon Rectum 34:744–747

96. Corman ML (2005) Colon and rectal surgery, 5th edn. Lippincott Williams & Wilkins, Philadelphia
97. Parks AG (1975) Anorectal incontinence. J R Soc Med 68:681–690
98. Oliveira L, Pfeifer J, Wexner SD (1996) Physiological and clinical outcome of anterior sphincteroplasty. Br J Surg 83:502–505
99. Fleshman JW, Dreznik Z, Fry RD, Kodner IJ (1991) Anal sphincter repair for obstetric injury: manometric evaluation of functional results. Dis Colon Rectum 34:1061–1067
100. Fleshman JW, Peters WR, Shemesh EI et al (1991) Anal sphincter reconstruction: anterior overlapping muscle repair. Dis Colon Rectum 34:739–743
101. Tjandra JJ, Han WR, Goh J et al (2003) Direct repair vs. overlapping sphincter repair: a randomized controlled clinical trial. Dis Colon Rectum 46:937–943
102. Zorcolo L, Covotta L, Bartolo DC (2005) Outcome of anterior sphincter repair for obstetric injury: comparison of early and late results. Disc Colon Rectum 48:524–531
103. Vaizey CJ, Norton C, Thornton MJ et al (2004) Long-term results of repeat anterior anal sphincter repair. Disc Colon Rectum 47:858–863
104. Halverson AL, Hull TL (2002) Long-term outcome of overlapping anal sphincter repair. Dis Colon Rectum 45:345–348
105. Barisic GI, Krivokapic ZV, Markovic VA, Popovic MA (2006) Outcome of overlapping anal sphincter repair after 3 months and after a mean of 80 months. Int J Colorectal Dis 21:52–56
106. Gutierrez AB, Madoff RD, Lowry AC et al (2004) Long-term results of anterior sphincteroplasty. Dis Colon Rectum 47:727–732
107. Rasmussen O, Puggaard L, Christiansen J (1999) Anal sphincter repair in patients with obstetric trauma: age affects outcome. 42:193–195
108. Simmang C, Birnbaum EH, Kodner IJ et al (1994) Anal sphincter reconstruction in the elderly:does advancing age affect outcome? Dis Colon Rectum 37:1065–1069
109. Engel AF, Kamm MA, Sultan AH et al (1994) Anterior anal sphincter repair in patients with obstetric trauma. Br J Surg 81(8):1231–1234
110. Felt-Bersma RJ, Cuesta MA, Koorevaar M (1996) Anal sphincter repair improves anorectal function and endosonographic image. A prospective clinical study. Dis Colon Rectum 39(8):878–885
111. Nikiteas N, Korsgen S, Kumar D, Keighley MR (1996) Audit of sphincter repair. Factors associated with poor outcome. Dis Colon Rectum 39(10):1164–1170
112. Ternent CA, Shashidharan M, Blatchford GJ (1997) Transanal ultrasound and anorectal physiology findings affecting continence after sphincteroplasty. Dis Colon Rectum 40(4):462–467
113. Engel AF, van Baal SJ, Brummelkamp WH (1994) Late results of anterior sphincter plication for traumatic faecal incontinence. Eur J Surg 160(11):633–636
114. Chew S, Rieger N (2004) Transperineal repair of obstetric-related anovaginal fistula. ANZ J Obstet Gynecol 44:68–71
115. Venkatesh KS, Ramanujan PS, Larson DM, Haywood MA (1989) Anorectal complications of vaginal delivery. Dis Colon Rectum 41:1141–1146
116. Rahman MS, Al-Suleiman SA, Rahman J (2003) Surgical treatment of rectovaginal fistula of obstetric origin: a review of 15 years' experience in a teaching hospital. J Obstet Gynaecol 23:607–610
117. Khanduja KS, Yamashita HJ, Wise WE Jr et al (1994) Delayed repair of obstetric injuries of the anorectum and vagina: a stratified surgical approach. Dis Colon Rectum 37:344–349

Obstetric Lesions: The Gynaecologist's Point of View

30

Eddie H.M. Sze, Maria Ciarleglio

Repair of Third- and Fourth-degree Perineal Lacerations: Introduction

Data from the obstetrical literature show that about 0.4–3.7% of all vaginal deliveries result in a third- or fourth-degree perineal laceration [1, 2]. Rarely, the reported incidence can go as high as 20–39% [3, 4]. When a third- or fourth-degree perineal laceration occurs during vaginal delivery, the standard repair is to approximate the torn ends of the anal sphincter using two to six interrupted mattress or figure-of-eight stitches and close the vaginal and perineal tissues in layers. Postpartum, the patient is typically put on a soft diet and given a stool softener for 7–10 days. This method of repair is described in the latest edition of *Williams Obstetrics* [5], the newest edition of Gabbe et al. [6], and numerous other obstetrical textbooks.

This end-to-end method of repair seems to be very effective in restoring the function of the torn anal sphincter. Studies from the early and mid-1960s showed that women who sustained a third- or fourth-degree perineal laceration rarely, if ever, experienced any significant complication postpartum [3, 4]. Consequently, anal sphincter tear during vaginal delivery was not regarded as a major complication [3]. However, this absence of complication was based on the finding that very few patients complained of anal incontinence postpartum. In addition, these early studies did not state whether the investigators ever asked their patients about anal function postpartum or even saw most of these women for follow-up [3, 4]. In contrast, more recent studies found that women who sustained a third- or fourth-degree perineal laceration during vaginal delivery often develop anal incontinence (to flatus, liquid, and solid stool) postpartum. Four cohort studies demonstrated that within 12 months postpartum, 17–44% of women who had a third- or fourth-degree perineal laceration were incontinent to flatus and up to 17% had fecal incontinence (Table 1) [7–10]. These rates are significantly higher than in women who delivered during the same time period but did not have an anal sphincter tear. With longer duration of follow-up, the outcome is even worse. After 4–30 years, 38–63% of women with third–or fourth–degree perineal laceration had anal incontinence (Table 2) [1, 8, 11–13]. Although the majority were still incontinent to flatus, the proportion that had fecal incontinence had increased significantly. In addition, anal incontinence was more severe among women who had a third- or fourth-degree perineal laceration than those who delivered with an intact sphincter (Table 3) [12–14].

Table 1. Prevalence of anal incontinence after an anal sphincter tear

Reference	Degree of tear vs. control	Number	Flatus incontinence	Fecal incontinence	Follow-up
Zetterstrom et al. [7]	3rd/4th	46	39%	2%	9 months
	Control	574	14%	1%	
Pollack et al. [8]	3rd/4th	36	44%	0%	9 months
	Control	206	24%	1%	
Crawford et al. [9]	3rd/4th	35	17%	6%	9 - 12 months
	Control	35	3%	3%	
Borello-France et al. [10]	3rd/4th	335	23%	17%	6 months
	Control	319	18%	8%	

Table 2. Long-term outcome after an anal sphincter tear

Reference	Degree of tear vs. control	Number	Flatus incontinence	Fecal incontinence	Duration of follow-up
Wagenius et al. [13]	3rd/4th	186	33%	25%	4 years
	Control	348	15%	9%	
Pollack et al. [8]	3rd/4th	36	53%	11%	5 years
	Control	206	31%	5%	
Haadem et al. [1]	3rd/4th	41	22%	46%	18 years
	Control	38	3%	5%	
Faltin et al. [12]	3rd/4th	259	46%	14%	19 years
	Control	281	37%	5%	
Nygaard et al. [11]	3rd/4th	29	31%	7%	30 years
	Episiotomy	89	43%	18%	

Etiology of Incontinence

Many investigators believed that this deterioration in anal continence after a third- or fourth-degree perineal laceration is caused by neurological injury sustained during the sphincter tear, because pelvic neuropathy is frequently found in women with anal incontinence [15–17]. Since this type of neurological injury is usually not amenable to medical or surgical therapy, obstetricians believed that there is very little they can do to ensure that their patient will maintain continence after sustaining a third- or fourth-degree perineal laceration.

In the early 1990s, an investigator from Great Britain published a small study that involved 34 women who sustained a third-degree perineal laceration during vaginal delivery. Eighty-five percent of the women in this small study had a persistent tear in their anal sphincter 2–22 months after their third-degree perineal laceration was repaired [18]. This finding demonstrated that 85% of anal sphincter repairs had failed. The failed repair usually involved both the internal and the external anal sphincters. Other investigators subsequently reported that 54–91% of their anal sphincter repair failed (Table 4) [10, 18–21]. The presence of a failed repair is an important risk factor for developing anal incontinence postpartum. Data from seven studies revealed that approximately 55% of subjects who failed anal sphincter repair were incontinent postpartum [10, 18–23]. In contrast, only 20% of those who had a successful repair were incontinent. These findings demonstrated that anal sphincter repair outcome plays an important role in determining whether a woman will maintain continence after sustaining a third- or fourth-degree perineal laceration.

Table 3. Severity of anal incontinence after an anal sphincter tear

Reference	Degree of tear vs. control	Number	Degree/type of incontinence and quality of life (QOL) scores		Duration of follow-up
			Severe incontinence	Very severe incontinence	
Faltin et al. [12]	3rd/4th	445	13%	4%	18 years
	Control	445	8%	1%	
			Fecal incontinence	Affected QOL	
Wagenius et al. [13]	3rd/4th	186	25%	30%	4 years
	Control	348	9%	10%	
			Median (range[a]) flatus incontinence score	Median (range[a]) fecal incontinence score	
Fornell et al. [14]	Partial AST	33	4 (1–6)	4 (1–4)	10 years
	Complete AST	7	2 (1–4)	2 (1–6)	
	Control	19	5 (3–6)	6 (2–6)	

AST anal sphincter tear
[a] 1 = severe problem, 6 = no problem

Table 4. Prevalence of persistent defect after anal sphincter repair

Reference	Number	Interval	Number with persistent defect			
			EAS	IAS	EAS+IAS	Total
Sultan et al. [18]	34	2–22 months	5	1	23	29 (85%)
Poen et al. [21]	40	1–11 years	23	0	12	35 (88%)
Gjessing et al. [20]	35	1–5 years				19 (54%)
Nielsen et al. [19]	24	3–18 months	13	1	0	14 (58%)
Borello-France et al. [10]	22	12 months	13	1	6	20 (91%)

EAS external anal sphincter, *IAS* internal anal sphincter

Overlapping Repair

The high rate of failed repair associated with the end-to-end approximation suggests that it is an ineffective method of repairing torn anal sphincters. Investigators have tried different repairs and various other ancillary therapies to improve the surgical outcome. One frequently suggested approach was to abandon the end-to-end approximation in favor of the overlapping repair. Although obstetricians primarily use the end-to-end approximation, some investigators believe that this technique is inherently incapable of repairing the torn anal sphincter because the sphincter muscle and capsule are just not strong enough to hold the sutures in an end-to-end configuration. In contrast, colorectal surgeons generally favor the overlapping repair. This method, originally described in the early 1970s by Sir Allen Park, distributes the tension on the sutures over a larger area to reduce the likelihood that they will tear through the sphincter muscle and capsule [24].

Two small case series seemed to suggest that the overlapping repair has a lower failure rate than end-to-end approximation [25, 26]. Two British investigators used the overlapping technique to repair 32 anal sphincters torn during vaginal delivery [25]. After 20 weeks, the authors reported that their subjects had a lower incontinence rate (40% vs. 8%) and fewer failed repairs (85% vs. 15%) than historical controls (repaired with end-to-end approximation). A Swedish study found only one (3%) failed repair among 30 cases of third- and fourth-degree perineal lacerations that were repaired with the overlapping technique at 24 months postpartum [26].

In contrast, data from controlled studies were less encouraging. A group of investigators from the Dublin Maternity Hospital compared the end-to-end and overlapping methods in a prospective study. One hundred and fifty-four women with third- or fourth-degree perineal laceration were repaired with either the end-to-end or overlapping method, depending on the obstetrician's preference. After 3 months, the percent with a small persistent defect [47/84 (54%) vs. 33/67 (49%)], a large persistent defect [27/87 (31%) vs. 24/67 (36%)], and a successful repair [13/87 (15%) vs. 10/67 (15%)] were similar between the two methods [27]. In addition, the two surgical repairs were equally efficacious in preserving anal continence, evidenced by the similar proportion that developed incontinence [36/67 (54%) vs. 46/87 (53%)] and the median incontinence score [Cleveland Clinic Florida Fecal Incontinence (CCF-FI) score: 1/20 (range: 0–5) vs. 2/20 (range: 0–16)] [28].

The same group of investigators subsequently compared the end-to-end and overlapping repairs in a randomized controlled trial [29]. Again, the proportion that had a small persistent defect [50/57 (88%) vs. 42/55 (78%), $p = 0.27$], a large persistent defect [3/57 (5%) vs. 3/57 (5%), $p = 0.45$], and a successful repair [4/57 (7%) vs. 6/55 (11%), $p = 0.70$] were similar between the two methods after 3 months. In addition, the two types of repair were equally effective in preserving anal continence postpartum. The proportion of patients who developed anal incontinence [27/55 (49%) vs. 33/57 (58%), $p = 0.46$] and the median incontinence score [modified Wexner score: 0/20 (range: 0–13) vs. 2/20 (range: 0–14), $p = 0.20$] [28] were also similar between the two types of repair.

Findings from the Dublin studies were later confirmed by a small randomized controlled trial from the University of New Mexico [30]. The latter study also found that the overlapping method is no more effective in repairing the torn anal sphincter or preserving continence than the end-to-end method. The proportions that had failed repair [4/15 (27%) vs. 1/11 (9%), $p > 0.10$], had flatus incontinence [4/15

(27%) vs. 3/11 (27%)], and had fecal incontinence [1/15 (7%) vs. 3/11 (27%)] were similar between the end-to-end and the overlapping methods at 4 months.

Interestingly, the New Mexico study was much more successful in repairing the torn internal and external anal sphincters using either the end-to-end or the overlapping method than other studies, including earlier data from the same investigators [31]. Eleven (73%) of 15 women in the end-to-end group and 10 (91%) of 11 in the overlapping group had intact external and internal anal sphincters at 4 months postpartum. Findings from this study may have been affected by its small sample size ($n = 41$), problem with randomization, and the 37% of subjects who did not return for follow-up.

In 2006, a group of investigators from Great Britain published a third randomized controlled trial that compared the end-to-end with the overlapping method [32]. They found that the outcome was similar between the two methods at 3 and 6 months postpartum. However, after 1 year, more women in the end-to-end group had developed anal incontinence (0/27 vs. 5/25, $p = 0.009$) and more severe incontinence [median Wexner incontinence score: 1/20 (range 0–9) vs. 0/20 (range 0–5), $p = 0.05$] than subjects in the overlapping group. Although these differences were statistically significant, clinical significance was less certain because the median Wexner incontinence score was 1/20 for the end-to-end repair and 0/20 for the overlapping repair. Also, the scores for all four components (mean life style, coping/behavior, depression/self-perception, and embarrassment) of the Fecal Incontinence Quality of Life (FIQOL) scale [33] were similar.

The British study had another interesting finding [32]. More women whose torn anal sphincter was repaired with the overlapping method experienced improvement in their incontinence during the study period [17/27 (63%) vs. 9/25 (36%), $p = 0.01$], whereas more subjects that had end-to-end approximation developed an exacerbation of incontinence [0/27 vs. 4/25 (16%), $p = 0.01$]. This finding is perplexing, as both repairs have been shown in several studies to have a similar failure rate at 3–4 months postpartum [29, 30, 32]. Although the exacerbation of incontinence may be due to a difference in the 1-year outcome between the two repairs, the improvement in incontinence is difficult to explain because a failed repair is not likely to heal itself. A possible explanation is that this study did not have a sufficient sample size, which resulted in an unequal distribution of subjects with flatus and fecal incontinence between the overlapping and end-to-end repairs. As about 11% of flatus incontinence would resolve spontaneously during the first 18 months postpartum but a similar percent of fecal incontinence would exacerbate during the same period, the insufficient sample size could result in a discrepancy between the two surgical outcomes [34]. However, the British study did not compare the condition of the repaired anal sphincters or differentiate between subjects with flatus and fecal incontinence or the extent of improvement and exacerbation of incontinence after 1 year. Whether the observed differences were due to a type I error or the two repair methods need to be further evaluated in a larger study remains unclear.

After reviewing the available data, one must conclude that the overlapping technique is no more effective in repairing the torn anal sphincter or preserving continence postpartum than the end-to-end method.

Internal Anal Sphincter

As all fourth-degree perineal lacerations and a significant number of third-degree tears involved the internal anal sphincter, some investigators have proposed that obstetricians should specifically look for, and repair when present, a torn internal sphincter. The function of the internal anal sphincter is to maintain a constant tone in the anal canal, and repairing it would theoretically reduce the risk of developing passive incontinence.

Two British investigators attempted to identify and repair torn internal anal sphincter in 27 cases of third-degree perineal laceration [25]. After an average follow-up of 20 (range: 7–34) weeks, only two (7%) women developed flatus incontinence. Internal anal sphincter repair probably did not contribute to this study outcome, as four (33%) of the 12 repairs failed and eight (40%) of the 20 torn internal sphincters were not identified despite the investigators' concerted effort.

A group of Norwegian investigators also attempted to identify and repair torn internal anal sphincters among 30 cases of third- and fourth-degree perineal lacerations [26]. These investigators were unable to identify one (6%) of the 18 torn internal sphincters, and two (12%) of the 17 repairs failed. After a median follow-up of 34 (range: 12–63) months, five patients (17%) complained of flatus incontinence, and two (7%) had developed fecal incontinence.

Although findings from these two studies appear promising, data from two small uncontrolled series are insufficient to determine whether repairing the torn internal sphincter would help retain anal continence after a third- or fourth-degree perineal laceration.

Consult a Specialist

Recently, several studies from Scandinavia reported that obstetricians in their hospital were encouraged to routinely consult a colorectal surgeon to repair third- and fourth-degree perineal lacerations [35–37].

In a Norwegian study, two colorectal surgeons repaired 30 cases of third- and fourth-degree perineal lacerations using the overlapping method [36]. After 24 months, one (3%) external sphincter and two (6%) internal sphincter repairs failed. In addition, they also failed to identify one (3%) internal sphincter tear. In another small study, two British urogynecologists repaired 27 anal sphincters torn during vaginal delivery [25]. After 20 weeks, four (15%) of the 27 external sphincter and four (33%) of the 12 internal sphincter repairs failed. These investigators also failed to identify eight (40%) of the 20 torn internal anal sphincters. Although these outcomes look very favorable, findings from two small uncontrolled series are insufficient to establish that colorectal surgeons or urogynecologists would have more success than obstetricians in repairing third- and fourth-degree perineal lacerations.

Operating Room

In European countries, third- and fourth-degree perineal lacerations are frequently repaired under general or regional anesthesia in the operating room [1, 2, 7, 8, 10, 13, 14, 19–21, 23, 25–27, 29, 32]. The operating room provides superior lighting, appropriate equipment, and better exposure. In addition, general or regional anesthesia relaxes the patient and sphincter muscle tone. This allows the operator to retrieve the torn ends of the anal sphincter that had retracted into its fibrous capsule and perform the repair without tension. Investigators found that anal sphincter repair performed under such optimal conditions still has a 54–91% failure rate (Table 4) [10, 18–21].

In contrast, anal sphincter tear in the United States is frequently repaired in the birthing room under local or regional anesthesia with less lighting and exposure. However, there are very little data evaluating the outcome of repairs performed in the birthing room. Investigators from the University of New Mexico were much more successful in repairing torn internal and external anal sphincters in the delivery room using either the end-to-end or the overlapping method than their European counterparts [30]. As previously noted, the New Mexico study had only 41 patients, and 15 (37%) did not return for follow-up. Whether anal sphincter repair performed in the operating room under regional or general anesthesia has a better outcome than those repaired in the birthing room needs to be objectively evaluated in a larger study.

Bowel Confinement

Another approach that has been used to improve surgical outcome is bowel confinement. Many obstetricians routinely order a soft diet and a stool softener for women who had an anal sphincter repair, whereas others prefer a laxative or a constipating agent. These regimens are intended to lessen tension on the sutures during bowel movement and allow the torn ends of the anal sphincter to heal together. However, there are very little data that show whether bowel confinement affects the outcome of anal sphincter repair. A study from Dublin randomized 105 patients who had a third-degree perineal laceration to either 3 days of codeine followed by 4 days of laxative or 7 days of laxative [37]. After 3 months, the median incontinence score was similar between the two groups [Wexner incontinence score: 1/20 (range: 0–8) vs. 0/20 (range: 0–9), $p = 0.096$].

Current data show that the only available treatment that would increase a woman's chance of maintaining anal continence after sustaining a third- or fourth-degree perineal laceration is a successful repair. However, there are no guidelines available to help obstetricians consistently perform a successful repair.

Childbirth after a Third-degree Tear

Third- and fourth-degree perineal lacerations occur three to seven times more frequently among nulliparas than multiparas [27, 38, 39]. Consequently, many women who had an anal sphincter tear would want to have more children. Vaginal delivery after an anal sphincter tear has frequently been cited as a major risk factor for developing a new and more severe anal incontinence [8, 14, 21, 38]. As we do not know how to effectively repair a torn anal sphincter, and a significant number of failed repairs would develop incontinence, obstetricians are naturally reluctant to subject women who had a prior third- or fourth-degree perineal laceration to the stress of another vaginal birth. In addition, about 7.5–10.5% of women who had a prior third- or fourth-degree perineal laceration would develop a recurrent sphincter tear during subsequent vaginal delivery. These findings have led some investigators to propose that women with a prior third- or fourth-degree tear should have elective cesarean for all subsequent births [40]. However, there are very few studies that objectively evaluate the effect of vaginal delivery or elective cesarean on the anal function of these women.

Current data have not clearly delineated the effect of vaginal delivery on the anal function of women who had already sustained a third-degree sphincter tear. A prospective study from Sweden followed 34 primiparas who had a prior third-degree perineal laceration and two who had a prior fourth-degree anal sphincter tear [8]. Among the nine subjects who had no subsequent delivery after the anal sphincter tear, 44% were incontinent at 9 months and at 5 years postpartum. In contrast, the prevalence of anal incontinence among 27 subjects with at least one additional vaginal delivery had increased from 44% at 9 months to 56% at 5 years ($p = 0.009$).

A second Swedish study prospectively followed for 10 years 23 women who had a third-degree perineal laceration [14]. Four women had at least two additional vaginal deliveries, 13 had one subsequent vaginal birth, and six had no additional birth. The only difference among the three groups was that women with two or more additional vaginal deliveries had more severe flatus incontinence, whereas the severity of fecal incontinence was similar.

A group of Danish investigators followed 72 women who had a third-degree perineal laceration for 2–4 years. Four (24%) of the 17 women who had a subsequent vaginal delivery after the anal sphincter tear developed new or more severe flatus incontinence. Eight (15%) of 55 with no additional birth developed flatus incontinence and nine (16%) sustained fecal incontinence [38].

In contrast to the previous two findings, this study suggests that subsequent vaginal delivery has a protective effect on the anal function of women who had a prior third-degree perineal laceration. However, findings from all three studies may have been affected by their small sample size, inclusion of subjects with superficial and partial third- and fourth-degree tears, and those that had subsequent cesarean delivery.

Findings from retrospective studies also vary as to whether vaginal birth after a third-degree perineal laceration is associated with a higher or lower rate of anal incontinence. A Swiss study found that women with no additional delivery after a third-degree perineal laceration experienced anal incontinence more frequently than those who had one or at least two subsequent vaginal births [10/49 (20%) vs. 4/60 (7%) vs. 1/20 (5%), $p = 0.03$) [41]. In contrast, a group of Scandinavian investigators found that the prevalence of anal incontinence was higher among women who had a vaginal birth after sustaining a third-degree perineal laceration than those who had no further delivery [24/43 (56%) vs. 23/67 (34%), risk ratio (RR) = 1.6, 95% confidence interval (CI): 1.1–2.5] [21]. A probable reason for this discrepancy is that both studies included women of different parity who sustained either a partial or complete anal sphincter laceration with and without extensions into the anal mucosa, and the possible inclusion of women with recurrent sphincter tear or cesarean during subsequent deliveries [21, 35, 41–47]. All of these factors have been shown to affect anal continence and, consequently, may have altered the study outcome.

A third retrospective study from East Carolina University included only women who sustained a complete third-degree perineal laceration during their first childbirth and did not have cesarean, repeat anal sphincter tear, or operative vaginal delivery during subsequent births [48]. Among women who had 0, 1, and at least 2 additional vaginal deliveries after the sphincter tear, the prevalence of anal incontinence [11/65 (17%), 11/67 (16%), and 12/40 (30%), $p = 0.179$] and the severity of incontinence (mean Pescatori score: 3.2±1.4, 3.5±1.1, and 3.2±1.4, $p = 0.846$) [49] were similar. In addition, the proportion that had severe incontinence, defined as having a Pescatori score of 5 or 6 points out of a maximum of 6 and that the incontinence had a severe effect on the subject's daily activities and quality of life, were also similar (2/65, 1/67, and 2/40, $p = 0.811$). However, this retrospective study probably did not have sufficient sample size to detect the observed difference. Also, it did not use a validated system to grade incontinence severity or to measure the effect of incontinence on quality of life. These data suggest that the effect of subsequent vaginal birth on the anal function of women who had a prior third-degree perineal laceration has not been established.

Childbirth after a Fourth-degree Tear

There are very few studies evaluating the effect of vaginal birth on women's anal function after a fourth-degree perineal laceration. However, findings from available studies are fairly consistent. A Swiss study reported that women who had one or at least two vaginal deliveries after a fourth-degree perineal laceration developed fecal incontinence more frequently than those who had no subsequent birth [7/25 (28%) vs. 2/9 (22%) vs. 0/14, $p = 0.04$] [41]. Although the prevalence of anal incontinence was similar [20/52 (38%) vs. 14/60 (23%) vs. 10/36 (28%), $p = 0.208$], the East Carolina study found that women who had at least two additional vaginal deliveries after a fourth-degree sphincter tear developed severe incontinence more frequently than those who had no or one subsequent delivery [4/36 (11%) vs. 0 vs. 0, $p = 0.002$] [50]. Thus, existing data suggest that vaginal delivery after a fourth-degree perineal laceration probably increases the prevalence and/or severity of anal incontinence.

Elective Cesarean after an Anal Sphincter Tear

Although elective cesarean for all births after a third- or fourth-degree perineal laceration has been widely advocated as the method to prevent the occurrence of a new or more severe incontinence, there is very little evidence to support the effectiveness of this prophylactic measure. Elective cesarean has a rather limited protective effect on the anal function. The International Randomized Term Breech Trial found that at 3 months postpartum, only mild flatus incontinence was more prevalent among the planned vaginal delivery than the planned cesarean group (33/58 vs. 20/61, $p = 0.008$) [51]. The prevalence of flatus incontinence (66/616 vs. 59/606, $p = 0.64$), severe flatus incontinence (1/61 vs. 2/58, $p = 0.481$), fecal incontinence (5/619 vs. 9/607, $p = 0.29$), and mild fecal incontinence (2/4 vs. 7/9, $p = 0.353$) were similar between the two groups. The reason for this limited protective effect is that anal incontinence that develops during childbirth occurs primarily during antepartum [52, 53]. Whether elective cesarean would prevent the occurrence of a new and/or more severe incontinence during subsequent childbirth among women who had a prior anal sphincter tear has not been studied.

Conclusion

Third- and fourth-degree perineal lacerations are major complications of vaginal birth. Repair of the torn anal sphincter frequently fails, which predisposes these women to develop incontinence. At the present time, there is no available method that can consistently repair the torn sphincter and restore its function. To achieve the best possible outcome, current evidence suggests that third- and fourth-degree perineal lacerations probably should be repaired in the operating room under general or regional anesthesia, preferably by someone with expertise in this area.

Elective cesarean for all births has been widely advocated as the prophylactic method to prevent the occurrence of a new or more severe incontinence among women who had a prior third- or fourth-degree perineal laceration. Although vaginal delivery after a fourth-degree perineal laceration has been associated with a higher prevalence and more severe incontinence, the effect of subsequent vaginal birth on the anal function of women who had a prior third-degree perineal laceration has not been established. In addition, whether elective cesarean would protect the anal function of women who had a prior third- or fourth-degree perineal laceration during subsequent childbirth also has not been established. Consequently, there is no evidence to suggest that elective cesarean would prevent the occurrence of a new or more severe incontinence during childbirth among women who had a prior third- or fourth-degree perineal laceration.

References

1. Haadem K, Gudmundsson S (1997) Can women with intraprtum rupture of anal sphincter still suffer aftereffects two decades later. Acta Obstet Gynecol Scand 76:601–603
2. Jander C, Lyrenas S (2001) Third and fourth degree perineal tears. Predictor factors in a referral hospital. Acta Obstet Gynecol Scand 80:229–234
3. O'Leary JL, O'Leary JA (1965) The complete episiotomy. Analysis of 1224 complete lacerations, sphincterotomies, and episiproctomies. Obstet Gynecol 25:235–240
4. Sieber EH, Kroon JD (1962) Morbidity in the third degree laceration. Obstet Gynecol 19:677–680
5. Cunningham FG, Leveno KJ, Bloom SL et al (eds) (2005) Williams Obstetrics, 22nd edn. McGraw-Hill, New York
6. Gabbe SG, Niebyl JR, Simposn JL (eds) (2002) Obstetrics, normal and problem pregnancies, 4th edn. Churchill Livingston, Philadelphia
7. Zetterstrom J, Lopez A, Anzen B et al (1999) Anal sphincter tears at vaginal delivery: Risk factors and clinical outcome of primary repair. Obstet Gynecol 94:21–28
8. Pollack J, Nordenstam J, Brismar S et al (2004) Anal incontinence after vaginal delivery: A five year prospective cohort study. Obstet Gynecol 104: 1397–1402
9. Crawford LA, Quint EH, Pearl ML (1993) Incontinence following rupture of the anal sphincter during delivery. Obstet Gynecol 82:527–531
10. Borello-France D, Burgio KL, Richter HE et al (2006) Fecal and urinary incontinence in primiparous women. Obstet Gynecol 108:863–872
11. Nygaard IE, Rao SSC, Dawson JD (1997) Anal incontinence after anal sphincter disruption: A 30-year retrospective study. Obstet Gynecol 89:896–901
12. Faltin DL, Otero M, Petignat P et al (2006) Women's health 18 years after rupture of the anal sphincter during childbirth: I. Fecal incontinence. Am J Obstet Gynecol 194:1255–1259
13. Wagenius J, Laurin J (2003) Clinical symptoms after anal sphincter rupture: A retrospective study. Acta Obstet Gynecol Scand 82:246–250
14. Fornell EU, Matthiesen L, Sjodhl R et al (2005) Obstetric anal sphincter injury ten years after: subjective and objective long term effects. BJOG 112:312–316
15. Parks AG, Swash M, Urich H (1977) Sphincter denervation in anorectal incontinence and rectal prolapse. Gut 18:656–665
16. Bartolo DEC, Jarratt JA, Read MG et al (1983) The role

of partial denervation of the puborectalis in idiopathic fecal incontinence. Br J Surg 70:664–667
17 Kiff ES, Swash M (1984) Slowed conduction in the pudendal nerves in idiopathic fecal incontinence. Br J Surg 71:614–616
18. Sultan AH, Kamm MA, Hudson CN et al (1994) Third degree obstetric anal sphincter tears: risk factors and outcome of primary repair. BMJ 308:887–891
19. Nielsen MB, Hauge C, Rasmussen OO et al (1992) Anal endosonographic findings in the follow-up of primary sutured sphincteric ruptures. Br J Surg 79:104–106
20. Gjessing H, Backe B, Sahlin Y (1998) Third degree obstetric tears: outcome after primary repair. Acta Obstet Gynecol Scand 77:736–740
21. Poen AC, Felt-Bersma RJF, Strijers RLM et al (1998) Third-degree obstetric perineal tear: long term clinical and functional results after primary repair. Br J Surg 85:1433–1438
22. Belmonte-Montes C, Hagerman G, Vega-Yepez PA et al (2001) Anal sphincter injury after vaginal delivery in primiparous females. Dis Colon Rectum 44:1244–1248
23. Norderval S, Oian P, Revhaug A et al (2005) Anal incontinence after obstetric sphincter tears: Outcome of anatomic primary repair. Dis Colon Rectum 48:1055–1061
24. Parks AG, McPartlin JF (1971) Late repairs of injuries of the anal sphincter. Proc R Soc Med 64:1187–1189
25. Sultan AH, Monga AK, Kumar D et al (1999) Primary repair of obstetric anal sphincter rupture using the overlap technique. BJOG 106:318–323
26. Kairaluoma MV, Raivio P, Aarnio MT et al (2004) Immediate repair of obstetric anal sphincter rupture: Medium-term outcome of the overlap technique. Dis Colon Rectum 47:1358–1363
27. Fitzpatrick M, Fynes M, Cassidy M et al (2000) Prospective study of the influence of parity and operative technique on the outcome of primary anal sphincter repair following obstetric injury. Eur J Obstet Gynecol Reprod Biol 89:159–163
28. Jorge J, Wexner SD (1993) Etiology and management of fecal incontinence. Dis Colon Rectum 36:77–79
29. Fitzpatrick M, Behan M, O'Connell PR et al (2000) A randomized clinical trial comparing primary overlap with approximation repair of third-degree obstetric tears. Am J Obstet Gynecol 183:1220–1224
30. Garcia V, Rogers R, Kim SS et al (2005) Primary repair of obstetric anal sphincter laceration: A randomized trail of two surgical techniques. Am J Obstet Gynecol 192:1697–1701
31. Kammerer-Doak DN, Wesol AB, Rogers RG et al (1999) A prospective cohort study of women after primary repair of obstetric anal sphincter laceration. Am J Obstet Gynecol 181:1317-1323
32. Fernando RJ, Sultan AH, Kettle C et al (2006) Repair techniques for obstetric anal sphincter injury. Obstet Gynecol 107:1261–1268
33. Rockwood TH, Church JM, Fleshman JW et al (2000) Fecal incontinence quality of life scale: quality of life instrument for patients with fecal incontinence. Dis Colon Rectum 43:9–16
34. Nazir M, Stien R, Carlsen E et al (2003) Early evaluation of bowel symptoms after primary repair of obstetric perineal rupture is misleading. An observational cohort study. Dis Colon rectum 46:1245–1250
35. Norderval S, Nsubuga D, Bjelke C et al (2004) Anal incontinence after obstetric sphincter tears: incidence in a Norwegian county. Acta Obstet Gynecol Scand 83:989–994
36. Kairaluoma MV, Raivio P, Aarnio MT et al (2004) Immediate repair of obstetric anal sphincter rupture: Medium-term outcome of the overlap technique. Dis Colon Rectum 47:1358–1363
37. Mahony R, Behan M, O'Herlihy C et al (2004) Randomized, clinical trial of bowel confinement vs. laxative use after primary repair of a third-degree obstetric anal sphincter tear. Dis Colon Rectum 47:12–17
38. Tetzschner T, Sorenson M, Gunnar L et al (1996) Anal and urinary incontinence in women with obstetric anal sphincter rupture. BJOG 103:1034–1040
39. Spydalaug A, Trogstad LIS, Skrondal A et al (2005) Recurrent risk of anal sphincter laceration among women with vaginal deliveries. Obstet Gynecol 105:307–313
40. McKenna DS, Ester JB, Fischer JR (2003) Elective cesarean delivery for women with a previous anal sphincter rupture. Am J Obstet Gynecol 189:1251–1256
41. Sangalli MR, Floris L, Faltin D et al (2000) Anal incontinence in women with third or fourth degree perineal tears and subsequent vaginal deliveries. Aust N Z J Obstet Gynecol 3:244–248
42. Ryhammer AM, Bek KM, Laurberg S (1995) Multiple vaginal deliveries increase the risk of permanent incontinence of flatus and urine in normal premenopausal women. Dis Colon Rectum 38:1206–1209
43. Nichols CM, Lamb EH, Ramakrishnan V (2005) Differences in outcome after third- versus fourth-degree perineal laceration repair: A prospective study. Am J Obstet Gynecol 193:530–536
44. Fynes M, Donnelly VS, O'Connell PR et al (1998) Cesarean delivery and anal sphincter injury. Obstet Gynecol 92:496–500
45. Peleg D, Kennedy CM, Merrill D et al (1999) Risk of repetition of a severe perineal laceration. Obstet Gynecol 93:1021–1024
46. Payne TN, Carey JC, Rayburn WF (1999) Prior third- or fourth-degree perineal tears and recurrence risks. Inter J Gynecol Obstet 64:55–57
47. Sorensen M, Tetzschner T, Rasmussen OO et al (1993) Sphincter rupture in childbirth. Br J Surg 80:392–394
48. Sze EHM (2005) Anal incontinence among women with one versus two complete third-degree perineal lacerations. Inter J Gynecol Obstet 90:213–217
49. Pescatori M, Anastasio G, Bottini C et al (1992) New grading and scoring for anal incontinence. Dis Colon Rectum 35:482–487
50. Sze EHM (2005) Prevalence and severity of anal incontinence in women with and without additional vaginal deliveries after a fourth-degree perineal laceration. Dis Colon Rectum 48:66–68
51. Hannah ME, Hannah WJ, Hodnett ED et al (2002) Outcomes at 3 months after planned cesarean versus planned vaginal delivery for breech presentation at term. JAMA 287:1822–1831
52. Chaliha C, Kalia V, Stanton SL et al (1999) Antenatal prediction of postpartum urinary and fecal incontinence. Obstet Gynecol 94:689–694
53. Chaliha C, Sultan AH, Bland JM et al (2001) Anal function: Effect of pregnancy and delivery. Am J Obstet Gynecol 185:427–432

Neurogenic Fecal Incontinence

31

Giuseppe Pelliccioni, Osvaldo Scarpino

Introduction

Fecal incontinence, according to the most used definition, is the "involuntary loss of the stool or soiling at a socially inappropriate time or place" [1]. It is an important health issue that strongly affects patient quality of life and restricts their social activities. It is a common problem, with prevalence ranging from 2.2% to 15% in the community and up to 40% in nursing homes [2]. The prevalence of fecal incontinence in neurological patients is higher than in the general population. Many neurological disorders are associated with fecal incontinence, and this chapter is a review of the current clinical knowledge regarding the pathogenesis and clinical findings. When considering the possible effects of central and peripheral neurological lesions on fecal continence, it is important to keep in mind that continence depends on intact neural pathways and normal function of the cerebral, spinal, and cauda equina centers, and peripheral nerves. It should be remembered, however, that signs, symptoms, and gastrointestinal dysfunction may differ from expectations by virtue of incomplete neuronal lesions, coexisting involvement of supraspinal or spinal centers, or damage to the distal parts of the autonomic or somatic innervation of the pelvic floor sphincter muscles.

Functional Anatomy and Physiology

Fecal continence is a complex function that requires coordinated responses in the pelvic floor sphincter muscles and abdominal and anorectal muscles. Consequently, fecal incontinence occurs when the normal anatomy or physiology of the anorectal unit is disrupted. In most cases, different pathophysiological mechanisms are involved in the pathogenesis of fecal incontinence, resulting in multifactorial etiology [3]. Physiological interaction of rectal motility and sensation with the tonic activity of smooth and striated muscle is complex and incompletely understood. Neural control of the colon can be separated into the intrinsic and the extrinsic colonic nervous systems.

The intrinsic enteric system (ENS) consists of nerve-cell bodies and endings that are located between the circular and the longitudinal muscle coats. The ENS is comprised of an outer myenteric or Auerbach's plexus that regulates smooth-muscle activity and an inner submucosal Meissner's plexus that influences the absorptive and secretory functions of the enteric mucosa. The ENS can function in isolation, without input from the brain or spinal cord.

The extrinsic system innervates the gut and acts as a modulator of visceral activity through sympathetic, parasympathetic, and somatic functions. The sympathetic inhibitory innervation of the gastrointestinal tract works by noradrenergic neurons on the enteric nerves and originates in the thoracolumbar spinal cord (T5–L2). The sympathetic fibers, leaving the spinal cord, pass through the paravertebral ganglia to relay in the celiac and mesenteric ganglia, terminating with postganglionic fibers on the enteric system. Sympathetic activity generally hyperpolarizes smooth-muscle cells, thereby reducing colorectal motility. Parasympathetic outflow to the colon is divided into cranial (vagus nerve fibers) and sacral divisions. The vagus nerve innervates the foregut and midgut, and the pelvic nerves innervate the descending and sigmoid colons and the anorectum. Parasympathetic activity inducing depolarization of smooth muscle increases the overall activity of the gastrointestinal tract by promoting peristalsis and increasing colorectal motility.

The internal anal sphincter (IAS), regulated by the sympathetic nerves, provides most of the resting anal pressure and during voluntary squeeze is reinforced by the tonic activity of the external anal sphincter (EAS). Fecal continence requires the ability to maintain resting IAS tone and EAS contraction in response to increased intra-abdominal pressure, rectal distension, and rectal contraction. The IAS is composed of smooth muscle arranged in inner circular and outer longitudinal layers. The EAS is composed of striated voluntary muscle closely related to the puborectalis (PR) muscle. The PR muscle originates at the pubis, wraps around the junction of the lower rectum and the anal canal, and plays an important role in fecal continence and in physiological defecation. Relaxation of the PR is, in fact, necessary for normal bowel emptying.

Although the colon and the pelvic floor sphincter muscles are peripherally innervated by the autonomic nervous system, voluntary cortical control is an essential feature of their physiological behavior. Whereas clinical information is defined in relation to the cortical control of the bladder, much less is known about cerebral determinants of bowel function. The medial prefrontal area and the anterior cingulate gyrus seem to represent two of the most important cortical centers that modulate bowel function, mediating voluntary control through spinal pathways. In particular, frontal-lobe lesions of the inferior and medial surfaces are associated with fecal and urinary incontinence [4].

The EAS is innervated by axons of the somatic neurons originating from the anterior horns of the S2–S4 spinal cord (Onuf's nucleus) via the pudendal nerves. Its course through the pelvic floor makes the pudendal nerve vulnerable to stretch injury, particularly during vaginal delivery.

Normal functions related to the pelvic organs, such as urination, defecation, and ejaculation, involves coordination between the different organ systems [5]. Experimental studies shown that distension of urinary bladder both inhibits colonic contractions and produces simultaneous contraction of the anal sphincter [6, 7]. The reverse also occurs: the urinary system is inhibited during defecation. Neural mechanisms underlying the interactions between the various pelvic organs are likely mediated by both the peripheral and central nervous systems. It is hypothesized that there must be some sort of viscerovisceral convergence within the central nervous system (CNS), both in the spinal cord itself and supraspinally.

Sensory perception from pelvic floor, anal canal, and rectal wall plays an essential role in defecation and in maintaining fecal continence. The afferent pathway involved in the perception of rectal filling, the preliminary event of defecation, is poorly understood. Rectal sensitivity arises from mechanoreceptors situated in the superficial and deep layers of the rectal wall and from the stimulation of nerve endings at the anal transitional zone [8, 9]. Recent animal models confirmed the presence of intraganglionic laminar nerve ending receptors specialized for mechanical distension in the myenteric plexus of the rectal wall [10]. The superficial receptors travel to the autonomic presacral ganglia, whereas the deep receptors project to the lumbar cord. Rectal distension is most likely transmitted along the S2–S4 parasympathetic pathway. When this innervation is absent (i.e., in paraplegics or traumatic sacral lesions), rectal filling is perceived as a minor sensation of discomfort.

Pelvic nerves are the main sensory pathways from the rectum; some sensory information is also conveyed in the sympathetic hypogastric nerves to the thoracolumbar spinal cord. Sensory information from the anal canal, perineum, and urethra is carried almost exclusively by the pudendal nerves. Pudendal nerve block induces, in fact, a loss of sensation in genital perianal skin and EAS weakness but does not affect rectal sensation [11].

Little is known about the cortical processing of anorectal sensation. The differences between rectal and anal sensation relate both to the differences in peripheral innervation and cortical representation. Unlike somatic sensation strongly represented in the primary somatosensory cortex, visceral sensation is primarily represented in the secondary somatosensory cortex. Furthermore, other cortical areas, such as prefrontal cortex and paralimbic and limbic areas (in particular, anterior insular cortex, amygdala, and cingulated cortex) contribute to the affective and cognitive components of rectal sensation [12, 13].

Fecal Incontinence in Disease Mainly Affecting the Brain

Loss of control of the ascending and descending pathways induced by lesions in the CNS may present with urinary and fecal incontinence. Any supraspinal lesion of brain, brainstem, and spinal cord rostral to the sacral Onuf's nucleus–including cerebrovascular disease, hydrocephalus, intrinsic or extrinsic tumors, traumatic head injury, multiple sclerosis, Parkinson's disease (PD) and other neurodegenerative diseases, and spinal cord injury (SCI)–may affect voiding and fecal continence.

Furthermore, in most patients with neurological disease, colorectal dysfunction is frequently caused by a combination of lesions of the central or peripheral nervous systems, altered dietary habits, immobility, or use of different drugs. The effects of fecal incontinence in nonneurological and in neurological patients are very severe and are associated with a reluctance to leave home [14]. Kamm pointed out that fecal incontinence is, in fact, a more common reason than dementia for seeking placement in a nursing home [15]. However, Andrew and Nathan stated that in patients with bladder and bowel disturbances as a result of frontal-lobe lesions, defecation was affected much less often than micturition [4]. A particular type of fecal incontinence consisting of an inappropriate context more than an involuntary emptying of the bowel is described in frontotemporal dementia or in vascular or traumatic frontal encephalopathy. A mixed pattern of urgency and involuntary emptying of the bowel and bladder in inappropriate context can occur in multifocal vascular or inflammatory disorders.

Stroke and Cerebrovascular Disease

Fecal incontinence is a common complication after stroke and affects about 30–40% of patients in the acute phase and 11% at 3 and 12 months [16–18]. The occurrence of bowel and urinary symptoms is related to the size of vascular lesion; in particular, fecal incontinence is associated with the severity of the stroke [18]. Large ischemic frontoparietotemporal lesions can induce a higher incidence of urinary and bowel symptoms than can frontal injury alone. In the Copenhagen Stroke Study, patients with fecal incontinence in the first week after stroke were significantly more frequently women and more often had a history of former stroke comorbidity of other disabling diseases than patients without fecal incontinence [18]. The same study reported that lesions in patients with fecal incontinence were significantly more often due to a hemorrhage, were larger in size, and more often involved the cerebral cortex than those in patients without fecal incontinence. Patients with fecal incontinence also had significantly lower scores on the initial Barthel Index and Scandinavian Stroke Scale (SSS) [19].

Age, diabetes mellitus, severity of stroke (initial SSS score and diameter of lesion) and comorbidity of other disabling disease are significant risk factors for fecal incontinence [18]. Urinary and fecal incontinence appear to be a powerful indicator for poor prognosis in ischemic stroke [20]. Patients who develop fecal incontinence have a higher risk of death within 6 months compared with those who remain continent; furthermore, severe disability and institutionalization frequently occur among stroke survivors [18, 21–23]. Fecal incontinence is also linked with mortality. Harari et al. have shown that 36% of patients with initial fecal incontinence compared with 4% of continent patients had died at 3 months after stroke and 20% of 3-month survivors with fecal incontinence versus 8% of those continent at 3 months had died by 1 year [16].

Functional urinary and bowel disorders can result from a large cortical hemispheric lesion that interrupts the central, frontally dependent pathways for urinary and bowel storage and voiding [24]. In the acute phase of the illness, 30–40% of large ischemic stroke patients develop fecal incontinence within 2 weeks; however, this symptom tends to improve along with neurological signs. After a 6-month follow-up, between 3% and 9% of patients remain incontinent [25].

Harari et al. [16] have also provided some indication of the impact of fecal incontinence on other adverse outcomes. Incontinent patients were more likely to be in long-term care (28% vs. 6%) and to receive district nurse services (20% vs. 11%) than continent patients at 3 months. This suggests that fecal incontinence in stroke survivors may increase the risk of institutionalization and the need for nursing support in the community. It is presumed that incontinence is a predicting factor for poor prognosis for different reasons: the same lesion might cause neurogenic bowel and bladder dysfunction in addition to cognitive or motor impairment; moreover, fecal and urinary incontinence may induce marked psychological problems that hamper functional recovery.

Parkinson's Disease and Parkinsonian Syndromes

The majority of patients with PD or parkinsonian syndromes–in particular, multiple system atrophy (MSA)–complains of gastrointestinal and pelvic organ dysfunction. Stocchi et al [26] reported a similar occurrence of altered bowel frequency and defecation in PD and MSA patients. Gastrointestinal symptoms in PD include gastroparesis and constipation as a result of decreased bowel movement frequency and defecation difficulty. In all patients, these disorders became manifest or worsened after the onset of neurologic symptoms. The most striking features of bowel dysfunction in PD patients were constipation and difficulty in expulsion [27]. The prevalence of constipation in PD patients is high: more than 50% suffer from moderate to severe constipation [27, 28]. PD patients are reported to have prolonged colorectal transit time and paradoxical contraction of the PR muscle on defecation [29, 30]. Difficulty in defecation is a very common symptom in PD, occurring in 67–94% of patients; constipation is present in 29–77% of patients compared with 13% of age-matched controls [31]. Singaram et al. [32] reported a reduction of dopamine-containing neurons in immunostaining of biopsied submucosa and colonic musculature and the presence of Levy bodies in the myenteric plexus of the colon. These findings suggest that prolonged transit time and constipation in PD patients may depend not only on central but also on peripheral dopamine reduction in the colon.

The most frequent anorectal manometric findings by Stocchi et al. [26] in MSA patients were low resting anal pressure, reduced voluntary anal contractility, and a paradoxical anal contraction or insufficient anal relaxation during straining; the same impairments have been reported by Edwards et al. in PD patients [28]. Abnormal straining is an important cause of constipation in both PD and MSA patients and frequently is involved in the pathogenesis of outlet-type constipation. Therefore, anorectal manometric variables do not differentiate PD from MSA patients.

Sakakibara et al. [27] reported that fecal incontinence in PD patients commonly occurred together with urinary incontinence, but there was no significant relation between sexual dysfunction and bladder or bowel dysfunction. Although much less common than constipation, fecal incontinence may also occur in MSA patients, which does not seem to be related with the presence of voiding dysfunction and, in particular, urinary incontinence. A low resting anal tone is not a typical finding in MSA and PD patients, and only some patients have marked sphincter hypotonia involved in facilitating fecal incontinence [26].

Fecal Incontinence in Spinal Cord Disease

Multiple Sclerosis, Myelopathies, and Spinal Cord Injury

Multiple sclerosis (MS) is a progressive neurologic disease that results from multiple demyelinating lesions within the CNS and that shows a variety of clinical presentations and courses determined by the location and number of the same lesions. Bladder and bowel dysfunction is the third most important discomfort in MS patients after spasticity and fatigue [33, 34]. Genitourinary dysfunctions in MS patients frequently occur due to the spinal involvement, with an incidence of 78% [35–38]. Bowel-related disorders in MS patients are very common. The prevalence of bowel dysfunction, fecal incontinence, and/or constipation is reported to be between 52% and 66% [39–41]. Hinds et al. [42] found that 51% of 280 MS patients experienced fecal incontinence; it occurred at least weekly in 25%. The authors also demonstrated a strong correlation between fecal incontinence and the duration of MS and degree of disability [42]. Conversely, Chia et al. [39] found no correlation between the presence of bowel dysfunction and disease duration, patients' age, Disability Status Scale, and Kurtzke score.

The discrepancy in these studies may be explained with the variety of underlying central and peripheral pathogenesis of fecal incontinence in MS patients. MS leads to fecal incontinence by medullary dysfunction and in particular by conus medullaris lesions, causing weakness and denervation of the pelvic floor striated sphincter muscles [43]. Changes in bowel function among MS patients are in many ways similar to those described for SCI patients. However, due to the multiple lesions within the CNS, many patients have a combination of supraconal and conal lesions. Loss of voluntary control of the EAS muscle may also occur as a consequence of MS plaques affecting the central pelvic floor motor control pathway. Glick et al. [44] suggest that fecal incontinence can also occur by alteration of colonic motility with the generation of high intracolonic pressures due to reduction or interruption of the normal cortical inhibition of colonic motor activity. Most studies have also shown that anorectal sensibility [45], anal squeeze pressure [45–48], and anal resting pressure are reduced in MS patients. The rectal wall is also hyperirritable with reduced compliance, and all these issues may result in fecal incontinence [45, 49, 50].

Bowel and anorectal dysfunction resulting in fecal incontinence and severe constipation are common complications of SCI [51–56]. Bowel dysfunctions and in particular fecal incontinence are the most important factor affecting not only acute rehabilitation treatment following SCI but also both long-term quality of life [57, 58] and chronic treatment for bowel care [59, 60]. Immediately after acute SCI, patients are in spinal shock, and all sensory perceptions, motor functions, and reflex activity below the level of the spinal cord lesion are lost or reduced. Spinal shock with temporary loss of spinal reflexes lasts for a variable period of time. Krogh et al. reported that in most patients, spinal shock affects the rectum for less than 4 weeks [61]. Colorectal problems can be a cause of morbidity immediately after SCI, and these problems become more frequent with increasing time after injury [57].

Between 27% and 90% of SCI patients complain of symptoms of neurogenic bowel dysfunctions due to the lack of nervous control [51, 62]. Two types of colon dysfunctions and complications may arise, depending on the level of the spinal injury: upper motor neuron bowel (UMNB) dysfunctions and lower motor neuron bowel (LMNB) dysfunctions [63–65]. UMNB dysfunction results from a spinal cord lesion above the conus medullaris, whereas LMNB or areflexic bowel results from a lesion affecting the parasympathetic cell bodies in the conus medullaris and the cauda equina [63]. The main differences between the two clinical pictures consist of the presence of spinal-cord-mediated reflex peristalsis and the functional integrity of the pudendal nerve in UMNB, whereas in LMNB, no spinal-cord-mediated reflex peristalsis occurs, and there is slow stool propulsion. Due to the complete or incomplete EAS muscle denervation on electromyography (EMG) examination, there is increased risk for fecal incontinence. The levator ani muscles lack tone, reducing the rectal angle and causing the lumen of the rectum to open [66]. The EAS and pelvic muscles are flaccid, and there is no reflex response to increased intra-abdominal pressure. The loss of parasympathetic control and reflex innervation of the IAS means a further reduction in resting anal tone and leads to fecal incontinence [55]. Only the myenteric plexus coordinates colonic segmental peristalsis, and a dryer stool and rounder stool shape can occur. In UMNB or hyperreflexic bowel, voluntary EAS muscle control is discontinued; however, connections between the spinal cord and the colon remain intact, with the presence of reflex coordination and stool propulsion. There is increased colonic wall and anal tone. The EAS muscle remains tight, thereby retaining stool and inducing constipation and fecal retention [63, 67].

The majority of SCI patients, 42–95%, suffer from constipation, and two thirds need to induce defecation by digital stimulation of the anal canal or rectum or to empty their rectum digitally [51, 53, 68]. Patterns of gut dysmotility have been described for different levels and degrees of SCI. Rajendra et al. demonstrated that lesions above T1 result in delayed mouth-to-caecum time, but lesions below this level show normal transit times to the caecum and markedly delayed transit times beyond the ileocaecal valve [69]. Keshavarzian et al. [70] showed a slowed transit throughout the whole colon in patients with spinal cord lesions above the lumbar region, a delay in part due to loss of colonic compliance. The lack of compliance leads to functional obstruction, increased transit times, abdominal distension, bloating, and discomfort [55]. Regarding the frequency of defecation, Yim et al. revealed that patients with UMNB emptied their bowels about three times a week, whereas LMNB patients did so about twice a day, with a high risk of fecal incontinence due to lax EAS muscle mechanism [64]. To avoid incontinence, the LMNB group tended to perform their bowel care program about twice a day, but despite this frequent care program, they experienced fecal incontinence 2.61 times per month. This suggests that CNS modulates and regulates colonic motility and that loss of the descending inhibitory pathway from CNS produces an increased colonic activity and decreased compliance [71].

The most common cause of neuropathic bowel in children is myelodysplasia, in particular spina bifida, that results in both constipation and fecal incontinence. Lie et al. found that bowel dysfunctions are present in approximately 78% of children aged 4–18 years with spina bifida, and lack of bowel control is found to be as stressful as bladder dysfunction and more stressful than impairment of motor function [72]. Typical changes in myelodysplasia include poor voluntary sphincter function and poor anorectal sensibility. Left-colon motility is usually disturbed, whereas IAS tone is normal or near normal. At least half of the patients with myelodysplasia suffer from fecal incontinence, and 90% need assistance to maintain bowel function [72]. The majority of patients with spina bifida also may have hydrocephalus that results in intellectual deficits potentially contributing to fecal incontinence. In a series of 109 adults with myelodysplasia, Malone et al. [73] found that 55% had regular fecal soiling. The type of bowel dysfunction is dependent on the myelodysplasia level. In high-thoracic or thoracolumbar-meningomyelocele is relatively rare, the colonic transit time is very slow, voluntary sphincter function and rectal sensibility are missing, and patients are prone to fecal loading [74]. In most patients, the myelomeningocele is lumbosacral or sacral, resulting in a lesion of the conus medullaris or cauda equina. Patients with lumbosacral lesions show slow left-colonic transit time, resulting in pellet-like stools evacuated with the help of the gastrocolic reflex; fecal loading is uncommon. The main functional problem in these patients is the automatic event of bowel emptying, and careful timing of rectal stimulation can induce bowel emptying with some degree of voluntary control. Many patients with sacral lesions usually are ambulant with normal mobility and have some, but never normal, anorectal sensation and voluntary sphincter activity. Agnarsson et al. found that in children with lumbosacral or sacral myelomeningocele, rectal compliance is normal [75]. Patients with spina bifida and damage to the S2–S4 sacral roots present reduced resting and squeeze pressure in the anal canal that induce fecal incontinence [76]. In addition, patients with spina bifida may also develop a tethered cord syndrome, which is associated with a worse bowel function that does not seem to improve after surgery [77].

Cauda Equina and Lumbosacral Plexus Disorders

Lumbar and sacral nerve roots arise from the conus medullaris, the terminal part of spinal cord, forming a nerve bundle within the spinal canal called the cauda equina. The destinations for these roots are the lumbar and sacral plexuses, leaving the cauda equina at their specific neural foramina. Because of the differential growth of the vertebral column compared with the spinal cord, the conus medullaris is located at the L1 level. Acute injuries to cauda equina are mostly caused by sudden central disk herniation or, with minor frequency, by trauma, vertebral collapse due to metastatic infiltration, or extradural hematoma. Extrinsic tumors, including metastases, usually present with pain before neurological signs develop.

The incidence and prevalence of cauda equina lesions are not known, but it is estimated that they constitute from 1% to 5% of spinal pathology [78]. Cauda equina compression is an acute emergency that may develop as a sudden major disk prolapse in a patient with a long history of sciatica or of previous lumbar or sacral laminectomy, sometimes postoperatively following disk excision with hemorrhage at the operative site. The disk usually involved is L4–L5, but herniations at other levels can occur, inducing a similar syndrome. The clinical picture is characterized by weakness and sensory loss in the lower limbs, buttocks, and perineum, usually with marked impairment of bladder, bowel, erectile, and ejaculatory function. Symptoms and signs vary depending on the nerve roots involved, the size and position of the disk herniated, and the dimension of the spinal canal. The patient complains usually a loss of sensation and burning pain in the perineum, with a characteristic "saddle" distribution, weakness of hip extension and abduction with sparing of hip flexion and quadriceps movement, a patulous anal sphincter, and loss of the anal wink and bulbocavernosus reflexes. A marked impairment of the normal sensation of filling of the bladder and anorectum is also present, resulting in retention of feces and urine, with overflow and defecation and micturition inability. Anal motor response to coughing and anal squeeze response to volitional activity are absent. Lumbosacral computed tomography (CT) scanning and particularly magnetic resonance imaging (MRI) are the urgent diagnostic imaging techniques of choice to define acute cauda equina syndrome and to perform early decompression surgery. The disk, in this case, should be urgently removed surgically within 48 h for a good outcome [79]. Delays of surgical treatment lessen the chance of good recovery of bowel, bladder, and sexual function.

Fecal Incontinence in Peripheral Neuropathies

Many patients affected by "idiopathic" fecal incontinence have evidence of either a neurogenic or muscular injury, and some patients remain truly idiopathic without clear identifiable cause for sphincteric dysfunction. The peripheral nervous system is divided into the somatic and autonomic portions with sensory and motor nerve fibers. Autonomic nerve fibers normally supply the gastrointestinal, bladder, sexual, and cardiovascular functions. Neuropathies can be functionally selective so that sensory, motor, or autonomic function can be involved separately or in various combinations. Disease process consists of generalized polyneuropathies, with symmetric distribution on the two sides of the body, or focal and multifocal neuropathies in which involvement is localized. Focal and multifocal neuropathies involving the nerves of the pelvis and the polyneuropathies with autonomic impairment commonly induce bowel, bladder, and sexual dysfunction.

Diabetes mellitus is the most common cause of polyneuropathy in developed countries. Diabetic neuropathy is a chronic symmetrical sensorimotor polyneuropathy that usually begins after years of hyperglycemia and is frequently associated with autonomic neuropathy and bowel, bladder, and sexual dysfunction. Severe diabetic autonomic neuropathy (DAN) is almost always associated with insulin-dependent diabetes. Symptoms of autonomic involvement include impairment of sweating and of vascular reflexes, constipation, nocturnal diarrhea and fecal incontinence, atonic bladder, sexual impotence, and occasionally postural hypotension. The pathogenetic mechanism of the constipation is uncertain, but autonomic neuropathy causing parasympathetic denervation is likely to be implicated. Diarrhea typically occurs at night or after meals, is a more troublesome complication of diabetes, and may be an isolated symptom of autonomic dysfunction. It is usually chronic, but it is intermittent and alternates with bouts of constipation or normal bowel movements. Reduced resting anal tone induced by sympathetic autonomic neuropathy and loss of rectal sensation may play a role in the nocturnal fecal incontinence [80]. The upper gastrointestinal tract symptoms that consist of heartburn, dysphagia, and bloating may sometimes occur in diabetic patients in addition to bowel dysfunctions.

Neuropathy due to deposition of amyloid–a proteinaceous substance in different tissues and in particular in peripheral nerve–can occur in patients with benign plasma-cell dyscrasia or in multiple myeloma, Waldenstrom's macroglobulinemia, or non-Hodgkin's lymphoma [81]. The neuropathy is of the small-fiber type, with a predominant loss of pain and temperature sensation early in the course of the illness and a later involvement of motor functions and sensory modalities subserved by large myelinated fibers. Autonomic involvement is another early characteristic of amyloidotic neuropathy. Anhidrosis, loss of papillary light reflexes, vasomotor paralysis with orthostatic hypotension, and alternating diarrhea and constipation are frequent in the course of the illness. Amyloidosis can also present with reduced urinary flow and infrequent voiding with reduced bladder contractility and an increased postvoiding urine volume. Uncoordinated contractions of the small bowel have been demonstrated in patients affected by familiar amyloidotic neuropathy, mainly resulting in diarrhea, but sometimes constipation may alternate with diarrhea. Diarrhea and steatorrhea are prominent in primary amyloidosis.

Constipation or, occasionally, paralytic ileus and bladder dysfunction with urine retention occurs in 20–30% of patients affected by Guillain-Barré syndrome [82]. This inflammatory disease occurs in all ages and both genders. A mild respiratory or gastrointestinal infection, surgical procedure, or viral exanthemas precede the symptoms by 1–3 weeks in 70–80% of patients. The major clinical manifestation is weakness of proximal and distal muscles of the limbs, trunk, and intercostals, and neck muscles, which evolves symmetrically over a period of several days. The weakness can progress to total motor paralysis, with death from respiratory failure. The hyperactivity or hypoactivity of sympathetic and parasympathetic fibers can induce severe disturbances of autonomic function. Sinus tachycardia and less often bradycardia with cardiac arrhythmias, fluctuating hypertension and hypotension, loss of sweating ability, or facial flushing are frequent in the course of the disease.

Vitamin B12 deficiency may arise from inadequate oral intake, deficiency of intrinsic factors, various malabsorption disorders, resection of the stomach, or terminal ileum, inducing various neurological symptoms including peripheral neuropathy, myelopathy, altered mental status, and optic neuropathy [83]. Subacute combined degeneration of the spinal cord and distal peripheral neuropathy are the main neurological consequences of vitamin B12 deficiency. Most patients with pernicious anemia and neurological dysfunction show, therefore, a mixed myelopathic or neuropathic clinical picture. Symmetrical numbness and paraesthesia of lower limbs and gait ataxia are the commonest presenting complaints. Weakness is sometimes found but is always accompanied by sensory lower-limb abnormalities. A small number of patients have symptoms of autonomic dysfunction with fecal and urinary incontinence.

Fecal Incontinence in Myopathies

Anal sphincter function in myopathies has been investigated infrequently. In myotonic dystrophy, most patients suffer from diarrhea and abdominal cramps. Different studies showed widespread abnormalities of gastrointestinal motility in myotonic dystrophy, involving the esophagus and small and large intestines [84–87]. Dysphagia is a prominent symptom in myotonic dystrophy patients, with a reported prevalence of 25–85% in different series. Impaired pharyngeal contraction, myotonia of the tongue and pharynx, gastric and small-bowel dilation, megacolon, and abnormal anal sphincter contractions have been reported [88–90]. Abercrombie et al. illustrated degeneration of smooth-muscle cells and fibrosis in the IAS and loss of striated muscle fibers in the EAS and puborectalis muscles [91]. EMG data confirm EAS involvement, with reduced numbers of motor units, myotonia, and myopathic features without neurogenic lesions. Digital and manometric anorectal examination show poor resting tone and low squeeze pressure in the anal canal and reduced rectal compliance.

Constipation and diarrhea are frequent in most muscular dystrophies; these clinical features have been particularly investigated in Duchenne's dystrophy, where colonic transit time is commonly increased [92]. Altered motility of the small and large intestines has been described in other muscular dystrophies [93]. Atrophy and fibrosis of the intestinal smooth muscles possibly reflect the diffuse muscle-dystrophic process. Chronic constipation from immobility is believed to contribute to bowel dysfunctions, which include abdominal pain, distension, and vomiting. Acute gastric dilation, gastric perforation, and, rarely, peritonitis may occur [94].

Dysfunction of the smooth muscles at several levels of the gastrointestinal tract in myasthenia gravis is well known, and about 33% of patients complain of significant fatigable dysphagia [95, 96]. Mastication and swallowing difficulties worsen as a meal progresses, in particular at the end of the day. Myasthenia gravis can also present with a clinical picture of fecal and urinary incontinence [97].

Neurophysiologic Investigations

Neurophysiological examination of patients with fecal incontinence usually follows surgical and clinical evaluation and, almost always, other endoscopic, manometric, ultrasound, and MRI investigations able to diagnose the most important causes of fecal incontinence [98]. These different investigations can identify focal morphological lesions to the IAS and EAS muscle [99–101], location of neoplastic lesions [102], capacity and compliance of the rectum, reflex activity, reduced sensation of the anorectum, and IAS and EAS muscle dysfunctions [103].

With the advent of neurophysiological techniques available to evaluate anorectal disorders, a more detailed understanding of the neurogenic pathophysiological mechanisms underlying fecal incontinence is evolving. Clinical history and neurological examination should be performed to propose a diagnosis of neurogenic bowel dysfunction and to plan further electrophysiological tests [98, 104]. Although clinical neurophysiologic investigations and concentric needle EMG are performed worldwide, their application to pelvic floor disorders is limited to a few centers. No consensus statement for a standardized approach to anorectal neurogenic disorders has been reached, and the role of different tests has not yet been clearly defined. Extensive neurophysiological investigations should be performed in any patient with anorectal disorders of suspected central or peripheral neurogenic etiology. These tests include concentric needle EMG of different pelvic floor muscles, measurement of sacral reflex latency (pudendoanal and bulbocavernosus reflex) induced by electrical stimulation, pudendal somatosensory-evoked potentials (SEP) after electrical stimulation of the anal canal, and motor-evoked potentials (MEP) from EAS muscles by transcranial and lumbosacral magnetic stimulation.

A short clinical assessment should precede the neurophysiological tests, along with a history of the patient's complaints. Usually the main symptoms described are pain variably located in the low back and perineal and sacral areas, paresthesias, leg weakness, erectile dysfunction, and bladder and bowel disturbances. Scoring systems for symptoms of fecal incontinence are used and have been validated against the severity of the bowel disorder [105]. The Cleveland Clinic Florida Fecal Incontinence (CCF-FI) scoring system is one of the most recognized method for quantifying the degree of symptoms in patients undergoing neurological sphincter assessment [106].

A clinical neurological examination is performed with special attention to the status of the lower limbs and the perineal and buttock areas, particularly looking for signs of pyramidal and peripheral nervous system lesions [107]. Examination usually includes anal sphincter tone, strength in the S1–S2 innervated muscles (gastrocnemius, gluteal muscles), sensation extending from the soles of the feet to the perianal area, and presence of anal and bulbocavernous reflexes. Anal reflex is induced by pricking or scratching the perianal skin area, whereas bulbocavernosus reflex is evoked by a nonpainful clitoral or gland squeeze [108, 109]. Clinically elicited reflexes may be extinguished by mild or severe nerve lesions, whereas the same reflexes can be recorded neurophysiologically, though with a prolonged latency and reduced amplitude, also in almost complete nerve lesions [110].

Concentric needle EMG is the most important neurophysiologic test in the evaluation of patients with suspected neurogenic etiology of bowel dysfunction [107]. EMG assessment for the pelvic floor and EAS muscle is mainly indicated to determine: (1) the presence of pathological spontaneous activity, fibrillation potentials and positive sharp waves, and denervation of muscle fibers, (2) presence of muscle-fiber reinnervation [111–114], (3) normal mild continuous tonic contraction in the EAS and puborectalis muscles [115] and adequate contraction or relaxation during squeeze or straining, and (4) recruitment pattern and motor-unit-potential (MUP) waveform [116]. The most important parameters in the analysis of MUP are amplitude, duration, area, number of phases and turns, and firing rate that can be automatically evaluated by advanced EMG systems provided with special software analysis.

Examination of the EAS muscle holds the central position in Podnar's and Vodusek's algorithm for electrodiagnostic evaluation of the sacral nervous system [104]. With the patient in a comfortable lateral position with knees and hips flexed, after grounded electrically at the thigh, a standard concentric needle EMG electrode is inserted into the subcutaneous portion of the EAS muscle to a depth of 3–5 mm under the mucosa, 1 cm from the anal orifice [66, 104, 117, 118]. Both left and right halves of the subcutaneous EAS muscle must be examined separately, starting on the side with the clinical evidence of sphincter dysfunction (episiotomy scar tissue, patulous anus). If partial or complete atrophy of the subcutaneous EAS muscle is appreciated, a concentric needle electrode can be introduced 1- to 3-cm deeper through the skin to evaluate spontaneous activity, recruitment pattern, and functional contractile capacity of the deeper EAS and 4- to 5-cm deeper for examination of the PR muscle. In the presence of fibrosis, there is a loss of contractile capacity of pelvic floor muscles, and consequently, no spontaneous activity or MUP is recognized. When the needle advances in the EAS muscle, continuous firing of low-threshold MUP is normally appreciated, and during a brief period of relaxation, the presence of spontaneous activity, fibrillation, or jasper potentials can be recorded. EMG recordings from the EAS were performed at rest and during squeezing, coughing, and straining that simulates rectal evacuation. In healthy subjects, squeeze and cough increase the MUP recruitment pattern, whereas strain decreases or inhibits MUP firing. Needle examination of the bulbocavernosus muscles is indicated when no EMG signals are recorded in the subcutaneous or deeper EAS muscles [119].

Sacral reflexes evaluate the functional status of the afferent neural fibers of the clitoris or penis, the S2–S4 sacral intraspinal segments, and the efferent pathways to EAS and bulbocavernosus muscles [108, 110, 120]. The central circuit at the spinal level is complex and probably involves many sacral interneurons. These sacral reflexes, named pudendoanal reflex and bulbocavernosus reflex, reveal, in fact, two components with different thresholds at the electrical stimulation: a first component with a shorter latency, probably oligosynaptic, and a second component with a longer latency, typical for a polysynaptic response. A latency delay of these reflexes may be of localizing neurological value. Only the largest myelinated, fastest fibers convey the neurophysiological signals traveling in the afferent limb of these reflexes. Many disorders of bowel and anorectal function are the result of unmyelinated fiber dysfunction; therefore, conduction in these fibers is not tested by these procedures [121].

Scalp recording of pudendal SEP is a method for evaluating the afferent sensory pathway and is used in investigating central and peripheral neurological diseases. Cortical responses can be evoked by mechanical stimulation (balloon distension of the rectum) [122] or by electrical stimulation of the rectosigmoid colon [123], the rectum [122, 124, 125], and the anal canal [126]. All these anatomical structures are innervated by the inferior branches of the pudendal nerve. Pudendal SEP are recorded by surface electrodes placed on the scalp 2-cm behind the vertex over the cortical representation of the pelvic region. A first positive peak can be recorded in normal subjects at about 42 ms using a stimulus intensity of two to four times the sensory threshold. Later negative and positive peaks show a large variability in amplitude between individuals.

Transcranial magnetic stimulation (TMS) is a neurophysiological technique that permits activation of the cortical motor areas without causing patient discomfort; therefore, it is widely used to study the central motor pathways in normal subjects [127] and neurological patients [128]. TMS is also applied to study the corticospinal pathway to the EAS muscle [129–131]. The EAS MEP after TMS have a mean latency of about 27 ms in the resting state and 23 ms during facilitation, a functional condition of mild contraction of the pelvic floor muscles. The intensity of TMS necessary to obtain an MEP in the EAS muscle is much higher than the intensity to elicit an MEP in the limbs. This fact can be explained by the cortical representation of the anogenital area that is localized deep within the motor strip in the interhemispheric fissure. The magnetic stimulation applied over the lower lumbar spine is known to activate the lumbosacral ventral roots at their exit from the vertebral canal [132]. Latency of the motor response is approximately 6 ms [131]. Corticospinal abnormalities detected by this method in patients with neurogenic bladder and bowel disorders have been reported [133–137].

The different types of MEP abnormalities, i.e., responses with decreased amplitude or delayed latency, may imply the axonal or demyelinative impairment underlying the different clinical pathological conditions. TMS might improve the understanding of different pelvic floor dysfunctions; however, a rigorous electrophysiological technique and standardized methods will be required.

The inferior rectal branches of the pudendal nerve can be electrophysiologically evaluated by measuring pudendal nerve terminal motor latency (PNTML), which is the technique most often used for neurologic assessment in patients with idiopathic neurogenic anorectal incontinence [118]. The PNTML technique was first described in 1984 by Kiff and Swash [138, 139]. PNTML is determined by recording anal sphincter motor potential evoked by stimulation of the pudendal nerve with a special surface electrode assembly fixed to a gloved index finger (St. Mark's electrode) near the ischial spine through the rectal wall. The test owes its popularity to different studies showing abnormal latencies in various clinical situations [140–146]. More recently, however, the PNTML clinical value has been questioned, and two consensus statements, uroneurological and gastroenterological, did not propose this test for evaluating patients with bladder and bowel dysfunction [119, 147]. In particular, the American Gastroenterological Association (AGA) medical position statement concluded that PNTML cannot be recommended for evaluating patients with fecal incontinence because: (1) PNTML has a poor correlation with clinical symptoms and histologic findings, (2) the technique does not discriminate between muscle weakness caused by pudendal nerve injury and muscle injury in patients with fecal incontinence, (3) there is a lack of test sensitivity and specificity for detecting EAS muscle weakness, (4) it is considered to be an operator-dependent technique, and (5) the test does not predict surgical outcome [147].

Conclusions

Fecal incontinence affects both genders and all age groups and is a common symptom in patients with several different neurological diseases. It often influences their quality of life and induces a devastating effect on their social activities. Knowledge of the neuronal mechanisms underlying colorectal and anal sphincter function is useful in evaluating the different impairments occurring in each neurological disorder.

In patients with suspected neurogenic bowel disorders and in particular those with fecal incontinence, electrodiagnostic techniques should be considered in planning diagnostic workup, treatment, and management.

References

1. Lamah M, Kumar D (1999) Fecal incontinence. Dig Dis Sci 44:2488–2499
2. Nelson RL (2004) Epidemiology of fecal incontinence. Gastroenterology 126:S3–S7
3. Rao SS (2004) Pathophysiology of adult fecal incontinence. Gastroenterology 126:S14–S22
4. Andrew J, Nathan PW (1964) Lesions on the anterior frontal lobes and disturbances of micturition and defaecation. Brain 87:233–262
5. Kaddumi EG, Hubscher CH (2006) Convergence of multiple pelvic organ inputs in the rat rostral medulla. J Physiol 572:393–405
6. Bouvier M, Grimaud JC (1984) Neuronally mediated interactions between urinary bladder and internal anal sphincter motility in the cat. J Physiol 346:461–469
7. Bouvier M, Grimaud JC, Abysique A (1990) Effects of stimulation of vesical afferents on colonic motility in cats. Gastroenterology 98:1148–1154
8. Duthie HL, Gairns FW (1960) Sensory nerve-endings and sensation in the anal region of man. Br J Surg 47:585–595
9. Rogers J (1992) Testing for and the role of anal and rectal sensation. Baillieres Clin Gastroenterol 6:179–191
10. Lynn PA, Olsson C, Zagorodnyuk V et al (2003) Rectal intraganglionic laminar endings are transduction sites of extrinsic mechanoreceptors in the guinea pig rectum. Gastroenterology 125:786–794
11. Frenckner B, Euler CV (1975) Influence of pudendal block on the function of the anal sphincters. Gut 16:482–489
12. Hobday DI, Aziz Q, Thacker N et al (2001) A study of the cortical processing of ano-rectal sensation using functional MRI. Brain 124:361–368
13. Grundy D, Al-Chaer ED, Aziz Q et al (2006) Fundamentals of neurogastroenterology: basic science. Gastroenterology 130:1391–1411
14. Norton C (1996) Faecal incontinence in adults. 1: Prevalence and causes. Br J Nurs 5:1366–1368, 1370–1374
15. Kamm MA (1998) Faecal incontinence. BMJ 316:528–532
16. Harari D, Coshall C, Rudd AG, Wolfe CD (2003) New-onset fecal incontinence after stroke: prevalence, natural history, risk factors, and impact. Stroke 34:144–150
17. Baztan JJ, Domenech JR, Gonzalez M (2003) New-onset fecal incontinence after stroke: risk factor or consequence of poor outcomes after rehabilitation? Stroke 34:e101–102
18. Nakayama H, Jorgensen HS, Pedersen PM et al (1997) Prevalence and risk factors of incontinence after stroke. The Copenhagen Stroke Study. Stroke 28:58–62
19. Scandinavian Stroke Study Group (1985) Multicenter trial of hemodilution in ischemic stroke-background and study protocol. Stroke 16:885–890
20. Wade DT, Hewer RL (1985) Outlook after an acute stroke: urinary incontinence and loss of consciousness compared in 532 patients. Q J Med 56:601–608
21. Ween JE, Alexander MP, D'Esposito M, Roberts M (1996) Incontinence after stroke in a rehabilitation setting: outcome associations and predictive factors. Neurology 47:659–663
22. Patel M, Coshall C, Rudd AG, Wolfe CD (2001) Natural history and effects on 2-year outcomes of urinary incontinence after stroke. Stroke 32:122–127
23. Taub NA, Wolfe CD, Richardson E, Burney PG (1994) Predicting the disability of first-time stroke sufferers at 1 year. 12-month follow-up of a population-based cohort in southeast England. Stroke 25:352–357
24. Gelber DA, Good DC, Laven LJ, Verhulst SJ (1993) Causes of urinary incontinence after acute hemispheric stroke. Stroke 24:378–382
25. Robain G, Chennevelle JM, Petit F, Piera JB (2002) [Incidence of constipation after recent vascular hemiplegia: a prospective cohort of 152 patients]. Rev Neurol 158:589–592
26. Stocchi F, Badiali D, Vacca L et al (2000) Anorectal function in multiple system atrophy and Parkinson's disease. Mov Disord 15:71–76
27. Sakakibara R, Shinotoh H, Uchiyama T et al (2001) Questionnaire-based assessment of pelvic organ dysfunction in Parkinson's disease. Auton Neurosci 92:76–85
28. Edwards LL, Quigley EM, Harned RK et al (1994) Characterization of swallowing and defecation in Parkinson's disease. Am J Gastroenterol 89:15–25
29. Mathers SE, Kempster PA, Swash M, Lees AJ (1988) Constipation and paradoxical puborectalis contraction in anismus and Parkinson's disease: a dystonic phenomenon? J Neurol Neurosurg Psychiatry 51:1503–1507
30. Edwards LL, Quigley EM, Harned RK et al (1993) Defecatory function in Parkinson's disease: response to apomorphine. Ann Neurol 33:490–493
31. Edwards LL, Quigley EM, Pfeiffer RF (1992) Gastrointestinal dysfunction in Parkinson's disease: frequency and pathophysiology. Neurology 42:726–732
32. Singaram C, Ashraf W, Gaumnitz EA et al (1995) Dopaminergic defect of enteric nervous system in Parkinson's disease patients with chronic constipation. Lancet 346:861–864
33. Bauer HJ, Firnhaber W, Winkler W (1965) Prognostic Criteria In Multiple Sclerosis. Ann N Y Acad Sci 122:542–551
34. Crayton H, Heyman RA, Rossman HS (2004) A multimodal approach to managing the symptoms of multiple sclerosis. Neurology 63:S12–18
35. Miller H, Simpson CA, Yeates WK (1965) Bladder Dysfunction In Multiple Sclerosis. Br Med J 5445:1265–1269
36. Andersen JT, Bradley WE (1976) Abnormalities of detrusor and sphincter function in multiple sclerosis. Br J Urol 48:193–198
37. Blaivas JG, Bhimani G, Labib KB (1979) Vesicourethral dysfunction in multiple sclerosis. J Urol 122:342–347
38. Bennett N, O'Leary M, Patel AS et al (2004) Can higher doses of oxybutynin improve efficacy in neurogenic bladder? J Urol 171:749–751
39. Chia YW, Fowler CJ, Kamm MA et al (1995) Prevalence of bowel dysfunction in patients with multiple sclerosis and bladder dysfunction. J Neurol 242:105–108
40. Bakke A, Myhr KM, Gronning M, Nyland H (1996)

Bladder, bowel and sexual dysfunction in patients with multiple sclerosis-a cohort study. Scand J Urol Nephrol Suppl 179:61–66
41. Rosenblum D, Saffir M (1998) The natural history of multiple sclerosis and its diagnosis. Phys Med Rehabil Clin N Am 9:537–549
42. Hinds JP, Eidelman BH, Wald A (1990) Prevalence of bowel dysfunction in multiple sclerosis. A population survey. Gastroenterology 98:1538–1542
43. Swash M, Snooks SJ, Chalmers DH (1987) Parity as a factor in incontinence in multiple sclerosis. Arch Neurol 44:504–508
44. Glick ME, Meshkinpour H, Haldeman S et al (1982) Colonic dysfunction in multiple sclerosis. Gastroenterology 83:1002–1007
45. Waldron DJ, Horgan PG, Patel FR et al (1993) Multiple sclerosis: assessment of colonic and anorectal function in the presence of faecal incontinence. Int J Colorectal Dis 8:220–224
46. Sorensen M, Lorentzen M, Petersen J, Christiansen J (1991) Anorectal dysfunction in patients with urologic disturbance due to multiple sclerosis. Dis Colon Rectum 34:136–139
47. Jameson JS, Rogers J, Chia YW et al (1994) Pelvic floor function in multiple sclerosis. Gut 35:388–390
48. Nordenbo AM, Andersen JR, Andersen JT (1996) Disturbances of ano-rectal function in multiple sclerosis. J Neurol 243:445–451
49. Weber J, Grise P, Roquebert M et al (1987) Radiopaque markers transit and anorectal manometry in 16 patients with multiple sclerosis and urinary bladder dysfunction. Dis Colon Rectum 30:95–100
50. Haldeman S, Glick M, Bhatia NN et al (1982) Colonometry, cystometry, and evoked potentials in multiple sclerosis. Arch Neurol 39:698–701
51. Glickman S, Kamm MA (1996) Bowel dysfunction in spinal-cord-injury patients. Lancet 347:1651–1653
52. Krogh K, Mosdal C, Laurberg S (2000) Gastrointestinal and segmental colonic transit times in patients with acute and chronic spinal cord lesions. Spinal Cord 38:615–621
53. Krogh K, Nielsen J, Djurhuus JC et al (1997) Colorectal function in patients with spinal cord lesions. Dis Colon Rectum 40:1233–1239
54. Lynch AC, Anthony A, Dobbs BR, Frizelle FA (2000) Anorectal physiology following spinal cord injury. Spinal Cord 38:573–580
55. Lynch AC, Antony A, Dobbs BR, Frizelle FA (2001) Bowel dysfunction following spinal cord injury. Spinal Cord 39:193–203
56. Lynch AC, Wong C, Anthony A et al (2000) Bowel dysfunction following spinal cord injury: a description of bowel function in a spinal cord-injured population and comparison with age and gender matched controls. Spinal Cord 38:717–723
57. Stone JM, Nino-Murcia M, Wolfe VA, Perkash I (1990) Chronic gastrointestinal problems in spinal cord injury patients: a prospective analysis. Am J Gastroenterol 85:1114–1119
58. Randell N, Lynch AC, Anthony A et al (2001) Does a colostomy alter quality of life in patients with spinal cord injury? A controlled study. Spinal Cord 39:279–282
59. Stone JM, Wolfe VA, Nino-Murcia M, Perkash I (1990) Colostomy as treatment for complications of spinal cord injury. Arch Phys Med Rehabil 71:514–518
60. Kelly SR, Shashidharan M, Borwell B et al (1999) The role of intestinal stoma in patients with spinal cord injury. Spinal Cord 37:211–214
61. Krogh K, Mosdal C, Gregersen H, Laurberg S (2002) Rectal wall properties in patients with acute and chronic spinal cord lesions. Dis Colon Rectum 45:641–649
62. Kirk PM, King RB, Temple R et al (1997) Long-term follow-up of bowel management after spinal cord injury. SCI Nurs 14:56–63
63. Stiens SA, Bergman SB, Goetz LL (1997) Neurogenic bowel dysfunction after spinal cord injury: clinical evaluation and rehabilitative management. Arch Phys Med Rehabil 78:S86–102
64. Yim SY, Yoon SH, Lee IY et al (2001) A comparison of bowel care patterns in patients with spinal cord injury: upper motor neuron bowel vs lower motor neuron bowel. Spinal Cord 39:204–207
65. Benevento BT, Sipski ML (2002) Neurogenic bladder, neurogenic bowel, and sexual dysfunction in people with spinal cord injury. Phys Ther 82:601–612
66. Bartolo DC, Jarratt JA, Read NW (1983) The use of conventional electromyography to assess external sphincter neuropathy in man. J Neurol Neurosurg Psychiatry 46:1115–1118
67. Staas WE Jr, Nemunaitis G (1989) Management of reflex sweating in spinal cord injured patients. Arch Phys Med Rehabil 70:544–546
68. De Looze D, Van Laere M, De Muynck M et al (1998) Constipation and other chronic gastrointestinal problems in spinal cord injury patients. Spinal Cord 36:63–66
69. Rajendran SK, Reiser JR, Bauman W et al (1992) Gastrointestinal transit after spinal cord injury: effect of cisapride. Am J Gastroenterol 87:1614–1617
70. Keshavarzian A, Barnes WE, Bruninga K et al (1995) Delayed colonic transit in spinal cord-injured patients measured by indium-111 Amberlite scintigraphy. Am J Gastroenterol 90:1295–1300
71. Glick ME, Meshkinpour H, Haldeman S et al (1984) Colonic dysfunction in patients with thoracic spinal cord injury. Gastroenterology 86:287–294
72. Lie HR, Lagergren J, Rasmussen F et al (1991) Bowel and bladder control of children with myelomeningocele: a Nordic study. Dev Med Child Neurol 33:1053–1061
73. Malone PS, Wheeler RA, Williams JE (1994) Continence in patients with spina bifida: long term results. Arch Dis Child 70:107–110
74. Rintala RJ (2002) Fecal incontinence in anorectal malformations, neuropathy, and miscellaneous conditions. Semin Pediatr Surg 11:75–82
75. Agnarsson U, Warde C, McCarthy G et al (1993) Anorectal function of children with neurological problems. I: Spina bifida. Dev Med Child Neurol 35:893–902
76. Arhan P, Faverdin C, Devroede G et al (1984) Anorectal motility after surgery for spina bifida. Dis Colon Rectum 27:159–163
77. Levitt MA, Patel M, Rodriguez G et al (1997) The teth-

ered spinal cord in patients with anorectal malformations. J Pediatr Surg 32:462–468
78. Shapiro S (1993) Cauda equina syndrome secondary to lumbar disc herniation. Neurosurgery 32:743–746; discussion 746–747
79. Gleave JR, MacFarlane R (1990) Prognosis for recovery of bladder function following lumbar central disc prolapse. Br J Neurosurg 4:205–209
80. Wald A, Tunuguntla AK (1984) Anorectal sensorimotor dysfunction in fecal incontinence and diabetes mellitus. Modification with biofeedback therapy. N Engl J Med 310:1282–1287
81. Kyle RA (1995) Monoclonal gammopathy of undetermined significance (MGUS). Baillieres Clin Haematol 8:761–781
82. Zochodne DW, Ramsay DA, Saly V et al (1994) Acute necrotizing myopathy of intensive care: electrophysiological studies. Muscle Nerve 17:285–292
83. Healton EB, Savage DG, Brust JC et al (1991) Neurologic aspects of cobalamin deficiency. Medicine 70:229–245
84. Nowak TV, Anuras S, Brown BP et al (1984) Small intestinal motility in myotonic dystrophy patients. Gastroenterology 86:808–813
85. Nowak TV, Ionasescu V, Anuras S (1982) Gastrointestinal manifestations of the muscular dystrophies. Gastroenterology 82:800–810
86. Yoshida MM, Krishnamurthy S, Wattchow DA et al (1988) Megacolon in myotonic dystrophy caused by a degenerative neuropathy of the myenteric plexus. Gastroenterology 95:820–827
87. Harper PS (1979) Myotonic dystrophy, major problems in neurology, Vol. 9. Saunders, Philadelphia, pp 1–324
88. Brunner HG, Hamel BC, Rieu P et al (1992) Intestinal pseudo-obstruction in myotonic dystrophy. J Med Genet 29:791–793
89. Eckardt VF, Nix W (1991) The anal sphincter in patients with myotonic muscular dystrophy. Gastroenterology 100:424–430
90. Chaudhry V, Umapathi T, Ravich WJ (2002) Neuromuscular diseases and disorders of the alimentary system. Muscle Nerve 25:768–784
91. Abercrombie JF, Rogers J, Swash M (1998) Faecal incontinence in myotonic dystrophy. J Neurol Neurosurg Psychiatry 64:128–130
92. Perkin GD, Murray-Lyon I (1998) Neurology and the gastrointestinal system. J Neurol Neurosurg Psychiatry 65:291–300
93. Leon SH, Schuffler MD, Kettler M, Rohrmann CA (1986) Chronic intestinal pseudoobstruction as a complication of Duchenne's muscular dystrophy. Gastroenterology 90:455–459
94. Bensen ES, Jaffe KM, Tarr PI (1996) Acute gastric dilatation in Duchenne muscular dystrophy: a case report and review of the literature. Arch Phys Med Rehabil 77:512–514
95. Khan OA, Campbell WW (1994) Myasthenia gravis presenting as dysphagia: clinical considerations. Am J Gastroenterol 89:1083–1085
96. Kluin KJ, Bromberg MB, Feldman EL, Simmons Z (1996) Dysphagia in elderly men with myasthenia gravis. J Neurol Sci 138:49–52
97. Berger AR, Swerdlow M, Herskovitz S (1996) Myasthenia gravis presenting as uncontrollable flatus and urinary/fecal incontinence. Muscle Nerve 19:113–114
98. Podnar S (2003) Electrodiagnosis of the anorectum: a review of techniques and clinical applications. Tech Coloproctol 7:71–76
99. Sultan AH, Kamm MA, Hudson CN et al (1993) Anal-sphincter disruption during vaginal delivery. N Engl J Med 329:1905–1911
100. Enck P, von Giesen HJ, Schafer A et al (1996) Comparison of anal sonography with conventional needle electromyography in the evaluation of anal sphincter defects. Am J Gastroenterol 91:2539–2543
101. Stoker J, Bartram CI, Halligan S (2002) Imaging of the posterior pelvic floor. Eur Radiol 12:779–788
102. Hussain SM, Stoker J, Schutte HE, Lameris JS (1996) Imaging of the anorectal region. Eur J Radiol 22:116–122
103. Rao SS (1997) Manometric evaluation of defecation disorders: Part II. Fecal incontinence. Gastroenterologist 5:99–111
104. Podnar S, Vodusek DB (2001) Protocol for clinical neurophysiologic examination of the pelvic floor. Neurourol Urodyn 20:669–682
105. Vaizey CJ, Carapeti E, Cahill JA, Kamm MA (1999) Prospective comparison of faecal incontinence grading systems. Gut 44:77–80
106. Jorge JM, Wexner SD (1993) Etiology and management of fecal incontinence. Dis Colon Rectum 36:77–97
107. Fowler CJ (2001) A neurologist's clinical and investigative approach to patients with bladder, bowel and sexual dysfunction. In: Fowler CJ (ed) Neurology of bladder, bowel, and sexual dysfunction. Elsevier, Boston, pp 1–6
108. Pedersen E, Klemar B, Schroder HD, Torring J (1982) Anal sphincter responses after perianal electrical stimulation. J Neurol Neurosurg Psychiatry 45:770–773
109. Swash M (1982) Early and late components in the human anal reflex. J Neurol Neurosurg Psychiatry 45:767–769
110. Vodusek DB, Janko M, Lokar J (1983) Direct and reflex responses in perineal muscles on electrical stimulation. J Neurol Neurosurg Psychiatry 46:67–71
111. Podnar S (2004) Criteria for neuropathic abnormality in quantitative anal sphincter electromyography. Muscle Nerve 30:596–601
112. Podnar S, Fowler CJ (2004) Sphincter electromyography in diagnosis of multiple system atrophy: technical issues. Muscle Nerve 29:151–156
113. Podnar S, Mrkaic M (2002) Predictive power of motor unit potential parameters in anal sphincter electromyography. Muscle Nerve 26:389–394
114. Podnar S, Vodusek DB, Stalberg E (2002) Comparison of quantitative techniques in anal sphincter electromyography. Muscle Nerve 25:83–92
115. Floyd WF, Walls EW (1953) Electromyography of the sphincter ani externus in man. J Physiol 122:599–609
116. Swash M (1992) Electromyography in pelvic floor disorders. In: Henry MM, Swash M (eds) Coloproctology and the pelvic floor. Butterworth Heinemann, Oxford, pp 184–195
117. Stryker SJ, Daube JR, Kelly KA et al (1985) Anal

sphincter electromyography after colectomy, mucosal rectectomy, and ileoanal anastomosis. Arch Surg 120:713–716
118. Cheong DM, Vaccaro CA, Salanga VD et al (1995) Electrodiagnostic evaluation of fecal incontinence. Muscle Nerve 18:612–619
119. Fowler CJ, Benson JT, Craggs MD et al (2002) Clinical neurophysiology. In: Abrams P, Cardozo L, Khoury S, Wein A (eds) Incontinence. 2nd International Consultation on Incontinence. Plymbridge Distributors, Plymouth, pp 389–424
120. Ertekin C, Reel F (1976) Bulbocavernosus reflex in normal men and in patients with neurogenic bladder and/or impotence. J Neurol Sci 28:1–15
121. Fowler CJ (1995) Pelvic floor neurophysiology. In: Clinical neurophysiology. Butterworth Heinemann, Oxford, pp 233–252
122. Loening-Baucke V, Anderson RH, Yamada T, Zhu YX (1995) Study of the afferent pathways from the rectum with a new distention control device. Neurology 45:1510–1516
123. Frieling T, Enck P, Wienbeck M (1989) Cerebral responses evoked by electrical stimulation of rectosigmoid in normal subjects. Dig Dis Sci 34:202–205
124. Loening-Baucke V, Read NW, Yamada T (1992) Further evaluation of the afferent nervous pathways from the rectum. Am J Physiol 262:G927–933
125. Meunier P, Collet L, Duclaux R, Chery-Croze S (1987) Endorectal cerebral evoked potentials in human. Int J Neurosci 37:193–196
126. Delechenault P, Leroi AM, Bruna T et al (1993) Cerebral potentials evoked by electrical stimulation of the anal canal. Dis Colon Rectum 36:55–60
127. Barker AT, Jalinous R, Freeston IL (1985) Non-invasive magnetic stimulation of human motor cortex. Lancet 1:1106–1107
128. Rothwell JC, Hallett M, Berardelli A et al (1999) Magnetic stimulation: motor evoked potentials. The International Federation of Clinical Neurophysiology. Electroencephalogr Clin Neurophysiol Suppl 52:97–103
129. Opsomer RJ, Caramia MD, Zarola F et al (1989) Neurophysiological evaluation of central-peripheral sensory and motor pudendal fibres. Electroencephalogr Clin Neurophysiol 74:260–270
130. Ertekin C, Hansen MV, Larsson LE, Sjodahl R (1990) Examination of the descending pathway to the external anal sphincter and pelvic floor muscles by transcranial cortical stimulation. Electroencephalogr Clin Neurophysiol 75:500–510
131. Pelliccioni G, Scarpino O, Piloni V (1997) Motor evoked potentials recorded from external anal sphincter by cortical and lumbo-sacral magnetic stimulation: normative data. J Neurol Sci 149:69–72
132. King PJL, Chiappa KH (1989) Motor evoked potentials. In: Chiappa KH (ed) Evoked potentials in clinical medicine. Raven Press, New York, pp 509–561
133. Mathers SE, Ingram DA, Swash M (1990) Electrophysiology of motor pathways for sphincter control in multiple sclerosis. J Neurol Neurosurg Psychiatry 53:955–960
134. Del Carro U, Riva D, Comi GC et al (1993) Neurophysiological evaluation in detrusor instability. Neurourol Urodyn 12:455–462
135. Gunnarsson M, Ahlmann S, Lindstrom S et al (1999) Cortical magnetic stimulation in patients with genuine stress incontinence: correlation with results of pelvic floor exercises. Neurourol Urodyn 18:437–444; discussion 444–435
136. Brostrom S, Frederiksen JL, Jennum P, Lose G (2003) Motor evoked potentials from the pelvic floor in patients with multiple sclerosis. J Neurol Neurosurg Psychiatry 74:498–500
137. Jennum P, Neerup Jensen L, Fenger K et al (2001) Motor evoked potentials from the external anal sphincter in patients with autosomal dominant pure spastic paraplegia linked to chromosome 2p. J Neurol Neurosurg Psychiatry 71:561–562
138. Kiff ES, Swash M (1984) Slowed conduction in the pudendal nerves in idiopathic (neurogenic) faecal incontinence. Br J Surg 71:614–616
139. Kiff ES, Swash M (1984) Normal proximal and delayed distal conduction in the pudendal nerves of patients with idiopathic (neurogenic) faecal incontinence. J Neurol Neurosurg Psychiatry 47:820–823
140. Snooks SJ, Badenoch DF, Tiptaft RC, Swash M (1985) Perineal nerve damage in genuine stress urinary incontinence. An electrophysiological study. Br J Urol 57:422–426
141. Snooks SJ, Setchell M, Swash M, Henry MM (1984) Injury to innervation of pelvic floor sphincter musculature in childbirth. Lancet 2:546–550
142. Jones PN, Lubowski DZ, Swash M, Henry MM (1987) Relation between perineal descent and pudendal nerve damage in idiopathic faecal incontinence. Int J Colorectal Dis 2:93–95
143. Smith AR, Hosker GL, Warrell DW (1989) The role of pudendal nerve damage in the aetiology of genuine stress incontinence in women. Br J Obstet Gynaecol 96:29–32
144. Smith AR, Hosker GL, Warrell DW (1989) The role of partial denervation of the pelvic floor in the aetiology of genitourinary prolapse and stress incontinence of urine. A neurophysiological study. Br J Obstet Gynaecol 96:24–28
145. Gilliland R, Altomare DF, Moreira H Jr et al (1998) Pudendal neuropathy is predictive of failure following anterior overlapping sphincteroplasty. Dis Colon Rectum 41:1516–1522
146. Bakas P, Liapis A, Karandreas A, Creatsas G (2001) Pudendal nerve terminal motor latency in women with genuine stress incontinence and prolapse. Gynecol Obstet Invest 51:187–190
147. Barnett JL, Hasler WL, Camilleri M (1999) American Gastroenterological Association medical position statement on anorectal testing techniques. American Gastroenterological Association. Gastroenterology 116:732–760

Diabetes

32

Marie-France Kong, Michael Horowitz

Introduction

It is now recognised, albeit relatively recently, that chronic gastrointestinal symptoms represent a clinically important problem in a substantial number of people who have type 1 or type 2 diabetes [1, 2]. Whereas the amount of information relating to anorectal function in diabetes is limited, it is clear that faecal incontinence occurs relatively frequently [1, 3, 4] and is often overlooked as a cause of morbidity.

Prevalence and Epidemiology

In an early study, Feldman and Schiller reported that faecal incontinence occurred in 20% of 136 unselected diabetic outpatients referred to a tertiary centre [1]. About half of the diabetic patients with diarrhoea had faecal incontinence when specifically asked. Interestingly, 10% of the cohort claimed to have had episodes of faecal incontinence without chronic diarrhoea. The prevalence of disordered defecation appears to be less prevalent among patients with diabetes attending secondary referral centres [5, 6], where constipation has been reported in about 20% and faecal incontinence in about 9% [6]. There is little information about the prevalence of disordered defecation in diabetic patients managed in the community by primary care physicians, although faecal incontinence is a common problem in the community, with a prevalence of 2–15% [7]. Whereas age, gender, physical incapacity, and impaired general health have been established as risk factors for faecal incontinence in community studies, an association with diabetes has not been clearly established [8]. There is also no formal information about the prevalence of faecal incontinence in type 1 compared with type 2 diabetes.

Faecal incontinence in diabetics is probably unrecognised by clinicians in the majority of cases. Enck et al. reported a systematic underestimation of faecal incontinence in that only 5% of patients with faecal incontinence, irrespective of the underlying cause, had incontinence symptoms noted in their medical charts [9]. It is likely that the lack of recognition of faecal incontinence reflects both the patient's failure to volunteer the information, perhaps because of embarrassment, and the reluctance of medical practitioners to ask about it, perhaps because they feel that little can be done for such patients. Whereas the relative importance of the two factors is unknown, it appears certain that diabetic patients frequently fail to report disturbances in defecation, even when symptoms are severe, whether this is in a primary, secondary, or tertiary care setting. This has been shown to be the case with erectile dysfunction in diabetics. Faecal incontinence may, however, result in dramatic behavioural and personality changes, with patients becoming socially withdrawn and reluctant to leave their homes. Hence, it is essential that health care professionals become proactive and ask directed questions about faecal incontinence as part of a routine medical history if this information is not volunteered. Faecal incontinence also cannot be predicted by the presence of disordered motility in other regions of the gut, for example, gastroparesis, which occurs in perhaps 40% of patients with long-standing type 1 or type 2 diabetes.

Defecation disorders appear to occur more frequently in patients who have peripheral and/or autonomic neuropathy. Faecal incontinence has been reported to occur in 18% of secondary referrals with clinical evidence of peripheral diabetic neuropathy [10], and constipation was more common in patients with autonomic neuropathy than in those without [11]. In 16 diabetic patients with chronic diarrhoea, the onset of faecal incontinence occurred about the same time as diarrhoea (approximately 10 years after the initial diagnosis of diabetes) in 12 patients and within 6 years of the onset of diarrhoea in the other four [12]. All of these patients had extragastrointestinal manifestations of autonomic neuropathy. However, as chronic disorders of defecation occur relatively frequently in the normal population, with an increased prevalence in the elderly [13–15], it would be incorrect to suggest that such disturbances in colonic functions are inevitably caused by diabetes per se. For example, irritable bowel syndrome, which is more common in women, may be a risk factor for faecal incontinence [16]. There is only limited data about the prevalence of irritable bowel syndrome in the diabetic population, and it is probable that patients in the community who have been "labelled" as suffering from irritable bowel syndrome actually have faecal incontinence. Irritable bowel syndrome has strong associations with emotional upset, and it is possible that the emotional stress of coping with diabetes increases the propensity to irritable bowel syndrome.

A recent longitudinal study evaluating lower gastrointestinal symptoms in (predominantly type 2) diabetes suggested that although the prevalences of abdominal pain, constipation, diarrhoea, and faecal incontinence were essentially stable over time, symptom turnover was common and characterised by resolving symptoms in 50% of subjects and emerging symptoms in the remainder. Turnover was 8% for faecal incontinence [17, 18].

Pathophysiology of Anorectal Dysfunction in Diabetes: Effects of Autonomic Dysfunction and Hyperglycaemia

Many studies of anorectal function in diabetes have substantial limitations: the techniques used were often suboptimal, only isolated aspects of anorectal function were evaluated, and no account was taken of the potential impact of acute or chronic glycaemia. A number of factors, including autonomic neuropathy, glycaemic control, and psychiatric comorbidity, may potentially influence the development and/or regression of gastrointestinal symptoms, including incontinence, in diabetes.

As mentioned, anorectal dysfunction is more common in patients with diabetes complicated by neuropathy [10, 11]. Diabetic microangiopathy impairs nerve conduction and synaptic transmission [19]; 24–30% of type 1 patients have clinical evidence of peripheral neuropathy and 17% have evidence of autonomic neuropathy [20]. The prevalence of diabetic neuropathy is related to age, duration of diabetes, and glycaemic control [21]. Because those tests that evaluate gastrointestinal autonomic function directly have substantial limitations, measurements of cardiovascular function are often used as a surrogate, although there is only a weak correlation between diabetic autonomic neuropathy diagnosed from cardiovascular tests and disturbances in motility in other regions of the gastrointestinal tract [6, 22, 23]. In a study by Erckenbrecht et al. [23], stool frequency and stool continence, basal and squeeze anal sphincter pressures, and continence to rectally infused isotonic saline solution (1,500 ml) were prospectively evaluated in 12 incontinent and 15 continent patients with diabetes and related to quantitative measures of autonomic neuropathy, as assessed by heart rate variation in response to breathing, the pupillary reflex response to light, and quantitative measures of peripheral neuropathy as assessed by nerve conduction velocity and sensitivity to vibration. Incontinent patients as a group exhibited decreased basal and squeeze anal sphincter pressures and reduced continence for fluid compared with continent controls. The degree of incontinence correlated well with the maximal volume of retained rectally infused saline solution, but not with basal or squeeze anal sphincter pressures or with the severity of autonomic or peripheral neuropathy. The authors, accordingly, suggested that a generalised dysfunction of the autonomic or peripheral nervous system does not play a major role in the pathogenesis of faecal incontinence in diabetes. Blood glucose levels were not measured in this study. In contrast, Talley et al. [17] suggested that turnover of gastrointestinal symptoms in diabetes was related to autonomic neuropathy in that those with clinical evidence of autonomic neuropathy were more likely to report chronic symptoms of abdominal pain and faecal incontinence as opposed to fluctuating symptoms. However, objective measures of autonomic neuropathy were not performed. Glycaemic control did not seem to predict symptom change.

Whereas disordered defecation induced by diabetes mellitus has hitherto been believed to result from irreversible damage to autonomic nerves, there is now persuasive evidence that reversible changes in gastrointestinal motility may result from acute alterations in the blood glucose concentration [24, 25]. For example, the rate of gastric emptying is slowed by acute hyperglycaemia [24] and accelerated by hypoglycaemia [26]. It is likely that some of the abnormalities in anorectal motility observed in diabetic patients reflect the effects of hyperglycaemia rather than diabetes per se, particularly in view of observations relating to the effects of acute hyperglycaemia on anorectal motor and sensory function in healthy subjects [27–31] and diabetes [32]. Acute elevation of the blood glucose level to about 12 mmol/l has been shown to inhibit internal and external anal sphincter function in normal subjects, as evidenced by an increased number of spontaneous anal relaxations and a reduction in squeeze pressure (Fig. 1) (which would predispose to incontinence), whereas rectal sensitivity and compliance were increased [27]. In contrast, Chey et al. [28] reported that both the perception of rectal distension and the rectoanal

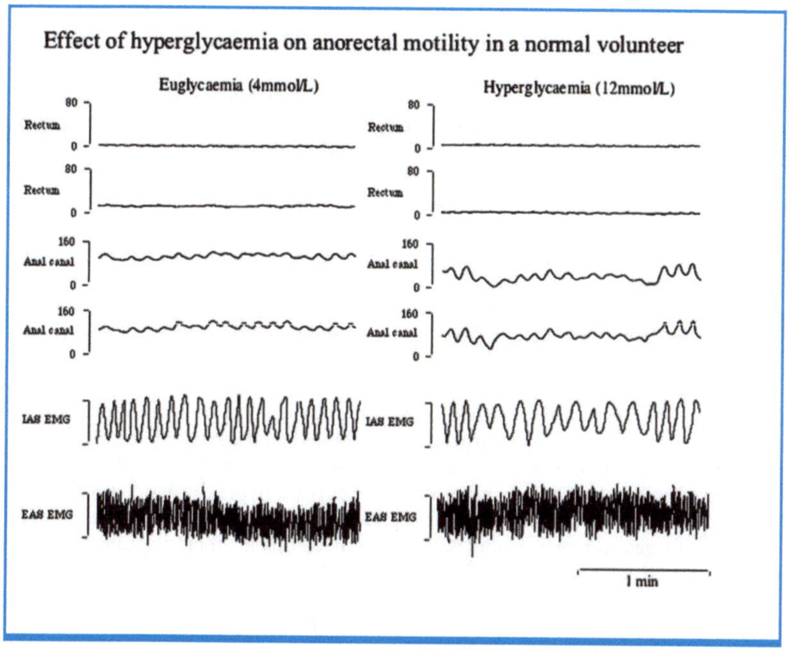

Fig. 1. Recordings of basal pressures in the rectum and anal canal and electrical activity of the internal (IAS) and external (EAS) anal sphincters in a healthy subject during euglycaemia (blood glucose 4 mmol/l) and hyperglycaemia (blood glucose 12 mmol/l). Hyperglycaemia is associated with a reduction in anal sphincter pressures and instability of the IAS. Data from [27]

inhibitory reflex were blunted by hyperglycaemia (blood glucose 15 mmol/l) in normal subjects. Russo et al. [30] established that the central processing of rectal distension (as assessed by measurement of cortical evoked potentials) is affected by hyperglycaemia in healthy subjects, consistent with other observations that indicate that the perception of a number of sensations arising from the gastrointestinal tract is modulated by acute hyperglycaemia [25]. The apparently discrepant effects of acute hyperglycaemia on anorectal function may well reflect the methodology used [28]. The gastrocolonic response has been shown to be blunted by hyperglycaemia in healthy subjects [31]. Accordingly, it is clear that acute elevations of blood glucose have the capacity to induce reversible changes in anorectal function and the perception of rectal distension in healthy subjects.

Only one study has hitherto evaluated the effects of hyperglycaemia on anorectal motility in diabetes. Anorectal motility and sensation was evaluated in eight patients with type 1 and ten patients with type 2 diabetes whilst the blood glucose concentration was stabilised at either 5 mmol/l or 12 mmol/l [32]. Eight healthy subjects were also studied under euglycaemic conditions. In diabetic subjects, hyperglycaemia was associated with reductions in maximal and plateau anal squeeze pressures and the rectal pressure/volume relationship (compliance) during barostat distension without any effect on the perception of rectal distension. Apart from a reduction in rectal compliance and a trend for an increased number of spontaneous anal sphincter relaxations, there were no differences between the patients studied during euglycaemia and healthy subjects. Thus, although the available data are limited in patients with diabetes, as in healthy subjects, acute hyperglycaemia inhibits external anal sphincter function and decreases rectal compliance, potentially increasing the risk of faecal incontinence.

It is now well established that the risk of both the development and progression of microvascular complications of diabetes–that is, retinopathy, nephropathy, and neuropathy–is greater in patients with poorly controlled diabetes [33, 34]. Therefore, it is likely that irreversible changes in anorectal motility may occur as a result of chronically poor glycaemic control [35, 36]. Studies of the effects of both acute and chronic glycaemia on anorectal function in diabetes are required to address these issues. It should also be recognised that hyperglycaemia and autonomic dysfunction are related. For example, acute hyperglycaemia affects cardiovascular autonomic function [37].

Mechanisms of Faecal Incontinence in Diabetes

As discussed elsewhere in this volume, defecation involves close integration of the peripheral autonomic and enteric nerves. Therefore, it is reasonable to infer that ischaemic or toxic damage to these nerves caused by diabetes can lead to disorders of defecation that will vary according to the site and type of nerve(s) that are affected. As mentioned, it is important to not attribute the disturbances in defecation that occur in patients with diabetes as necessarily complications of diabetes; for example, patients with diabetes are also at risk for cognitive and mobility impairment, faecal retention, and obstetric trauma. It has been suggested that when anxiety and depression are taken into account, no specific gastrointestinal symptom is significantly associated with autonomic neuropathy [38].

Faecal incontinence may be provoked by irresistible colonic propulsion and secretion, but it usually also implies a measure of dysfunction in the anorectal apparatus for maintaining continence. This might include weakness of the striated musculature of the puborectalis and external anal sphincter, a reduction in internal sphincter tone, a reduction in rectal sensitivity (so that the subject fails to detect the arrival of faecal material), or failure of rectoanal coordination (so that the patient fails to contract the striated muscles in sufficient time to prevent leakage).

Patients with long-standing diabetes are apparently more likely to be affected by nocturnal faecal incontinence than are nondiabetics with faecal incontinence, which may reflect neuropathy involving the sympathetic nerve supply. The colon is normally relatively quiescent during sleep, probably as a result of tonic activity in the sympathetic efferent nerves to the colon [39], which reduces propulsion, facilitates fermentation, and increases absorption. Damage of the sympathetic nerves supplying the colon by diabetic microvascular disease could result in mass movements at times when they would not normally occur. Therefore, events such as the delivery of meal contents into the caecum and the build-up of fermentation gases could readily generate colonic mass movements, which would rapidly distend the rectum, causing unrecognised relaxation of the internal anal sphincter and thus faecal incontinence. This is particularly important at night when there is no conscious augmentation of external sphincter contraction in response to rapid entry of faeces into the rectum. Under those conditions, the last barrier protecting continence is the tone of the internal sphincter.

As discussed, the majority of studies evaluating anorectal function in diabetes have not taken the potential impact of acute changes in blood glucose into account. Physiological studies have shown that internal sphincter tone is reduced in diabetes, and the internal anal sphincter is also markedly unstable (Fig. 2) [40]. Both abnormalities may be related to neuropathic damage to the sympathetic nerves [41]. Rectal compliance is also impaired, which is likely to be indicative of damage to the enteric nerves, although it should be recognised that ultrastructural degeneration of smooth muscle has been reported in visceral smooth muscle specimens from the stomach of diabetic patients [42]. It would also not be surprising if diabetes was associated with changes in the biomechanical characteristics of anorectal smooth muscle; chronic hyperglycaemia is known to result in functional alterations and tissue damage and proposed mechanisms include nonenzymatic glycation of proteins, with irreversible formation and deposition of reactive advanced glycation end products in the tissues and increased oxidative stress [43].

Impairment of neural function caused by diabetic microvascular disease can to a lesser or greater extent affect all the mechanisms involved in the maintenance of faecal incontinence. So whether an individual develops faecal incontinence or not is likely to be dependent on the interplay between all of these mechanism. Physiological studies have shown that cohorts of patients with long-standing diabetes have an abnormally low anal tone, weak squeeze pressures, and impaired rectal sensation [44–46]. Anal sensitivity may also be impaired [47, 48], although it has also been suggested that perception and nociception are well preserved in diabetics, even in those with evidence of neuropathy [48]. In a study of 11 patients with diabetes and faecal incontinence and 20 healthy controls, Sun et al. [40] found that nine of the 11 patients had impaired rectal sensitivity. During rectal distension, four patients showed no anal relaxation, and in the remainder, relaxation occurred at an abnormally high threshold. Accordingly, these abnormalities frequently coexist and may be associated with other changes that could threaten continence, in particular, the chronic diarrhoea that occurs in up to 20% of patients. Faecal incontinence in patients with diabetes is also often associated with urinary incontinence [49], which may be attributable to damage to the pudendal nerve supplying the pelvic floor muscles. Diabetes is known to lead to a progressive prolongation of the pudendal nerve terminal motor latency (PNTML), with consequent weakening of the external anal sphincter [50].

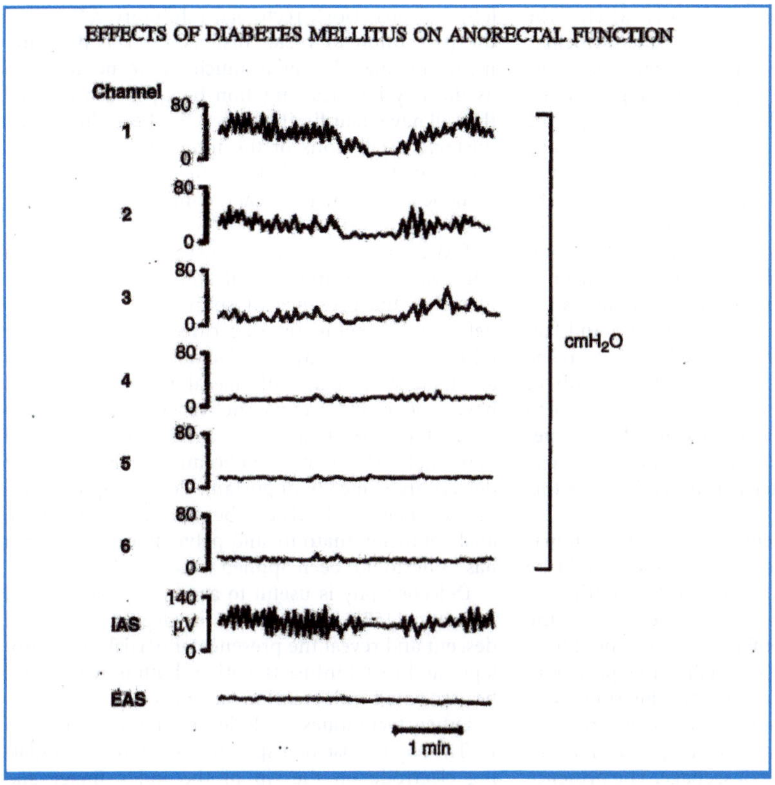

Fig. 2. Basal recording of anorectal pressure from ports situated 0.5, 1.0, 2.0, 2.5 and 4.5 cm from the anal verge (channels 1–5) and from a rectal balloon (channel 6) 6–11 cm from the anal verge, and electrical activity of internal (IAS) (raw) and external anal sphincter (EAS) (integrated) in a type-1 patient with faecal incontinence. Note that the anal pressure oscillations and the pressure reduction during spontaneous anal relaxation are associated with changes in electrical activity of the *IAS* but not the *EAS*; and the anal pressure is lowest during spontaneous anal relaxation. Reprinted with permission from [40]

Women with poor glycaemic control tend to give birth to large babies and are more likely to experience long and difficult labours and require assisted delivery with forceps or ventouse [51]. Inevitably, such women are more liable to suffer from obstetric complications, such as traumatic disruption of the anal sphincter or weakness of the pelvic floor, leading to chronic stretching of the pudendal nerve.

Clinical Assessment

As with all cases of faecal incontinence, a comprehensive history including documentation of potential sphincter injury and thorough physical examination are essential. Many techniques have been employed to elucidate the pathophysiology of faecal incontinence, but the majority of them are used primarily as research tools. The objective of clinical assessment is to characterise the type and severity of faecal incontinence, including awareness of the desire to defecate prior to incontinence, and to identify conditions that may respond to specific treatment, particularly risk factors for anorectal injury. It also provides the opportunity to establish rapport with the patient. The severity of faecal incontinence and its impact on quality of life can be evaluated by specific scales [52]. Anorectal manometry, anal endosonography, measurements of pudendal nerve latency studies, and electromyography are part of the standard evaluation.

Patients are likely to suffer from faecal incontinence and seepage if their faeces are liquid. Profuse amounts of stool, as associated with viral gastroenteritis or infectious colitis, may overwhelm the sphincter mechanism and lead to incontinence. Thus, patients with severe diarrhoea who pass large amounts of liquid motion require investigation and treatment of their diarrhoea before any specific investigations of anorectal function, because in many cases, the incontinence will cease to be a problem if the diarrhoea is treated satisfactorily. Faecal incontinence associated with faecal impaction and overflow incontinence is well described [53]. Incomplete emptying of the rectum can lead to overflow incontinence, as liquid stool passes by the inspissated faecal mass. An association between constipation and faecal incontinence has been reported. This may be caused by pelvic nerve damage in this group of patients [54]. For this reason, it is important not to miss faecal impaction with overflow and identify specific neurological causes of incontinence. It is also important to identify obstetric trauma, because this can be treated surgically.

Inspection of the perineum and digital examination of the anorectum are essential and should be performed in all patients with faecal incontinence before enemas or laxatives are given. With the patient lying in the left lateral position, he/she should be asked to bear down. Normally, the perineum descends no more than a centimetre. Bearing down may also reveal the existence of rectal prolapse, which is frequently associated with sphincter weakness and is a frequent cause of seepage. The presence of obvious external haemorrhoids is also a common cause of anal seepage of mucus. Digital examination of the rectum is a useful and simple means of assessing resting anal tone and the strength of the conscious contraction.

Proctoscopy and/or sigmoidoscopy (with or without biopsy) should be performed to exclude not only haemorrhoids, fistulas, and fissures, but also solitary rectal ulcers, proctitis, inflammatory bowel disease, and tumours. The remaining colon should be evaluated, usually by colonoscopy, to exclude proximal contributory pathology. Importantly, partially obstructing colorectal cancers may result in a change in bowel habit and incontinence secondary to partial obstruction. There are no specific findings on clinical examination to indicate anorectal dysfunction caused by diabetes.

Clinical investigation might include anorectal manometry, endoanal ultrasonography (EAUS), and X-ray defecography [55]. Anorectal manometry will quantify the impact of sphincter injury on sphincter function. This painless, 10-min, outpatient examination requires no bowel preparation and measures both resting and sphincter canal tone (internal anal sphincter activity), squeeze pressure (external anal sphincter activity) in four quadrants (anterior, right, left, and posterior), rectoanal inhibitory reflex, and the perception of rectal distension. The measurements obtained depend as much on the method used as the physiological function being measured, and they all have their limitations. It has been shown that unstable oscillations of the internal anal sphincter tone and electrical activity occur more frequently in diabetic patients with faecal incontinence than in any other group [40].

EAUS has been used with increasing frequency to noninvasively examine anal sphincter integrity. It identifies the presence of sphincter thinning or a defect in the sphincter ring caused by obstetric or other trauma [55, 56]. EAUS should be conducted in all diabetic women with faecal incontinence who have undergone vaginal deliveries and have low sphincter pressures. Both EAUS and anorectal manometry should be used because not all sphincter defects are clinically important. Pelvic magnetic resonance imaging (MRI) can be used to visualise both anal sphincter anatomy and pelvic floor motion but has hitherto not been applied widely in diabetics.

Defecography is useful to assess the dynamics of defecation [57]. It can assess the degree of perineal descent and reveal the presence of partial rectal prolapse and rectal intussusception, both of which may be associated with faecal incontinence.

Other techniques include the measurement of PNTML by the use of a special glove with a stimulating electrode on the tip of the index finger and recording electrodes at the base of the finger [58] [electromyography (EMG)], but its value is questionable. Needle EMG is recommended when there is clinical suspicion of a proximal neurogenic lesion.

Treatment

The treatment of faecal incontinence in patients with diabetes is largely symptomatic. Despite the absence of clear-cut data, tight glycaemic control should be recommended, as it may slow, stop, or even reverse the neuropathic process and prevent the adverse effects of acute hyperglycaemia on anorectal function [27–30, 32, 59]. In most cases, this level of glycaemic control is, however, not achievable without the use of insulin and a concomitant increased incidence of hypoglycaemia. The risks of the latter are substantial, particularly in those patients with impaired awareness of hypoglycaemia. A number of agents, including aldose reductase inhibitors, may be effective in the treatment of diabetic autonomic and peripheral neuropathy [60], but there is no information about their effects on anorectal function.

Management should be tailored to clinical manifestations. The major aim of treatment of faecal incontinence is to improve symptoms to a level where there is minimal impact on lifestyle, and it is important to point out that patients may only rarely be "cured". Many patients may not seek help because they think that little can be done and wrongly consider incontinence to be the "natural" result of getting old or childbirth. The majority of patients are unaware of the association between faecal incontinence with diabetes. As discussed, many physicians are also pessimistic about the options for these patients, other than antidiarrhoeal agents and diapers, and perhaps for this reason, fail to enquire specifically about faecal incontinence. Occasionally, diarrhoea and incontinence will remit spontaneously, but permanent remission seems to be unusual.

When diabetic diarrhoea is complicated by faecal incontinence, the first priority is to bring the diarrhoea under control and, subsequently, ascertain whether the patient has a treatable cause for incontinence. Certain conditions that occur with increased frequency in patients with diabetes, including coeliac disease, pancreatic insufficiency, and bacterial overgrowth of the small intestine, must be excluded. Coeliac disease in particular is easily overlooked and can be excluded by taking jejunal biopsies. Pancreatic insufficiency must be considered and should be excluded by measurement of faecal fat and appropriate pancreatic function tests, or by a trial of oral pancreatic enzyme therapy. Bacterial overgrowth can be diagnosed by a hydrogen breath test or suspected by improvement of the diarrhoea by a short course of broad-spectrum antibiotics (ampicillin, tetracycline). Other causes of diarrhoea that must be excluded are irritable bowel syndrome, laxative abuse, rectal prolapse, and abnormalities in bile salt metabolism.

It seems reasonable to try to control diarrhoea with antidiarrhoeal drugs in the hope that the continence mechanisms will be better able to cope with a smaller volume of more solid stool. Opiate-like antidiarrhoeal agents (such as loperamide, diphenoxylate, and codeine phosphate) increase stool consistency and decrease stool frequency and are the first-line agents for treatment of diarrhoea. They inhibit the local nervous reflexes responsible for both intestinal propulsion and secretion and increase the tone of the internal anal sphincter [61]. Loperamide is the most potent of these and, unlike codeine phosphate, does not cross the blood–brain barrier. As many as 12 tablets of loperamide (8 mg tds) may be taken daily without unwanted side effects. It is important to exclude the possibility that diarrhoea is related to intestinal stasis with bacterial overgrowth, as loperamide may potentially exacerbate this.

Rapid intestinal transit sufficient to cause diarrhoea is often associated with bile acid absorption. Bile acids stimulate colonic secretion and propulsion and may exacerbate symptoms of urgency and faecal incontinence. Cholestyramine, a bile acid binding agent, is sometimes dramatically effective in stopping diarrhoea that is associated with urgency and faecal incontinence and resistant to loperamide and opiate-like antidiarrhoeal agents. Condon et al. [62] treated six patients with watery postvagotomy diarrhoea and four with intractable diabetic diarrhoea with cholestyramine. The diarrhoea responded completely to therapy. Thus, it was suggested that the mechanism of diarrhoea is similar in both disorders and is due to neuropathy of the hepatic fibres of the vagus nerve, which results in distension of the gallbladder, contraction of which expels increased quantities of bile salts, which swamp the reabsorptive capacity of the small intestine and induce diarrhoea by direct action on the colon. It is essential that the patient be instructed to take cholestyramine half an hour before meals and that the dose is titrated with the size of the meal because bile acids are released whilst a meal is ingested. The patient is usually started on a small dose of two sachets (8 g) before dinner in the evening and one (4 g) before lunch, and the physician should involve the patient in finding the most appropriate dose according to his/her pattern of eating and the response to treatment.

Octreotide can reduce stool volume and frequency in high-volume diabetic diarrhoea when conventional antidiarrhoeal agents have failed. Its therapeutic benefit appears to be predominantly related to a marked increase in mouth to caecum transit time [63].

The α 2-adrenergic agonists, such as clonidine, have been advocated and shown to be effective in the management of diabetic diarrhoea [64], as there is evidence that diabetic diarrhoea and nocturnal incontinence may be related to sympathetic neuropathy. Clonidine artificially restores sympathetic tone, enhancing salt and water absorption and reducing propulsive contractions [65]. Fedorak et al. [65] reported the empirical treatment of three patients with "idiopathic diarrhoea" after other treatments had failed. The patients had had poorly controlled type 1 diabetes for 6–15 years complicated by peripheral sensory neuropathy, retinopathy, and gastroparesis. In each patient, stool volume was substantially reduced by clonidine. The clonidine was given orally at a dose of 0.1 mg every 12 h and increased to 0.5 or 0.6 mg every 12 h over the next 72 h. Diarrhoea recurred when the clonidine was withdrawn but remitted when it was reintroduced. Clonidine also modulates colonic motor and sensory function in healthy subjects [66]. It also seems probable that clonidine may help to restore internal anal sphincter stability and tone, although this has yet to be tested.

Clonidine should always be considered in the management of patients with nocturnal incontinence. The doses used are comparable with those employed in the treatment of hypertension. It should be remembered that special care and attention must be paid to treating patients with autonomic neuropathy and postural hypotension. However, in the three patients described by Fedorak et al. [65], clonidine did not worsen existing postural hypotension and did not induce it when it was not present; moreover, symptoms of gastroparesis were not aggravated.

Faecal impaction with overflow is usually treated by examination using digital extraction and enemas, followed by a regular regime of bulk laxatives and toilet training [67]. Biofeedback training (operant reconditioning) is a useful method for treating incontinence of all types. However, to our knowledge the efficacy of this treatment has not been formally evaluated in patients with diabetes. It is usually the first line of treatment if medical therapy fails, especially in patients with mild to moderate faecal incontinence and in some severe cases. However, in a controlled study of biofeedback for faecal incontinence, Norton et al. [68] reported that neither pelvic floor exercises nor biofeedback was superior to standard care supplemented by advice and education (~50% improvement in both groups). The exact mechanism of action of biofeedback is poorly understood, and it has been suggested that patient–therapist interaction and patient coping strategies may be more important in improving continence than performing exercises or receiving physiological feedback. Much of the research associated with biofeedback also recognises the need for patient compliance, and this is critical to success.

When medical therapy is unsuccessful and symptoms remain disabling, a surgeon knowledgeable about faecal incontinence should be consulted. As already mentioned, obstetric causes for faecal incontinence may well be more common in patients with diabetes and can be treated by surgery. However, the results of postanal repair are often poor if perineal descent has resulted in severe neuropathic weakness of the sphincter or the pudendal neuropathy caused by compression and tension is exacerbated by diabetic microangiopathy. The common denominator between the medical and surgical treatment groups is the necessity of pretreatment physiologic assessment. It is the results of these tests that permit optimal therapeutic assignment. For example, PNTML is the most important predictor of functional outcome. However, even the most experienced examiner's digit cannot assess PNTML. In the absence of pudendal neuropathy, sphincteroplasty is an excellent option.

Sacral nerve stimulation has been reported to greatly improve continence and quality of life in selected patients with morphologically intact or repaired sphincter complex, offering a treatment for patients in whom treatment options are limited [69]. As far as we are aware, the effects of sacral nerve stimulation in diabetic patients have not been studied. A permanent colostomy may be the only reasonable solution when a patient is troubled from continuous soiling that does not respond to treatment.

People with diabetes have a higher prevalence of emotional problems [70]. Diabetes has been reported to double the risk of depression compared with those without the disorder [71], and the chances of becoming depressed increase as diabetes complications worsen. Depression leads to poorer physical and mental functioning, and thus a person is less likely to follow a required diet or medication plan. Some patients may live in fear of losing their sight or their legs or of going on dialysis, and it is important for the physician to recognise this and address this appropriately whilst at the same time treating their patient faecal incontinence.

References

1. Feldman M, Schiller LR (1983) Disorders of gastrointestinal motility associated with diabetes mellitus. Ann Intern Med 98:378–384
2. Horowitz M, Fraser R (1994) Disordered gastric motor function in diabetes mellitus. Review. Diabetologia 37:543–551
3. Goyal RK, Spiro HM (1971) Gastrointestinal manifestations of diabetes mellitus. Med Clin North Am 55:1031–1044
4. Camilleri M (1996) Gastrointestinal problems in diabetes. Endocrinol Metab Clin North Am 25:361–378
5. Rundles R (1945) Diabetic neuropathy; general review with report of 125 cases. Medicine 24:111–160
6. Horowitz M, Maddox AF, Wishart JM et al (1991) Relationships between oesophageal transit and solid and liquid gastric emptying in diabetes mellitus. Eur J Nucl Med 18:229–234
7. Nelson RL (2004) Epidemiology of fecal incontinence. Gastroenterology 126:S3–S7
8. Kalantar JS, Howell S, Talley NJ (2002) Prevalence of faecal incontinence and associated risk factors. An underdiagnosed problem in the Australian community? Med J Aust 176:54–57
9. Enck P, Bielefeldt K, Rathmann W et al (1991) Epidemiology of faecal incontinence in selected patient groups. Int J Colorectal Dis 6:143–146
10. Martin M (1958) Diabetic neuropathy: a clinical study of 150 cases. Brain 76:594–624
11. Maxton DG, Whorwell PJ (1991) Functional bowel symptoms in diabetes-the role of autonomic neuropathy. Postgrad Med J 67:991–993
12. Schiller LR, Santa Ana CA, Schmulen AC et al (1982) Pathogenesis of fecal incontinence in diabetes mellitus: evidence for internal-anal-sphincter dysfunction. N Engl J Med 307:1666–1671

13. Drossman DA, Li Z, Andruzzi E et al (1993) US householder survey of functional gastrointestinal disorders: prevalence, sociodemography and health impact. Dig Dis Sci 38:1569–1580
14. Thompson WG, Heaton KW (1980) Functional bowel disorders in apparently healthy people. Gastroenterology 79:283–288
15. Talley NJ, O'Keefe EA, Zinsmeister AR, Melton LJ (1992) Prevalence of gastrointestinal symptoms in the elderly: a population-based study. Gastroenterology 102:895–901
16. Drossman DA (1989) What can be done to control incontinence associated with the irritable bowel syndrome? Am J Gastroenterol 84:355–357
17. Talley NJ, Howell S, Jones MP, Horowitz M (2002) Predictors of turnover of lower gastrointestinal symptoms in diabetes mellitus. Am J Gastroenterol 97:3087–3094
18. Bytzer P, Talley NJ, Hammer J et al (2002) GI symptoms in diabetes mellitus are associated with both poor glycemic control and diabetic complications.
19. Schmidt RE, Beaudet LN, Plurad SB, Dorsey DA (1997) Axonal cytoskeletal pathology in aged and diabetic human sympathetic autonomic ganglia. Brain Res 769:375–383
20. Flynn MD, O'Brien JA, Corall RJ (1995) The prevalence of autonomic and peripheral neuropathy in insulin-treated diabetic subjects. Diabet Med 12:310–313
21. Tesfaye S, Stevens LK, Stephenson JM et al (1996) Prevalence of diabetic neuropathy and its relation to glycaemic control and potential risk factors. The Euro Diab IDDM complications study. Diabetologia 39:1377–1384
22. Horowitz M, Harding PE, Maddox A et al (1986) Gastric and oesophageal emptying in insulin-dependent diabetes mellitus. J Gastroenterol Hepatol 1:97–113
23. Erckenbrecht JF, Winter HJ, Cicmir I et al (1988) Faecal incontinence in diabetes mellitus: is it correlated to diabetic autonomic or peripheral neuropathy? Z Gastroenterol 26:731–736
24. Fraser R, Horowitz M, Maddox A et al (1990) Hyperglycaemia slows gastric emptying in type 1 (insulin-dependent diabetes mellitus). Diabetologia 30:675–680
25. Rayner CK, Samsom M, Jones K, Horowitz M (2001) Relationships of upper gastrointestinal motor and sensory function with glycaemic control. Diabetes Care 24:371–381
26. Schvarcz E, Palmer M, Aman J et al (1993) Hypoglycaemia increases the gastric emptying rate in patients with type 1 diabetes mellitus. Diabet Med 10:660–663
27. Russo A, Sun WM, Sattawatthamrong Y et al (1997) Acute hyperglycaemia effects anorectal motor and sensory function in normal subjects. Gut 41:494–499
28. Chey WD, Kim M, Hasler WI, Owyang C (1998) Hyperglycaemia alters perception of rectal distension and blunts the rectoanal inhibitory reflex in healthy volunteers. Gastroenterology 108:1700–1708
29. Azvar E, Ersoz O, Karisik E et al (1997) Hyperglycaemia-induced attenuation of rectal perception depends on pattern of rectal balloon inflation. Dig Dis Sci 42:2206–2212
30. Russo A, Smout AJPM, Kositchaiwat C et al (1999) The effect of hyperglycaemia on cerebral potentials evoked by rapid rectal distension in healthy humans. Eur J Clin Invest 29:512–518
31. Sims MA, Hasler WL, Chey WD et al (1995). Hyperglycaemia inhibits mechanoreceptor-mediated gastrocolonic responses and colonic peristaltic reflexes in healthy humans. Gastroenterology 108:350–359
32. Russo A, Botten R, Kong M-F et al (2004) Effects of acute hyperglycaemia on anorectal motor and sensory function in diabetes mellitus. Diabet Med 21(2):176–182
33. DCCT Research Group (1993) The effect of intensive treatment of diabetes on the development and progression of long-term complications in insulin-dependent diabetes mellitus. N Engl J Med 329:977–986
34. UKPDS Study Group (1998) Effect of intensive blood-glucose control with metformin on complications in overweight patients with type 2 diabetes. UKPDS 34. Lancet 352:854–865
35. Allen C, Shen G, Palta M, Lotz B et al (1997) Long-term hyperglycaemia is related to peripheral nerve changes at a diabetes duration of 4 years. The Wisconsin Diabetes Registry. Diabetes Care 20:1154–1158
36. Greene D (1986) A sodium-pump defect in diabetic peripheral nerve corrected by sorbinil administration: relationship to myoinositol metabolism and nerve conduction slowing. Metab Clin Exp 35(4 Suppl 1): 60–65
37. Yeap BB, Russo A, Fraser RJ et al (1996) Hyperglycemia affects cardiovascular autonomic nerve function in normal subjects. Diabetes Care 19:880–882
38. Clouse RE, Lustman PJ (1989) Gastrointestinal symptoms in diabetic patients: lack of association with neuropathy. Am J Gastroenterol 84:868–872
39. Narducci F, Bassotti G, Gaburri M, Morelli A (1987) Twenty-four-hour manometric recording of colonic motor activity in healthy man. Gut 28:17–25
40. Sun WM, Katsinelos P, Horowitz M, Read NW (1996) Disturbances in anorectal function in patients with diabetes mellitus and faecal incontinence. Eur J Gastroenterol Hepatol 8:1007–1012
41. Speakman CTM, Hoyle CHV, Kamm MA et al (1990) Adrenergic control of the internal anal sphincter is abnormal in patients with idiopathic faecal incontinence. Br J Surg 77:1342–1344
42. Ejskjaer NT, Bradley JL, Buxton-Thomas MS et al (1999) Novel surgical treatment and gastric pathology in diabetic gastroparesis. Diabet Med 16:488–495
43. Singh R, Barden A, Mori T, Beilin L (2001) Advanced glycation end-products: a review. Diabetologia 44:129–146
44. Rogers J, Levy DM, Henry MM, Misiewicz JJ (1988) Pelvic floor neuropathy: a comparative study of diabetes mellitus and idiopathic faecal incontinence. Gut 29:756–761
45. Wald A, Tunuguntla AK (1984) Anorectal sensorimotor dysfunction in fecal incontinence and diabetes mellitus. Modification with biofeedback therapy. N Engl J Med 310:1282–1287
46. Rogers J, Henry MM, Misiewicz JJ (1988) Combined sensory and motor deficit in primary neuropathic faecal incontinence. Gut 29:5–9
47. Aitchison M, Fisher BM, Carter K et al (1991) Impaired anal sensation and early diabetic faecal incontinence.

Diabet Med 8:960–963
48. Sarna S, Erasmus LP, Haslbeck M, Holzl R (1994) Visceral perception and gut changes in diabetes mellitus. Neurogastroenterol Motil 6:85–94
49. Nakanishi N, Tatara K, Naramura H et al (1997) Urinary and faecal incontinence in a community-residing older population in Japan. J Am Geriat Soc 45:215–219
50. Pinna-Pintor M, Zara GP, Falletto E et al (1994) Pudendal neuropathy in diabetic patients with faecal incontinence. Int J colorectal Dis 9:105–109
51. Kuhl C, Hornness PU, Anderson O (1985) Etiology and pathophysiology of gestational diabetes mellitus. Diabetes 34:66–70
52. McHorney CA, Ware JJ, Raczek AE (1993) The MOS 36-Item Short-Form Health Survey (SF-36): II. Psychometric and clinical tests of validity in measuring physical and mental health constructs. Medical Care 31:247–263
53. Wald A (1997) Fecal incontinence: three steps to successful management. Geriatrics 52:49–52
54. Read NW, Celik AF, Katsinelos P (1995) Constipation and incontinence in the elderly. J Clin Gastroenterol 20:61–70
55. Rao SSC, Sun WM (1997) Current techniques of assessing defecation dynamics. Dig Dis Sci 15(Suppl 1):64–77
56. Sun WM, Rao SS (2001) Manometric assessment of anorectal function. Gastroenterol Clin N Am 30:15–32
57. Mahieu P (1984) Defaecography. I. Description of a new procedure and results in normal patients. Gastrointest Radiol 9:247–251
58. Kiff ES, Swash M (1984) Slowed conduction in the pudendal nerves in idiopathic (neurogenic) faecal incontinence. Br J Surg 71:614–616
59. Kawagishi T, Nishizawa Y, Emoto M et al (1997) Gastric myoelectrical activity in patients with diabetes. Role of glucose control and autonomic nerve function. Diabetes Care 20:848–854
60. Guigliano D, Marfella R, Quatraro A et al (1993) Tolrestat for mild diabetic neuropathy. A 52-week, randomized, placebo-controlled trial. Ann Intern Med 118:7–11
61. Sun WM, Read NW, Verlinden M (1997) Effects of loperamide oxide on gastrointestinal transit time and anorectal function in patients with chronic diarrhoea and faecal incontinence. Scand J Gastroenterol 32:34–38
62. Condon JR, Robinson V, Suleman MI, Fan VS, McKeown MD (1976) The cause and treatment of postvagotomy diarrhoea. Br J Surg 62:309–312
63. Murao S, Hirata K, Ishida T, Takahara J (1999) Severe diabetic diarrhea successfully treated with octreotide, a somatostatin analogue. Endocr J 46:477–478
64. Schiller LR, Santa Ana CA, Morawski SG, Fordtran JS (1985) Studies of the anti-diarrhoeal action of Clonidine. Gastroenterology 89:982–988
65. Fedorak R, Field M, Chang E (1985) Treatment of diabetic diarrhoea with Clonidine. Ann Intern Med 102:197–199
66. Bharucha AE, Camilleri M, Zinsmeister AR, Hanson RB (1997) Adrenergic modulation of human colonic motor and sensory function. Am J Physiol 273:G997–1006
67. Bartolo DCC, Sun WM (1997) Colorectal and anorectal motor dysfunctions. In: Shearman DJ, Finlayson NC, Camilleri M (eds). Diseases of the gastrointestinal tract and liver, 3rd edn. Churchill Livingstone, New York, pp 1315–1341
68. Norton C, Chelvanayagam S, Wilson-Barnett J et al (2003) Randomized controlled trial of biofeedback for fecal incontinence. Gastroenterology 125:1320–1329
69. Matzel KE, Kamm MA, Stosser M et al (2004) Sacral spinal nerve stimulation for faecal incontinence: multicentre study. Lancet 363:1270–1276
70. Van der Does FE, De Neeling JN, Snoek FJ et al (1996) Symptoms and well-being in relation to glycaemic control in type 2 diabetes. Diabetes Care 19:204–210
71. Anderson RJ, Lustman PJ, Clouse RE et al (2000) Prevalence of depression in adults with diabetes: a systematic review. Diabetes 49(Suppl 1):A64

Fecal Incontinence in Elderly and Institutionalized Patients

33

Arnold Wald

Introduction

At any age, fecal incontinence is one of the most devastating of all nonfatal illnesses, resulting in considerable embarrassment, anxiety, and social isolation to those who suffer from it. So embarrassing is it that individuals with incontinence frequently do not volunteer this complaint to their physicians and must be asked directly about fecal incontinence [1]. The physician should also be aware that patients might complain of "diarrhea," which may be a euphemism for fecal incontinence.

Background and Prevalence

The presence of fecal incontinence is especially problematic for the elderly and institutionalized individuals, in whom the prevalence of incontinence is higher than that of the general adult population and which is equally prevalent in both men and women (Table 1). Among ambulatory persons ≥65 years, the frequency of incontinence has ranged from 3.7 to 27% [2–5] depending upon whether defining criteria encompass mild and infrequent soiling or just the most frequent and severe (Table 1). Incontinence is most often associated with chronic diarrhea, multiple health problems, and poor self-perceived health [6]. In hospitalized elderly, the prevalence of incontinence ranges from 10 to 25% [7]. More than half of all elderly patients in long-term care facilities suffer from fecal incontinence, in part related to the high prevalence of dementia and delirium in such settings [8–10]. Incontinence in residents in long-term facilities and those who are institutionalized for cognitive or psychiatric reasons is associated with poor overall health, increased mortality, and significantly increased expenditures for health care [11, 12]. "Double incontinence" (both urinary and fecal) is a major cause of institutionalization in the elderly [9, 10, 13].

Table 1. Prevalence of fecal incontinence in elderly populations[a]

Population	Prevalence
Age ≥65 years (community)	3.7–27%
Hospitalized patients	10–25%
Nursing home	>50%
Hospitalization with dementia	>80%

[a] See text for references

Risk Factors and Causes of Fecal Incontinence

As with persons of all ages, fecal incontinence in elderly individuals has multiple etiologies and requires careful assessment of each patient. Following is a partial list of causes of fecal incontinence in the elderly:

- Decreased rectal sensation
  - Fecal impactions
  - Megarectum
  - Diabetes mellitus
- Decreased reservoir capacity
  - Radiation
  - Surgical resection
  - Ischemia
  - Inflammation
- Impaired anal sphincter/puborectalis function
  - Spinal cord lesions
  - Pudendal neuropathy
  - Trauma, surgery
- Functional impairment
  - Dementia, delirium, confusion
  - Weakness, immobility, instability
  - Depression, psychosis
- Other
  - Diarrhea
  - Inadequate toilet arrangements

In ambulatory intact elderly patients, causation is similar to that in the general adult population and requires an assessment similar to that of younger adults [7]. It should be the philosophy of all health care workers that fecal incontinence is not a normal consequence of the aging process but often occurs as a result of structural or functional impairment of continence mechanisms and/or alteration of stool consistency and delivery. It is also useful to recall that fecal continence requires the ability to sense rectal filling and impending defecation, appropriate responses of the anal sphincters and puborectalis muscle to prevent unwanted defecations, the ability of the distal colon and rectum to store fecal material for variable periods of time, and motivation by the individual to remain continent [14]. Abnormalities of any one or several of these must be considered as potential causes of incontinence in a patient of any age.

In contrast to ambulatory elderly individuals, factors other than impaired continence mechanisms become more important in the institutionalized or hospitalized patient. These factors include lack of motivation associated with cognitive dysfunction or behavioral maladaptation. The possibility of acute or chronic obstipation with fecal impaction leading to overflow incontinence must always be considered in the appropriate clinical setting [12]. Immobility, inadequate toileting arrangements, use of constipating medications, and diarrhea due to infections, medications, or inflammation must also be carefully assessed for. For example, the use of patient trunk restraints was found to be the most important cause for the development of incontinence in nursing homes, even after adjusting for the major reasons why restraints were implemented [15]. Clearly, restraints prevent access to toilet facilities and represent a remedial cause of incontinence in this population.

A frequent cause of fecal incontinence in the institutionalized or otherwise functionally impaired patient is fecal impaction, either with or without megarectum. In these patients, anal sphincter pressures are generally normal and are no different before and after disimpaction [16]. Two critical abnormalities are frequently encountered. First, there is impaired rectal sensation so that the rectums of recently disimpacted patients require distension with much higher volumes before patients perceive fullness or desire to defecate [17]. Second, patients are unable to perceive rectal volumes that are sufficiently large to inhibit the resting tone of the internal anal sphincter. Thus, liquid stool is able to seep around the impaction and pass through the decreased sphincter pressures of the anal canal, resulting in spurious diarrhea. Failure to identify an impaction may lead to the inappropriate prescription of antidiarrheal agents, which will exacerbate the problem.

Evaluation and Management

A wide array of diagnostic tests is available to assess anorectal structure and function in selected patients with fecal incontinence [14]. Diagnostic tests often illuminate underlying pathophysiology and provide a greater understanding of causation. It has been argued that such information should lead to more rational decision making when choosing among treatment options. It is therefore appropriate to ask whether in an elderly patient with fecal incontinence the standard of care should include validated and often informative manometric and imaging studies of the anorectum. In most elderly and institutionalized patients, such tests are often not necessary [18]. In my opinion, the vast majority of these patients can be managed satisfactorily with a careful history and a directed physical examination that includes digital rectal examination and a focused exam involving the perineum, lower extremities, and back. This is certainly so in patients with overflow incontinence, those with decreased colorectal storage capacity, and those with minor soiling associated with internal anal sphincter weakness. In some of the remaining patients in whom the cause of fecal incontinence is not apparent or in whom surgery may provide remediation, studies of anorectal structure and function may provide useful information about appropriate management. This should not include most elderly patients, including those who are functionally intact and living at home.

Overflow Incontinence

Fecal impaction with overflow incontinence may occur in patients of all ages but is disproportionately seen in those with dementia, psychosis, and the elderly, especially those who are institutionalized. This diagnosis should always be considered in a clinical setting in which there is frequent or constant seepage of liquid stools. Diagnosis is confirmed by a digital rectal examination (if the impaction is in the low rectum) or by an abdominal X-ray that demonstrates fecal loading in a patient who is incontinent of diarrheal stools (Fig. 1). Treatment consists of disimpaction, thorough colon cleansing, and a bowel-retraining regimen, together with periodic bowel emptying depending upon clinical circumstances (see below). The latter is critically important because of the high recurrence rate in patients without appropriate follow-up measures [19]. There is no indication for diagnostic anorectal studies in such patients.

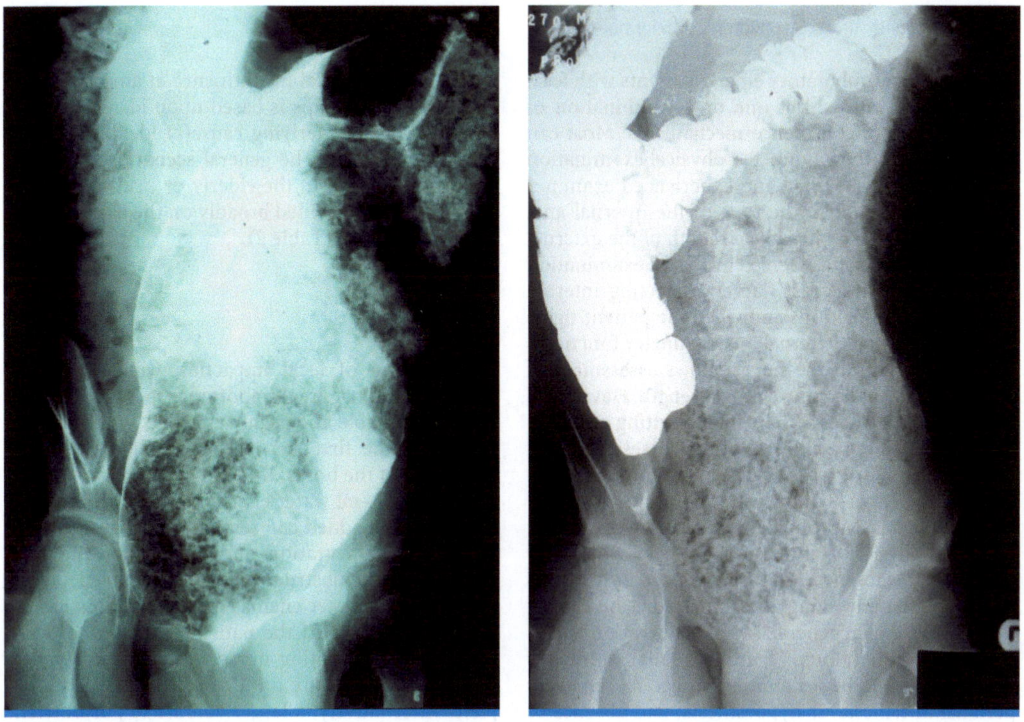

Fig. 1. Large rectum and left colon filled with impacted stool in a patient who is incontinent of liquid stool ("spurious diarrhea")

Reservoir Incontinence

Impaired rectal and/or colonic storage capacity is another cause of chronic fecal incontinence. This entity is frequently suggested by the patient's history and may in some patients require confirmation by an endoscopic evaluation. Some of the more frequently encountered causes in elderly patients are inflammatory bowel diseases involving the colon and rectum, proctectomy, and radiation proctopathy leading to fibrosis. Treatment consists of anti-inflammatory drugs for inflammatory bowel diseases in an effort to reverse inflammation; in the absence of a reversible condition, dietary fiber restriction with antidiarrheal agents helps minimize stool volume and regulate delivery (see below). Anorectal physiological tests are generally unnecessary in this clinical situation.

Minor Soiling with Normal Bowel Habits

Another important group of patients is frequently composed of healthy older men and women who present with minor soiling or seepage in the presence of normal bowel habits. This does not involve incontinence of solid stool but, rather, "spotting" of underclothes by persistent soiling of the perianal area. Digital anorectal examination often suggests decreased anal canal tone at rest, strong voluntary contraction of the external anal sphincter and puborectalis muscle, and absence of fecal impaction, mucosal, or hemorrhoidal prolapse and other perianal conditions that can produce minor soiling. This clinical scenario is consistent with isolated weakness or dysfunction of the internal anal sphincter. A history of lateral internal sphincterotomy, i.e., for anal fissure, should alert the physician to this diagnosis, but in most patients, internal anal sphincter dysfunction is idiopathic and appears to be associated with aging- related fibrosis [20]. The use of a simple anal cotton plug as an absorbent barrier can often alleviate this embarrassing problem (see below). Formal physiological testing is rarely necessary.

Incontinence with Anorectal Sphincteric Abnormalities

The remaining ambulatory elderly patients with fecal incontinence will exhibit one or a combination of abnormalities of continence mechanisms. Most can be ascertained when a directed physical examination is performed by a skilled and experienced examiner [14, 18]. For example, the tone of the internal anal sphincter and the contractile strength of the external anal sphincter can be assessed by digital examination of the anal canal at rest (largely reflecting internal anal sphincter function) and when the patient tightens the anal canal (external anal sphincter function). Deeper insertion of the finger allows assessment of puborectalis muscle contraction strength. Having the patient bear down, especially in a squatting or dorsal lithotomy position, allows optimal assessment for rectal prolapse or excessive descent of the perineum, suggesting weakness of the pelvic floor muscles. Only impaired rectal sensation cannot be assessed by conventional physical examination; however, this rarely occurs in the absence of other evidence of a neurologic disorder involving the spinal cord or central nervous system. In general, sacral denervation is suggested by a patulous ("gaping") anal sphincter observed when the examining finger is removed, perianal anesthesia or hypoesthesia, and absence of anal sphincter contractions ("anal wink") with mild stroking of the perianal skin.

Management Principles

Management of fecal incontinence at any age and in all population groups is based upon identifying and correcting the underlying cause(s) identified at the initial assessment. The general scenarios associated with incontinence in the elderly or institutionalized persons may be divided broadly on the basis of clinical presentations (Table 2).

Overflow Incontinence

Identification of fecal impaction with or without megarectum is of great importance, because remediation is available and highly effective [7, 19]. Disimpaction is the first step and often includes digital fracturing of the bolus. If the impaction is very hard, a 500- to 750-ml water enema with 1–2 tablespoons of mineral oil added can serve to soften the bolus to facilitate fragmentation and passage of the fecal bolus. Once the obstructive mass is removed, larger-volume warm-water enemas may be administered to cleanse the colon. If the patient is unable to do so independently, visiting nurses may be employed to provide enemas daily until colon cleansing is complete. Alternatively, a larger volume of polyethylene glycol (PEG) electrolyte solution may be given orally as 240 ml every 30 min until the rectal contents are

Table 2. Management of fecal incontinence in elderly or institutionalized persons

Causes	Management
Overflow	Disimpaction Colon evacuation Periodic defecation with laxatives/enemas if necessary
Reservoir	Low-fiber diet Loperamide Periodic defecation with or without laxatives
Isolated internal anal sphincter weakness	Loperamide as needed Anal cotton plug
Anal sphincter impairment	Loperamide Surgery? Sacral nerve stimulation?
Behavioral/dementia	Prompted defecation or loperamide with regular laxatives, suppositories, or enemas three times a week
General measures	Skin care Pads Odor control Caregiver support

free of stool. On occasion, gastrografin enemas are useful for this purpose and also serve to exclude obstructive colon disease. If the colon in such patients is not effectively emptied, impaction recurrence is quite high.

As mentioned earlier, such patients are prone to reimpaction because of underlying rectal sensation impairment, megarectum, or predisposing causes of constipation. Thus, habit training with laxatives should be started to ensure periodic defecation. This involves regularly scheduled attempts to defecate with the assistance of small amounts of osmotic laxatives, such as PEG-containing solutions. Oral or rectal stimulant laxatives are given if there is no defecation for 3 days. Fiber supplements are not helpful and only add to the fecal load. With appropriate attention to detail, recurrent impactions should be effectively prevented.

Reservoir Incontinence

This clinical situation is generally identified by clinical history and examination. If a treatable cause of reduced colorectal storage capacity such as ulcerative colitis is not present, treatment strategies should incorporate reduction of stool volume by decreasing dietary fiber and alteration of stool delivery with antidiarrheal agents such as loperamide and diphenoxylate with atropine [21]. Evacuation of the colon once or twice per week with oral laxatives prevents stool buildup in these patients.

Internal Anal Sphincter Weakness (Minor Soiling)

If patients report normal bowel habits with minor seepage, the best approach is to employ an anal cotton pledget to occlude the anal canal. This is held in place by the gluteal muscles and tissues and serves as a physical and absorbent barrier to anal seepage, somewhat analogous to a vaginal tampon. The use of a narrow panty liner serves as a contingency mechanism and prevents underwear staining. This is particularly useful for ambulatory persons and has the added advantage of being inexpensive and readily available. This device is often effective for patients with minor seepage due to anal cushion defects, i.e., after hemorrhoidectomy or fistula in ano.

Diarrhea/Loose Stools

On occasion, diarrhea may overwhelm normal continence mechanisms, but in the elderly, altered stool delivery and increased stool liquidity may also breach mild sphincter dysfunctions that are subclinical because of underlying constipation or simply normal firm stool. Identification and treatment of acute diarrhea in the elderly who are especially prone to *Clostridium difficile* infections or who are more susceptible to bacterial diarrheas because of gastric achlorhydria caused by disease or use of medications such as proton pump inhibitors is too extensive to review comprehensively here [13]. Additional causes of loose stools in the elderly include microscopic colitis (diagnosed only by colonic biopsies), bile-salt-induced diarrheas occurring after cholecystectomy, bacterial overgrowth syndromes [22], and diarrheagenic medications. Normalizing stool delivery by treating specific disorders with the use of antidiarrheal agents such as loperamide often ameliorates fecal incontinence [21]. Adequate doses and timing are important, i.e., 2–4 mg 30 min before meals or prior to social occasions to avoid accidents outside the home. The coexistence of diarrhea predominant or mixed irritable bowel syndrome (IBS) may be especially troublesome in the elderly; in patients with these forms of IBS, the cautious use of tricyclic agents with reduced receptor affinity for receptors producing unwanted side effects such as nortriptyline, imipramine, and desipramine may be helpful [23, 24].

Incontinence in Persons with Dementia or Psychiatric Illness

Incontinence may occur in patients with dementia or psychiatric illness for three main reasons:

1. Patients with advanced dementia may lose neurological control of bowel and bladder functions.
2. Behavioral disturbances impair the social impetus to reach a toilet in an appropriate and timely way. These may involve impaired memory, expressive or receptive aphasia, or complete apathy.
3. Comorbid conditions that remain unrecognized in a psychotic or demented individual.

Management of such patients requires careful analysis of possible causative or contributing factors and attempts to correct them. These include simplifying access to toilets, using clothing that is easily undone, creating a secure and familiar environment, preventing constipation, and avoiding medications that can cause diarrhea [15, 25, 26].

Incontinence in the Independently Functioning Elderly

Fecal incontinence in independently functioning adults of all ages may be associated with one or a combination of rectal sensory and continence muscle abnormalities. In addition to conservative measures focused on changes in stool consistency and delivery, other therapies have been recommended [27]. These therapies include surgical repair of disrupted anal sphincter muscles, and pelvic floor training and biofeedback for compliant and cognitively intact patients who are not candidates for surgery. Sacral nerve stimulation is a new and hopeful approach for selected patients who fail other forms of therapy.

Pelvic Floor Training and Biofeedback

Both pelvic floor training and biofeedback have been reported to be effective in many patients with fecal incontinence associated with impaired functioning of the puborectalis muscle and/or the external anal sphincter. In contrast to pelvic floor retraining, which is directed exclusively at reeducating weakened or impaired muscles, biofeedback often employs techniques to alter rectal sensation and sphincter muscle responsiveness to intrarectal stimuli such as balloon distension. However, the biofeedback literature does not reflect a unified mechanistic approach. There appears to be a general consensus that improvement of thresholds of perception of rectal sensation and the synchronization of external anal sphincter contractions to rectal distension are important factors associated with improvement [28]. In contrast, increased striated muscle strength and endurance after biofeedback training have not been shown consistently.

There is widespread agreement that biofeedback is effective in many patients who fulfill entry criteria, and it has no adverse consequences. However, the biofeedback literature has been plagued by methodological inadequacies, few long-term follow-up studies, and absence of consistent and validated outcomes. There is no consensus concerning which components of biofeedback are important, including the critical role of the patient–therapist relationship [28]. To address these issues, a recent study examined critical components of the biofeedback process by randomizing 171 patients with fecal incontinence into four therapeutic groups [29]. Slightly more than 50% of patients reported clinical improvement on an intention-to-treat analysis. However, there were no differences between patients who received only advice from nurse therapists about strategies to reduce incontinence, those who received both advice and verbal instructions about sphincter exercises, those who received advice together with a hospital-based biofeedback program, and those who received both hospital and home biofeedback. At present, the evidence for using instrument-based training is insufficient, but the value of dedicated and trained individuals to work with patients cannot be overstated [29].

Surgery

Anal sphincteroplasty has been performed for many years and is based on the straightforward premise of repairing an anatomically disrupted anal sphincter complex. The use of anal sonography to demonstrate anal sphincter disruptions has largely replaced the more invasive and painful electromyographic (EMG) mapping of the external sphincter. Although studies have reported short-term improvement of fecal continence in up to 85% of patients following surgery, long-term follow-ups have been disappointing [30]. In three recent representative series, full continence after sphincteroplasty was maintained in only 28% of patients after a mean follow-up of 40 months and in only 11–14% of patients followed for over 69 months. Suggested predictive factors for treatment failure include the presence of an internal anal sphincter defect, prolongation of pudendal nerve terminal motor latencies (PNTML), external anal sphincter atrophy as demonstrated by pelvic magnetic resonance imaging (MRI), and the presence of IBS with diarrhea predominance. In the absence of demonstrable anal sphincter defects, the efficacy of surgery to correct abnormalities of the pelvic floor, such as anterior levatorplasty, postanal repair, and total pelvic floor repair, is unproven. A Cochrane Review concluded that there was insufficient evidence to determine whether clinically important differences between various alternative procedures existed to guide clinical practice [31]. These procedures cannot be recommended for patients of any age with neurogenic incontinence or in the absence of structural defects.

Sacral Nerve Stimulation

Sacral spinal nerve stimulation is a new therapeutic approach for patients with fecal incontinence that is associated with structurally intact anal sphincters. This technique is an extension of the successful use of this modality for urinary voiding and continence disorders, with the realization that stimulating electrodes implanted into pelvic floor muscles are prone to infection, migration, and fibrous tissue reactions. The procedure involves the following three phases:

1. Location of sacral spinal nerves by percutaneous probing with a needle electrode to identify the nerve root that maximally stimulates anal sphincter contraction.
2. Temporary placement of an electrode to chronically stimulate the nerve root identified as the most efficient during acute testing.
3. Permanent implantation of a neurostimulator for chronic therapeutic stimulation.

In patients who successfully complete the first two phases, clinical improvement of fecal incontinence has been confirmed in both short- and long-term studies [32]. Clinical parameters include substantial decrease in episodes of stool incontinence and significant improvement of quality-of-life parameters, as assessed by validated quality-of-life questionnaires, for periods ranging from 6 months to more than 5 years. Objective physiologic changes include increases in both resting and squeeze pressures, increased squeeze durations, decreased thresholds of rectal sensation, and increased time of retention of a saline load. A multicenter study in the United States is currently in progress.

Conclusions

Fecal incontinence in the elderly is a socially devastating disorder with numerous potential etiologies. Appropriate management begins with a detailed history and physical examination that either reveal the probable cause or determine that additional diagnostic studies to elucidate pathophysiology may be required. A large array of therapeutic options is available, many with little evidence to support efficacy, but together, they allow most incontinent patients to be managed effectively.

References

1. Johanson JF, Lafferty J (1996) Epidemiology of fecal incontinence: the silent affliction. Am J Gastroenterol 91:33–36
2. Kok AL, Voorhorst FJ, Burger CW et al (1992) Urinary and fecal incontinence in community-residing elderly women. Age Ageing 21:211–215
3. Talley NJ, O'Keefe EA, Zinsmeister AR, Melton LJ 3rd (1992) Prevalence of gastrointestinal symptoms in the elderly: a population-based study. Gastroenterology 102:895–901
4. Roberts RO, Jacobsen SJ, Reilly WT et al (1999) Prevalence of combined fecal and urinary incontinence: a community based study. J Am Geriatr Soc 47:837–841
5. Bharucha AE, Zinsmeister AR, Locke GR et al (2005) Prevalence and burden of fecal incontinence: a population based study in women. Gastroenterology 129:42–49
6. Goode PS, Burgio KL, Halli AD et al (2005) Prevalence and correlates of fecal incontinence in community-dwelling older adults. J Am Ger Soc 53:629–635
7. Wald A (1990) Constipation and fecal incontinence in the elderly. Gastroenterol Clin North Am 19:405–418
8. Chassagne P, Landrin I, Neveu G et al (1999) Fecal incontinence in the institutionalized elderly: incidence, risk factors, and prognosis. Am J Med 106:185–190
9. Nelson R, Furner S, Jesudason V (1998) Fecal incontinence in Wisconsin nursing homes: prevalence and associations. Dis Colon Rectum 41:1226–1229
10. O'Donnell BF, Drachman DA, Barnes HJ (1992) Incontinence and troublesome behaviors predict institutionalization in dementia. J Geriatr Psychiatry Neurol 5:45–52
11. Borrie MJ, Davidson HA (1992) Incontinence in institutions: costs and contributing factors. CMAJ 147:322–328
12. Tobin GW, Brocklehurst JC (1986) Fecal incontinence in residential homes for the elderly: prevalence, aetiology and management. Age Ageing 15:41–46
13. Tariq SH, Morley JE, Prather CM (2003) Fecal incontinence in the elderly patient. Am J Med 115:217–227
14. Bharucha AE (2003) Fecal incontinence. Gastroenterology 124:1672–1685
15. Nelson RL, Furner SE (2005) Risk factors for the development of fecal and urinary incontinence in Wisconsin nursing home residents. Maturitas 52(1):26–31
16. Read NW, Abouzekry L, Read MG et al (1985) Anorectal function in elderly patients with fecal impactions. Gastroenterology 89:959–966
17. Read NW, Abouzekry L (1986) Why do patients with fecal impaction have fecal incontinence? Gut 27:283–287
18. Wald A (2006) Anorectal manometry and imaging are not necessary in patients with fecal incontinence. Am J Gastroenterol 101(12):2681–2683
19. Chassagne P, Jego A, Gloc P et al (2000) Does treatment of constipation improve fecal incontinence in institutionalized elderly patients? Age Ageing 29:159–164
20. Klosterhalfen B, Offner F, Topf N et al (1990) Sclerosis of the internal anal sphincter—a process of aging. Dis Colon Rectum 33:606–609
21. Read M, Read NW, Barber DC, Duthie HL (1982) Effects of loperamide on anal sphincter function in patients complaining of chronic diarrhea and fecal incontinence and urgency. Dig Dis Sci 27:807–814
22. Riordan SM, McIver CJ, Wakefield D et al (1997) Small intestinal bacterial overgrowth in the symptomatic elderly. Am J Gastroenterol 92:47–51
23. Wald A (2002) Psychotropic agents in irritable bowel syndrome. J Clin Gastroenterol 35:553–557
24. Santoro GA, Estan BZ, Pryde A, Bartolo DC (2003) Open study of low-dose amitriptyline in the treatment of patients with idiopathic fecal incontinence. Dis Colon Rectum 43:1676–1682
25. Potter J, Wagg A (2005) Management of bowel problems in older people: an update. Clin Med 3:289–295
26. Ouslander JG, Simmons S, Schnelle J et al (1996) Effects of prompted voiding on fecal continence among nursing home residents. J Am Geriatr Soc 44:424–428
27. Cheung O, Wald A (2004) Review article: Management of pelvic floor disorders. Aliment Pharmacol Ther 19:481–495
28. Wald A (2003) Biofeedback for fecal incontinence. Gastroenterology 125:1533–1535
29. Norton C, Chelvanayregam S, Wilson-Barnett J et al (2003) Randomized controlled trial of biofeedback for fecal incontinence. Gastroenterology 125:1320–1329
30. Madoff RD (2004) Surgical treatment options for fecal incontinence. Gastroenterology 126:S48–54
31. Bachoo P, Brazzelli M, Grant A (2000) Surgery for fecal incontinence in adults. Cochrane Electronic Library (2):CD001757
32. Matzel KE, Kamm MA, Stosser M et al (2004) Sacral spinal nerve stimulation for fecal incontinence: multicenter study. Lancet 363:1270–1276

34 Pelvic Radiotherapy

Soeren Laurberg, Mette M. Soerensen

Introduction

Radiation injury is a well-known complication after external radiotherapy of cancers within the pelvic cavity. Radiation therapy might be the primary treatment for such cancers (prostate, uterine, cervical, bladder, and anal cancers), or it might be combined with surgery (rectal cancer).

Side Effects of Pelvic Radiation Therapy

Radiotherapy can cause both acute and chronic sequelae. Side effects can be related to functional impairment (bladder, sexual, and bowel), pain and local fractures. If the small bowels are included, this might lead to strictures, fistulation, and increased risk of adhesions requiring surgical management. Furthermore, radiotherapy might increase the risk of postoperative cardiopulmonary problems and secondary malignancy. This chapter focuses on the risk of long-term fecal incontinence when radiation (or chemoradiation) is used as a single modality or combined with surgery.

Interpretation of Risk of Fecal Incontinence after Pelvic Radiotherapy

The interpretation of the risk and the degree of fecal incontinence after pelvic radiotherapy is difficult for several reasons. First, the classification of fecal incontinence strongly depends on the method used. Second, chronic radiation damage progresses with time, and the risk and degree of fecal incontinence is therefore directly related to the observational period. Third, not only the total dose but also the fractionation scheme, the number of fields, and the total irradiated volume will influence the risk of fecal incontinence. Thus, the commonly used preoperative neoadjuvant fractionation scheme of 5×5 Gy before surgery for rectal cancer is equivalent to a biological dose of approximately 50 Gy when fractions of 1.8–2 Gy is used. Fourth, with modern techniques with shielding and use of many fields, the dose to structures near the target field is reduced. Finally, the anal sphincters are now excluded from the radiation field whenever possible. It is therefore likely that the risk of fecal incontinence using modern radiation therapy will be less than the risk with traditional methods.

For rectal cancer, surgery has also improved, with much more focus on sparing the autonomic nerves [1] and with reconstruction of a neorectum when total mesorectal excision is combined with a coloanal anastomosis [2, 3]. As both surgery and radiotherapy have improved, it is likely that modern combination of surgery and radiotherapy will create fewer functional problems [3, 4]. However, this must be evaluated in high-quality prospective observational studies.

Fecal Incontinence and Rectal Cancer

Surgery Alone

It is well established that surgical resection of the rectum with anastomosis can lead to the anterior resection syndrome in about 25–50% of patients after traditional restorative resection [3]. This syndrome is characterized by urgency, frequent bowel movements, and some degree of fecal incontinence. The syndrome is related to the loss of rectal reservoir function, and it is more frequent after a total mesorectal excision. If a small neorectal reservoir is constructed, either using a colonic J-pouch or the Baker type side-to-end anastomosis, the symptoms will be less severe [3]. The functional bowel problems are most pronounced initially, decrease within the first year, and then become stable. This is in contrast to the deficits after adjuvant therapy, which progress with time.

Surgery and Long-Course Postoperative Radiotherapy

The risk of fecal incontinence after postoperative radiotherapy for rectal cancer has been studied in a randomized Danish trial where patients with Dukes B

Table 1. Adverse effects of adjuvant postoperative radiotheraphy and surgery only on bowel function. Reprinted with permission from Elsevier [6]

	No radiotherapy (n = 44)	Radiotherapy (n = 49)	*P*
Patients			
Median age	73 (73–90)	77 (42–90)	ns
Male/female	15/29	22/27	ns
Duke B/C	36/8	32/17	ns
Low/high resection	32/12	27/22	ns
Years since surgery	13 (11–17)	14 (11–17)	ns
Symptoms	%	%	
Stool frequency ≥5 /day	2	18	< 0.001
Loose/liquid stool	2	25	0.024
Fecal urgency	12	41	0.003
Fecal incontinence	5	49	< 0.001
Use of pads	0	26	< 0.001
Differentiated stool/gas	95	77	0.014
Impaired social function	15	29	0.893
Antidiarrhoea medication	11	25	0.132
Abdominal pain	14	27	0.208
Tenesmus	3	13	0.122

Figures in parentheses are ranges.

and C cancers were randomized to surgery with or without postoperative radiotherapy (50 Gy) [5, 6]. In this trial, the addition of postoperative radiotherapy was followed by a substantially increased risk of bowel problems, with a high risk of multiple defecations per day, urgency, fecal incontinence, and use of pads (Table 1). Similar impaired anal function has been described in other non-randomized and randomized studies [7].

The physiological studies suggest that the high

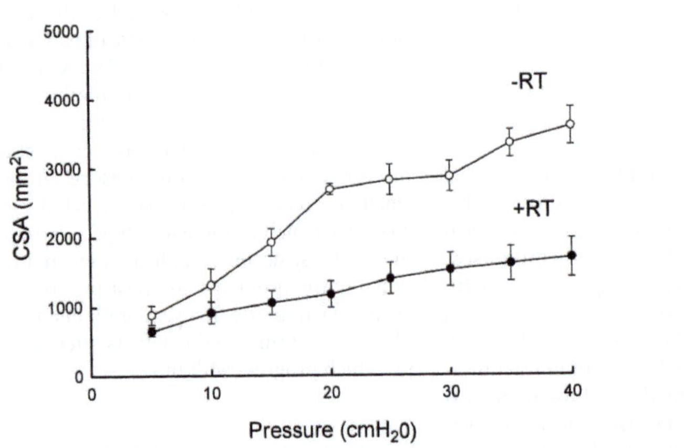

Fig. 1. Pressure/cross-sectional area (CSA) relationship in patients treated with adjuvant radiotherapy (+RT) and patients treated with surgery alone (–RT) (p=0.0001). Reprinted with permission from [5]

risk of fecal incontinence after postoperative radiotherapy was due to a substantial reduction in rectal capacity and distensibility [5] (Fig. 1). In addition, there was a reduction in anal sphincter function, with a reduction in squeeze pressure and a thinning of the internal anal sphincter.

Strength and Limitation of the Danish Study

The main strength of the Danish study is that it was a randomized study, and the functional deficits were classified without knowledge of whether the patients had radiotherapy. The observational period was long, and it was therefore possible to describe the long-term detrimental effects of radiotherapy. However, the study also has several limitations, as old-fashion irradiation and surgery was used. The radiation field included the sphincter in all cases. It is therefore likely that the study overestimated the risk of long-term anorectal dysfunction with modern techniques.

Surgery Combined with Short-Course Preoperative Radiotherapy

The risk of fecal incontinence after preoperative short-course radiotherapy (5x5 Gy) has been studied in both Swedish [8, 9] and Dutch trials [4, 10]. Patients with respectable rectal cancer were randomized to surgery alone or surgery combined with preoperative radiotherapy. In both trials, the addition of short-course radiotherapy reduced the risk of local recurrence [4, 10, 11], and in the Swedish trial, survival was improved. However, the addition of short-course radiotherapy substantially increased the risk of bowel problems, with a higher risk of fecal incontinence, urgency, and use of pads (Table 2) [12, 13]. Furthermore, radiotherapy decreased sexual function in both men and women [11, 14].

In the Dutch trial, this substantial increase in risk of fecal incontinence had no or only minor effect on health-related quality of life [4]. Overall perceived health, measured by the visual analog scale (VAS), did not differ significantly between irradiated patients and patients without radiotherapy [4, 10]. However, impaired social life because of bowel dysfunction was more frequent in irradiated patients compared with surgery alone [4, 10, 13, 15]. It is notable that patients with a stoma were more satisfied with their bowel function than were patients without a stoma, whether they had received radiotherapy or not [10].

Strength and Limitation of the Swedish and the Dutch Studies

The main strength of these studies was their randomized design. However, suboptimal irradiation therapy was used, and the radiation field included the sphincter in the majority of cases. Thus, it is likely that risk of long-term anorectal dysfunction is less with modern treatment. Compared with the study using postoperative radiotherapy, the functional deficit was apparently less. This should, however, be interpreted with caution. One reason for the difference might be that the outcome was evaluated differently. Another possibility is that the observational period was longer in the Danish study, and the Danish technique was more "old-fashioned" [1, 5, 6].

However, theoretically, it is likely that preoperative adjuvant therapy would cause less functional problems than postoperative therapy. First, the radiation-induced damage might be greater when performed after surgery. Second, with postoperative

Table 2. Adverse events and symptoms in patients treated with and without preoperative radiotherapy

	Radiotherapy ($n = 65$)	No radiotherapy ($n = 74$)	P**
Any adverse event	45 (69)	32 (43)	0.002
Cardiovascolar disease	23 (35)	14 (19)	0.032
Venous thromboebolism	4 (6)	5 (7)	0.823
Faecal incontinence*	12 (57)	11 (26)	0.013
Small-bowel obstruction	19 (29)	13 (18)	0.074
Urinary incontinence	29 (45)	20 (27)	0.023
Incomplete bladder emptying	17 (26)	13 (18)	0.193
Fractures (all types)	11 (17)	6 (8)	0.118
Hip and pelvic fractures	3 (5)	1 (1)	0.227

Values in parentheses are percentages. *Assessed only in patients who had anterior resection. **Fisher's exact test. Reproduced with permission from [12]

radiotherapy, the rectal remnant or neorectum is irradiated, and this irradiation might severely impair the function of the reservoir, leading to a narrow rigid conduit. With preoperative adjuvant therapy, the neorectum would be outside the irradiated field, and with low anastomosis, there would be no irradiated rectum remnant. This is supported by Welsh et al. [16]. Preoperative short-course irradiation had little effect on risk of fecal incontinence in patients with anastomosis <6 cm from the anal verge, though the risk of incontinence was much higher than with a high anastomosis. In the latter patients, neoadjuvant short-course irradiation increased the risk of fecal incontinence, suggesting that irradiation of a rectal remnant might increase the risk of fecal incontinence after preoperative radiotherapy.

Long-Course Preoperative (Chemo)Radiotherapy for Rectal Cancer

It is now generally accepted that preoperative radiotherapy is more effective than postoperative radiotherapy and that the addition of chemotherapy decreases the risk of local recurrence [17–19]. Unfortunately, description of the functional deficit following long-course chemoradiation has not been studied scientifically. Therefore, we do not know the effect of long-course chemoradiation on function. However, the addition of chemotherapy might potentially increase the risk of side effects. On the other hand, the larger fractions that are used in short-course radiation, 5×5 Gy, may induce more damage to the normal tissue.

Only one study has compared short-course radiotherapy with long-course preoperative chemoradiation [20]. There were no significant difference in survival and risk of local recurrence, but functional problems have not yet been evaluated in the Polish trial [20].

Conclusion: Pelvic Radiotherapy for Rectal Cancer

There is no doubt that the addition of (chemo)radiation increases the risk of fecal incontinence and other sequelae. On the other hand, this treatment modality decreases the risk of local recurrence and may also increase survival [11]. Further studies are needed to clarify which rectal cancer patient needs neoadjuvant therapy and how functional outcome can be improved by improving the quality of both radiotherapy and surgery. Hopefully, in the future, we will have much more specific methods to select patients who will benefit from neoadjuvant therapy and identify patients with the highest risk of functional problems.

Fecal Incontinence Associated with Radiotherapy for other Cancers

Several studies have shown that radical radiotherapy for both prostate cancer and bladder cancer is associated with an increased risk of fecal incontinence [21–24]. After 2 years, bowel frequency, fecal urgency, and fecal incontinence were increased in 50%, 47%, and 26% of patients, respectively [24]. These functional deficits were associated with a reduction in resting anal pressures, squeeze pressure, and rectal compliance [24].

With a medium observation time of 29 months after radical radiotherapy for urinary bladder cancer, about 55% of the patients experienced impairment in bowel function, including urgency, incontinence, and use of pads [22]. These changes had a moderate or severe impact on the performance of daily activity in 29% of patients. Physiological studies suggest that the impaired function, also for bladder cancer, is due to a combination of sphincter weakness and changes in rectal function.

For patients with cervical cancer treated with surgery and external radiotherapy, overall bowel dysfunction was the most important source of distress of any degree in a Swedish study [25]. In an Australian study, ten out of 15 patients who had pelvic irradiation for a gynecological cancer had urgency of defecation, and four suffered from fecal incontinence [26]. This dysfunction was also associated with reduction in anal canal pressures and changes in rectal function. There is a relationship between late anorectal dysfunction and dose-volume parameters from the rectum and anal canal [27].

Interpretation of Studies

All the studies were observational studies. They all show that late anorectal dysfunction was common and related to a change in rectal function and weaknesses of the anal sphincters. The changes progressed with time. The studies suggest that pelvic irradiation fields should be optimized, excluding the anal canal from the high-dose volume and applying rectal shielding whenever possible.

Treatment of Fecal Incontinence after Pelvic Radiotherapy

There is little knowledge on how to treat fecal incontinence in these patients, and patients have, in general, been treated empirically with constipating agencies or suppositories. Two new treatment modalities, however, may be attractive to use in these patients:

transanal irrigation and percutaneous nerve evaluation (PNE)/sacral nerve stimulation (SNS).

Transanal Irrigation

This conservative management has proven very effective in certain groups of patients with bowel problems [28], with improvement in incontinence, constipation, and quality of life in a randomized trial on spinal cord patients [29, 30]. Small observational studies also suggest that this treatment can be very effective in patients with irradiation-related fecal incontinence [31] (Fig. 2).

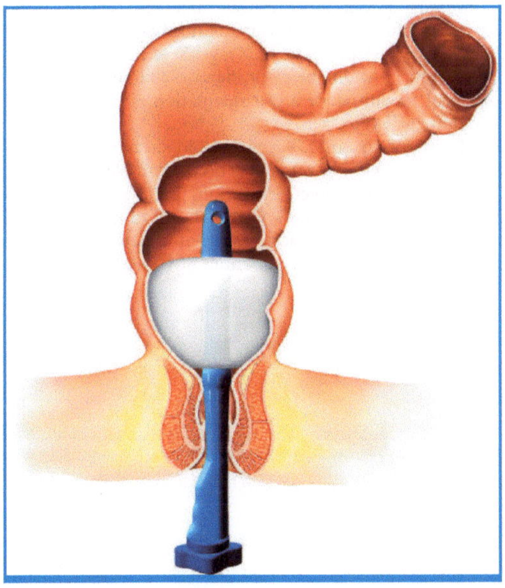

Fig. 2. Transanal irrigation

PNE/SNS

Sacral nerve stimulation has been shown repeatedly to be a very effective treatment modality for various patient groups with fecal incontinence [32]. Small observational studies suggest that this can be very effective in patients with incontinence after pelvic irradiation. Further studies are, however, needed to evaluate the effectiveness of this treatment and how it influences the physiology in these patients.

References

1. Havenga K, Maas CP, DeRuiter MC et al (2000) Avoiding long-term disturbance to bladder and sexual function in pelvic surgery, particularly with rectal cancer. Semin.Surg.Oncol 18:235–243
2. Engel J, Kerr J, Schlesinger-Raab A et al (2003) Quality of life in rectal cancer patients: a four-year prospective study. AnnSurg 238:203–213
3. Hallbook O, Sjodahl R (2000) Surgical approaches to obtaining optimal bowel function. Semin Surg Oncol 18:249–258
4. Marijnen CA, van de Velde CJ, Putter H et al (2005) Impact of short-term preoperative radiotherapy on health-related quality of life and sexual functioning in primary rectal cancer: report of a multicenter randomized trial. J Clin Oncol 2023(9):1847–1858
5. Lundby L, Krogh K, Jensen VJ et al (2005) Long-term anorectal dysfunction after postoperative radiotherapy for rectal cancer. Dis Colon Rectum 48:1343–1349
6. Lundby L, Jensen VJ, Overgaard J, Laurberg S (1997) Long-term colorectal function after postoperative radiotherapy for colorectal cancer. Lancet 350(9077):564
7. Frykholm GJ, Glimelius B, Pahlman L (1993) Preoperative or postoperative irradiation in adenocarcinoma of the rectum: final treatment results of a randomized trial and an evaluation of late secondary effects. Dis Colon Rectum 36(6):564–572
8. Pollack J, Holm T, Cedermark B et al (2006) Long-term effect of preoperative radiation therapy on anorectal function. Dis Colon Rectum 49:345–352
9. Folkesson J, Birgisson H, Pahlman L et al (2005) Swedish Rectal Cancer Trial: Long Lasting Benefits from Radiotherapy on Survival and Local Recurrence Rate. J Clin Oncol 23(24):5644–5649
10. Peeters KC, van de Velde CJ, Leer JW et al (2005) Late side effects of short-course preoperative radiotherapy combined with total mesorectal excision for rectal cancer: increased bowel dysfunction in irradiated patients-a Dutch colorectal cancer group study. J Clin Oncol 23(25):6199–6206
11. Ortholan C, Francois E, Thomas O et al (2006) Role of radiotherapy with surgery for T3 and resectable T4 rectal cancer: evidence from randomized trials. Dis Colon Rectum 49(3):302–310
12. Pollack J, Holm T, Cedermark B et al (2006) Late adverse effects of short-course preoperative radiotherapy in rectal cancer. Br J Surg 93:1519–1525
13. Dahlberg M, Glimelius B, Graf W, Pahlman L (1998) Preoperative Irradiation Affects Functional Results After Surgery for Rectal Cancer. Dis Colon Rectum 41(5):543–549
14. Yoshihiro M (2006) Function Preservation in rectal cancer surgery. Int J Clin Oncol 11:339–343
15. Vironen JH, Kairaluoma M, Aalto AM, Kellokumpu IH (2006) Impact of functional results on quality of life after rectal cancer surgery. Dis Colon Rectum 49(5):568–578
16. Welsh FKS, McFall M, Mitchell G, Miles WFA et al (2002) Pre-operative short-course radiotherapy is associated with faecal incontinence after anterior resection. Colorectal Disease 5:563–568

17. Bosset JF, Collette L, Calais G et al; EORTC Radiotherapy Group Trial 22921 (2006) Chemotherapy with preoperative radiotherapy in rectal cancer. N Engl J Med 355(11):1114–1123
18. Urso E, Serpentini S, Pucciarelli S et al (2006) Complications, functional outcome and quality of life after intensive preoperative chemoradiotherapy for rectal cancer. Eur J Surg Oncol 32(10):1201–1208
19. Glynne-Jones R, Grainger J, Harrison M et al (2006) Neoadjuvant chemotherapy prior to preoperative chemoradiation or radiation in rectal cancer: should we be more cautious?. Br J Cancer 94(3):363–371. Review
20. Bujko K, Nowacki MP, Nasierowska-Guttmejer A et al (2006) Long-term results of a randomized trial comparing preoperative short-course radiotherapy with preoperative conventionally fractionated chemoradiation for rectal cancer. Br J Surg 93(10):1215–1223
21. Kushwaha RS, Hayne D, Vaizey CJ et al (2003) Physiologic changes of the anorectum after pelvic radiotherapy for the treatment of prostate and bladder cancer. Dis Colon Rectum 46(9):1182–1188
22. Fokdal L, Hoyer M, Meldgaard P, von der Maase H (2004) Long-term bladder, colorectal, and sexual functions after radical radiotherapy for urinary bladder cancer. Radiother Oncol 72(2):139–145
23. Kneebone A, Mameghan H, Bolin T et al (2004) Effect of oral sucralfate on late rectal injury associated with radiotherapy for prostate cancer: A double-blind, randomized trial. Int J Radiat Oncol Biol Phys 60(4): 1088–1097
24. Yeoh EE, Holloway RH, Fraser RJ et al (2004) Anorectal dysfunction increases with time following radiation therapy for carcinoma of the prostate. Am J Gastroenterol 99(2):361–369
25. Bergmark K, Avall-Lundqvist E, Dickman PW et al (2002) Patient-rating of distressful symptoms after treatment for early cervical cancer. Acta Obstet Gynecol Scand 81(5):443–450
26. Yeoh E, Sun WM, Russo A et al (1996) A retrospective study of the effects of pelvic irradiation for gynecological cancer on anorectal function. Int J Radiat Oncol Biol Phys 35(5):1003–1010
27. Fokdal L, Honoré H, Hoyer M, von der Maase H (2005) Dose-volume histograms associated to long-term colorectal functions in patients receiving pelvic radiotherapy. Radiother Oncol 74(2):203–210
28. Gosselink MP, Darby M, Zimmerman DD et al (2005) Long-term follow-up of retrograde colonic irrigation for defaecation disturbances. Colorectal Dis 7:65–69
29. Christensen P, Bazzocchi G, Coggrave M et al (2006) A randomized, controlled trial of transanal irrigation versus conservative bowel management in spinal cord-injured patients. Gastroenterology 131:738–747
30. Christensen P, Olsen N, Krogh K et al (2003) Scintigraphic assessment of retrograde colonic washout in fecal incontinence and constipation. Dis Colon Rectum 46:68–76
31. Iwama T, Imajo M, Yaegashi K, Mishima Y (1989) Self washout method for defecational complaints following low anterior rectal resection. Jpn J Surg 19:251–253
32. Jarrett ME, Mowatt G, Glazener CM et al (2004) Systematic review of sacral nerve stimulation for faecal incontinence and constipation. Br J Surg 91:1559–1569

Double Incontinence

Mauro Cervigni, Albert Mako, Franca Natale

Introduction

Double incontinence (DI) is the concomitant presence of urinary and anal incontinence in the same subject. This condition is widely underreported due to social stigma and embarrassment. In fact, women who suffer from both diseases have greater impairment regarding their physical and psychosocial well-being than do women suffering from isolated urinary incontinence (UI) or fecal incontinence (FI) [1], resulting in social isolation and reduced quality of life [2]. Few studies have evaluated the prevalence of DI. The different results of these studies depend on the method utilized for data collection and on the demographic features of the study population. Table 1 shows the prevalence of DI reported by various authors [3–9].

A significant association between urinary and anal incontinence was found in patients with pelvic floor disorders [adjusted odds ratio (OR) 4.6; 95% confidence interval (CI) 1.9–11.2] [10]. Particularly, this association was found in women with concomitant UI and pelvic organ prolapse (POP) who have a higher incidence of anal incontinence (OR 2.72; 95% CI 1.2–6.1) with respect to patients with UI or POP only [11]. A recent paper found that FI is associated with UI but not with POP [12]. Roberts et al. [6], in a cross-sectional, community-base study, found a 9.4% incidence of DI. Jackson et al. [13] reported 9% of subjects with both symptoms in their study. Other authors found the prevalence of FI in women with UI ranged from 26% to 35% [14, 15]. Lacima et al. [16] reported 80% of stress urinary incontinence (SUI) in women with FI. MacLennan et al. [17] compared the risk of UI and FI in women and men. They showed that for women the risk is 11.7 and 1.6 times greater, respectively, than for men.

Table 1. Prevalence of double incontinence

Authors	Prevalence
Khullar et al. [3]	15%
Gordon et al. [4]	29%
Leroi et al. [5]	29%
Roberts et al. [6]	9.4%
Meschia et al. [7]	20%
Soligo et al. [8]	20%
Griffiths et al. [9]	8.4%

Classification of Incontinence

UI is classified on the basis of the standardization of the International Continence Society [18]. The following can be distinguished:

1. Urodynamic stress incontinence (USI): involuntary leakage of urine during increased abdominal pressure in the absence of a detrusor contraction.
2. Detrusor overactivity (DO): involuntary detrusor contraction during the filling phase that may be spontaneous or provoked and that can cause irritative bladder symptoms such as frequency, urgency, urge incontinence, or nocturia.
3. Mixed incontinence (MI): a combination of both stress and urge incontinence.

Urodynamics is mandatory to make these diagnoses.

There is no such clear classification for FI. In fact, anal incontinence can be divided in two subgroups, distinguished only by clinical features:

1. Urge incontinence: loss of feces due to the inability to suppress an urgency to defecate.
2. Passive incontinence: loss of feces without the patient's awareness.

Several studies show that patients with external sphincter dysfunction have fecal urge incontinence, whereas dysfunction of the internal sphincter causes passive incontinence [19].

It has been clearly demonstrated that the pathophysiology of DI is connected with an alteration of the sphincteric components, but recently, the attention of the authors has also focused on smooth-muscle motility disorders [20]. Moreover, in patients with DI, there is a higher prevalence of posterior vaginal wall descent [8]. It has been established that rectocele may be associated with anal incontinence for many reasons, including complete rectal prolapse and rectoanal intussusception [21]. But it is important to note that the association between rectocele and anal incontinence is more evident in the subgroup with urge FI [8].

Factors Associated with Pelvic Floor Dysfunction

Among the factors regarded as associated with DI, we can mention childbirth-associated external anal sphincter injury, pregnancy, advanced age, menopause, collagen disorders, and some neurological diseases (multiple sclerosis and Parkinson's disease).

Pregnancy has an important association with FI and DI [22]. Davis et al. [23] reported that nearly two out of three women who had third-degree perineal tears at delivery refer with UI and/or FI; meanwhile, Fenner et al. [24] found a higher incidence of FI associated with fourth-degree and perineal laceration. At 2–4 years after delivery, the prevalence of DI in women with obstetric anal sphincter injury was 18% [25].

Pathophysiology of Double Incontinence

Numerous studies suggest a common etiology for the development of UI, FI, and POP. These are due to damage to the muscles and connective tissue of the pelvic floor and to pudendal nerve injury [26, 27]. The presence of crossed reflexes between the bladder, urethra, and anorectum in animal studies could explain the contemporary association of UI and FI [28]. There exist vesicoanal and urethroanal reflex arcs that are probably mediated within the spinal cord. Distention or irritation of the bladder or urethra causes a reflex increase in internal [29] and external sphincter activity [30].

Neuropathic Trauma of the Pudendal Nerve

One of the hypotheses that try to explain the pathophysiological mechanism of DI is neuropathic trauma of the pudendal nerve. Vaginal delivery may cause partial denervation of the pelvic floor in most nulliparous women. In fact, the pudendal nerve terminal motor latency (PNTML) measured 48–72 h after delivery who increases in women delivered vaginally compared with nulliparous women [31]. Different studies have demonstrated that multiparity, forceps delivery, increased duration of the second stage of labor, third-degree perineal tear, and high birth weight are also important factors leading to pudendal nerve damage [32, 33]. A recent paper reported the experience of a Spanish group who tested the hypothesis that pudendal nerve neuropathy was a more frequent lesion in patients with DI compared to patients with isolated FI. They found no statistically significant difference of bilateral or unilateral prolonged PNTML between two groups ($p = 0.3$), so they concluded that pudendal neuropathy is not a distinct characteristic of patients with DI [34].

Parity

It is generally accepted that parity is a strong predictor of pelvic floor damage and in a recent article, vaginal delivery was clearly considered as a risk factor for stress incontinence [35]. Vaginal delivery may initiate damage to the continence mechanism by direct injury to the pelvic floor muscles or damage to their motor innervation or both. Additional denervation may occur with aging, resulting in functional disability many years after the initial trauma. There seem to exist four major mechanisms by which vaginal delivery might contribute to the increased risk of incontinence among women:

1. Injury to connective tissue supports by the mechanical process of vaginal delivery.
2. Vascular damage to the pelvic structures as the result of compression by the presenting part of the fetus during labor.
3. Damage to the pelvic nerves and/or muscles as the result of trauma during parturition.
4. Direct injury during labor and delivery.

The physiological changes produced by pregnancy may make women more susceptible to injury from these pathophysiological processes. Peschers et al. [36] showed that pelvic floor muscle strength is significantly reduced 3–8 days postpartum in women following vaginal birth but not in women after cesarean delivery. Six to 10 weeks later, palpation and vesical-neck elevation on perineal ultrasound do not show any significant differences to antepartum values, whereas intravaginal pressure on perineometry remains significantly lower in primiparas but not in multiparas. Therefore, pelvic floor muscle strength is impaired shortly after vaginal birth but for most women it returns within 2 months. In a few women, this is severe and is associated with UI and FI. For some women, it is likely to be the first step along a path leading to prolapse and/or incontinence.

There is also electromyographic (EMG) evidence of reinnervation in the pelvic floor muscles after vaginal delivery in 80% of women. Mainly, women who have a long, active, second stage of labor and heavier babies show the most EMG evidence of nerve damage [36]. An elevation in perineal body position as well as a decrease in the area of the urogenital hiatus and of the levator hiatus at 2 weeks postpartum suggests a return of normal levator ani geometry after vaginal delivery in most women [37]. Women with three or more deliveries are more likely to have incontinence and excessive pelvic floor descent [38].

Role of Epidural Anesthesia

Regional anesthesia for the relief of labor pain has become more popular over the past 20 years. Some studies suggest that epidural analgesia, by enabling relaxation of the pelvic floor, leads to greater control of delivery of the fetal head and consequently fewer perineal lacerations [39], but prolongation of the second stage of labor may also increase the incidence of pudendal nerve damage [40, 41]. Robinson et al. [42] recently examined the relationship between epidural analgesia and perineal damage and found that the rate of significant perineal injury was higher with epidural analgesia (16.1%) than with increased use of operative intervention.

Episiotomy

Episiotomy is a widely performed intervention in childbirth despite equivocal scientific evidence might regarding its benefit. Routine episiotomy avoid spontaneous uncontrolled tears and long-term relaxation of the pelvic floor, but these advantages are difficult to substantiate. There is a widespread assumption that it may do more harm than good [43]. In fact, there is no evidence that either first- or second-degree perineal tears cause long-term consequences [44]. Moreover, a growing body of evidence suggests that episiotomy offers no protection against third- and forth-degree tears, which are associated with adverse sequelae. An overview by Myers-Helfgott and Helfgott [45] emphasized the absence of scientific evidence to support a role for liberal elective episiotomy in the reduction of third-degree lacerations during childbirth. Indeed, several reports have implicated routine episiotomy in the genesis of major perineal and anal sphincter tears, even after checking for confounding variables [46]. In particular, midline episiotomy is associated with significantly higher rates of third- and fourth-degree perineal tears than are mediolateral episiotomies [47]. Therefore, midline episiotomy is not considered effective in protecting the perineum and sphincters during childbirth and may impair anal continence [48]. Coats et al. [49] in a randomized controlled trial of 407 women, found that with midline episiotomy, 11.6% of patients experienced lacerations of the anal canal versus 2% who experienced these complications in association with mediolateral episiotomies. This association was compounded when instrumental delivery was employed, with anal sphincter injury rates of 50% reported with the use of midline episiotomy and forceps. Therefore, midline episiotomy is not effective in protecting the perineum and sphincters during childbirth and should be restricted to specified fetal-maternal indications [50, 51]. In spite of these data, midline episiotomy is still bewilderingly widespread, presumably because it is perceived to heal better and cause less postnatal discomfort. Policies of restrictive episiotomy appear to have a number of benefits compared with routine episiotomy. There was less posterior perineal trauma, less suturing, fewer complications, and no difference for most pain measures and severe vaginal or perineal trauma, although there was an increased risk of anterior perineal trauma with restrictive episiotomy [52, 53].

Women who have episiotomies have a higher risk of FI at 3 and 6 months postpartum compared with women with an intact perineum. Compared with women with a spontaneous laceration, episiotomy triples the risk of FI at 3 months and 6 months postpartum and doubles the risk of flatus incontinence at 3 months and 6 months postpartum. A nonextending episiotomy (second-degree surgical incision) triples the risk of FI and doubles the risk of flatus incontinence postpartum compared with women who have a second-degree spontaneous tear.

Obstetric Injury

Obstetric injury is one of the most important causes of FI and DI. After instrumental extraction, the risk for anal incontinence is multiplied from 1.94 to 7.2 times [54, 55]. However, few randomized control trials evaluate functional signs after instrumental extraction. Johanson et al. [56] found no significant differences regarding anal and UI 5 years postpartum (forceps vs. vacuum). MacArthur et al. [57] found that the use of forceps was associated with an increased risk for anal incontinence 10 months postpartum and with 4% of new anal incontinence.

Forceps

Anal incontinence seems to occur more frequently after forceps than after spontaneous delivery. Sultan et al. [58] demonstrated that forceps delivery was associated with significantly more damage to the anal sphincter. Numerous retrospective studies demonstrated that forceps is an independent risk factor for sphincter damage [59–61]. On the contrary, two prospective studies found no correlation between sphincteric injury and the use of forceps [62, 63]. In a recent study, forceps was not considered and independent risk factor, confounding for heavier babies and mediolateral episiotomy [64].

Vacuum

Tetzschner et al. [25] found that vacuum deliveries were associated with an increased risk for prolongation of PNTML and the development of UI. Postpartum pudendal neuropathy returned to normal in more than one half of women within 8 weeks postpartum; however, multiparous women show a greater tendency toward more severe and permanent nerve injury when compared with nulliparous women [65]. This could be only the first step that later may lead to incontinence or POP. Fornell et al. [66] found a lower risk of UI after vacuum extraction, and they postulated that the downward traction in a correctly performed vacuum extraction could possibly protect the anterior vaginal wall and increase the risk of anal sphincter rupture. On the contrary, the risk of anal sphincter rupture was low in vaginal delivery [67].

Chronic Straining

Chronic straining is well known to cause perineal descent. Stretch injury to the pudendal nerve that happens with perineal descent is associated with prolonged terminal motor latencies [68], both in the pudendal nerve and its perineal branch, which innervates the urethra [69]. Denervation is associated with an increase in fiber density of the external anal sphincter [70] that has been shown to occur in women with stress UI as well [71].

Hysterectomy

Hysterectomy seems to be associated with incontinence and defecation by digitation due to pelvic nerve injury [72, 73].

Chronic Bronchitis

Chronic bronchitis shows a strong link with FI and UI, and it may weaken the pelvic floor through denervation of connective tissue and of musculature [74].

Instrumental Delivery and Cesarean Section in the Second Stage of Labor

Although the majority of women have a spontaneous vaginal delivery, a significant proportion fails to progress in the second stage of labor. Therefore, it is necessary to choose between a potentially difficult instrumental vaginal delivery and cesarean section at full dilatation, each with inherent risks. Liebling et al. compared two groups of women: in the first group, a cesarean section at full dilatation was performed; the women of the second group underwent an instrumental delivery. This study demonstrated that cesarean section appears to offer some protection against urinary tract morbidity but less than elective cesarean section. Probably this is due to neuronal damage that occurred when the woman reached full dilatation [75].

Connective Tissue Disease

Connective tissue disease has been suggested as a possible cause of DI. In fact, benign joint hypermobility disease may cause increased perineal descent, which may lead to pudendal neuropathy and consequently to UI and FI [76].

Role of Smooth Visceral Motility Disorders

It has been demonstrated that women with lower urinary tract dysfunction suffer more frequently from bowel disorders than does the general female population [3, 4]. There are important correlations between irritable bowel syndrome and postpartum anal incontinence. UI is the greatest risk factor for FI, followed by loss of ability to perform daily activities, tube feeding, physical restraints, diarrhea, dementia, impaired vision, and constipation [77]. Various papers have demonstrated that detrusor overactivity is associated more frequently with anal incontinence with respect to SUI [3], and this is true particularly for women who complain of anal urgency and anal urge incontinence. Soligo et al. [8] found that women with anal urge incontinence showed a higher score for UI on the visual analog scale (VAS) and a higher frequency of urodynamic detrusor overactivity with respect to women with passive anal incontinence. This subgroup also complained of concomitant disorders of colonic motility. These findings suggest a role of a common visceral motility disorder in DI.

To clarify the role of visceral motility in the development of urge anal incontinence, the use of pancolonic manometry was suggested. Herbst et al. [78], utilizing this exam, found high-pressure colic waves in three women with urge incontinence. They concluded that these high-pressure waves, identical to those occurring in healthy subjects, could cause incontinence only in the presence of an impaired sphincter response. Shafik et al. [79], utilizing rectometrography, postulated that uninhibited rectum might be a cause of FI in patients with normal anal pressure and sphincteric mechanism. They concluded that the rectum did not adapt, as in the control group, to the distension, but responded with contraction. Therefore, FI in these patients appears to be a consequence of the unstable or uninhibited rectum. These data support the hypothesis that an impaired function of smooth visceral muscles could be one reason for the development of DI in the group with urge urinary and anal incontinence.

Instrumental Evaluation

Urodynamic evaluation of the urinary tract is essential to differentiate stress and detrusor activity as the cause of incontinence. Anal manometry and endoanal three-dimensional (3D) ultrasound are the baseline test evaluations for FI. Pudendal nerve terminal evaluation and proctography are performed as needed. Magnetic resonance imaging (MRI) has been used for studying the pelvic floor anatomy in normal and problematic women. MRI detected more levator hernias, although the clinical significance remains unclear [80]. The International Consultation on Incontinence (ICI) considers MRI as not indicated for the routine evaluation of UI or pelvic prolapse [81].

Treatment

Pelvic floor muscle training (PFMT) practiced during pregnancy has proven protective effect against the development of UI. Nulliparous women who received PFMT at 20 weeks gestation were significantly less likely to have UI at 6 weeks and 6 months postpartum [82]. At 10 months postpartum, UI incidence decreased in 19% of women who received PFMT compared with 2% in the control group [83]. However, in a Cochrane Review, there were no sufficient data to determine the effect of physical therapies in preventing UI during pregnancy [84]. PFMT is an effective therapy for the treatment of UI and FI [85, 86]. Electrical stimulation and biofeedback are other well-established conservative treatments. A randomized controlled study shows a significant improvement in anal continence in women who had electrical stimulation compared with PFMT and biofeedback [87].

The choice of surgical technique depends on the type of UI. In women with SUI and anal sphincter defects, a midurethral sling or colposuspension and a sphincteroplasty can be performed concomitantly. Ross et al. [88] reported 46 cases of combined overlapping sphincteroplasty and laparoscopic colposuspension with 89% cure of UI and 82% of FI at 1-year follow-up.

Sacral nerve neuromodulation (SNM) acts by stimulating the S3 sacral nerve roots using an implanted electrode. SNM is effective in the treatment of both urge UI [89] and FI [90].

Artificial sphincter and bulking agents have been used with poor results for the treatment of DI.

References

1. Fialkow MF, Melville JL, Lentz GM et al (2003) The functional and psychosocial impact of faecal incontinence in women with urinary incontinence. Am J Obstet Gynecol 189:127–129
2. Sailer M, Bussen D, Debus ES et al (1998) Quality of life in patients with benign anorectal disorders. Br J Surg 85:1716–1719
3. Khullar V, Damiano R, Toozs-Hobson P, Cardozo L (1998) Prevalence of urinary incontinence among women with urinary incontinence. BJOG 105:1211–1213
4. Gordon D, Groutz A, Goldman G et al (1999) Anal incontinence: prevalence among female patients attending a urogynecologic clinic. Neurourol Urodyn 18:199–204
5. Leroi AM, Weber J, Menard et al (1999) Prevalence of anal incontinence in 409 patients investigated for stress urinary incontinence. Neurourol Urodyn 18:579–590
6. Roberts RO, Jacobsen SJ, Reilly WT et al (1999) Prevalence of combined fecal and urinary incontinence: a Community based study. J Am Geriart Soc 47:837–841
7. Meschia M, Buonaguidi A, Pifarotti P et al (2002) Prevalence of anal incontinence in women with symptoms of urinary incontinence and genital prolapse. Obstet Gynecol 100:719–723
8. Soligo M, Salvatore S, Milani R et al (2003) Double incontinence in urogynecologic practice: a new insight. Am J Obstet Gynecol 189:438–443
9. Griffiths AN, Makam A, Edwards GJ (2006) Should we actively screen for urinary and anal incontinence in the general gynecology outpatients setting? J Obstet Gynecol 26:442–444
10. Jackson SL, Weber AM, Hull TL et al (1997) Fecal incontinence in women with urinary incontinence and pelvic organ prolapse. Obstet Gynecol 89:423–427
11. Nichols CM, Gill EJ, Nguyen T et al (2004) Anal sphincter injury in women with pelvic floor disorders. Obstet Gynecol 104:690–696
12. Jelovsek JE, Barber MD, Paraiso MFR, Walters MD (2005) Functional bowel and anorectal disorders in patients with pelvic organ prolapse and incontinence. Obstet Gynecol 193:2105–2111

13. Jackson SL, Weber A, Hull TL et al (1997) Fecal incontinence in women with urinary incontinence and pelvic organ prolapse. Obstet Gynecol 89:423–427
14. Caputo RM, Benson JT (1992) Idiopathic fecal incontinence. Curr Opin Obstet Gynecol 4:565–570
15. Snooks SJ, Barnes PRH, Swash M (1984) Damage to the innervation of the voluntary anal and periurethral sphincter musculature in incontinence: An electrophysiological study. J Neurol Neurosurg Psychiatry 47:1269–1273
16. Lacima G, Espuna M, Pera M et al (2002) Clinical, urodynamic, and manometric findings in women with combined urinary and fecal incontinence. Neurourol Urodyn 21:464–469
17. MacLennan AH, Taylor AW, Wilson DH, Wilson D (2000) The prevalence of pelvic floor disorders and their relationship to gender, age, parity, and mode of delivery. Br J Obstet Gynaecol 107:1460–1470
18. Abrams P, Cardozo L, Fall M et al (2002) The standardization of terminology of the lower urinary tract function: report from the standardization sub-committee of the International Continence Society. Neurourol Urodyn 21:167–178
19. Engel AF, Kamm MA, Bartram CI, Nicholls RJ (1995) Relationship of symptoms in faecal incontinence to specific sphincter abnormalities. Int J Colorect Dis 10:152–155
20. Manning J, Eyers AA, Korda A et al (2001) Is there an association between fecal incontinence and lower urinary tract dysfunction? Dis Colon Rectum 44:790–798
21. Marti MC, Roche B, Deleaval J (1999) Rectocele: value of video defecography in section of treatment policy. Colorectal Dis 1:324–329
22. Nelson RL (2004) Epidemiology of faecal incontinence, advancing in treatment of faecal and urinary incontinence through research, trial design, outcome measures and research priorities. Gastroenterology 126:S175–S179
23. Davis K, Kumar D, Stanton SL et al (2003) Symptoms and anal sphincter morphology following primary repair of third-degrees tears. Br J Surg 90:1573–1579
24. Fenner DE, Genberg B, Brahna P et al (2003) Fecal and urinary incontinence after vaginal delivery with anal sphincter disruption in an obstetrics unit in the United States. Am J Obstet Gynecol 189:1543–1550
25. Tetzschner T, Sorensen M, Lose G, Christiansen J (1996) Anal and urinary incontinence in women with obstetric anal sphincter rupture Br J Obstet Gynaecol 105:1211–1213
26. Kiff ES, Swash M (1984) Slowed conduction in pudendal nerves in idiopathic faecal incontinentce. Br J Surg 71:614–616
27. Womack NR, Morrison JFB, Williams NS (1989) The role of pudendal nerve damage in the aetiology of idiopathic faecal incontinence. Br J Surg 96:29–32
28. Bouvier M, Grimaud JC, Salducci J, Gonella J (1984) Role of vesical afferent nerve fibres involved in the control of internal anal sphincter motility. J Auton Nerv Syst 10:243–245
29. Bouvier M, Grimaud JC (1984) Neuronally mediated interaction between urinary bladder and anal sphincter motility in cat. J Physiol 346:461–469
30. Thor KB, Muhlhauser MA (1999) Vesicoanal, urethroanal, and urethrovesical reflexes initiated by lower urinary tract irritation in the rat. Am J Physiol 277:R1002–R1012
31. Jorge JMH, Wexner SD (1993) Etiology and management of faecal incontinence. Dis Colon Rectum 36:77–97
32. Snooks SJ, Swash M, Henry MM, Setchel M (1986) Risk factors in childbirth causing damage to the pelvic floor innervation. Int J Colorectal Disease 1:20–24
33. Handa VI, Harris TA, Ostegard DR (1996) Protecting the pelvic floor: obstetric management to prevent incontinence and pelvic floor prolapse. Obstet Gynecol 88:470–478
34. Lacima G, Pera M, Valls-Sole J et al (2006) Electrophysiologic study and clinical findings in females with combined fecal and urinary incontinence: a prospective study. Dis Colon Rectum 49:353–359
35. Rortveit G, Daltveit AK, Hannestad YS et al (2003) Urinary incontinence after vaginal delivery or caesarean section. N Engl J Med 348:900–907
36. Peschers UM, Schaer GN, DeLancey JO, Schuessler B (1997) Levator ani function before and after childbirth. Br J Obstet Gynaecol 104:1004–1008
37. Tunn R, DeLancey JO, Howard D et al (1999) MR imaging of levator ani muscle recovery following vaginal delivery. Int Urogynecol J Plevic Floor Dysfunct 10:300–307
38. King J, Freeman R (1998) Is antenatal bladder neck mobility a risk factor for postpartum stress incontinence? Br J Obstet Genaecol 105:1300–1307
39. Abtibol MM (1997) Birth and human evolution: anatomical and obstetrical mechanism in primates. Bergin and Gravey, Westport
40. Rortveit G, Daltveit AK, Hannestad YS, Hunskaar S (2003) Vaginal delivery parameters and urinary incontinence: the Norwegian EPINCONT study. Am J Obstet Gynecol 189:1268–1274
41. Moerman ML (1982) Growth of the birth canal in adolescent girls. Am J Obstet Gynecol 143:528–532
42. Robinson JN, Norwitz ER, McElrath TF, Lieberman ES (1999) Epidural analgesia and third- or fourth-degree lacerations in nulliparas. Obstet Gynecol 94:259–262
43. Persson J, Wolner HP, Rydhstroem H (2000) Obstetric risk factors of for stress urinary incontintnce: a a population-based study. Obstet Gynecol 96:440–445
44. Stanton SL, Kerr-Wilson RR, Harris VG (1980) The incidence of urological symptoms in normal pregnancy. Br Jobstet Gynaecol 87:897–900
45. Myers-Helfgott MG, Helfgott AW (1999) Routine use of episiotomy in modern obstetrics. Should it be performed? Obstet Gynecol Clin North Am 26:305–325
46. Francis WJA (1960) The onset of stress incontinence. J Obstet Gynecol Br Emp 899–890
47. Viktup L, Lose G, Rolff M, Barfoed K (1992) The symptoms of stress incontinence caused by pregnancy or delivery in primiparas. Obstet Gynecol 79:945–949
48. Signorello LB, Harlow BL, Chekos, AK, Repke, JT (2000) Midline episiotomy and anal incontinence: retrospective cohort study. BMJ 320:86–90
49. Coats PM, Chan KK, Wilkins M, Beard RJ (1980) A comparison between midline and mediolateral episiotomies. Br J Obstet Gynaecol 87:408–412
50. Chaliha C, Sultan AH (2000) Midline episiotomy and anal incontinence. Training is needed in the recogni-

tion and repair of perineal trauma. BMJ 320:1601
51. Mills MS, Murphy DJ (2000) Midline episiotomy and anal incontinence. Results should be interpreted with caution in British context. BMJ 320:1601–1602
52. Carroli G, Belizan J (1999) Episiotomy for vaginal birth. Birth 26:263
53. Angioli R, Gomez-Marin O, Cantuaria G et al (2000) Severe perineal lacerations during vaginal delivery: the University of Miami experience. Am J Obstet Gynecol 182:1083–1085
54. MacArthur C, Glazener CM, Wilson PD (2001) Obstetric practice and faecal incontinence three months after delivery. BJOG 108:678–683
55. Donnely V, Fynes M, Campbell D et al (1998) Obstetrics events leading to anal sphincter damage. Obstet Gynecol 92:955–961
56. Johanson RB, Heycock E, Carter J et al (1999) Maternal and child health care after assisted vaginal delivery: five-years follow-up of a randomized controlled study comparing forceps and ventouse. Br J Obstet Gynaecol 106:544–549
57. MacArthur C, Bick DE, Keighley MR (1997) Faecal incontinence after childbirth. Br J Obstet Gynaecol 104:46–50
58. Sultan AH, Kamm MA, Hudson CN, Bartam CI (1993) Anal sphincter disruption during vaginal delivery. N Engl J Med 329:1905–1911
59. De Leeuw JW, Struijk PC, Vierhout ME et al (2001) Risk factors for third degree perineal ruptures during delivery. BJOG 108:383–387
60. Riskin-Mashiah S, O'Brian S, Wilkins IA (2002) Risk factors for severe perineal tear: can we do better? Am J Peinatol 19:225–234
61. Richter HE, Brumfield CG, Cliver SP et al (2002) Risk factor associated with anal sphincter treat: a comparison of primiparous patients, vaginal birth after caesarean deliveries, and patients with previous vaginal delivery. Am J Obstet Gynecol 187:1194–1198
62. Zetterstrom J, Lopez AM, Anzen Bo et al (1999) Anal sphincter tears at vaginal delivery: risk factor and clinical outcome of primary repair. Obstet Gynecol 94:21–28
63. Shiono P, Klebanoff MA, Carey JC (1990) Midline episiotomies: more harm than good? Obstet Gynecol 75:765–770
64. Andrews V, Sultan AH, Thakar R, Jones PW (2006) Risk factors for obstetric anal sphincter injury: a prospective study. Birth 32 (2):117–122
65. Jorge JMH, Wexner SD (1993) Etiology and management of faecal incontinence. Dis Colon Rectum 36.77–97
66. Fornell EU, Wingren G, Kiolhede P (2004) Factors associated with pelvic floor dysfunction with emphasis on urinary and fecal incontinence and genital prolapse: an epidemiological study. Acta Obstet Gynecol Scand 83:383–389
67. Fornell EK, Berg G, Halbook O et al (1996) Clinical consequences of anal sphincter rupture during vaginal delivery. J Am Coll Surg 183:553–558
68. Ho YH, Goh HS (1995) The neurophysiological significance of perineal descent. Int J Colorectal Dis 10:107–111
69. Amarenco G, Kerdraon J, Lanoe Y (1990) Perineal neuropathy due to stretching and urinary incontinence. Physiopathology, diagnosis and therapeutic implications. Ann Urol 24:463–466
70. Aanestad O, Flink R (1999) Urinary stress incontinence. A urodynamic and quantitative electromyographic study of perineal muscle. Acta Obstet Gynecol Scand 78:245–253
71. Anderson RS (1984) A neurogenic element to urinary genuine stress incontinence Br J Obstet Gynaecol 9:41–45
72. Thom DH, Brown JS (1998) Reproductive and hormonal risk factors for urinary incontinence in later life: a review of the clinical and epidemiologic literature. J Am Geriatr Soc 46:1411–1417
73. Parys BT, Woolfenden KA, Parsopns KF (1990) Baldder dysfunction after simple hysterectomy: urodynamic and neurological evaluation. Eur Urol 17:129–133
74. Uustal Fornell E, Wingren G, Kjolhede P (2004) Factors associated with pelvic floor dysfunction with emphasis on urinary and fecal incontinence and genital prolapse: an epidemiological study. Acta Obstet Gynecol Scand 83:383–389
75. Liebling RE, Swingler R, Patel R et al (2004) Pelvic floor morbidity up to one year after difficult instrumental delivery and a cesarean section in the second stage of labor: a cohort study. Am J Obstet Gynecol 191:4–10
76. Jha S, Arunkalaivanan AS, Situnayake RD (2006) Prevalence of incontinence in women with benign joint hypermobility syndrome. Int Urogynecol J Pelvic Floor Dysfunct 18(1):61–64
77. Lal M, MannCH, Callender R, Radley S (2003) Does Caesarean delivery prevent anal incontinence? Obstet Gynecol 89:61–66
78. Herbst F, Kamm MA, Morris GP et al (1997) Gastrointestinal transit and prolonged ambulatory colonic motility in health and faecal incontinence. Gut 41:381–389
79. Shafik A, Ahmed A (2001) The "uninhibited rectum": a cause of fecal incontinence. J Spinal Cord Med 24:159–163
80. Kauffman HS, Buller JL, Thompson JR et al (2001) Dynamic pelvic MR imaging and cystocolpoproctography alter surgical management of pelvic floor disorders. Dis Colon Rectum 44:1575–1583
81. Tubaro A, Artibani W, Bartram C et al (2005) Imaging and other investigations. In: Abrams P, Cardoza L, Khoury S, Wein A (eds) Incontinence: 3rd International Consultation on Incontinence. Plymouth, UK: Health Publication, pp 1397–98
82. Sampselle CM, Miller JM, Mims BM et al (1998) Effect of pelvic muscle exercise on transient incontinence during pregnancy and after birth. Obstet Gynecol 91:406–412
83. Meyer S, Hohlfield H, Achtari C, De Grandi P (2001) Pelvic floor education after vaginal delivery. Obstet Gynecol 97:673–677
84. Hay-Smith J, Herbison P, Morkved S (2003) Physical therapies for prevention of urinary and faecal incontinence in adult. In: Cochrane Library, Issue 4 Chichester UK: John Wiley and Sons
85. Berghmans LC, Hendrics HJ, Bo K et al (1998) Conser-

vative treatment of stress urinary incontinence: a systematic review of randomised clinical trial. Br J Urol 82:181–191
86. Enck P (1993) Biofeedback training in disordered defecation: a critical review. Dig Dis Sci 11:1953–1960
87. Fynes MM, Marshall K, Cassidy M et al (1999) A prospective randomised study comparing the effect of augmented biofeedback with sensory biofeedback alone on faecal incontinence after obstetric trauma. Dis Colon Rectum 42:753–761
88. Ross JW (2001) Laparoscopic Burch colposuspension and overlapping sphincteroplasty for double incontinence. JSLS 5:203–209
89. Latini JM, Alipour M, Kreder KJ (2006) Efficacy of sacral neuromodulation for symptomatic treatment of refractory urinary urge incontinence. Urology 67:550–553
90. Jarrett M (2004) Sacral nerve neuromodulation and fecal incontinence: indications, technique, and results. Minim Invasive Ther Allied Technol 13:230–236

Invited Commentary

Marco Soligo

Double incontinence (DI) is a very peculiar condition both in its pathogenesis and in its clinical presentation and treatment options. The chapter from Mauro Cervigni et al. clearly describes these controversial aspects and draws a clear picture of the condition. It is therefore very difficult to add any comment to it. I will thus approach the problem from a different perspective, i.e. from an everyday clinical basis.

From a practical point of view, what strikes me most about DI is the gap between the figures in epidemiological studies and the actual number of patients coming to our attention with a clinically relevant disorder. In fact, estimates of DI in urogynaecological settings average 20%, as shown in Table 1 of the chapter [1–7]. However, it must be said that these data result from a systematic bowel investigation in urogynaecological patients. Actually, we do not know how many symptomatic women within that group are really bothered by their symptoms.

In 2000, we presented our data aimed at identifying the self-reporting rate of anal symptoms in a urogynaecological setting. In a group of 167 consecutive women, an anal incontinence rate of 19.8% was observed. Only three (9.1%) of the 33 symptomatic women spontaneously complained of this symptom during the consultation [8]. How, then, can this be explained? The following are some possible answers:

- The anal symptom is really mild and the patient does not perceive it as a problem.
- The patient is embarrassed and reluctant to talk about anal disorder to anybody.
- The patient does not perceive the urogynaecologist as being the right person to talk to about anal dysfunctions.

Whatever the answer, the key point is to establish the epidemiology of clinically relevant DI. The literature available on this is very scarce, and further research is advisable. In the absence of clear data, the perception of a practising clinician is that survey studies overestimate the size of the problem. This perception is particularly true when the problem of anal incontinence is debated in an obstetrical setting. Generally speaking, obstetricians consider the problem to be much less frequent than data would imply. Why is this so? Once again, we can only make hypotheses:

- Obstetricians are not used to routinely investigating these aspects in their patients.
- Very few patients have a bothersome disorder.
- In many cases, the dysfunction begins many years after delivery, and obstetricians therefore miss the opportunity to see it.

So it is probably true that clinically evident anal incontinence after delivery is a rare finding.

However obstetricians only see the "tip of the iceberg". In fact, a damaged pelvic floor can develop a functional compensation, thus resulting in a symptom-free woman. Nevertheless, that woman is at higher risk for anal incontinence as a consequence of subsequent deliveries [9] and of aging. It is well known that DI represents a problem mainly in the elderly patient. Compared with women with only urinary incontinence, women with DI are significantly older (59.16±10.37 years vs. 55.8±12.28 years; $p= 0.013$) [7]. Even if obstetricians only see the tip of the iceberg, this is nevertheless a major health problem because of its great impact on quality of life, as we are referring to young, active, otherwise healthy women whose social life is severely restricted as a consequence of the disorder.

The authors of the chapter clearly emphasise the fact that obstetric injury can be considered the primary aetiological factor for DI. This should be taken into account when giving advice to symptomatic women with regard to further pregnancies and when policies for follow-up in puerperium need to be designed.

References

1. Khullar V, Damiano R, Toozs-Hobson P, Cardozo L (1998) Prevalence of urinary incontinence among women with urinary incontinence. BJOG 105:1211–1213
2. Gordon D, Groutz A, Goldman G et al (1999) Anal incontinence: prevalence among female patients attending a urogynecologic clinic. Neurourol Urodyn 18:199–204

3. Leroi AM, Weber J, Menard et al (1999) Prevalence of anal incontinence in 409 patients investigated for stress urinary incontinence. Neurourol Urodyn 18:579–590
4. Roberts RO, Jacobsen SJ, Reilly WT et al (1999) Prevalence of combined fecal and urinary incontinence: a community-based study. J Am Geriart Soc 47:837–841
5. Meschia M, Buonaguidi A, Pifarotti P et al (2002) Prevalence of anal incontinence in women with symptoms of urinary incontinence and genital prolapse. Obstet Gynecol 100:719–723
6. Soligo M, Salvatore S, Milani R et al (2003) Double incontinence in urogynecologic practice: a new insight. Am J Obstet Gynecol 189:438–443
7. Griffiths AN, Makam A, Edwards GJ (2006) Should we actively screen for urinary and anal incontinence in the general gynecology outpatients setting? J Obstet Gynecol 26:442–444
8. Soligo M, Salvatore S, Lalia M et al (2000) Self-reporting bowel symptoms during urogynaecological assessment. 30th International Continence Society Annual Meeting, Tampere, Finland 28–31 August 2000, p 340
9. Fynes M, Donnelly V, Behan M et al (1999) Effect of second vaginal delivery on anorectal physiology and faecal continence: a prospective study. Lancet 354(9183):983–986

36

Pediatric Fecal Incontinence

Marc A. Levitt, Richard A. Falcone Jr., Alberto Peña

Introduction

Fecal incontinence represents a devastating problem for all those who suffer from it. It often prevents a person from becoming socially accepted, which in turn provokes serious psychological sequelae. It is a problem that impacts more children than previously thought, affecting those born with anorectal malformations and Hirschsprung's disease as well as children with spinal cord problems or spinal injuries.

True fecal incontinence must be distinguished from overflow pseudoincontinence. Pediatric patients with true fecal incontinence include some surgical patients with anorectal malformations and Hirschsprung's disease and patient with spinal problems, either congenital or acquired. Those with pseudoincontinence are patients with potential for bowel control but who suffer from overflow or encopresis related to severe constipation.

Most patients who undergo an anorectal malformation repair suffer from some degree of functional defecation disorder, and all suffer from an abnormality in their fecal continence mechanism. Approximately 25% of patients are deficient enough in these mechanisms that they are fecally incontinent and cannot have a voluntary bowel movement. The others are capable of having voluntary bowel movements but may require treatment of an underlying dysmotility disorder, which manifests as constipation [1]. A small yet significant number of patients with Hirschsprung's disease (<5%) suffer from fecal incontinence. Patients with spinal problems or injuries can lack the capacity for voluntary bowel movements or have this ability only to varying degrees.

Patients with true fecal incontinence require an artificial method to keep them clean and in normal underwear, a regimen termed bowel management. Patients with pseudoincontinence require proper treatment of constipation. Understanding this major differentiation is the key to deciding on correct management.

Continence Mechanism

Fecal continence depends on three main factors: voluntary sphincter muscles, anal canal sensation, and colonic motility [1].

Voluntary Muscle Structures

In the normal patient, voluntary muscle structures are represented by the levators, the muscle complex, and the external sphincter. Normally, they are used only for brief periods when the rectal fecal mass reaches the anorectal area, pushed by the involuntary peristaltic contraction of rectosigmoid motility. This voluntary contraction occurs only in the minutes prior to defecation, and these muscles are used only occasionally during the rest of the day and night.

Patients with anorectal malformations have abnormal voluntary striated muscles with different degrees of hypodevelopment. Patients with spinal problems or injuries can have varying degrees of sphincter dysfunction. Voluntary muscles can be used only when the patient has the sensation that it is necessary to use them. To appreciate that sensation, the patient needs information that can only be derived from an intact anal sensory mechanism, a mechanism that many patients with anorectal malformations and spinal problems lack.

Anal Canal

Exquisite sensation in normal individuals resides in the anal canal. Except for patients with rectal atresia, most patients with anorectal malformations are born without an anal canal; therefore, sensation does not exist or is rudimentary. Patients with Hirschsprung's disease are born with a normal anal canal, but this can be injured if not meticulously preserved at the time of their colonic pull through. Patients with perineal trauma may have an injured or destroyed anal canal.

It seems that patients can perceive distention of the rectum, but this requires a rectum that has been properly located within the muscle structures, a surgical point quite important for patients undergoing pull-through procedures for an imperforate anus. This sensation seems to be a consequence of voluntary muscle stretching (proprioception). The most important clinical implication of this situation is that the patient may not feel liquid stool or soft fecal material, as it does not distend the rectum. Thus, to achieve some degree of sensation and bowel control, the patient must have the capacity to form solid stool. This point is quite relevant in children with ulcerative colitis who have undergone an ileoanal pull through. They may suffer from varying degrees of incontinence due to the incapacity to form solid stool. In the majority of cases, normal sphincter muscles and anal canal allow them to overcome this problem.

Bowel Motility

Perhaps the most important factor in fecal continence is bowel motility; however, its impact has been largely underestimated. In a normal individual, the rectosigmoid remains quiet for variable periods (1 to several days), depending on specific defecation habits. During that time, sensation and voluntary muscle structures are almost not necessary because the stool, if it is solid, remains inside the colon. The patient feels the peristaltic contraction of the rectosigmoid that occurs prior to defecation. The normal individual can voluntarily relax the striated muscles, which allows the rectal contents to migrate down into the highly sensitive area of the anal canal. There, the anal canal provides accurate information concerning stool consistency and quality. The voluntary muscles are used to push the rectal contents back up into the rectosigmoid and to hold them until the appropriate time for evacuation. At the time of defecation, the voluntary muscle structures relax.

The main factor that provokes rectosigmoid emptying is a massive involuntary peristaltic contraction sometimes helped by a Valsalva maneuver. Most patients with an anorectal malformation suffer from a disturbance of this sophisticated bowel motility mechanism. Patients who have undergone a posterior sagittal anorectoplasty or any other type of sacroperineal approach, in which the most distal part of the bowel was preserved, show evidence of an overefficient bowel reservoir (megarectum). The main clinical manifestation of this is constipation, which seems to be more severe in patients with lower defects [2]. Constipation that is not aggressively treated, in combination with an ectatic distended colon, eventually leads to severe constipation, and a vicious cycle ensues, with worsening constipation leading to more rectosigmoid dilation, leading to worse constipation. The enormously dilated rectosigmoid, with normal ganglion cells, behaves like a myopathic type of hypomotile colon [1].

Patients with anorectal malformation treated with techniques in which the most distal part of the bowel was resected behave clinically as individuals without a rectal reservoir. This is a situation equivalent to a perineal colostomy. Depending on the amount of colon resected, the patient may have loose stools. In these cases, medical management consisting of enemas plus a constipating diet and medications to slow down colonic motility is indicated. Patients with Hirschsprung's disease have undergone distal aganglionic colon resection, but it is their normal anal canal and sphincter mechanism that allows the vast majority of them to be continent despite the lack of a rectal reservoir. Amazingly, some patients with an injured anal canal and sphincters (perineal trauma) can be continent if their motility is normal, and the regular contraction of the rectosigmoid can be translated into a successful voluntary bowel movement.

True Fecal Incontinence

For patients with true fecal incontinence, the ideal treatment approach is a bowel management program consisting of teaching the patient and his or her parents how to clean the colon once daily so it stays completely clean for 24 h. This is achieved by keeping the colon quiet between enemas. These patients cannot have voluntary bowel movements and require an artificial mechanism to empty their colon: a daily enema. The program, although simplistic, is implemented by trial and error over a period of 1 week. The patient is seen by the physician each day, and an abdominal X-ray is taken so that the patient can be monitored on a daily basis for the amount and location of any stool left in the colon. Presence of stool in the underwear is also noted. The decision as to whether enema type and/or quality should be modified, as well as changes in diet and/or medication, can be made daily [3].

Which Pediatric Patients have True Fecal Incontinence?

In children with anorectal malformations, 75% who have undergone a correct and successful operation have voluntary bowel movements after the age of 3 years [2]. About half of these patients soil their underwear on occasion. Those episodes of soiling are usually related to constipation. When the constipation is properly treated, soiling frequently disappears. Thus, approximately 40% of all children with anorectal malformations have voluntary bowel movements and no soiling. In other words, they behave like normal children. Children with good bowel control still may suffer from temporary episodes of fecal incontinence, especially when they experience severe diarrhea.

Some 25% of all children suffer from real fecal incontinence, and they are the patients who need bowel management to keep them clean. As noted, certain patients with Hirschsprung's disease and those with spinal problems can suffer from true fecal incontinence. For these patients, similar principles of bowel management that have proven effective in treating patients with anorectal malformations [3] can be applied.

For children with anorectal malformations, the surgeon should be able to predict which ones may have a good functional prognosis and which ones may have a poor prognosis. Table 1 shows the most common indicators of good and poor prognoses. After the main repair and colostomy closure, it is possible to establish the functional prognosis (Table 2). Parents must be informed of their child's realistic chances for bowel control, thus avoiding needless frustration later. It is imperative to establish the functional prognosis of each child as early as possible, which sometimes is possible even in the newborn period, to avoid creating false expectations for the parents.

Once diagnosis of the specific anorectal defect is established, functional prognosis can be predicted. If the child's defect is of a type associated with good prognosis–such as a vestibular fistula, perineal fistula, rectal atresia, rectourethral bulbar fistula, or imperforate anus with no fistula–the child can be expected to have voluntary bowel movements by the age of 3 years. These children will still need supervision to avoid fecal impaction, constipation, and soiling.

If the child's defect is of the type associated with a poor prognosis–for example, a very high cloaca with a common channel longer than 3 cm, a recto-bladder-neck fistula, or if they have a very hypodeveloped sacrum–parents must understand that their child will most likely need a bowel management program to remain clean. This program should be implemented when the child is 3–4 years of age, before starting school. Children with rectoprostatic fistulas have an almost 50-50 chance of having voluntary bowel movements or of being incontinent. In these children, an attempt should be made to achieve toilet training by the age of 3 years. If this proves unsuccessful, bowel management should be implemented. Each summer, after school is finished, reattempts can be made to assess the child's ability to potty train.

In patients previously operated on for an imperforate anus with fecal incontinence, a reoperation to

Table 1. Prognostic signs for patients with anorectal malformations. From [4]

Good prognosis signs	Poor prognosis signs
- Good bowel movement pattern: 1–2 bowel movement per day – no soiling in between - Evidence of sensation when passing stool (pushing, making faces) - Urinary control	- Constant soiling and passing of stool - No sensation (no pushing) - Urinary incontinence, dribbling of urine

Table 2. Predictors of prognosis in patients with anorectal malformations. From [4]

Indicators of good prognosis for bowel control	Indicators of poor prognosis for bowel control
- Normal sacrum - Prominent midline groove (good muscles) - Some types of anorectal malformations: • Rectal atresia • Vestibular fistula • Imperforate anus without a fistula • Cloacas with a common channel <3 cm • Less complex malformations: perineal fistula	- Abnormal sacrum - Flat perineum (poor muscles) - Some types of anorectal malformations: • Rectobladder-neck fistula • Cloacas with a common channel >3 cm • Complex malformations

relocate a misplaced rectum with the hope of obtaining good bowel control should be considered if the child was born with a good sacrum, good sphincter mechanism, and a malformation with good functional prognosis. A redo posterior sagittal anorectoplasty can be performed, and the rectum can be relocated within the limits of the sphincter mechanism. Approximately 50% of children operated on under these very specific circumstances have significant improvement in bowel control [5].

Patients with fecal incontinence and a tendency toward constipation cannot be treated with laxatives but need bowel management. In fact, laxatives in such patients make their soiling worse. Such children are usually those born with a poor prognosis type of defect and severe associated defects (defect of the sacrum, poor muscle complex).

Children operated on for imperforate anus who suffer from fecal incontinence can be divided into two well-defined groups, each requiring individualized treatment plans. The first and larger group includes patients with fecal incontinence and a tendency toward constipation. The second group comprises fecally incontinent patients with a tendency toward loose stool. Patients with fecal incontinence after operations for Hirschsprung's disease and those with spinal disorders usually fall into the first group: those with a tendency toward constipation.

Children with Constipation (Colonic Hypomotility)

In these children, colon motility is significantly reduced. The basis of the bowel management program in these patients is to teach parents to clean the child's colon once a day with a suppository, an enema, or colonic irrigation. No special diet or medications are necessary. The fact that these children suffer from constipation (hypomotility) is helpful, as it helps them remain clean between enemas. The real challenge is to find an enema capable of completely cleaning the colon. Definitive evidence that the colon is truly empty following an enema requires a plain abdominal radiograph. Soiling episodes or "accidents" occur when there is incomplete bowel cleaning and feces that progressively accumulates.

Children with Loose Stools and Diarrhea

The great majority of children with anorectal malformations who suffer from this kind of problem were repaired before 1980 and the introduction of the posterior sagittal technique. During those years, the procedures frequently included rectosigmoid resection [6, 7], Therefore, this group of children has an overactive colon because they lack a rectal reservoir. Rapid stool transit results in frequent diarrhea episodes. This means that even when an enema cleans their colon rather easily, stool keeps passing fairly quickly from the cecum to the descending colon and anus. To prevent this, a constipating diet and/or medications to slow down the colon are necessary. Eliminating foods that further loosen bowel movements will help the colon slow down. A small subset of patients with Hirschsprung's disease behaves as though they have hypermotility and can be managed similarly.

The keys to success of this bowel management program are dedication and sensitivity from the medical team. The basis of the program is to clean the colon and keep it quiet, thus keeping the patient clean for the 24 h after the enema.

The program is an ongoing process that is responsive to the individual patient and differs for each child. It is usually successful within a week, during which time family, patient, physician, and nurse undergo a process of trial and error, tailoring the regimen to the specific patient. More than 95% of children who follow this program are artificially clean and dry for the whole day and can have a completely normal life. One should embrace the philosophy that it is unacceptable to send a child with fecal incontinence to school in diapers when his classmates are already toilet trained. Proper treatment to prevent this is perhaps more important than the surgical procedure itself.

The first step in the program is to perform a contrast enema study with hydrosoluble material. The study should never be done with barium, and it is also important to obtain a picture after contrast material evacuation. This study shows the type of colon: dilated (constipated) Figure 1 or nondilated (tendency toward loose stool) (Fig. 2).

The bowel management program is then implemented according to the patient's type of colon, and results are evaluated daily. Changes in enema volume and content are made until the colon is successfully cleaned. To achieve this, a daily abdominal X-ray is invaluable in determining whether the colon is empty.

There are different types of enema solutions: some are ready-made and can be bought in a drugstore, and some can be prepared at home based on water and salt (0.9% saline can be made by adding 2 teaspoons of salt to 960 ml of water). The use of phosphate enemas is most convenient, as they are available in a prepared vial. However, saline enemas are often just as effective, and some families find them easier and less expensive. Occasionally, children will complain of cramping with the phosphate enema but

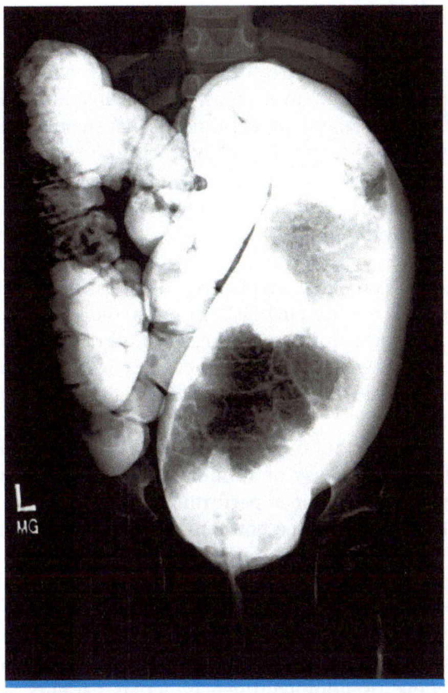

Fig. 1. Contrast enema of megarectosigmoid. Reprinted with permission from [1]

have no complaints with the saline one. Children older than 8 years or heavier than 30 kg may receive one adult phosphate enema daily (133 ml). Children between 3 and 8 years or between 15 and 30 kg may receive one pediatric phosphate enema (70 ml) daily. Children should never receive more than one phosphate enema a day because of the risk of phosphate intoxication, and others with impaired renal function should use these enemas with caution.

The enema administered on a regular basis should result in a bowel movement within 30–45 min, followed by a period of 24 h of complete cleanliness. If one enema is not enough to clean the colon (as demonstrated by an X-ray, or if the child keeps soiling), then the child requires a more aggressive treatment program, and saline solution is added to the phosphate one. If addition of the saline enema still produces inadequate results, then glycerin can be added. Administering the enema with a balloon catheter may help prevent enema leakage. The "right" saline enema is the one that can empty the child's colon and allow him or her to stay clean for the following 24 h. This can be achieved only by trial and error and learning from previous attempts.

Children with loose stool have an overactive colon and most often have no rectal reservoir. This means that even when an enema cleans their colon rather easily, new stool passes quickly from the cecum to the descending colon and anus. To prevent this, a constipating diet, bulking agents, and/or medications (such as loperamide) to slow down the colon are recommended. Eliminating foods that loosen bowel movements will help the colon move more slowly.

Parents are provided with a list of constipating foods to be given and a list of laxative foods to be avoided. The diet is rigid: banana, apple, baked bread, white pasta with no sauce, boiled meat, etc. Fried foods and dairy products must be avoided (Table 3). Most parents know which meals provoke loose stools and which ones constipate their child. To determine the right combination, the treatment starts with enemas, a very strict diet, and loperamide. Most children respond to this aggressive management within several days. The child should remain on a strict diet until clean for 24 h for 2–3 consecutive days. They can then choose one new food every 2–3 days, and the parent observes the effect on his or her colonic activity. If the child soils after eating a newly introduced food, that food must be eliminated. Over several months, the most liberal diet possible should be sought. If the child remains clean with a liberal

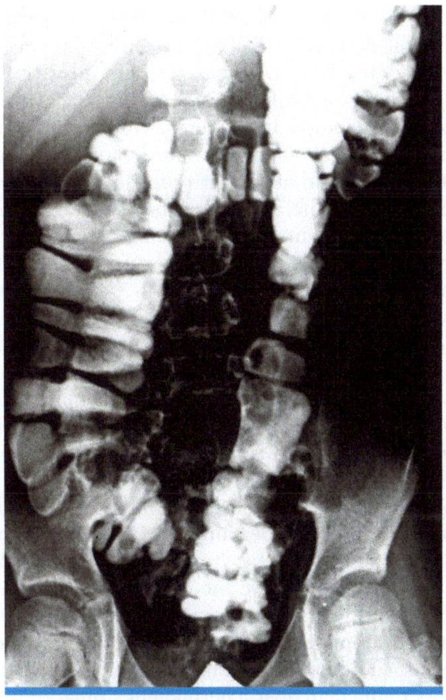

Fig. 2. Contrast enema in a patient with resected rectosigmoid. Reprinted with permission from [8]

Table 3. Constipating foods. From [4]

Constipating diet	
Avoid	**Encourage**
Milk or milk products	Apple Sauce
Fats	Apples without skin
Fried foods	Rice
Fruits	White bread
Vegetables	Bagels
Spices	Soft drinks
Fruit juices	Banana
French fries	Pasta
Chocolate	Pretzels
	Tea
	Potato
	Jelly (no jam)
	Boiled, broiled, baked
	Meat, chicken or fish

diet, medication can gradually be reduced to the lowest effective dose necessary to keep the child clean for 24 h.

In children in whom a successful bowel management program has been implemented, parents frequently ask if this program will be needed for life. The answer is "yes" for those patients born with no potential for bowel control. However, because we are dealing with a spectrum of defects, there are patients with some degree of bowel control. These patients are subjected to the bowel management program in order not to be exposed to embarrassing accidents of uncontrolled bowel movements. However, as time goes by, the child becomes more cooperative and more interested in his or her problem. It is conceivable that later in life, a child may be able to stop using enemas and remain clean, following a specific regimen of a disciplined diet with regular meals (three meals per day and no snacks) to provoke bowel movements at a predictable time. Every summer, children with some potential for bowel control can try to determine how well they can control their bowel movements without the help of enemas. This is done during vacations to avoid accidents at school, a time when they can stay home and try some potty training strategies.

For patients with a colostomy and no potential for bowel control, a key question is whether to perform a pull through or to leave the permanent stoma. We feel that if patients have the capacity to form solid stool, a pull through can be performed, with a daily enema to keep them clean. We believe that for these patients, successful bowel management gives a better quality of life than does a permanent stoma.

Most preschool and school-aged children enjoy a good quality of life while undergoing the bowel management program. However, when they reach puberty, many express a high degree of dissatisfaction. They feel that their parents are intruding on their privacy by giving them enemas. It is feasible but rather difficult for them to administer the enema themselves. For this specific group of children, an operation called a continent appendicostomy or a Malone procedure has been designed [9] whereby the appendix is connected to the umbilicus and through which the enema can be administered (Fig. 3). A valve mechanism is created that allows catheterization of the appendix for the enema fluid but avoids leakage of stool through it. If the child has lost his or her appendix, it is possible to create a new one from the colon. This procedure is known as a continent neoappendicostomy.

It is important to stress that the Malone procedure is just another way of administering an enema, and therefore, before it is performed, the child must be perfectly clean with a bowel management regimen.

Pseudoincontinence

It is vital to differentiate real fecal incontinence from overflow pseudoincontinence. As in patients with real fecal incontinence, the normal bowel control mechanism is deficient. Pseudoincontinence occurs when a patient behaves as if they are fecally incontinent, but they really have severe constipation and overflow soiling. Once the disimpaction is treated and the patient receives enough laxatives to avoid constipation, he or she becomes continent.

The colon absorbs water from the stool and serves a reservoir function. These processes depend on colonic motility, an area of physiology not well understood and for which treatments of problems are limited. In normal individuals, the rectosigmoid stores the stool and every 24–48 h develops active peristaltic waves indicating that it is time to empty. A normal individual feels this sensation and decides when to relax the voluntary sphincter mechanism.

If a child is fecally continent, then pseudoincontinence management involves treatment of constipation using laxatives, which help provoke peristalsis and overcome the dysmotility disorder. Patients who have undergone successful surgery for Hirschsprung's disease and for anorectal malformations (with a good prognosis type of anorectal defect) and have normal spines should be fecally continent.

Constipation in anorectal malformations is extremely common, particularly in the more benign types [10]. It is also common in patients following successful surgery for Hirschsprung's disease and occurs in a large group of patients considered to have idiopathic constipation [1]. When left untreated,

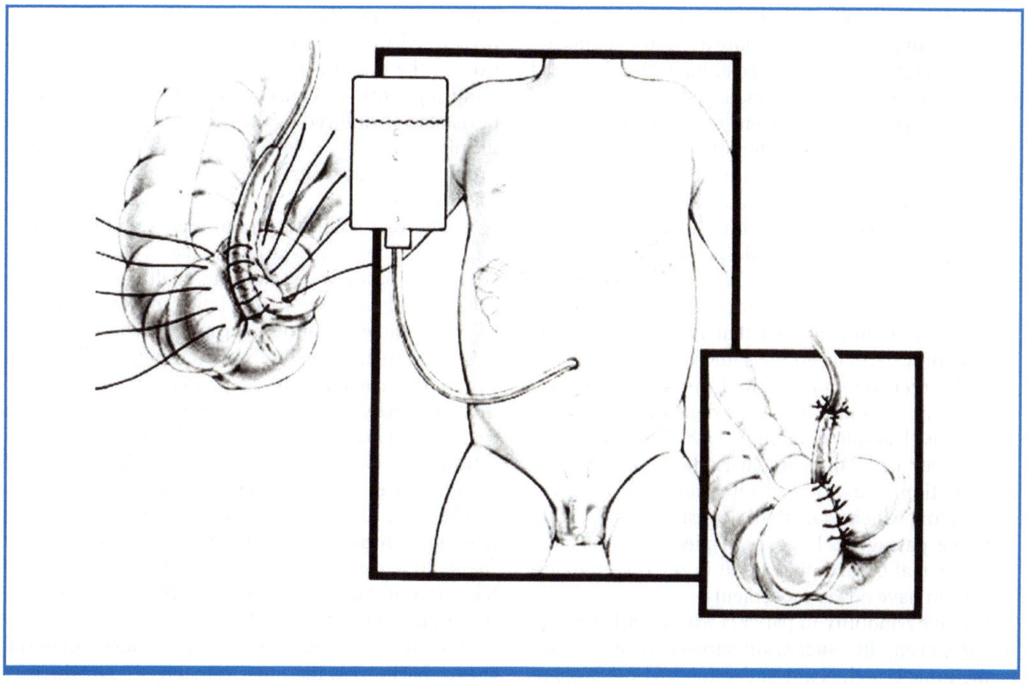

Fig. 3. Malone appendicostomy. Reprinted with permission from [9]

constipation can be extremely incapacitating and in its most serious forms can produce a form of fecal incontinence known as overflow pseudoincontinence. Diet impacts colonic motility, but its therapeutic value is negligible in the most serious forms of constipation. It is true that many patients with severe constipation suffer from psychological disorders, but a psychological origin cannot explain severe forms, as it is not easy to voluntarily retain the stool when an otherwise autonomous rectosigmoid peristalses. Passage of large, hard pieces of stool may provoke pain and make the patient behave as if they are stool retainers. This may complicate the problem, but it is not the original cause.

The clinician must decide which type of patient he or she is dealing with. Patients with good prognosis for bowel control are more likely to have constipation, and aggressive, proactive treatment of their constipation is the best approach. The child must be deemed capable of being fecally continent and have the capacity for voluntary bowel movements before initiating treatment for constipation.

Most of these patients suffer from different degrees of dilation of the rectum and sigmoid, a condition defined as megarectosigmoid (Fig. 1), due to a hypomotility disorder that interferes with complete rectosigmoid emptying [1]. These patients may be children born with a good prognosis type of anorectal defect and who underwent a technically correct operation but did not receive appropriate treatment for constipation. They therefore developed fecal impaction and overflow pseudoincontinence. These may also be children with severe idiopathic constipation who have a very dilated rectosigmoid.

Impaction needs to be removed with enemas and colonic irrigations to clean the megarectosigmoid. Subsequently, the constipation is treated with the administration of large doses of laxatives. Laxative dosage is increased daily until the right amount of laxative is reached to completely empty the colon every day. If medical treatment proves to be extremely difficult because the child has a severe megasigmoid and requires an enormous amount of laxatives to empty, the surgeon can offer a segmental resection of the colon. After the sigmoid resection, the amount of laxatives required to treat these children can be significantly reduced or even eliminated. Before performing this operation, it is mandatory to confirm that the child is definitely suffering from overflow pseudoincontinence rather than true fecal incontinence with constipation. Failure to make this distinction may lead to an operation in which a fecally incontinent constipated child is changed to one with a tendency to have loose stool, which will make them much more difficult to manage.

When children with anorectal malformations and Hirschsprung's disease are managed from the beginning with aggressive treatment of constipation, children with good prognosis should potty train without difficulty. When constipation is not managed properly and a patient presents after many years, they behave much like children with idiopathic constipation and have overflow pseudoincontinence.

Constipation in anorectal malformations is a self-perpetuating disease. A patient suffering from a certain degree of constipation that is not treated adequately only partially empties the colon, leaving larger and larger amounts of stool inside the rectosigmoid, which results in greater degrees of megasigmoid. It is clear that dilatation of a hollow viscus produces poor peristalsis, which explains the fact that constipation leads to fecal retention and thereafter megacolon, which exacerbates constipation. In addition, the passage of large, hard pieces of stool may produce anal fissures that result in reluctance by the patient to have bowel movements.

Colon dysmotility in patients with Hirschsprung's disease, even after successful surgery to remove the aganglionic bowel, is not understood. These patients do, however, benefit from proactive medical treatment of their constipation. The clinician must accept the fact that dysmotility is essentially incurable. It is, however, manageable, but requires careful life-long follow-up. Treatments cannot be given on a temporary basis, as once they are tapered or interrupted, constipation recurs.

Some clinicians treat such patients with colostomies or colonic washouts via a catheterizable stoma or button device and monitor the degree of colonic dilatation with contrast studies [11]. Once the distal colon regains a normal caliber, the physician assumes that the patient is cured, and the colostomy is closed or the washouts are discontinued. Unfortunately, symptoms quickly recur. We believe that washouts are really only for patients with true fecal incontinence who are incapable of having voluntary bowel movements and thus require a daily irrigation to empty. Patients with pseudoincontinence are capable of emptying their colon with the help of adequate doses of laxatives and thus do not need washouts.

Determining with which patient the clinician is dealing is the challenge. If the patient is incontinent, washouts with a bowel management regimen are appropriate. If the patient is continent, then aggressive constipation management after ensuring disimpaction is the treatment choice.

Fecal impaction is a stressful event of retained stool for several days or weeks, crampy abdominal pain, and sometimes tenesmus. When laxatives are prescribed to such a patient, the result is exacerbation of the crampy abdominal pain and sometimes vomiting. This is a consequence of increased colonic peristalsis (produced by the laxative) acting against a fecally impacted colon. Therefore, disimpaction, proven by X-ray, must precede initiation of laxative therapy.

Underwear soiling is an ominous sign of bad constipation. A patient who at an age of bowel control soils their underwear day and night and basically does not have spontaneous bowel movements may have overflow pseudoincontinence. These patients behave similarly to fecally incontinent individuals. When the constipation is treated adequately, the great majority of these pseudoincontinent children regain bowel control. Of course, this clinical presentation may also occur in a patient with true fecal incontinence. When uncertain, the physician can start a three-and-a-half to four-year-old child having trouble with potty training on a daily enema. Once the child is clean with this regimen and if he or she has the potential for bowel control, then a laxative program can be attempted.

A contrast enema with a hydrosoluble material (never barium) is the most valuable study, which in the constipated patient usually shows a megarectosigmoid with colon dilatation all the way down to the level of the levator mechanism (Fig. 1). There is usually a dramatic size discrepancy between a normal transverse and descending colon and the very dilated megarectosigmoid. Colon size guides laxative dosing, and it seems that the more localized the rectosigmoid dilation, the better the results of a sigmoid resection in reducing or eliminating the need for laxatives.

Rectal and colonic manometry may help in the evaluation of these patients; however, techniques that are more objective are required. Manometry is performed by placing balloons at different levels of the colon and recording contraction waves [12] or electrical activity [13]. Scintigraphy, a nuclear medicine study, is also being used to assess colonic motility [14]. These are sophisticated studies that do not yet help guide therapeutic decisions. The key information the surgeon needs to know is whether and where a colonic resection would provide benefit to the patient who requires enormous doses of laxatives to empty. Histologic studies of the colon in these patients mainly show hypertrophic smooth muscle and normal ganglion cells in the area of the dilated colon, but more sophisticated histopathologic investigations will hopefully soon yield more valuable results. Further investigations in this area will enhance our knowledge about colonic dysmotility in these patients and thereby guide therapy.

Treatment

Patients with anorectal malformations with potential for bowel control and severe constipation as well as patients with severe idiopathic constipation in whom dietary measures or gentle laxatives do not work require a more aggressive regimen. Drugs designed to increase colon motility are best, as opposed to medications that are only stool softeners. Softening the stool without improving colonic motility will likely make the patient worse, because with soft stool, patients no longer have control, whereas they do reasonably well with solid stool that allows them to feel rectal distension.

In many cases, the laxative regimen uses the same medications that have been tried previously, but the protocol is different in that the dosage is adapted to the patient's response. Response is monitored daily with an abdominal radiograph, and the laxative dose is adjusted if necessary. Almost always, the patient had previously received a lower dose than they need. Severe constipation is treated as follows:

Disimpaction

The disimpaction process is a vital and often neglected step. The routine includes administration of enemas three times a day until the patient is disimpacted. This is confirmed radiologically. If the patient remains impacted after 3 days, then he or she is given a balanced electrolyte solution via nasogastric tube in the hospital, and the enema regimen is continued. If this is unsuccessful, manual disimpaction under anesthesia may be necessary. It is important to remember not to prescribe laxatives to a fecally impacted patient. To do so may provoke vomiting and crampy abdominal pain. In addition, the patient will become reluctant to take laxatives because they are afraid of those symptoms.

Determining Laxative Requirement in a Disimpacted Patient

Once the patient has been disimpacted, an arbitrary amount of laxative is started, usually a senna derivative. The initial amount is based on information the parent gives about previous response to laxatives and the subjective evaluation of the megasigmoid on the contrast enema. The empiric dose is given, and the patient is observed for the next 24 h. If the patient does not have a bowel movement in the 24 h after receiving the laxative, it means the laxative dose was not enough and must be increased. An enema is also required to remove the stool produced during the previous 24 h. Stool in these extremely constipated patients should never remain in the rectosigmoid for more than 24 h.

The routine of increasing the amount of laxatives and giving an enema, if needed, is continued every night until the child has a voluntary bowel movement and completely empties the colon. The day that the patient has a bowel movement (which is usually with diarrhea), a radiograph should confirm that the bowel movement was effective, meaning that the patient completely emptied the rectosigmoid. If the patient passed stool but did not empty completely, the laxative dose must be increased.

As this condition covers a wide spectrum, patients may have laxative requirements much larger than the manufacturer's recommendation. Occasionally, in the process of increasing the amount of laxatives, patients throw up before reaching any positive effect. In these patients, a different medication can be tried. Some patients vomit all types of laxatives and are unable to reach the amount of laxative that produces a bowel movement that empties the colon. Such a patient is considered intractable and therefore a candidate for surgical intervention. Most of the time, however, the dosage that the patient needs in order to empty the colon completely, as demonstrated radiologically, can be achieved. At that dose, the patient should stop soiling because they are successfully emptying their colon each day, and because the colon is empty, they remain clean until the next voluntary bowel movement.

At this point, the patient and the parents have the opportunity to evaluate the quality of life attained with the treatment, understanding that this treatment will most likely be for life. For many of these patients, a sigmoid or rectosigmoid resection can provide symptomatic improvement leading to significant reduction in or complete elimination of laxatives.

Rectosigmoid Resection

For the last 14 years, we have been performing a sigmoid resection to treat select patients with severe constipation [15, 16]. The very dilated megarectosigmoid is resected, and the descending colon is anastomosed to the rectum. In a recent review of patients with anorectal malformations, 315 suffered from severe constipation, were fecally continent, but required significant laxative doses to empty their colon. Of these, 53 underwent a sigmoid resection. The degree of improvement varied. Following sigmoid resection, 10% of patients no longer required laxatives, had daily bowel movements, and no longer soiled; 30% decreased their laxative requirement by 80%; and the remaining 60% decreased their laxative requirement by 40%. These patients must be followed closely because the condition is not cured by the operation. The remaining rectum is most likely abnormal, and without careful observation and treatment of constipation, the colon can redilate.

A possible alternative could be to resect the rectosigmoid, including the rectum, down to the pectinate line in a similar manner used for patients with Hirschsprung's disease and anastomose the nondilated colon (which is assumed to have normal motility) to the rectum above the pectinate line. This is particularly applicable to the patient with idiopathic constipation who has normal sphincters and a normal anal canal. It should not be performed in patients with anorectal malformations, because this treatment eliminates the rectal reservoir, which may impact continence in some patients.

The most dilated part of the colon is resected because it is the most seriously affected. The nondilated part of the colon is assumed to have a more normal motility. Clearly, there must be a more scientific way to assess the dysmotile anatomy. Perhaps with the emergence of new colonic motility techniques, these studies will help with surgical planning. It does seem that patients who improve the most are those who have a more localized form of megarectosigmoid. Patients with more generalized dilation of the colon do not respond as well and may require a more extensive resection. Perhaps in the future, these observations can be corroborated, and results of resection can be better predicted by noninvasive modalities.

References

1. Peña A, Levitt MA (2002) Colonic inertia disorders. Curr Probl Surg 39:666–730
2. Peña A (1995) Anorectal malformations. Semin Pediatr Surg 4(1):35–47
3. Peña A, Guardino K, Tovilla JM et al (1998) bowel management for fecal incontinence in patients with anorectal malformations. J Pediatr Surg 33(1):133–137
4. Levitt MA, Peña A (2006) Treatment of fecal incontinence. In: Holschneider AM, Hutson JM (eds) Anorectal malformations in children: embryology, diagnosis, surgical treatment, follow-up. Springer, Berlin Heidelberg New York, p 379
5. Peña A, Hong AR, Midulla P, Levitt M (2003) Reoperative surgery for anorectal anomalies. Sem Pediatr Surg 12(2):118–123
6. Kiesewetter WB (1967) Imperforate anus II. The rationale and technique of the sacroabdominoperineal operation. J Pediatr Surg 2:106
7. Rehbein F (1967) Imperforate anus: experiences with abdomino-perineal and abdomino-sacro-perineal pull through procedures. J Pediatr Surg 2:99–105
8. Levitt MA, Peña A (2006) Treatment of chronic constipation and resection of the inert rectosigmoid. In: Holschneider AM, Hutson JM (eds) Anorectal malformations in children: embryology, diagnosis, surgical treatment, follow-up. Springer, Berlin Heidelberg New York, p 417
9. Levitt MA Soffer SZ, Peña A (1997) Continent appendicostomy in the bowel management fecal incontinent children. J Pediatr Surg 32:1630–1633
10. Peña A, Levitt MA (2005) Imperforate anus and cloacal malformations. In: Pediatric surgery, 4th edn. Ashcraft KW, Holder TM, Holcomb W (eds) WB Saunders, Philadelphia, pp 496–517
11. Marshall J, Hutson JM, Anticich N, Stanton MP (2001) Antegrade continence enemas in the treatment of slow-transit constipation. J Pediatr Surg 36:1227–1230
12. DeLorenzo C, Flores AF, Reddy SN, Hyman PE (1992) Use of colonic manometry to differentiate causes of intractable constipation in children. J Pediatr 120:690–695
13. Sarna SK, Bardakjian BL, Waterfall WE, Lind JF (1980) Human colonic electric control activity (ECA). Gastroenterology 78:1526–1536
14. Cook BJ, Lim E, Cook D et al (2005) Radionuclear transit to assess sites of delay in large bowel transit in children with chronic idiopathic constipation. J Pediatr Surg 40(3):478–483
15. Peña A, El-Behery M (1993) Megasigmoid-A source of pseudo-incontinence in children with repaired anorectal malformations. J Pediatr Surg 28:1–5
16. Levitt MA, Carney DE, Powers CJ et al (2003) Laparoscopically assisted colon resection for severe idiopathic constipation with megarectosigmoid. Journal of Pediatric Endosurgery & Innovative Techniques 7:285–289

SECTION V

Future Perspectives

Future Perspectives in Management and Research of Fecal Incontinence

37

Carlo Ratto, Angelo Parello, Lorenza Donisi, Francesco Litta, Giovanni B. Doglietto

Introduction

As a common denominator of all the clinical aspects treated in this book, there is the awareness of potential benefits derived from rational management of fecal incontinence (FI) and the need for further efforts to improve the effectiveness of traditional and new treatments. Indeed, although progress made in this field during the last few decades has been significant, the lack of detailed knowledge in the physiology of fecal continence far too frequently makes the application of therapeutic procedures empiric and pragmatic. Moreover, there are discrepancies between countries and regions in referring patients to centers dedicated to FI management. This causes different attitudes in performing a homogeneous diagnostic workup, in application of similar strict selection criteria to the variety of available treatments, and in reporting results of the applied therapies. Worldwide, national institutes for health inadequately support medical research on FI treatment, even though the social, economic, and clinical importance of FI to society has been very well recognized. On the other hand, research into FI is all too frequently sponsored only by companies with a commercial interest in the subject.

Nevertheless, a number of priorities have been identified. In 2002, the Consensus Conference "Advancing the Treatment of Fecal and Urinary Incontinence Through Research: Trial Design, Outcome Measures, and Research Priorities" [1], emphasized the fields of primary interest (Table 1) to improve knowledge and treatment of FI by further planning research programs. Representatives of all specialties involved in FI management contributed to this conference. Even if the goal of the conference to produce significant results in 5–10 years is very ambitious, the relevance of the priorities identified remains actual. Following the same schema of this book, the conference emphasized: (1) pathophysiological and behavioral aspects, (2) diagnostic problems, (3) treatment-related issues, and (4) aspects related to specific clinical conditions.

Pathophysiological and Behavioral Aspects

Further studies investigating pathophysiological mechanisms of FI is of crucial importance because progress will have an impact on both diagnostic and therapeutic strategies. Due to the possible multifactorial origin of FI and the existence of different clinical presentations, basic research into the influence played by each of the numerous factors involved in continence control can be of help [2]. Future studies must consider that the traditional assumption that women younger than 65 years of age are at maximum risk of FI because of obstetric trauma to anal sphincters or pudendal neuropathy is not true [3]. Prevalence of FI in men has been certainly underestimated. Also, other causative factors, different than those secondary to childbirth, have to be of primary interest, these being neuropathies (diabetes, multiple sclerosis, Parkinson's disease, spinal cord injury, systemic sclerosis, myotonic dystrophy, amyloidosis) and conditions related to idiopathic FI. Moreover, conditions affecting general health or ability to perform daily activities (stroke, immobility) are significantly related to FI. These features could explain why nursing home residence is the most prominent factor associated with FI in patients affected by the abovementioned diseases.

The real role of sphincter tears, recent or previous, in the development of FI is being rethought, not only in relation to the pathophysiological aspect but also to treatment strategy. Primary conditions and associated factors need to be elucidated in regard to whether a limited or extended (how long? how large?) lesion involving either or both internal and external anal sphincters has caused FI [4–6]. Relationships between sphincter integrity and anorectal sensorial perception should be deeply studied, because they probably are the interpretation key of positive effects recently observed using sacral nerve stimulation (SNS) in patients with iatrogenic FI. On the other hand, nontraumatic FI is worthy of special attention because of the complexity of patterns possibly involved. Studies with electrophysiological tech-

Table 1. Priorities for treatment-related research on fecal incontinence (modified from [1])

Research priorities
Randomized controlled trials
Biofeedback vs. education and medical management
Biofeedback strength training vs. sensory training
Combined biofeedback plus surgery vs. each alone
Combined biofeedback plus drugs vs. each alone
Sacral nerve stimulation vs. biofeedback or surgery
Development of novel treatments
Develop and test new drugs
Identify the most effective surgery for obstetric tears
Optimize existing therapies
Improve adherence and maintenance
Evaluate long-term outcomes of surgery
Identify psychological symptoms that predict who consults
Geriatric population
Practical treatments for frail/demented elderly
Evaluate assisted toileting in nursing homes
Diagnostic tests
Develop normative values for diagnostic tests
Compare history and physical examination with diagnostic tests in predicting pathophysiology and response to biofeedback
Evaluate electromyogram of external anal sphincter and puborectalis muscle for diagnosis of neurogenic fecal incontinence
Evaluate relationship of quality of life to fecal incontinence severity
Standardize evaluation of severity and quality of life
Further studies of pathophysiological mechanisms
Prevention
Determine which diagnostic tests predict obstetric injury
Longitudinal studies of relationship of fecal incontinence to functional gastrointestinal disorders
Prevent anatomic defects leading to surgery by modifying behaviors (e.g., straining or hard stools)
Patient concerns
Counter social stigma associated with fecal incontinence
Provide better patient education regarding risk factors
Pediatric gastroenterology
Randomized controlled trial of laxative regimens in pediatric fecal incontinence
Compare enemas with oral laxatives in pediatric fecal incontinence
Compare enemas with toilet training in functional nonretentive fecal soiling
Randomized controlled trial comparing appendicostomy, colostomy, sphincter reconstruction, and artificial bowel sphincter in spinal cord injury and anorectal malformations

niques, magnetic resonance imaging (MRI), and positron emission tomography (PET) could explain aspects of the correlation between the central nervous system (CNS) and targeted pelvic organs involved in fecal and urinary continence. This will contribute to a more rational application of SNS using adequate criteria for patient selection [7].

Behavior in relation to FI is of unique impact on a patient's lifestyle and quality of life (QoL). Coping mechanisms should be analyzed in different subgroups of patients according to their specific clinical conditions [8–10]. For this purpose, adequate methods to measure coping mechanisms and behavior related to FI severity should be found and used [11]. Unfortunately, each of the scales most often used to measure QoL [12–18] has its strengths and weaknesses. Efforts should be directed to validate these scales in translated versions in order to use comparable forms in different countries [19].

Also, social stigma associated with FI must be acknowledged and then addressed. Due to their reluctance to confess to this disabling disorder, patients often renounce or refuse any diagnosis and treatment. Moreover, depression and anxiety affecting a very large percentage of FI patients (larger than in urinary incontinent patients) increase alienation from family and friends and create social isolation, with a significant impact on the social costs attributable to the disease. All these factors should be detailed and evaluated. Thereafter, informative campaigns should be promoted and psychological measures standardized to support these patients. In particular, risk factors of FI must be illustrated to subjects who are potentially incontinent in order to motivate them to investigate their condition.

Diagnostic Problems

Related to prevention of FI, of primary importance is the identification of diagnostic tests predicting sphincter lesions, not only obstetric [20] but secondary to other surgical procedures. Moreover, the relationship of FI to other functional gastrointestinal disorders should be better investigated in order to delimitate this subgroup of patients and address specific treatments [2].

The lack of homogeneity in the diagnostic workup for FI should be solved. One measure could be the identification of reference centers in which all the basic diagnostic tools are available and procedures performed according to largely shared standards [21]. Efforts must be made to improve diagnostic accuracy of anorectal tests, and normative values for each diagnostic test should be provided according to patients' age and gender [22]. The actual difficulty of finding measurable physiological parameters predicting FI severity, as well as treatment outcome, should be overcome by specifically designed trials using standard procedures for anorectal manometry (ARM) plus rectal sensory assessment, endoanal ultrasound (EAUS), and anorectal electrophysiology (AREP) in order to definitely establish the diagnostic value of each diagnostic tool alone and together in a multimodal diagnosis [23]. A specific set of parameters should be identified for each condition as a minimum required standard [24–26]. Moreover, other procedures (MRI, contrast defecography, and MRI defecography) could be selectively used in specific clinical conditions. Due to the large - and often contrasting - amount of data available in the literature concerning the diagnostic and prognostic value of physiological parameters [27–29], an accurate revision is desirable with the aim of achieving consensus. It would be beneficial to relate diagnostic and prognostic parameters to specific treatment options in order to elucidate the therapeutic potentials of each.

Treatment-Related Issues

Randomized controlled trials (RCTs) demonstrating not only effectiveness but also therapeutic validation are needed concerning almost all of the available treatments (biofeedback, sphincteroplasty, medications). The 2002 Consensus Conference [1] highlighted the necessity to obtain evidence of potential benefits using different treatment combinations utilizing synergistic effects of combined therapies in comparison with a single approach. This concept remains an actuality: combination of biofeedback plus surgery vs. each alone, or combination of biofeedback plus medications vs. each alone could be useful comparisons. SNS frequently holds a central position in the therapeutic algorithm for treating an increasing variety of FI conditions (following failed behavioral therapies and preceding anal sphincter replacement operations); however, its role needs to be confirmed in RCTs designed in specific situations. From this perspective, it will be interesting to confirm the effectiveness of SNS both in FI patients with sphincter lesions already treated with overlapping sphincteroplasty and in those with untreated sphincter tears. This is according to the aim of future research to optimize existing therapies, improving adherence and maintenance, and evaluating long-term results of a certain approach. This pertains, in particular, to behavioral therapies [30] because they are often considered first-line therapy for FI, being safe, effective, and inexpensive; it will be interesting to establish the impact for patients of changing from behavioral therapy to surgery.

The most intriguing aspect for future research is the development of novel treatments. Of course, efforts will be directed to noninvasive (new drugs) or minimally invasive (bulking agents, miniaturized devices) procedures [31–33]. On the other hand, establishing correct indications for available treatments could allow identification of the most effective surgery for each FI condition [34, 35].

Aspects Related to Specific Clinical Conditions

A wide review of FI management in specific clinical conditions is presented in the previous chapters of this book. The 2002 Consensus Conference [1] highlighted the necessity to focus attention primarily on geriatric and pediatric patients. Concerning older subjects, it is very important to counterbalance attempts to cure with patient frailty. Therefore, physicians should identify an adequate treatment for each type of disability, including minimally invasive surgery (implant of new, effective bulking agents) and supportive measures (anal plugs). Nurse education should be directed to improving assistance to patients, both home and nursing home residents.

As to FI in pediatrics, randomized controlled studies will elucidate the value of enemas, laxatives, and toilet training in FI and fecal soiling. Moreover, indications and use of surgical approaches should be redefined in FI patients with anorectal malformations and spinal cord injury, and SNS may have a role in neurogenic FI.

Special consideration will be dedicated in the future to FI secondary to multimodal treatment (surgery and chemoradiotherapy) for rectal cancer in order to define the pathophysiologic contribution of the multiple factors involved and to establish correct indications to treatment.

Problems related to iatrogenic anal sphincter lesions have been widely discussed. This is a field with large perspectives toward changing the actual approach due on one hand to documentation of the possibility of sphincteroplasty failure [36, 37] and on the other hand, to success with emerging therapies, i.e., SNS. Further RCTs should determine pathophysiological factors due to sphincter tears, surgery timing (immediate or delayed), reconstruction modality (end to end or overlapping), and, importantly, indications and contraindications to surgery [38–41].

Central and peripheral neuropathies (including those diseases determining nerve dysfunctions) require concentrated investigation to establish specific patterns of pathophysiology useful to address treatment. In this regard, a significant decrease in aggressive treatments (sphincter replacement surgery) is anticipated in these conditions in the future, whereas the increasing use of therapies directly impacting pathophysiology (i.e., SNS) will be justified by pathophysiological evidence.

Finally, increased integration of knowledge and cooperation between coloproctologists, urologists, and gynecologists will improve the effectiveness of treatment of double fecal and urinary incontinence [42–43]. This condition requires an accurate multimodal diagnostic assessment. Treatment could provide rehabilitative procedures, surgery, or both: precise indications toward the behavioral approach, prosthetic/reconstructive surgery, or SNS need to be defined.

References

1. Whitehead WE, Wald A, Norton NJ (2004) Priorities for treatment research from different professional perspectives. Gastroenterol 126:S180–S185
2. Deutekom M, Dobben AC, Terra MP et al (2007) Clinical presentation of fecal incontinence and anorectal function: what is the relationship? Am J Gastroenterol 102:351–361
3. Nelson RL (2004) Epidemiology of fecal incontinence. Gastroenterology 126(1 Suppl 1):S3–7
4. Fitzgerald MP, Weber AM, Howden N et al (2007) Risk factors for anal sphincter tear during vaginal delivery. Obstet Gynecol 109:29–34
5. Richter HE, Fielding JR, Bradley CS et al (2006) Endoanal ultrasound findings and fecal incontinence symptoms in women with and without recognized anal sphincter tears. Obstet Gynecol 108:1394–1401
6. Thornton MJ, Lubowski DZ (2006) Obstetric-induced incontinence: a black hole of preventable morbidity. Aust NZ J Obstet Gynaecol 46:468–473
7. Gourcerol G, Gallas S, Michot F et al (2006) Sacral nerve stimulation in fecal incontinence: are there factors associated with success? Dis Colon Rectum 49:1–10
8. Trowbridge ER Morgan D, Trowbridge MJ et al (2006) Sexual function, quality of life, and severity of anal incontinence after anal sphincteroplasty. Am J Obstet Gynecol 195:1753–1757
9. Pla-Martì V, Moro-Valdezate D, Alos-Company R et al (2007) The effect of surgery on quality of life in patients with faecal incontinence of obstetric origin. Colorectal Dis 9:90–95
10. Hetzer FH, Hahnloser D, clavien PA et al (2007) Quality of life and morbidity after permanent sacral nerve stimulation for fecal incontinence. Arch Surg 142:8–13
11. Rockwood TH (2004) Incontinence severity and QOL scales for fecal incontinence. Gastroenterology 126 (1 Suppl 1):S106–113
12. Rockwood TH, Church JM, Fleshman JW et al (2000) Fecal Incontinence Quality of Life Scale: quality of life instrument for patients with fecal incontinence. Dis Colon Rectum 43:9–16
13. Rothbarth J, Bemelman WA, Meijerink WJ et al (2001) What is the impact of fecal incontinence on quality of life? Dis Colon Rectum 44:67–71
14. Eypasch E, Williams JI, Wood-Dauphinee S et al (1995) Gastrointestinal Quality of Life Index: development, validation and application of a new instrument. Br J Surg 82:216–222
15. Sakakibara R, Shinotoh H, Uchiyama T et al (2001) Questionnaire-based assessment of pelvic organ dysfunction in Parkinson's disease. Auton Neurosi 92:76–85
16. Wiesel PH, Norton C, Roy AJ et al (2000) Gut focused behavioural treatment (biofeedback) for constipation and faecal incontinence in multiple sclerosis. J Neurol Neurosurg Psychiatry 69:240–243
17. Bai Y, Yuan Z, Wang W et al (2000) Quality of life for children with fecal incontinence after surgically corrected anorectal malformation. J Pediatr Surg 35:462–464
18. Bug GJ, Kiff ES, Hosker G (2001) A new condition-specific health-related quality of life questionnaire for the assessment of women with anal incontinence. BJOG 108:1057–1067
19. Sperber AD (2004) Translation and validation of study instruments for cross-cultural research. Gastroenterology 126(1 Suppl 1):S124–128
20. Gearhart S, Hull T, Floruta C (2005) Anal manometric parameters: predictors of outcome following anal sphincter repair? J Gastrointest Surg 9:115–120
21. Prott G, Hansen R, Badcock C et al (2005) What is the optimum methodology for the clinical measurement of resting anal sphincter pressure? Neurogastroenterol Motil 17:595–599
22. Siprouidhis L, Al Abkari M, El Alaoui M et al (2005) Low rectal volumes in patients suffering from fecal

incontinence: what does it mean? Aliment Pharmacol Ther 22:989–996
23. Deutekom M, Terra MP, Dijkgraaf MGW et al (2006) Patients' perception of tests in the assessment of faecal incontinence. Br J Radiol 79:94–100
24. Rattan S (2005) The internal anal sphincter: regulation of smooth muscle tone and relaxation. Neurogastroenterol Motil 17(Suppl 1):50–59
25. Enck P, Hinninghofen H, Merlett R et al (2005) The external anal sphincter and the role of surface electromyography. Neurogastroenterol Motil 17(Suppl 1): 60–67
26. Azpiroz F, Fernandez-Fraga X, Merlett R et al (2005) The puborectalis muscle. Neurogastroenterol Motil 17(Suppl 1):68–72
27. Saranovic D, Barisic G, Krivokapic Z et al (2007) Endoanal ultrasound of anorectal diseases and disorders: technique, indications, results and limitations. Eur J Radiol 61:480–489
28. Mortele KJ, Fairhurst J (2007) Dynamic MR defecography of the posterior compartment: indications, techniques and MRI features. Eur J Radiol 61:462–472
29. Maglinte DDT, Bartram C (2007) Dynamic imaging of posterior compartment pelvic floor dysfunction by evacuation proctography: techniques, indications, results and limitations. Eur J Radiol 61:454–461
30. Dobben AC, Terra MP, Berghmans B et al (2006) Functional changes after physiotherapy in fecal incontinence. Int J Colorectal Dis 21:515
31. Maeda Y, Vaizey CJ, Kamm MA (2007) Long-term results of perianal silicone injection for faecal incontinence. Colorectal Dis 9:357–361
32. Ratto C, Parello A, Donisi L et al (2007) Anal Gatekeeper: a new bulking agent for patients with fecal incontinence. Abstract P18. In: Proceedings ASCRS 2007 Annual Meeting, June 2–6, Cervantes Convention Center at America's Center, St. Louis, MO, USA
33. Schrag HJ, Ruthmann O, Doll A et al (2006) Development of a novel, remote-controlled artificial bowel sphincter through microsystems technology. Artif Organs 30:855–862
34. Tillin T, Gannon K, Feldman RA et al (2006) Third-party prospective evaluation of patient outcomes after dynamic graciloplasty. Br J Surg 93:1402–1410
35. Ruthmann O, Fisher A, Hopt UT et al (2006) Dynamic graciloplasty vs artificial bowel sphincter in the management of severe fecal incontinence. Chirurg 77:926–938
36. Maslekar S, Gardiner AB, Duthie GS (2007) Anterior anal sphincter repair for fecal incontinence: good long-term results are possible. J Am Coll Surg. 204:40–46
37. Barisic GI, Krivokapic ZV, Markovic VA et al (2006) Outcome of overlapping anal sphincter repair after 3 months and after a mean of 80 months. Int J Colorectal Dis 21:52–56
38. Oberwalder M, Dinnewitzer A, Baig MK et al (2006) Do internal anal sphincter defects decrease the success rate of anal sphincter repair? Tech Coloproctol 10:94–97
39. Hayes J, Shatari T, Toozs-Hobson P et al (2006) Early results of immediate repair of obstetric third-degree tears: 65% are completely asymptomatic despite persistent sphincter defects in 61%. Colorectal Dis 9:332–336
40. Kairaluoma MV, Raivio P, Aarnio MT et al (2004) Immediate repair of obstetric anal sphincter rupture: medium-term outcome of the overlap technique. Dis Colon Rectum 47:1358–1363
41. Steele SR, Lee P, Mullenix PS et al (2006) Is there a role for concomitant pelvic floor repair in patients with sphincter defects in the treatment of fecal incontinence? Int J Colorectal Dis 21: 508–514
42. Kapoor DS, Thakar R, Sultan AH (2005) Combined urinary and faecal incontinence. Int Urogynecol J 16:321–328
43. Soligo M, Salvatore S, Milani R et al (2003) Double incontinence in urogynecologic practice: a new insight. Am J Obstet Gynecol 189:438–443

Subject Index

T

U

V

W

MIX
Papier aus verantwortungsvollen Quellen
Paper from responsible sources
FSC® C105338

If you have any concerns about our products,
you can contact us on
ProductSafety@springernature.com

In case Publisher is established outside the EU,
the EU authorized representative is:
Springer Nature Customer Service Center GmbH
Europaplatz 3, 69115 Heidelberg, Germany

Printed by Libri Plureos GmbH
in Hamburg, Germany